CLINIC.

CW01649497

BRITISH NATIONAL FORMULARY 1982

BRITISH NATIONAL FORMULARY

Number 3 (1982)

British Medical Association
and
The Pharmaceutical Society of Great Britain

Copyright 1982 © by the British Medical Association and The Pharmaceutical Society of Great Britain

Copies may be obtained through any bookseller or, in cases of difficulty, direct from the publishers:

British Medical Association
Tavistock Square
London WC1H 9JP, England

The Pharmaceutical Press
1 Lambeth High Street
London SE1 7JN, England

ISBN: 0 85369 142 8. ISSN: 0260–535X

All rights reserved. No part of this publication may be reproduced, stored in a retrieval system, or transmitted in any form or by any means—electronic, mechanical, photocopying, recording or otherwise—without the prior written permission of the joint copyright holders.

Typeset in Great Britain by Page Bros (Norwich) Ltd, Norwich, Norfolk, and printed and bound by Richard Clay (The Chaucer Press) Ltd, Bungay, Suffolk.

Joint Formulary Committee 1981–82

Chairman

O. L. Wade, MD, FRCP, Hon FRCPI

Deputy Chairman

J. P. Kerr, FPS

Committee Members

J. E. Balmford, FPS

M. Goodman, MRCS, LRCP, FRCGP, DObstRCOG

P. R. Greenfield, BA, MB, BChir, DObstRCOG

J. P. Griffin, PhD, MB, BS, BSc, MRCS, MRCP

C. R. Hitchings, BPharm, MSc, MPS

G. M. Mitchell, CStJ, MB, ChB, FPS

G. R. Tudhope, BSc, MD, FRCP, FRCP(E)

B. A. Wills, BPharm, PhD, FPS, CChem, FRSC

Joint Secretaries

A. Wade, BPharm, MPhil, FPS

F. O. Wells, MB, BS

Executive Editor

G. R. Brown, MBE, BPharm, BSc, FPS

Editorial Staff

K. B. K. Davis, MPS

Sheenagh M. Langtry, BSc, Dip Lib

Jasmine Miller, BSc, MPS

Executive Secretary

Joanna J. Brennand, BSocSc

Contents

Arrangement of Information

Arrangement of the text
The main text consists of classified notes on drugs and preparations used in the treatment of diseases and conditions. These notes are split into 15 chapters, each of which is related to a particular system of the human body or to another main subject (infections, vaccines etc.). Each chapter is divided into sections which begin with appropriate *notes for prescribers*. These notes are intended to provide information to doctors, pharmacists, nurses etc. to facilitate the selection of suitable treatment. The notes are followed by details of relevant drugs and preparations.

Guidance on prescribing
This chapter includes information on prescription writing, prescribing for children and elderly patients, and prescribing for patients with liver and kidney disease. Information is also given on adverse reactions, controlled drugs, and dependence.

Emergency treatment of poisoning
The main intention of this chapter is to provide information on the management of acute poisoning when first seen in the home, although certain aspects of hospital-based treatment are briefly mentioned.

Drugs
Drugs appear under their pharmacopoeial titles or British Approved Names. If there is a drug of choice, information on it is usually given first; otherwise the drugs are arranged alphabetically.

Preparations
These usually follow immediately after the drug which is their main ingredient. They are printed in text-sized type but those considered by the Committee to be less suitable for prescribing are described briefly in smaller type. Small type is also used for the entries describing foods for special diets and preparations for stoma care. Preparations are included under a non-proprietary title only if (a) they are marketed under such a title, (b) various proprietary products are available that comply with the non-proprietary description, or (c) they may be prepared extemporaneously.

Formulated preparations that are commonly prepared extemporaneously are described briefly in the relevant chapter and full formulae are given in the Formulary section.

Prices
The relative price bands (see inside cover) have been calculated whenever possible from the basic cost used in pricing National Health Service prescriptions dispensed in August 1981; these prices are based on the largest pack size in use in general practice pharmacies. Relative price bands are omitted from statements on (1) concentrates supplied as a dispensing aid and not usually prescribed as such; (2) items supplied without charge; and (3) items not generally available in the United Kingdom.

Diluents
The diluents indicated for certain creams, ointments, elixirs, and mixtures are intended to be used when lower strengths or doses are ordered, as indicated under 'General Information'.

Preface

A new type of British National Formulary was introduced in February 1981, and the scope of the book was considerably increased although it still remained a pocket book for those concerned with the prescribing, dispensing and administration of medicines. Earlier editions of the BNF included only those products that had the confidence of the Joint Formulary Committee, and consequently only a limited selection of the many drugs and preparations available were described in the book.

The basis of selection has now been changed and information is included on most products available to prescribers in the United Kingdom. The entries, coupled with the relevant notes for prescribers, are intended to help in the choice of appropriate treatment of each patient.

Most of the preparations now follow immediately after the notes for prescribers with which they are associated. It is considered that this arrangement will help in the selection process. A small formulary section has been retained for convenience in dispensing those formulated preparations that are commonly prepared extemporaneously.

Following the publication of the first and second editions of the new book, numerous comments and suggestions for improvement were received from doctors, pharmacists, nurses, and others and the Joint Formulary Committee would like to thank all those who have sent notes and suggestions. As a result, many changes have been made in the text, which has also been updated to include new products that have become available. In the preparation of this edition the information in Appendix 2 (intravenous additives) has been considerably expanded. Some of the entries in the smaller type size have been revised to include more detailed information, and it is intended to complete the revision of these entries for the next edition. A small section on stoma care and prescribing for patients with a stoma has been added to Chapter 1. The notes for prescribers in chapter 13 (drugs acting on the skin) have been expanded, particularly in the sections on emollients and barrier preparations, and preparations for wounds and ulcers. Information on the use of drugs in pregnancy and lactation is being collected for inclusion in a future edition.

Among the innovations that attracted much attention was the introduction of relative price bands. These indications of relative cost were generally welcomed but numerous suggestions for improvement have been made. The bands represent the relative basic cost of a typical prescription and enable prescribers to take into account the need to make the best use of available resources. Good prescribing requires careful consideration of the needs of the patient and the condition being treated; these factors may result in a limitation of choice; however where there is a choice of a number of suitable preparations to treat a particular disease or condition the price bands may be used in making a selection on a basis of cost. The Committee has investigated some alternative methods of indicating relative prices and has concluded that weekly treatment costs or prices based on a course of treatment are of limited application in a work of this nature and do not offer any real advantage over the present method. Only minor changes have been made in the pricing arrangements in this edition.

It should be emphasised that cost-effective prescribing must take into account other factors such as dose frequency and duration of treatment that affect the total cost. The use of more expensive drugs is also justified if it will result in better treatment of the patient or a reduction of the length of an illness or the time spent in hospital.

Arrangements have been made to revise the BNF twice yearly, and between issues numerous changes are made. All copies of the BNF Number 2 (1981) should therefore be withdrawn from use and replaced by BNF Number 3 (1982). Changes notified to us after December 31st, 1981 are included in a late changes section, page 381.

The BNF is still intended to be a pocket book for rapid reference and so cannot contain all the information necessary for prescribing and dispensing. The information should be supplemented as necessary from specialised publications. Manufacturers' data sheets prepared in accordance with the Medicines (Data Sheet) Regulations 1972 are available for most proprietary medicines and these should also be consulted. Less detail is given in the chapters on malignant disease and immunosuppression, and anaesthesia, as it is expected that those undertaking treatment will have specialised knowledge and will consult specialist literature.

The Joint Formulary Committee acknowledges the help of individuals and organisations that provided information or advised on specific matters. The principal contributors for this edition were L. Beeley, A. M. Breckenridge, J. W. Dundee, A. M. Geddes, D. F. N. Harrison, R. Hoffenberg, E. C. Huskisson, J. A. Innes, F. A. Jenner, R. Marks, R. G. Penn, A. E. Read, A. Richens, E. R. Tallett, G. N. Volans, and J. M. A. Whitehouse. The Committee also wishes to express its thanks to correspondents in the pharmaceutical industry who provided information and made numerous comments on points of detail, and to colleagues who have advised members of the committee and the editorial staff on specific matters.

Comments and constructive criticism will be welcome, and should be sent to the Executive Editor, British National Formulary, 1 Lambeth High Street, London SE1 7JN.

Guidance on Prescribing

General Information

TITLES AND ABBREVIATIONS. In general, titles of drugs and preparations should be written *in full.* Unofficial abbreviations should not be used as they may be misinterpreted; obsolete titles, such as Mist. Expect. and Mist. Tussis should not be used.

NON-PROPRIETARY TITLES. It is recommended that where non-proprietary titles are given, they should be used in prescribing. This will enable any suitable product to be dispensed, thereby saving delay to the patient and sometimes expense to the health service. The only exceptional circumstance is in those few instances (such as lithium carbonate tablets) where bioavailability problems are so important that it is desirable that, once treatment has been started, the patient should continue to be treated with the product of the same manufacturer; in such cases, the brand name should be used or the manufacturer should be stated.

Titles used as headings for monographs included in the Formulary section may be used freely in Great Britain and Northern Ireland but in other countries may be subject to restriction.

Many of the non-proprietary titles used in this book are titles of monographs in the European Pharmacopoeia, British Pharmacopoeia 1980 or British Pharmaceutical Codex 1973. In such cases the preparations must comply with the standard (if any) in the appropriate publication, as required by the Medicines Act (section 65).

PROPRIETARY TITLES. Names followed by the symbol® are or have been used as proprietary names in the United Kingdom. These names may in general be applied only to products supplied by the owners of the trade marks.

DOSES. The doses stated in the BNF are intended for general guidance and represent, unless otherwise stated, the usual range of doses that are generally regarded as being suitable for adults; unless otherwise indicated the quantities are those generally suitable for administration on one occasion.

DILUTION. When fractional doses are prescribed *liquid preparations* for oral use will be diluted with a suitable vehicle to dose-volumes of 5 ml or a multiple thereof, unless otherwise directed in the text. Dilution should be effected at the time of dispensing and such diluted preparations may be less stable than the original undiluted preparations. Where a complete recipe is given in the formulary section the diluent is the specified vehicle, otherwise the diluent specified in the text should be used.

In the case of *creams, ointments etc.*, where a complete recipe is available the diluent is the specified vehicle, otherwise only diluents specified in the text should be used.

STRENGTHS AND QUANTITIES. The strength or quantity to be contained in capsules, lozenges, tablets, etc. should be stated by the prescriber.

If a pharmacist receives an incomplete prescription for a systemically administered preparation other than a prescription for a controlled drug and he considers it would not be appropriate for the patient to return to the doctor, the following procedures will apply:

(a) an attempt must always be made to contact the prescriber to ascertain his intention;
(b) if the attempt is successful the pharmacist must, where practicable, subsequently arrange for details of quantity, strength where applicable, and dosage to be inserted by the prescriber on the incomplete form;
(c) where, although the prescriber has been contacted, it has not proved possible to obtain his written intention regarding an incomplete prescription, the pharmacist may endorse the form 'p.c.' (prescriber contacted) and add details of the quantity and strength where applicable of the preparation supplied, and of the dose indicated. The endorsement should be initialled and dated by the pharmacist;
(d) where the prescriber cannot be contacted and the pharmacist has sufficient information to make a professional judgment he may dispense a sufficient quantity of the preparation to complete up to 5 days' treatment; except that where a combination pack (i.e., a proprietary pack containing more than one medicinal product) or oral contraceptive is prescribed by name only, the smallest pack shall be dispensed. In all cases he must endorse the prescription 'p.n.c.' (prescriber not contacted) and indicate the quantity, the strength, where applicable, of the preparation supplied, and the dose, and initial and date the endorsement;
(e) if the pharmacist has any doubt about exercising discretion, an incomplete prescription must be referred back to the prescriber.

CONTROLLED DRUGS. A prescription for a controlled drug may not be dispensed by a pharmacist unless the requirements of Regulation 15 of the Misuse of Drugs Regulations, 1973 are met. He may not add to the prescription or otherwise exercise discretion on the quantity, dosage, or strength of the drug which is to be dispensed. All incomplete prescriptions must therefore be referred back to the prescriber.

NOTICE CONCERNING PATENTS. In the British National Formulary certain drugs have been included notwithstanding the existence of actual or potential patent rights. In so far as such substances are protected by Letters Patent, their inclusion in this Formulary neither conveys, nor implies, licence to manufacture.

HEALTH AND SAFETY. The British National Formulary is intended for the guidance of medical practitioners, pharmacists, dentists, nurses, and other workers who have the necessary training and experience to interpret the information it provides. It is intended as a reference book for the pocket, and should be supplemented by a study of more detailed publications when required.

When handling chemical or biological materials particular attention should be given to the possibility of allergy, fire, explosion, radiation, or poisoning. Some substances, including corticosteroids, antibiotics, phenothiazine derivatives, and many cytotoxic substances, are irritant or very potent and should be handled with caution. Contact with the skin and inhalation of dust should be avoided.

LABELLING OF CONTAINERS WITH THE NAME OF THE PREPARATION. The Councils of the British Medical Association and the Pharmaceutical Society have agreed that the name of the preparation should appear on the label unless the prescriber indicates otherwise.

1. Subject to the conditions of paragraphs 4 and 6 below, the name of the prescribed preparation is stated on the label of dispensed medicines unless the prescriber deletes the letters 'NP' which appear on National Health Service prescription forms.

2. The strength is also stated on the label in the case of tablets, capsules, and similar preparations that are available in different strengths.

3. If it is the wish of the prescriber that a description of the preparation such as 'The Sedative Tablets' should appear on the label, he should write the desired description on the prescription form.

4. The arrangement will extend to approved names, proprietary names or titles given in the BP, BPC, BNF, or DPF. The arrangement does not apply when a prescription is written so that several ingredients are given.

5. The name written on the label is that used by the prescriber on the prescription.

6. If more than one item is prescribed on one form and the prescriber does not delete the letters 'NP', each dispensed medicine is named on the label, subject to the conditions given above in paragraph 4. If the prescriber wants only selected items on such a prescription to be so labelled he will indicate this by deleting the letters 'NP' on the form and writing 'NP' alongside the medicines to be labelled.

7. When a prescription is written other than on a National Health Service prescription form the name of the prescribed preparation will be stated on the label of the dispensed medicine unless the prescriber indicates otherwise.

PRESCRIBING IN PREGNANCY. For many drugs there is not sufficient evidence to ensure that they are entirely harmless to the foetus, especially in the first trimester of pregnancy. Special care is therefore required in prescribing for pregnant patients. Medicines should be prescribed only when they are essential and in all cases the benefit of administering the medicine should be considered in relation to the risk involved.

Prescription Writing

Prescriptions should be written legibly in ink or typewritten, dated and signed by the prescriber, and the full name and address of the individual patient added. The age of the patient should preferably be stated, and is essential for children[1]. The following recommendations should be observed:

(a) For solids, quantities of 1 gram or more should be written as 1 g etc. Quantities less than 1 gram should be written in milligrams, for example 500 mg, not 0.5 g. Similar quantities less than 1 mg should be written in micrograms, for example 100 micrograms, not 0.1 mg. 'Micrograms' and 'nanograms' should **not** be abbreviated.

(b) When decimals are unavoidable a zero should be written in front of the decimal point where there is no other figure, for example 0.5 ml, not .5 ml.

(c) The term 'millilitre' (ml) is used in medicine and pharmacy, and cubic centimetre, c.c., or cm^3 should not be used.

(d) Dose and dose frequency should be stated. For liquid medicines, doses should be stated in terms of 5-ml quantities for the linctus or elixir type and for preparations for children, and 10-ml quantities for mixtures for adults. In the case of mixtures with a dose of 10 ml or more, the patient will be directed to take the dose with water unless the prescription states the contrary.
When doses other than 5 ml or 10 ml are prescribed, the liquid medicine will be diluted to provide a dose of 5 ml or 10 ml or a multiple thereof. Exception is made with certain preparations, which are measured by means of a pipette. The volume of liquid preparation prescribed should normally be 50, 100, 150, 200, 300, or 500 ml.

(e) Total quantities of solids prescribed should normally be selected from the range 25, 50, 100, 200, 300, and 500 grams.

(f) The use of abbreviations for names of drugs and preparations should be avoided.

(g) Ensure that the prescription contains the symbol 'NP' if the medicine is to be labelled with the name of the prescribed preparations.[2]

(h) The quantity to be supplied may be stated by indicating the *length of treatment required*, and in most cases the exact amount will be supplied.[3] This does not apply to items directed to be used as required, as it is not then possible to calculate the exact amount; in such cases the quantity to be supplied should be stated.

(i) Prescriptions written in accordance with these recommendations are acceptable for prescription-only medicines. For items marked **CD** refer to the instructions for writing prescriptions for controlled drugs.

1. This is a legal requirement in the case of prescription-only medicines.
2. The symbol 'NP' is printed on National Health Service prescription forms. It should be deleted by the prescriber if labelling with the name of the prescribed preparation is not required. For full details see under General Information.

Quantities of Preparations

The following list indicates the quantities of preparations suitable for various purposes.

Liquid Preparations

Adult Mixtures (10-ml dose)	200 ml (20 doses) 300 ml (30 doses)
Elixirs, Linctuses and Paediatric Mixtures (5-ml dose)	50 ml (10 doses) 100 ml (20 doses) 150 ml (30 doses)
Ear-drops, Eye-drops, and Nasal Drops	10 ml
Eye Lotions, Gargles, and Mouth-washes	200 ml
Inhalations and Sprays	25 ml
Liniments	100 ml

Dermatological Preparations

	Creams and Ointments	*Lotions*
Face	5 to 15 g	100 ml
Both hands	25 to 50 g	200 ml
Scalp	50 to 100 g	200 ml
Both arms or both legs	100 to 200 g	200 ml
Body	200 g	500 ml
Groins and genitalia	15 to 25 g	100 ml
Dusting-powders	50 to 100 g	
Paints	10 to 25 ml	

Hydrocortisone and other corticosteroid preparations should be applied sparingly; ointments are usually available in 15- and 30-g containers, and lotions in 20-ml containers.

3. The number of days' treatment should be inserted in the box provided on National Health forms.

Approximate Conversions and Units

lb	*kg*
1	0.45
2	0.91
3	1.36
4	1.81
5	2.27
6	2.72
7	3.18
8	3.63
9	4.08
10	4.54
11	4.99
12	5.44
13	5.90
14	6.35

Stones	*kg*
1	6.35
2	12.70
3	19.05
4	25.40
5	31.75
6	38.10
7	44.45
8	50.80
9	57.15
10	63.50
11	69.85
12	76.20
13	82.55
14	88.90
15	95.25

ml	*fl. oz (approx)*
50	1.8
100	3.5
150	5.3
200	7.0
500	17.6
1000	35.2

Mass

1 kilogram (kg)	= 1000 grams (g)
1 gram (g)	= 1000 milligrams (mg)
1 milligram (mg)	= 1000 micrograms
1 microgram	= 1000 nanograms
1 nanogram	= 1000 picograms

Volume

1 litre	= 1000 millilitres (ml)
1 millilitre	= 1000 microlitres
1 pint	≈ 568.3 ml

Other units

1 kilocalorie (kcal)	= 4186.8 joules (J)
1000 kilocalories (kcal)	= 4.1868 megajoules (MJ)
1 megajoule (MJ)	= 238.8 kilocalories (kcal)
1 millimetre of mercury (mmHg)	= 133.3 pascals (Pa)
1 kilopascal (kPa)	= 7.5 mmHg (pressure)

Prescribing for Children

Children differ from adults in their response to drugs. The first 30 days of life (neonate) is the most dangerous period and dosage must be calculated carefully. In neonates, the toxicity of drugs may be increased by delayed excretion, inefficient renal filtration, differing target organ sensitivity, inadequate detoxifying systems, and enzyme deficiencies.

Prescriptions must state the dose, frequency of administration, and age of the child.

It is particularly important that the strengths of capsules or tablets should be stated. Liquid preparations are particularly suitable for young children. However most liquid medicines for children contain sucrose which encourages dental decay.

When a prescription for a mixture is written for a child, if the dose ordered is smaller than 5 ml the preparation will normally be diluted with a suitable vehicle (such as syrup) so that the required dose is contained in 5 ml. The parent must be instructed to use the standard 5-ml spoon to measure the dose and not to heap up a viscous preparation.

Parents should also be advised not to add the dose of any medicine to the milk in the infant's feeding bottle or any other liquid contained in the feeder, since the drug may interact with the milk or liquid or the dosage may be reduced because not all the contents may be drunk.

Parents must also be warned to keep all medicines out of the reach of children in a safe locked place and no medicine should be left in a child's room. They should be advised to dispose of unused medicines by flushing them down a WC or returning them to the supplier for destruction. As an additional precaution, certain medicines may be supplied in child-resistant containers.

Dosage in Children

Paediatric doses are stated in the individual drug entries as far as possible, except where paediatric use is not recommended, as with tetracyclines, or where there are special hazards.

Doses are generally based on the following age ranges:

- first month (neonate)
- up to 1 year (infant)
- 1–5 years
- 6–12 years

Where a single dose is quoted for a given range, it applies to the middle of the age range and extrapolation is necessary to obtain doses for ages at the lower and upper limits.

Dose calculation. Children's doses are calculated from age, body-weight, or body-surface. Many formulae are used to calculate the dose for the child when only the adult dose is known. The most reliable methods are those based on body-surface.

Age is a convenient basis for commonly prescribed drugs with a high therapeutic index. The percentage of the adult dose is shown in the table below.

Body-weight can be used to calculate an approximate dose from the formula:

$$\frac{\text{Patient's weight in kg}}{70} \times \text{adult dose}$$

or

$$\frac{\text{Patient's weight in lb}}{150} \times \text{adult dose}$$

In general, children require a higher dose per kilogram body-weight than adults (usually twice the adult figure up to 4 months, 1½ times the adult figure up to 7 years), since they have a higher metabolic rate.

Certain problems may arise if the only criterion used for calculating paediatric dosage is body-weight. A common problem is the obese child who is overweight for his age and height. Calculation by body-weight would then result in a much larger dose being given than is really required. In such cases, therefore, doses should be calculated from an ideal weight obtained from a table relating height and age.

The table given below allows calculations to be made on the basis of age or weight. The dose calculated is suitable only for a child of average size. *It is not applicable to neonates.* Where new or potentially toxic drugs are used the table provides a useful starting dose but blood concentrations must be monitored throughout treatment and used as a guide to subsequent doses.

Age over	Body-weight kg	Body-weight lb	Body-surface m^2	Percentage of adult dose
4 weeks*	3.5	7.5	0.21	12.5
2 months*	4.5	10	0.28	15
4 months*	6.5	14	0.36	20
1 year	10	22	0.49	25
3 years	15	33	0.65	33
7 years	23	51	0.87	50
12 years	40	88	1.27	75
Adult	65	143	1.76	100

* In this table, the infant figures relate to full term and not preterm infants who may need reduced dosage according to their clinical condition.

Body-surface measurements are more accurate for calculation of paediatric doses than body-weight since many physical phenomena are more closely related to body-surface area. The average body-surface area of a 70-kilogram human is about 1.8 m^2. Thus, to calculate the dose for a child the following formula may be used:

Approximate dose for patient =

$$\frac{\text{surface area of patient (m}^2\text{)}}{1.8} \times \text{adult dose}$$

The formula provides only an approximate dose and is unreliable when applied to pre-term infants.

Body-surface may be calculated from height and weight by means of a table (for example *The Pharmaceutical Codex*, 11th Edition, London, Pharmaceutical Press, 1979) or a nomogram (for example, B. S. B. Wood, *A Paediatric Vademecum,* 9th Edition, London, Lloyd Luke, 1977).

Prescribing for the Elderly

Many elderly patients exhibit deterioration of body systems, metabolic deficiencies, and multiple pathology. As a result the number of adverse reactions to drugs in this age group is high and this must be taken into account when prescribing. It is advisable (but not essential) to indicate the patient's age on the prescription. Special care is necessary when more than one prescriber is involved in the patient's treatment. Moreover, self-medication with laxatives and analgesics (or even drugs prescribed for the spouse) may be an added complication. Careful drug-history taking is essential and the record of current therapy must be complete. A home visit may be necessary to achieve this.

DOSAGE. The efficacy of a drug depends on its absorption, metabolism, transport, and excretion as well as on end-organ sensitivity and all these factors may be affected. Consequently dosage must be adjusted to give the required effect and carefully monitored.

In assessing dosage it is advisable to assume that there is at least mild impairment of renal function. Repeat prescriptions should not be issued routinely until the dosage has been stabilised and even then treatment should be kept under review. It has been shown for example that many elderly patients do not need to be kept on digoxin forever.

PATIENT COMPLIANCE. Compliance with simple regimens involving one or two drugs is usually satisfactory, but when more complex schemes are involved compliance may prove a problem, particularly if memory and intellect are failing. Patients may need assistance or special supervision when many medicines have to be taken. Full directions should be written on all prescriptions and hence on the labels of the medicines. Combination products may seem to be a possible solution to the problem of compliance but may create problems by reducing the flexibility of dosage.

SYMPTOMATIC TREATMENT. Symptoms often require treatment but need careful evaluation; for example, sleeplessness may be due to nocturnal frequency. Sometimes symptoms represent a cry for help and may be alleviated by readjustment of the old person's environment or daily activities.

HARMFUL SIDE-EFFECTS. As a result of good prescribing many elderly patients are able to continue to live happily with their ailments well controlled. However, some drugs may precipitate or exaggerate changes or effects associated with ageing, for example hypothermia, and in some cases the patient's condition as a whole may actually improve if drug treatment is discontinued. Orthostatic hypotension may be induced by many different drugs such as diuretics, antidepressants, hypnotics, and tranquillisers, and an indication of this risk should be clearly incorporated in the patient's notes as one would for penicillin or aspirin sensitivity.

CONCLUSION. Many old people are still admitted to hospital because of inappropriate prescribing. If drugs do not seem to be having the desired effect and it has been confirmed that they are being taken correctly, they should be discontinued and the patient reassessed. Drug schedules should be kept as simple as possible and doses low but adequate.

Prescribing in Liver Disease

Liver disease may alter the response to drugs in several ways as indicated below. The Table may be used as a guide to treatment of patients with impaired liver function but is not exhaustive.

IMPAIRED DRUG METABOLISM. Metabolism by the liver is the main route of elimination for many drugs, but the hepatic reserve appears to be large and liver disease has to be severe before important changes in drug metabolism occur. Routine liver-function tests are a poor guide to the capacity of the liver to metabolise drugs, and in the individual patient it is not possible to predict the extent to which the metabolism of a particular drug may be impaired.

A few drugs, for example rifampicin and fusidic acid, are excreted in the bile unchanged and may accumulate in patients with cholestatic jaundice.

HYPOPROTEINAEMIA. The hypoalbuminaemia in severe liver disease is associated with reduced protein binding and increased toxicity of some highly protein-bound drugs such as phenytoin and prednisone.

REDUCED CLOTTING. Reduced hepatic synthesis of blood-clotting factors, indicated by a prolonged prothrombin time, increases the sensitivity to oral anticoagulants such as warfarin and phenindione.

HEPATIC ENCEPHALOPATHY. In severe liver disease many drugs can further impair cerebral function and may precipitate hepatic encephalopathy. These include all sedative drugs, narcotic analgesics, and those diuretics that produce hypokalaemia.

FLUID OVERLOAD. Oedema and ascites in chronic liver disease may be exacerbated by drugs that give rise to fluid retention. These include anti-inflammatory analgesics such as phenylbutazone and indomethacin, corticosteroids and corticotrophin, and carbenoxolone.

HEPATOTOXIC DRUGS. Hepatotoxicity is either dose-related or unpredictable (idiosyncratic). Drugs causing dose-related toxicity may do so at lower doses than in patients with normal liver function, and some drugs producing reactions of the idiosyncratic kind do so more frequently in patients with liver disease. These drugs should be avoided.

Table: Drugs to be avoided or used with caution in liver disease

Drugs	Comment
1: Gastro-intestinal system	
Antacids	In patients with fluid retention, avoid those containing large amounts of sodium, e.g. magnesium trisilicate mixture, Gaviscon®. Avoid those causing constipation, e.g. calcium compounds, as this can precipitate coma
Anti-emetics—see 4	
Carbenoxolone	Produces fluid retention and hypokalaemia
Cimetidine	More likely to produce confusional states in patients with liver disease
Diphenoxylate	May precipitate coma
2: Cardiovascular system	
Anticoagulants, oral	Avoid, especially if prothrombin time is already prolonged
Cholestyramine	Interferes with absorption of fat-soluble vitamins and may aggravate the malabsorption associated with primary biliary cirrhosis
Diuretics Bumetanide, Ethacrynic acid, Frusemide, Thiazides	Hypokalaemia may precipitate coma. A potassium-sparing diuretic should be used to prevent this
Lignocaine	Avoid—or reduce dose
Methyldopa	Avoid—idiosyncratic reactions more common in patients with liver disease
Propranolol, Labetalol	Reduce oral dose
3: Respiratory system	
Aminophylline	Reduce dose
Cough linctuses	Avoid those containing opiates, e.g. codeine, pholcodine

Table: Drugs to be avoided or used with caution in liver disease (*continued*)

Drugs	Comment
4: Central nervous system	
Analgesics	
Anti-inflammatory analgesics, Phenylbutazone, Ibuprofen, etc.	Increased risk of gastro-intestinal bleeding and can cause fluid retention
Aspirin	Increased risk of gastro-intestinal bleeding—avoid
Narcotic analgesics	Avoid—may precipitate coma
Paracetamol	Dose-related toxicity—avoid large doses
Antidepressants	Tricyclics are preferable to monoamine-oxidase inhibitors but sedative effects are increased. Iprindole and MAOIs may cause idiosyncratic hepatotoxicity
Antiepileptics	Phenobarbitone and primidone may precipitate coma. Phenytoin dose should be reduced to avoid toxicity
Anti-emetics	Avoid antihistamines and phenothiazines—may precipitate coma. Chlorpromazine is hepatotoxic
Hypnotics and sedatives, antipsychotics	All can precipitate coma. A small dose of lorazepam or oxazepam is probably the safest. The oral dose of chlormethiazole must be reduced. Chlorpromazine is hepatotoxic
5: Infections	
Bacampicillin	Avoid in severe liver disease—potentially toxic products of hydrolysis of ester may accumulate
Chloramphenicol	Increased risk of bone-marrow depression—avoid
Clindamycin	Reduce dose
Erythromycin estolate	May cause idiosyncratic hepatotoxicity
Fusidic acid	Impaired biliary excretion. May be increased risk of hepatotoxicity. Avoid or reduce dose
Isoniazid, Pyrazinamide	Idiosyncratic reactions more common in patients with liver disease—avoid
Niridazole	Increased CNS toxicity in patients with cirrhosis or portal-systemic shunts
Pivampicillin	as bacampicillin
Rifampicin	Impaired elimination. May be increased risk of hepatotoxicity. Avoid or reduce dose
Talampicillin	as bacampicillin
Tetracyclines	Dose-related toxicity by i/v route—avoid
6: Endocrine system	
Androgens and anabolic steroids (17α-alkyl derivatives)—Methyltestosterone, Fluoxymesterone, Methandienone, Norethandrolone, Oxymetholone, Stanozolol	Dose-related toxicity—avoid
Antidiabetic drugs	
Biguanides—Metformin, Phenformin	Avoid—increased risk of lactic acidosis
Sulphonylureas—Chlorpropamide, Tolbutamide	Avoid—increased risk of hypoglycaemia and can produce jaundice.
Corticosteroids	
Prednisolone, Prednisone	Side-effects are more common. Prednisolone is preferable to prednisone which has to be converted to prednisolone by the liver before it is active
7: Obstetrics and gynaecology	
Oral contraceptives	Increased risk in cholestatic liver disease and in patients with a history of pruritus or cholestasis during pregnancy—avoid
8: Malignant disease and immunosuppression	
Methotrexate	Dose-related toxicity—avoid in treatment of non-malignant conditions such as psoriasis
10: Musculoskeletal and joint disease	
Analgesics—see 4	

Prescribing in Renal Impairment

The use of drugs in patients with reduced renal function can give rise to problems for several reasons. Failure to excrete a drug or its metabolites may produce toxicity; sensitivity to some drugs is increased even if elimination is unimpaired; many side-effects are tolerated poorly by patients in renal failure; and some drugs cease to be effective when renal function is reduced. Many of these problems can be avoided by reducing the dose or by using alternative drugs.

Principles of dose adjustment in renal impairment

The level of renal function below which the dose of a drug must be reduced depends on whether the drug is eliminated entirely by renal excretion or is partly metabolised, and on how toxic it is.

For many drugs with only minor or no dose-related side-effects very precise modification of the dose regimen is unnecessary and a simple scheme for dose reduction is sufficient.

For more toxic drugs with a small safety margin dose schedules based on glomerular filtration rate should be used. For drugs where both efficacy and toxicity are closely related to blood concentrations the recommended schedules should be seen only as a guide to initial treatment, and subsequent treatment must be adjusted according to the clinical response and the serum concentration achieved.

The total daily maintenance dose of a drug can be reduced either by reducing the size of the individual doses or by increasing the interval between doses. For some drugs, if the size of the maintenance dose is reduced it will be important to give a loading dose if an immediate effect is required. This is because when a patient is given a regular dose of any drug it takes more than five times the half-life to achieve steady-state blood concentrations. As the plasma half-life of drugs excreted by the kidney is prolonged in renal failure it may take many days for the reduced dosage to achieve a therapeutic blood concentration. The loading dose should usually be the same size as the initial dose for a patient with normal renal function.

Nephrotoxic drugs should, if possible, be avoided in patients with renal disease because the consequences of nephrotoxicity are likely to be more serious when the renal reserve is already reduced.

Use of dosage table

Dose recommendations are based on the severity of renal impairment. This is expressed in terms of glomerular filtration rate (GFR), also known as the **creatinine clearance**. The serum-creatinine concentration can be used instead as a measure of renal function but is only a rough guide unless corrected for age, weight, and sex. Nomograms are available for making the correction and should be used where accuracy is important.

Renal impairment is arbitrarily divided into 3 grades:

Grade	*GFR*	*Serum creatinine (approx.)*
Mild	20–50 ml/min	150–300 μmol/litre
Moderate	10–20 ml/min	300–700 μmol/litre
Severe	< 10 ml/min	> 700 μmol/litre

Renal function declines with age, and many elderly patients have a glomerular filtration rate less than 50 ml/minute which may not be indicated by a change in serum creatinine. It is probably wise to assume at least mild impairment of renal function when prescribing for the elderly.

In the table, drugs are listed under the same body systems as the chapters and only those which require a reduction in dose, which are potentially harmful, or which are ineffective are mentioned.

Renal function should be checked before prescribing any drug which requires dose modification even when renal impairment is mild.

Table: Drugs to be avoided or used with caution in renal impairment

Drugs	GFR ml/minute	Dosage recommendations	Comments
1: Gastro-intestinal system			
Carbenoxolone	<10	Avoid	Causes fluid retention
Cimetidine	10–20 <10	600 mg daily 400 mg daily	Increased risk of confusional states
Gaviscon®	<10	Avoid	High sodium content
Magnesium trisilicate, Magnesium carbonate	<10	Avoid	Risk of magnesium toxicity. Magnesium trisilicate mixture and magnesium carbonate mixture also have high sodium content
Metoclopramide	<10	Avoid or use small dose	Increased risk of extrapyramidal reactions
2: Cardiovascular system			
Anti-arrhythmic drugs			
Disopyramide	20–50 10–20 <10	100 mg every 8 hours 100 mg every 12 hours 100 mg every 24 hours	
Procainamide	<50	Avoid or reduce dose	
Antihypertensive drugs			
Bethanidine, Debrisoquine, Guanethidine	<20	Avoid	Increased postural hypotension and decrease in renal blood flow
Diazoxide	<10	75–150 mg i/v	Increased sensitivity to hypotensive effect
Hydralazine	<10	Start with small dose	Increased hypotensive effect
Methyldopa	<10	Start with small dose	Increased sensitivity to hypotensive effect
Prazosin	<10	Start with small dose	Increased sensitivity to hypotensive effect
Beta-adrenoceptor blocking drugs			
Atenolol, Nadolol, Pindolol, Sotalol	<10	Reduce dose or use another beta-blocker	Excreted unchanged
Metoprolol, Propranolol	<10	Start with small dose	Higher blood concentrations after oral adminstration. May reduce renal blood flow and adversely affect renal function in severe renal failure
Digitalis preparations			
Digitoxin	<10	Max. 100 micrograms daily	Toxicity may be increased by electrolyte disturbances in severe renal failure
Digoxin	20–50	250 micrograms daily	as digitoxin
	10–20	125–250 micrograms daily	
	<10	Up to 125 micrograms daily	
Medigoxin	<50	Reduce by similar amount as for digoxin	as digitoxin

Table: Drugs to be avoided or used with caution in renal impairment (*continued*)

Drugs	GFR ml/minute	Dosage recommendations	Comments
Diuretics			
Acetazolamide	<10	Avoid	Causes metabolic acidosis
Amiloride, Spironolactone, Triamterene	20–50 <20	Monitor serum K^+ Avoid	High risk of hyperkalaemia in renal failure
Bumetanide	<20	May need high doses	
Ethacrynic acid	<10	Avoid	Ototoxic
Frusemide	<20	May need high doses	Deafness may follow rapid i/v injection
Thiazides and related diuretics (except metolazone)	<20	Avoid	Ineffective (metolazone remains effective at low GFR)
Miscellaneous			
Clofibrate	10–50 <10	Reduce dose Avoid	Myopathy and further deterioration in renal function
Sulphinpyrazone—see 10			
4: Central nervous system			
Antiepileptics			
Phenobarbitone, Primidone	<10	Avoid large doses	
Sulthiame	<20	Avoid	Produces a metabolic acidosis
Anti-inflammatory analgesics	<10	Avoid if possible	Fluid retention and deterioration in renal function
Aspirin	<10	Avoid	As above. Also increased risk of gastro-intestinal bleeding
Azapropazone, Diflunisal, Sulindac	<20	Avoid	Excreted by kidney
Hypnotics and sedatives, antipsychotics	<10	Start with small doses	Increased cerebral sensitivity
Amylobarbitone	<10	Reduce dose	Active metabolite accumulates
Narcotic analgesics			
Dextropropoxyphene, Pethidine	<10	Avoid	Increased CNS toxicity
Miscellaneous			
Amantadine	<50	Avoid	
Baclofen	<50	Use smaller doses	Excreted by kidney
Lithium	20–50	Avoid if possible or reduce dose and monitor carefully	
	<20	Avoid	
Nomifensine	<20	Avoid	Excreted by kidney
Phenazopyridine	<50	Avoid	Crystalluria, methaemoglobinaemia
5: Infections			
Aminoglycosides			
Amikacin, Gentamicin, Kanamycin, Streptomycin, Tobramycin	<50	Reduce dose Monitor blood concentrations	Ototoxic and nephrotoxic
Neomycin	<50	Avoid	Ototoxic and nephrotoxic

Table: Drugs to be avoided or used with caution in renal impairment (*continued*)

Drugs	GFR ml/minute	Dosage recommendations	Comments
Amphotericin	<50	Use only if no alternative	Nephrotoxic
Capreomycin	<50	Reduce dose	Neurotoxic and ototoxic
Cephalosporins			
Cefoxitin, Cefuroxime, Cephamandole, Cephazolin, Cephradine	<50	Reduce dose	
Cephalexin	<10	Max. 500 mg daily	
Cephaloridine, Cephalothin	<50	Avoid	Nephrotoxic
Chloramphenicol	<10	Avoid unless no alternative	Dose-related depression of haemopoiesis
Chloroquine—see 10			
Cinoxacin	<20	Avoid	Nausea, rashes
Colistin sulphomethate sodium	<50	Reduce dose	Nephrotoxic and neurotoxic
Co-trifamole	<10	Avoid	
Co-trimazine	<20	Avoid	
Co-trimoxazole	<10	Max. 960 mg daily	Rashes and blood dyscrasias
Cycloserine	<50	Avoid	
Ethambutol	<50	Reduce dose	Optic nerve damage
Flucytosine	<50	Reduce dose	
Hexamine mandelate, Hexamine hippurate	<20	Avoid	Ineffective
Isoniazid	<10	Max. 200 mg daily	Peripheral neuropathy
Lincomycin	<20	Use clindamycin instead	
Metronidazole	<20	Reduce dose for anaerobic infections	
Nalidixic acid	<20	Avoid	Nausea, vomiting, rashes, photosensitivity
Nitrofurantoin	<50	Avoid	Peripheral neuropathy
Penicillins			
Amoxycillin	<10	Reduce dose	Rashes more common
Ampicillin	<10	Max. 250 mg every 8 hours	Rashes more common
Bacampicillin	<10	Avoid	Potentially toxic products of hydrolysis of ester may accumulate
Benzylpenicillin	<10	Max. 6 g daily	Neurotoxicity
Carbenicillin	<20	Reduce dose	Neurotoxic. May produce bleeding diathesis. 1 g contains 5.4 mmol sodium
Ciclacillin	<50	Reduce dose	
Pivampicillin	<10	Avoid	as bacampicillin
Talampicillin	<10	Avoid	as bacampicillin
Piperazine	<10	Reduce dose	Neurotoxic
Sodium aminosalicylate	<50	Avoid	
Sulphadiazine	<10	Avoid	High risk of crystalluria
Other sulphonamides	<10	Ensure high fluid intake	Rashes and blood dyscrasias. Crystalluria is a risk

Table: Drugs to be avoided or used with caution in renal impairment (*continued*)

Drugs	GFR ml/minute	Dosage recommendations	Comments
Tetracyclines (except doxycycline and minocycline)	<50	Avoid—use doxycycline or minocycline if necessary	Anti-anabolic effect, increased blood urea, further deterioration in renal function
Trimethoprim	<10	Reduce dose	
Vancomycin	<50	Avoid parenteral use if possible	Ototoxic and nephrotoxic
6: Endocrine system			
Antidiabetic drugs			
Chlorpropamide	<50	Avoid	Use tolbutamide instead
Other sulphonylureas	<10	May need dose reduction	Increased risk of prolonged hypoglycaemia
Insulin	<10	May need dose reduction	Insulin requirements fall, and compensatory response to hypo-glycaemia is impaired
Metformin, Phenformin	<50	Avoid	Increased risk of lactic acidosis
Propylthiouracil	<50	Reduce dose	
8: Malignant disease and immunosuppression			
Azathioprine	<10	Reduce dose	
Bleomycin, Cyclophosphamide, Melphalan, Mercaptopurine, Procarbazine, Thioguanine	<20	Reduce dose	
Cisplatin	<10	Avoid	Nephrotoxic
Methotrexate	20–50 <20	Reduce dose Avoid	Accumulates. Also nephrotoxic
9: Nutrition and blood			
Potassium supplements	<20	Avoid routine use	High risk of hyperkalaemia
10: Musculoskeletal and joint disease			
Allopurinol	10–20	Max. 200 mg daily	Increased toxicity; rashes
	<10	Max. 100 mg daily	
Chloroquine	20–50 10–20 <10	Max. 75 mg daily Max. 50 mg daily Avoid	Applies only to prolonged use
Colchicine	<10	Avoid	
Gold (sodium aurothiomalate)	<50	Avoid	Nephrotoxic
Penicillamine	<50	Avoid if possible or reduce dose	Nephrotoxic
Probenecid	<20	Avoid	Ineffective and toxicity increased
Sulphinpyrazone	<20	Avoid	Ineffective as a uricosuric
15: Anaesthetics			
Neuromuscular blocking drugs			
Fazadinium, Gallamine	<20	Avoid	Prolonged paralysis
Alcuronium, Pancuronium, Tubocurarine	<20		Large or repeated doses can produce prolonged paralysis

Adverse Reactions to Drugs

Almost any drug may produce unwanted or unexpected adverse reactions. Some of these like anaphylactic shock, blood dyscrasias, jaundice due to liver damage, cardiac arrhythmias, or exfoliative dermatitis may be a hazard to life. Not only is the incidence of drug reactions often not known but it is likely that there are many reactions which are not at present recognised as due to drugs. Doctors are asked to help research in this field by reporting all serious or fatal illnesses thought to be due to drugs and any unexpected reactions to The Medical Assessor, The Committee on Safety of Medicines, Market Towers, 1 Nine Elms Lane, London SW8 5NQ. Telephone: 01-720 2188.

There is no need to report well known adverse effects of older and established drugs such as rashes with penicillin or dry mouth with atropine but serious or unusual reactions should be reported even with these older drugs.

Preparations indicated by the sign ▼ are newer preparations for which the CSM requests that *all* suspected adverse reactions should be reported even if they are apparently minor ones such as rashes or gastro-intestinal upsets.

A supply of yellow prepaid postcards for reporting suspected adverse reactions is available from the above address.

Prevention of adverse reactions

1. Never use any drug unless there is a good indication. If the patient is pregnant do not use a drug unless the need for it is imperative.
2. It is very important to recognise allergy and idiosyncrasy as causes of adverse drug reactions. Ask the patient if he has had previous reactions.
3. Ask the patient if he is already taking other drugs and remember that drug interactions may occur.
4. Remember that age, hepatic disease, or renal disease may alter the metabolism or excretion of drugs, so that they may need to be prescribed in much smaller doses than usual. Pharmacogenetic factors may also be responsible for variations in the rate of metabolism of drugs, notably isoniazid and the tricyclic antidepressants. Appropriate dose adjustments may be necessary to compensate for these variations.
5. Always prescribe as few drugs as possible and give very clear instructions to the elderly or any patient likely to misunderstand complicated instructions.
6. When possible use a drug with which you are familiar. Be especially on the watch for adverse reactions if you use a new drug.
7. If serious adverse reactions are liable to occur warn the patient.

It is often wise to ask the patient to carry a card with information about his treatment, especially if it is to be long continued. Standard cards are available for oral anticoagulant treatment (section 2.8.2), monoamine-oxidase inhibitors (section 4.3.2), and corticosteroids (section 6.3.4).

Controlled Drugs and Drug Dependence

Prescriptions for controlled drugs

Preparations which are subject to the prescription requirements of the Misuse of Drugs Regulations 1973 are distinguished throughout the British National Formulary by the symbol **CD** (Controlled Drugs). The principal legal requirements relating to medical prescriptions are listed below.

Prescriptions ordering Controlled Drugs subject to prescription requirements must be *signed* and *dated*[1] by the prescriber and give his *address*. The prescription must always state *in the prescriber's own handwriting* (unless the prescriber has been specially exempted from this requirement) in ink or otherwise so as to be indelible:

1. The name and address of the patient
2. In the case of a preparation, the form and where appropriate the strength of the preparation
3. The total quantity of the drug or preparation, or the number of dose units, *in both words and figures*
4. The dose

A prescription may order a Controlled Drug to be dispensed by instalments; the amount of the instalments and the intervals to be observed must be specified.[2] 'Repeat' prescriptions are **not** permitted.

1. A prescription is valid for 13 weeks from the date stated thereon

2. A special form, FP10HP(ad), in Scotland HBP(A), is available to certain doctors in the National Health Service for prescribing cocaine, diamorphine, or methadone by instalments. Forms FP10 and FP10HP, in Scotland GP10 and HBP, are valid for supply on only **one** occasion

It is an offence for a doctor to issue an incomplete prescription and a pharmacist is **not** allowed to dispense a Controlled Drug unless all the information required by law is given on the prescription. Failure to comply with the regulations concerning the writing of prescriptions will result in inconvenience to patients and delay in supplying the necessary medicine.

Drug dependence related to misuse of drugs

The prevalence of drug dependence and misuse in Great Britain, particularly amongst young people, continues to give cause for concern to teachers, social workers, and the police, as well as doctors.

The most serious drugs of addiction are **diamorphine** (heroin), **morphine,** and the **synthetic narcotics.** The likelihood that the dose will be increased is considerable, psychic dependence is common, and the withdrawal syndrome may be severe.

Dependence on **amphetamine** is less serious and now less common that it used to be. It has been shown that the incidence of dependence and misuse of the amphetamines was related to the extent to which they were prescribed. As a result of the campaign run by doctors with the intention of reducing the prescribing of amphetamines, their use has fallen very markedly and many combination products containing amphetamines have been withdrawn from the market. There has been a similar campaign against **barbiturates**. The only indication for barbiturates (apart from their use in epilepsy or anaesthesia) is severe intractable insomnia.

Cannabis (Indian hemp) has no valid medicinal use and cannot be prescribed by doctors (except under licence from the Home Secretary). Its use is illegal but has become widespread in certain sections of society.Cannabis is a mild hallucinogen. It is seldom accompanied by a desire to increase the dose and withdrawal symptoms are unusual. **Lysergide** (lysergic acid diethylamide, LSD) is a much more potent hallucinogen. Its use can lead to severe psychotic states in which life may be at risk.

The Misuse of Drugs Act, 1971

This Act was passed in 1971 to provide more flexible and more comprehensive control over the misuse of drugs of all kinds than was possible under the earlier Dangerous Drugs Act. The Act prohibits certain activities in relation to 'Controlled drugs', in particular their manufacture, supply and possession. The penalties applicable to offences involving the different drugs are graded broadly according to the *harmfulness attributable to a drug when it is misused* and for this purpose the drugs are defined in the following three classes.

Class A includes: cocaine, dextromoramide, diamorphine (heroin), dipipanone, methadone, morphine, opium, pethidine, phencyclidine, lysergide (LSD), and class B substances when prepared for injection
Class B includes: oral amphetamines, cannabis, cannabis resin, codeine, ethylmorphine, methylphenidate, phenmetrazine, and pholcodine
Class C includes: certain drugs related to the amphetamines such as benzphetamine and chlorphentermine, and pipradrol

The Misuse of Drugs Regulations 1973 define the classes of person who are authorised to supply and possess controlled drugs while acting in their professional capacities and lay down the conditions under which these activities may be carried out. In the regulations drugs are divided into four schedules each specifying the requirements governing such activities as import, export, production, supply, possession, prescribing, and record keeping which apply to them.

Notification of Addicts

The Misuse of Drugs (Notification of and Supply to Addicts) Regulations 1973 require a medical practitioner to notify the Chief Medical Officer, Drugs Branch, Queen Anne's Gate, London SW1H 9AT of any person he considers, or has reasonable grounds to suspect, is addicted to any of the following substances:

Cocaine	Methadone
Dextromoramide	Morphine
Diamorphine	Opium
Dipipanone	Oxycodone
Hydrocodone	Pethidine
Hydromorphone	Phenazocine
Levorphanol	Piritramide

Dipipanone is only legally available as Diconal® Tablets. Dipipanone is addictive and its popularity amongst addicts has increased over the past few years and is causing some concern. Doctors and others should be suspicious of young people who ask for it, especially as temporary residents.

Particulars to be notified to the Chief Medical Officer are:

Name and address
Sex
Date of birth
National Health Service number
Date of first attendance
Name or names of drug or drugs to which the patient is or is suspected of being addicted

The notification must be made within seven days of first becoming aware that the patient may be an addict and only the particulars of which the practitioner has knowledge need be notified immediately; the remainder may be notified at a later date. Notification should be confirmed annually if the patient is still being treated by the practitioner. Notified information is incorporated in an Index which is maintained in the Home Office and any doctor may refer to this Index for information about a person under his care; in fact, it is good medical practice to check all new cases of addiction or suspected addiction with the Index before prescribing or supplying controlled drugs since this is a safeguard against addicts obtaining supplies simultaneously from two or more doctors. Enquiries can be made either in writing to the Chief Medical Officer or, preferably, by telephone 01-213 5141, 4274 or 6083. To keep notified information confidential, such enquiries are normally answered by means of a return telephone call. It should be noted that the reply will come from lay staff who are not qualified to give guidance on the clinical handling of cases.

The preceding paragraph applies only to medical practitioners in England, Scotland, and Wales. In Northern Ireland notification should be sent to the Chief Medical Officer, Department of Health and Social Services, Dundonald House, Belfast BT4 3SF, and any enquiries about the Northern Ireland Regulations or addicts should be made to that Department, also at Dundonald House, telephone number 0232 63939 extension 2874.

Prescribing of diamorphine (heroin) and cocaine for addicts

The Misuse of Drugs (Notification of and Supply to Addicts) Regulations also provide that only medical practitioners who hold a special licence issued by the Home Secretary may prescribe diamorphine or cocaine for addicts; other practitioners must refer any addict who requires these drugs to a treatment centre. General practitioners and other doctors may still prescribe heroin and cocaine for patients (including addicts) for relief of pain due to organic disease or injury without a special licence. Whenever possible the addict will be introduced by a member of staff from the treatment centre to a pharmacist whose agreement has been obtained and whose pharmacy is conveniently sited for the patient. Prescriptions for weekly supplies will be sent to the pharmacy by post and will be dispensed on a daily basis as indicated by the doctor. If any alterations of the arrangements are requested by the addict, the pharmacist **must** contact the treatment centre to ensure that such alteration is acceptable.

Prescribing drugs likely to cause dependence or misuse

The prescriber has three main responsibilities. The first is to see that he does not create dependence by introducing drugs to patients without sufficient reason. In this context, the proper use of the morphine-like drugs is well understood. The dangers of other controlled drugs are less clear because recognition of dependence is not easy and its effects, and those of withdrawal, are less obvious. Consequently, divergent views are held. Perhaps the most notable result of uninhibited prescribing is that there is a very large number of patients in the country taking tablets which do them neither much good nor much harm, but who are committed to them indefinitely because they cannot readily be stopped.

The second is to see that the patient does not gradually increase the dose of a drug, given for good medical reasons, to the point where dependence becomes more likely. This tendency is seen especially with the barbiturates and also with other hypnotics and tranquillisers, including the benzodiazepines. The prescriber should keep a close eye on the amount he prescribes to prevent patients from accumulating stocks that would enable them to arrange their own dosage or even that of their families and friends. A minimal amount should be prescribed in the first instance, or when seeing a new patient for the first time.

The third is for the prescriber to see that he is not being used as an unwitting source of supply for addicts. This manoeuvre is often attempted by addicts to narcotic analgesics and they may be very skilled, plausible, and persistent in attaining their ends.

The methods include visiting more than one doctor, fabricating stories to substantiate demands, and forging prescriptions. A doctor should therefore be wary of prescribing for strangers and he may be able to get information about suspected opiate addicts from the Drugs Branch of the Home Office or in Northern Ireland from the Drugs Branch, Department of Health and Social Services (*see* above).

Patients under temporary care should be given only small supplies of drugs unless they present an unequivocal letter from their own doctors. Doctors should remember that their own patients may be doing a collecting round with other doctors, especially in hospitals. It is sensible to decrease dosages steadily or to issue weekly or even daily prescriptions for small amounts if it is apparent that dependence is occurring.

The stealing and misuse of prescription forms could be minimised by the following precautions:

(a) lock up prescription pads whenever possible and avoid leaving them unattended if called away from the consulting room;
(b) draw a diagonal line across the blank part of the form under the prescription;
(c) write the quantity in words and figures when prescribing drugs prone to abuse; this is obligatory for controlled drugs (see Prescriptions for Controlled Drugs, above);
(d) alterations are best avoided but if any are made they should be clear and unambiguous; add initials against altered items;
(e) if prescriptions are left for collection they should be left in a safe place in a sealed envelope.

Preparations used in the treatment of drug dependence

CD Methadone Mixture 1 mg/ml, methadone hydrochloride 1 mg/ml (see Formulary). Price 100 ml = **B**. Used in replacement and maintenance treatment.
Note: this preparation is 2½ times the strength of methadone linctus.

Preparations used in the treatment of alcoholism

Disulfiram (Antabuse®) and **citrated calcium carbimide** (Abstem®) are used as an adjunct to the treatment of alcoholism. They give rise to extremely unpleasant systemic reactions after the ingestion of even small amounts of alcohol because they lead to accumulation of acetaldehyde in the body. Reactions include flushing of the face, throbbing headache, palpitations, tachycardia, nausea, vomiting, and, with large doses of alcohol, cardiac arrhythmias, hypotension, and collapse. Even the small amounts of alcohol included in many oral medicines may be sufficient to precipitate a reaction. It may be advisable for patients to carry a card warning of the danger of administration of alcohol.

For use of chlormethiazole in withdrawal treatment see section 4.1.1 and for use of benzodiazepines see section 4.1.2.

Abstem® (Lederle)
Tablets, citrated calcium carbimide 50 mg. Price 20 tabs = **E**
Dose: 50 mg twice daily

Antabuse 200® (Weddel)
Tablets, scored, disulfiram 200 mg. Price 20 tabs = **B**
Dose: initially 800 mg daily, reducing to 100–200 mg daily

Emergency Treatment of Poisoning

These notes deal with the management of acute poisoning when first seen in the home and although brief mention is given to certain aspects of hospital-based treatment, it is recommended that the reader refers to other sources for further information. The notes are divided into the following subsections.

General measures
- **1** Respiratory function
- **2** Shock
- **3** Hypothermia
- **4** Cardiac arrhythmias
- **5** Removal of poison from the stomach
- **6** Oral adsorbents
- **7** Active elimination techniques
- **8** Hospital admission

Notes on some common poisons
- **9** Amphetamine and related drugs
- **10** Aspirin and other Salicylates
- **11** Barbiturates and other Sedatives
- **12** Iron salts
- **13** Lithium salts
- **14** Morphine and other Narcotic Analgesics
- **15** Paracetamol
- **16** Paracetamol with Dextropropoxyphene
- **17** Phenothiazine derivatives
- **18** Tricyclic Antidepressants
- **19** Carbon Monoxide
- **20** Sulphur Dioxide, Chlorine, Phosgene, Ammonia
- **21** Snake and Insect Bites
- **22** Paraquat
- **23** Antidotes to other poisons

General measures

1. Respiratory function

Respiratory function is often impaired and requires immediate attention. All comatose patients are liable to obstruction by the tongue falling back and this can be avoided by holding the jaw forward, turning the patient semiprone or inserting an oropharyngeal airway. Drowsy and comatose patients are liable to inhale vomit; this risk is minimised with the patient positioned semiprone and head down. In the unconscious patient no attempt at passing a stomach tube should be made unless the lungs have been protected from aspiration by the passage of a cuffed endotracheal tube.

Most poisons that impair consciousness also depress respiration. This may not be very obvious if the rate is normal, yet the depth may be inadequate. Assistance may be needed according to circumstances by mouth to mouth or Ambu bag inflation or by one of the methods of 'artificial' respiration. Oxygen is not a substitute for ventilation, though it should be given in the highest concentration possible in poisoning with carbon monoxide and irritant gases.

Respiratory stimulants do not help and are **potentially dangerous**.

2. Shock

Shock is due to expansion of the venous capacitance bed causing a relative or absolute deficiency of intravascular volume and is most common in severe barbiturate poisoning. A systolic blood pressure of less than 80 mmHg impairs blood flow to the brain and kidneys and may result in permanent organ damage. The patient should be carried head downwards on a stretcher and nursed in this position in the ambulance. Oxygen should be given to correct any hypoxia and an intravenous infusion should be set up if at all practicable. Vasoconstrictors have now been abandoned as they may further decrease the blood supply to essential organs, despite increasing arterial blood pressure. Fluid depletion without hypotension is also common after prolonged coma and after aspirin poisoning on account of vomiting, sweating and hyperpnoea.

Fits should be stopped by intravenous diazepam or intramuscular paraldehyde. These drugs may further depress respiration and necessitate assistance.

Contaminated clothes, especially with organophosphorus compounds should be stripped off, wearing rubber gloves, and the patient washed with soap and water.

3. Hypothermia

Hypothermia is common in the elderly who have been in coma for some hours from the effects of barbiturates or phenothiazines. It is not obvious in such circumstances, but can be detected by a low-reading rectal thermometer. It is best treated by wrapping the patient in blankets to conserve his own heat. Hot-water bottles cause burns.

4. Cardiac arrhythmias

Cardiac arrhythmias may occur in acute poisoning, notably with the tricyclic antidepressants, but often respond to correction of hypoxia or acidosis. Persistent life-threatening ventricular arrhythmias that have been confirmed by emergency electrocardiography may require treatment with lignocaine hydrochloride 50 to 100 mg intravenously. Supraventricular arrhythmias are seldom immediately life-threatening and drug treatment is best withheld until the patient reaches hospital.

5. Removal of poison from the stomach

Removal of poison from the stomach is a contentious subject; the dangers of emptying the stomach have to be balanced against the toxicity of the ingested poison which must be considered in terms of quantity of poison ingested, severity of poisoning likely to result, and the time that has elapsed since ingestion. It can thus be seen that no action is needed if the risk of toxicity is small or the patient presents too late.

Emptying the stomach by **gastric lavage** or **emesis** is of doubtful value if attempted more than 4 hours after ingestion. However, a worthwhile recovery of salicylates can be achieved up to 24 hours and tricyclics (which delay gastric emptying) up to 8 hours. The chief danger of gastric aspiration and lavage is inhalation of stomach contents, and nothing should be attempted in drowsy or comatose patients unless the airway can be protected by a cuffed tube. Tubes should **not** be passed after corrosive poisoning.

Petroleum products are more dangerous in the lung than in the stomach and therefore removal from the stomach is not advised because of the risk of inhalation.

On balance therefore gastric lavage is almost never practical or desirable before the patient reaches hospital.

Emesis induced by using ipecacuanha (Paediatric Ipecacuanha Emetic Mixture, equivalent in strength to ipecacuanha syrup USP or Adelaide Children's Hospital formula) is favoured in children and may also be effective in adults. This may be given safely in the home providing that the patient is fully conscious and that the poison ingested is neither caustic nor a petroleum distillate. (Dosage is 10 ml from 6 to 18 months, 15 ml in older children, 30 ml in adults, repeated after 20 minutes if emesis has not occurred.) Pharyngeal stimulation may be effective if used immediately after ingestion of a poison in children.

All the other substances which have been recommended as **emetics** (such as sodium chloride, copper sulphate, apomorphine, or mustard) are **unreliable** and dangerous and should not be used.

Ipecacuanha Emetic Mixture, Paediatric, total alkaloids (as emetine) 14 mg/10 ml (see Formulary). Price 100 ml = **A**
Dose: see notes above

6. Oral adsorbents

In theory, absorption of a poison from the gut may be reduced by adsorption on to other substances taken by mouth. The old 'Universal Antidote' was potentially toxic in its own right but activated charcoal is safe and there is experimental evidence which suggests that it is particularly useful for the prevention of absorption of poisons which are toxic in small amounts, for example antidepressants. The dose is 5 or 10 g in water. A convenient effervescent formulation is available.

CHARCOAL, ACTIVATED
(Charcoal)
Indications: adsorption of potent poisons
Dose: *by mouth,* 5 to 50 g as a thick suspension in water

Charcoal Powder. Price 50 g = **B**
Medicoal® (Lundbeck)
Granules, effervescent, charcoal 5 g/sachet. Price per sachet = **B**
Dose: adults and children, 5–10 g in 100 ml water, repeated at intervals of 20 minutes, to a max. of 50 g

7. Active elimination techniques

Active elimination techniques may be of value in removing poisons that have already been absorbed from the gut. These are obviously only practicable in hospital and in fact are needed for only a small number of patients who are severely poisoned with a limited number of poisons.

Examples include:
- Forced Alkaline Diuresis for salicylates and phenobarbitone
- Forced Acid Diuresis for amphetamines and quinine
- Haemodialysis for salicylates and phenobarbitone
- Charcoal Haemoperfusion for medium- and short-acting barbiturates

8. Hospital admission

Hospital admission is generally advisable for all patients who show any symptoms of poisoning. Patients who appear well should also be referred if they have taken a poison with a delayed action such as salicylates, iron, paracetamol, tricyclic antidepressants, paraquat, and diphenoxylate with atropine. A note should be sent of what is known and has been done, together with a specimen of any vomit.

The identity of the poison and the size of the dose is often impossible to establish with any precision. Fortunately this is usually not very important because there are few poisonings that have specific antidotes, e.g. narcotic analgesics and iron, and few cases that require active removal of the drug. All others are dealt with by treating the clinical state as it presents. Nevertheless, knowledge of the type of poisoning does help in anticipating the course of events. Patients' reports may be little help, as they are confused or can only say they have taken an undefined amount, possibly of mixed drugs. Parents may think a child has taken something which might be poisonous. They may exaggerate or underplay the risks out of anxiety or guilt. Sometimes symptoms are due to an illness such as appendicitis. Accidents may arise from a large number of domestic and industrial products the contents of which are not generally known. Information can be obtained from the poisons information services at the following telephone numbers.

National Poisons Information Service

Belfast	0232 40503
Cardiff	0222 492233
Dublin	0001 745588
Edinburgh	031-229 2477
London	01-407 7600

Other Centres

Leeds	0532 32799
Manchester	061-795 7000
Newcastle	0632 325131

Laboratory analysis may help in the diagnosis and management of a small number of cases. Information on the available services can be obtained from the National Poisons Information Centre in London.

Notes on some common poisons

9. Amphetamine and related drugs

These cause wakefulness, excessive activity, psychotic states, and hypertension followed by exhaustion, convulsions, hyperthermia, and coma. The early stages can be controlled by chlorpromazine or barbiturates. Later, tepid sponging, anticonvulsants, and artificial respiration may be needed. Amphetamine excretion can also be increased by forced acid diuresis.

10. Aspirin and other Salicylates

Large amounts may lie unabsorbed in the stomach for several hours. The chief features are hyperpnoea, tinnitus, and sweating. Coma is uncommon except in children. There are complicated and altering metabolic disturbances, and patients are often more ill than is at first apparent. Gastric aspiration and lavage should be performed in all cases. Treatment must be in hospital where plasma salicylate, pH, and electrolytes can be measured. Fluid losses are replaced and forced alkaline diuresis should be considered when the plasma salicylate is greater than 50 mg/100 ml (500 mg/litre) in adults or 30 mg/100 ml (300 mg/litre) in children.

11. Barbiturates and other Sedatives

These are unpredictably absorbed but drowsiness and coma develop quickly. The duration and depth of cerebral depression vary greatly with the drug, the dose, and the tolerance of the patient. The severity of poisoning is often greater with a large dose of short- or medium-acting barbiturate than with the longer-acting phenobarbitone. The benzodiazepines seldom cause more than a prolonged but reversible period of unconsciousness unless the patient has chronic airway disease or emphysema, when death can occur. Respiratory depression, shock and circulatory failure, and hypothermia may have to be dealt with. Forced alkaline diuresis may be considered in severe phenobarbitone poisoning and a high urine output should in any case be maintained.

12. Iron salts

Poisoning is seen chiefly in children who swallow tablets that have been left about. The symptoms are gastro-intestinal irritation, dehydration, and later, damage to the liver and the nervous system. Mortality is reduced with intensive and specific therapy. The effective antidote is **desferrioxamine**, which produces a chelate with iron. The stomach should be emptied at once, preferably by inducing vomiting, as this is quickest and will get rid of tablets. Gastric lavage in hospital should follow as soon as possible, using desferrioxamine mesylate solution 2 g to 1 litre. A solution of 10 g of desferrioxamine mesylate in 50 ml water should be left in the stomach. Absorbed iron can also be chelated by an intramuscular injection of 2 g of desferrioxamine mesylate in 10 ml of water.

DESFERRIOXAMINE MESYLATE

Indications: removal of iron from the body in poisoning; chronic iron overload, as in haemolytic anaemia or haemochromatosis, see section 9.1.3

Side-effects: pain at site of intramuscular injection, anaphylactic reactions when intravenous injections are given too rapidly

Dose: in iron poisoning, *by mouth* after gastric lavage, 5–10 g in 50–100 ml of liquid

By intramuscular injection, 2 g in 8–12 ml of water for injections

By continuous intravenous infusion, up to 15 mg/kg/hour with a max. in 24 hours of 80 mg/kg

Desferal® (Ciba)

Injection, powder for reconstitution, desferrioxamine mesylate. Price 500-mg vial = **D**

13. Lithium salts

Most cases of lithium intoxication occur as a complication of long-term therapy and are caused by reduced excretion of the drug due to a variety of factors including deterioration of renal function, infections, dehydration, and co-adminstration of diuretic drugs. Acute deliberate overdoses may also occur and may exhibit a delayed onset of symptoms (12 hours or more) due to delayed entry of lithium into the tissues and the effects of sustained-release formulations.

The early clinical features are non-specific and may include apathy and restlessness which could be confused with mental changes due to the patient's depressive illness. Vomiting, diarrhoea, ataxia, weakness, dysarthria, muscle twitching, and tremor may follow. Severe poisoning is associated with convulsions, coma, renal failure, electrolyte imbalance and hypotension.

The usual therapeutic lithium concentrations are within the range of 0.6 to 1.2 mmol/litre. Lithium concentrations in excess of this range are likely to cause toxicity. Plasma lithium concentrations in excess of 2.2–2.5 mmol/litre are usually associated with serious toxicity and such cases may need treatment with forced alkaline diuresis or dialysis (if there is renal failure). Otherwise treatment is supportive with special regard to electrolyte balance, renal function, and control of convulsions.

14. Morphine and other Narcotic Analgesics

These cause varying degrees of coma, with hypoventilation and pinpoint pupils. The specific antidote naloxone is indicated if there is coma or dangerous bradypnoea. **Naloxone** is short-acting and 0.4 to 1.2 mg is given intravenously, repeated as required according to the state of breathing and degree of consciousness. Earlier antidotes such as nalorphine are also partial agonists and thus can depress respiration themselves. Their use has been discontinued.

NALOXONE HYDROCHLORIDE

Indications: overdosage with morphine-like compounds

Cautions: pregnancy, physical dependence on narcotics, large narcotic overdosage

Dose: by subcutaneous, intramuscular, or intravenous injection, 400 micrograms repeated once or twice at intervals of 2–3 minutes if respiratory function does not improve; CHILD 5–10 micrograms/kg

Narcan® (Winthrop)

Injection, naloxone hydrochloride 400 micrograms/ml. Price 1-ml amp = **F**

Narcan Neonatal® (Winthrop)

Injection, naloxone hydrochloride 20 micrograms/ml. Price 2-ml amp = **E**

15. Paracetamol

This can cause severe liver damage, often fatal, occurring up to several days after taking as little as 20 to 30 tablets (10 to 15 g). It can occur without jaundice. Less frequent complications are renal failure, cardiac damage, generalised bleeding, and hypoglycaemia. The use of antidotes such as **methionine**, **acetylcysteine**, or **cysteamine** is dictated by the plasma-paracetamol concentration and affords protection to the liver if given within 10 to 12 hours of ingestion. Treatment should be given to all patients who have plasma concentrations above a line (drawn on log/linear paper) joining the points 200 mg/litre at 4 hours and 60 mg/litre at 10 hours.

Ideally the patient should be seen in hospital as soon as possible but, if it is believed that a serious overdose has occurred, treatment in the home is feasible. An emetic may be given up to 4 hours after the paracetamol was ingested and the first dose of the antidotes methionine (2.5 g by mouth) or acetylcysteine (150 mg/kg intravenously over 15 minutes) can be given within 10 to 12 hours of ingestion of the paracetamol.Initiation of treatment should be based on clinical findings. The need for continued therapy may be reviewed in accordance with plasma paracetamol determinations; concentrations greater than 200 mg/litre at 4 hours or 60 mg/litre at 10 hours after the overdose are considered evidence that treatment should be continued. Cysteamine (mercaptamine) is not available in commerce but supplies are available from some poison centres. It is used in the same way as acetylcysteine but is more toxic.

METHIONINE

Indications: treatment of paracetamol overdosage

Dose: by mouth, 2.5 g initially, followed by further doses of 2.5 g every 4 hours depending on the plasma paracetamol concentration

Methionine Tablets, methionine 250 mg. Price 20 tabs = **C**

ACETYLCYSTEINE

Indications: treatment of paracetamol overdosage

Dose: by intravenous injection, initially 150 mg/kg over 15 minutes, followed by 50 mg/kg in 500 ml dextrose intravenous infusion (5%) over 4 hours and 100 mg/kg in 1000 ml dextrose intravenous infusion (5%) over 16 hours, adjusted according to the plasma-paracetamol concentration

Parvolex® (DF)

Injection, acetylcysteine 200 mg/ml. Price 10-ml amp = **E**

16. Paracetamol with Dextropropoxyphene

These drugs (in Distalgesic® etc.) are now frequently taken in overdosage. The initial presentation is one of acute narcotic overdosage with coma, respiratory depression, and pinpoint pupils. Such patients may die before reaching hospital unless adequately treated by resuscitation and administration of **naloxone** as antidote. Toxic effects due to the paracetamol content may develop later and require treatment as indicated for that drug (above).

17. Phenothiazine derivatives

There is less disturbance of consciousness and respiratory depression than with other sedatives. Hypotension, hypothermia, sinus tachycardia, and other cardiac arrhythmias may complicate poisoning and dystonic reactions can occur with small doses, and convulsions in severe cases. Drugs to control arrhythmias, dystonic reactions, and convulsions may be needed.

18. Tricyclic Antidepressants

These cause dryness of the mouth, coma of varying degree, hypothermia, hyperreflexia, convulsions, respiratory failure, and various cardiac arrhythmias. Dilated pupils, ileus, and urinary retention are commonly noted. The onset of symptoms may be delayed and hospital admission is advisable. Symptomatic treatment and activated charcoal by mouth may reasonably be given in the home before transfer.

19. Carbon Monoxide

The diagnosis may be obvious from the circumstances, but the clinical appearance is not always classical. Suicidal patients may have swallowed poisons as well. Immediate treatment is essential and the person should be removed into the fresh air, the airway cleared and artificial ventilation given. Oxygen (100%) should be administered as soon as available. Artificial respiration should be continued until adequate spontaneous breathing starts, or stopped only after persistent and efficient treatment of cardiac arrest has failed. About half the carbon monoxide will have been removed by one hour's ventilation in air, and most of it if oxygen is used. Admission to hospital is desirable because of complications which may arise after a delay of some hours or days. There may be a relapse into coma from cerebral oedema, which can be treated with corticosteroids or an intravenous infusion of mannitol.

20. Sulphur Dioxide, Chlorine, Phosgene, Ammonia

The immediate effect of all except phosgene is coughing and choking. The danger is pulmonary oedema, which may develop suddenly many hours after the irritation has subsided. Severe dyspnoea, cyanosis, and death may occur. Patients should be kept under observation and selected patients given 100% oxygen and mechanical ventilation if necessary. Corticosteroids are helpful.

21. Snake and Insect Bites

SNAKE BITE. Acute poisoning due to venomous snakes is extremely rare in the United Kingdom and the only venomous snake is the adder. The bite may cause local and systemic effects. The local effects include a mild inflammatory reaction with pain and swelling. Systemic effects include agitation, restlessness, abdominal colic, diarrhoea, and vomiting. Death is unlikely except in the case of a very weak debilitated person who receives a large amount of venom.

Only a minority of patients needs specific antivenom: severe systemic symptoms (persistent or recurrent hypotension, polymorphonuclear leucocytosis, electro-encephalographic abnormalities, or renal failure) should be present before antivenom is given. Two ampoules of Zagreb antivenom should be used (for adults and children) diluted with 2 to 3 volumes of sodium chloride intravenous infusion 0.9% and repeated in 1 to 2 hours if there is no clinical improvement.

For slight or moderate poisoning (local pain and swelling, possibly vomiting and diarrhoea) symptomatic treatment only is required. The site should be cleaned, covered with a dry dressing, and immobilised. Injections of benzylpenicillin and antitetanus immunoglobulin injection should be given. A sedative may be necessary and an antihistamine may be given by injection for its sedative and antihistamine effects.

INSECT BITES. Stings from ants, wasps, bees, and hornets cause some local pain and swelling but seldom cause severe toxicity. If the bite is in the mouth or on the tongue there may be marked swelling which may cause respiratory distress. The stings from these insects may usually be treated by cleansing the area, applying a cooling lotion, and giving an antihistamine by mouth. In severe cases of allergic reaction an intravenous injection of hydrocortisone 100 mg may be life-saving.

22. Paraquat

The concentrated liquid paraquat which is supplied to farmers and horticulturists is extremely toxic; it contains approximately 20% of active substance. The granular preparation available for domestic use is much weaker and the granules are dissolved in water prior to application. There have been few deaths following ingestion of the granular material but poisoning with the concentrated liquid is much more serious. Acute toxicity may show either a local or systemic effect.

The **local** effect is usually seen as irritation of the cornea and conjunctiva after accidental splashing of the eyes. With copious washing of the eye and the instillation of either sulphacetamide sodium or antibiotic eye-drops, healing should occur but it may be a long process. Skin irritation and blistering can occur from contact both with the concentrated and diluted forms. There is no significant absorption from intact skin. The inhalation of spray, mist, or dust containing paraquat may cause nose bleeding and sore throat.

If the concentrated solution is swallowed, **systemic** effects such as painful ulceration of the tongue, lips, and fauces may appear in a few hours along with nausea, sweating, and vomiting. There may also be tremors and convulsions. Some days after ingestion there may be dyspnoea with pulmonary oedema due to proliferative alveolitis and bronchiolitis. Acute renal failure may also occur.

Treatment should be started immediately and a qualitative test of the urine will confirm the diagnosis. Further samples of urine should be examined to monitor the excretion. The best method of testing the severity of poisoning is, however, to measure the plasma-paraquat concentrations and this can be arranged through the National Poisons Information Centres (see section 8 above).

The stomach should be emptied by careful gastric lavage and 500 ml of a suspension containing 30 g of fullers earth and 5 g of magnesium sulphate in each 100 ml of water left in the stomach. Oral administration of 200–500 ml fullers earth suspension should be repeated over a period of 24 hours and magnesium sulphate given as required to eliminate the adsorbent from the gastro-intestinal tract. Supportive therapy as necessary is also required. Forced diuresis combined with charcoal haemoperfusion may also be used. If respiratory difficulties arise oxygen therapy should be avoided since this may cause more damage to the lungs. If oxygen is administered it should be mixed with nitrogen to give an oxygen tension of 50–70 mmHg.

23. Antidotes to other poisons

A number of preparations are available for use as an aid in the removal of poisons other than those mentioned above, i.e. **cyanides** (dicobalt edetate, sodium nitrite and thiosulphate) and **heavy metals** (dimercaprol, disodium edetate, penicillamine).

DICOBALT EDETATE

Indications: poisoning with cyanides
Side-effects: transient fall in blood pressure, increased pulse rate, and vomiting

Dose: by intravenous injection 600 mg in 40 ml solution, followed by 50 ml of dextrose intravenous infusion (50%)

Kelocyanor® (Rona)
Injection, dicobalt edetate 300 mg/20 ml. Price 20-ml amp = **D**

DIMERCAPROL

(BAL)

Indications: poisoning by antimony, arsenic, bismuth, gold, mercury, thallium
Side-effects: malaise, nausea, vomiting, lachrymation, burning sensation, constriction of throat and chest, increase in blood pressure; rarely serious in normal dosage
Dose: 2.5–3 mg/kg up to 6 times daily

Dimercaprol Injection, dimercaprol 50 mg/ml. Price 2-ml amp = **B**

PENICILLAMINE

Indications: poisoning, particularly by copper and lead
Cautions: blood and urine examinations required
Side-effects: allergic reactions, nausea, anorexia, leucopenia, thrombocytopenia, proteinuria, nephrotic syndrome
Dose: by mouth, 0.5 to 1.5 g daily; CHILD up to 5 years 150 mg twice daily, 6 to 12 years 300 mg twice daily

Preparations
See section 10.1.3

SODIUM CALCIUMEDETATE

Indications: poisoning by heavy metals, especially lead
Cautions: impaired renal function
Side-effects: nausea, cramp; in overdosage renal damage
Dose: by intravenous infusion, in sodium chloride intravenous infusion (0.9%) or dextrose intravenous infusion (5%), up to 40 mg/kg twice daily

Ledclair® (Sinclair)
Injection, sodium calciumedetate 200 mg/ml. Price 5-ml amp = **D**
Cream, sodium calciumedetate 10%. Price 50 g = **E**. For lesions and skin sensitivity due to contact with heavy metals

---

SODIUM NITRITE

Indications: poisoning with cyanides
Side-effects: flushing and headache due to vasodilatation

Sodium Nitrite Injection, sodium nitrite 3% (30 mg/ml) in water for injections.
Dose: 10 ml by intravenous injection during 3 minutes, followed after 5 minutes by 50 ml of sodium thiosulphate injection

---

SODIUM THIOSULPHATE

Indications: poisoning with cyanides

Sodium Thiosulphate Injection, sodium thiosulphate 50% (500 mg/ml) in water for injections.
Dose: see above under Sodium Nitrite Injection

Classified Notes on Drugs and Preparations

1: Drugs acting on the GASTRO-INTESTINAL SYSTEM

The drugs and preparations in this chapter are described under the following sections:

1.1 Antacids
1.2 Antispasmodics
1.3 Ulcer-healing drugs
1.4 Antidiarrhoeal drugs
1.5 Treatment of chronic diarrhoeas
1.6 Laxatives
1.7 Rectal and colonic drugs
1.8 Stoma care
1.9 Drugs affecting intestinal secretions

1.1 Antacids

1.1.1 Official and simple proprietary antacids
1.1.2 Compound proprietary antacids
1.1.3 Other antacids

The antacids retain an important place in the treatment of gastro-intestinal disease. They are a simple, often effective, treatment for many dyspepsias and provide symptomatic relief in conditions such as peptic ulcer, gastritis, and oesophageal reflux with heartburn.

Doses are given between meals and at bedtime for symptomatic relief, but additional doses may be required at hourly intervals or less frequently. As antacids interfere with the absorption of many drugs they should not be taken with other medicines. Drug interactions: see Appendix 1.

High doses of antacids such as 200 to 300 ml of **aluminium hydroxide** mixture daily in divided doses at frequent intervals will promote ulcer healing but such treatment is inconvenient to the patient. Large doses may also be useful in treating haemorrhage from erosive gastritis. The choice of antacid preparation depends on personal preference and convenience. Magnesium trisilicate and aluminium hydroxide are as effective as many proprietary mixtures. Liquid preparations are more effective than solids. Antacids with a high sodium content (for example magnesium trisilicate mixture) should be avoided in patients whose dietary sodium intake needs to be restricted as in conditions such as hepatic and heart failure or pregnancy.

Antacids may be divided into 2 main groups according to their water solubility. **Aluminium glycinate** and **hydroxide** and **magnesium carbonate**, **hydroxide**, and **trisilicate** are insoluble in water and have a slow prolonged action (calcium and bismuth compounds are also insoluble but are considered in section 1.1.3). Magnesium salts tend to be laxative.

Sodium bicarbonate being water-soluble acts quickly but its effect is transient, and prolonged use may cause systemic alkalosis and renal damage. It is the only soluble antacid that is clinically useful.

1.1.1 Official and simple proprietary antacids

ALUMINIUM HYDROXIDE

Indications: dyspepsia

Aluminium Hydroxide Tablets, dried aluminium hydroxide 500 mg (low Na^+). Price 20 tabs = **B**
Dose: 1–2 tablets chewed when required

Aluminium Hydroxide Mixture (gel), about 4% w/w Al_2O_3 in water (low Na^+). Diluent water for preparations, life of diluted mixture 14 days. Price 100 ml = **A**
Dose: 5–15 ml when required

Alu-Cap® (Riker)
Capsules, green/red, dried aluminium hydroxide 475 mg (low Na^+). Price 20 caps = **C**
Dose: 1 capsule when required

Aludrox® (Wyeth)
Tablets, aluminium hydroxide 375 mg (low Na^+). Price 20 tabs = **B**
Dose: 2 tablets chewed when required
Gel, aluminium hydroxide mixture (see above). Price 100 ml = **A**

MAGNESIUM SALTS (ANTACID)

Indications: dyspepsia
Cautions: renal impairment
Side-effects: diarrhoea

Magnesium Carbonate Mixture (see Formulary). Contains about 9 mmol Na^+/10 ml. Price 200 ml = **A**
Dose: 10–20 ml when required

Magnesium Carbonate Mixture, Aromatic, (see Formulary). Contains about 6 mmol Na^+/10 ml. Price 200 ml = **A**
Dose: 10–20 ml when required

Magnesium Hydroxide Mixture, magnesium oxide (hydrated) about 550 mg/10 ml (low Na^+). Do not store in a cold place. Price 100 ml = **A**
Dose: 5–10 ml when required

Magnesium Trisilicate Tablets, Compound, magnesium trisilicate 250 mg, dried aluminium hydroxide 120 mg (low Na^+). Price 20 tabs = **A**
Dose: 1–2 tablets chewed when required

Magnesium Trisilicate Mixture (see Formulary). Contains about 6 mmol Na^+/10 ml. Price 200 ml = **B**
Dose: 10–20 ml when required

Magnesium Trisilicate Powder. (Low Na^+). Price 20 g = **A**
Dose: 0.5–2 g in liquid when required

Magnesium Trisilicate Oral Powder, Compound, magnesium trisilicate 250 mg, chalk 250 mg, heavy magnesium carbonate 250 mg,

sodium bicarbonate 250 mg/g. Contains about 3 mmol Na^+/g. Price 20 g = **A**
Dose: 1–5 g in liquid when required

SODIUM BICARBONATE

Indications: rapid relief of dyspepsia
Cautions: patients on a sodium-restricted diet
Side-effects: eructation due to liberated carbon dioxide and, with prolonged use, alkalosis
Dose: 1–5 g when required

Sodium Bicarbonate Tablets, Compound (Soda Mint Tablets), sodium bicarbonate 300 mg. Contains about 4 mmol Na^+/tab. Price 20 tabs = **A**
Dose: 2–6 tablets sucked when required

1.1.2 Compound proprietary antacids

A number of multi-ingredient preparations are available but they are not usually any more effective than simple preparations.

Other ingredients are often found in compound preparations. **Dimethicone** has an antifoaming action and is claimed to relieve flatulence but its value in treating dyspepsia is uncertain. **Alginates** are added to protect the mucosa and reduce the incidence of gastro-intestinal reflux.

Details of compound proprietary antacid preparations are shown in the table.

Table: Compound Proprietary Antacids

Name and Manufacturer	Presentation Diluent	Antacids	Other Ingredients	Dose	Price
Actal® (Winthrop)	Tablets	1 tablet = 5 ml mixture	—	1–2 tablets chewed or sucked when required	20 tabs = **A**
	Suspension (=mixture) Diluent 1	alexitol sodium 360 mg/5 ml	(low Na^+)	5–10 ml when required	100 ml = **B**
Actonorm® (Wallace Mfg)	Gel (=mixture)	dried aluminium hydroxide 220 mg, magnesium hydroxide 100 mg/5 ml	activated dimethicone 25 mg/5 ml	5–20 ml when required	100 ml = **B**
Alcin® (R&C)	Tablets	anhydrous sodium magnesium aluminium silicate and basic magnesium aluminate co-prepared mixture 360 mg	(1 mmol Na^+/ tablet)	1–2 tablets chewed or sucked when required	20 tabs = **A**
Altacite® (Roussel)	Tablets	hydrotalcite 500 mg	—	2 tablets; CHILD (6–12 years) 1 tablet, chewed when required	20 tabs =**C**
	Suspension (=mixture) Diluent 2	hydrotalcite 500 mg/ 5 ml	—	10 ml; CHILD (6–12 years) 5 ml, when required	100 ml = **C**
Altacite Plus®	Tablets	hydrotalcite 500 mg	activated dimethicone 250 mg	2 tablets; CHILD (8–12 years) 1 tablet, chewed when required	20 tabs = **C**
	Suspension (=mixture) Diluent 2	hydrotalcite 500 mg/ 5 ml	activated dimethicone 125 mg/5 ml	10 ml; CHILD (8–12 years) 5 ml, when required	100 ml = **C**

Table: Compound Proprietary Antacids *(continued)*

Name and Manufacturer	Presentation Diluent	Antacids	Other Ingredients	Dose	Price
Andursil® (Geigy)	Tablets	aluminium hydroxide-magnesium carbonate co-dried gel 750 mg	activated dimethicone 250 mg	1–2 tablets when required	20 tabs = **B**
	Suspension (=mixture) Diluent 2	Al_2O_3 200 mg (as aluminium hydroxide mixture), magnesium hydroxide 200 mg, aluminium hydroxide-magnesium carbonate co-dried gel 200 mg/5 ml	activated dimethicone 150 mg/5 ml	5–10 ml when required	100 ml = **B**
Antasil® (Stuart)	Tablets	dried aluminium hydroxide 400 mg, magnesium hydroxide 400 mg	activated dimethicone 250 mg (low Na^+)	1–2 tablets chewed or sucked when required	20 tabs = **C**
	Liquid (=mixture)	dried aluminium hydroxide 400 mg, magnesium hydroxide 400 mg/5 ml	activated dimethicone 150 mg/5 ml (low Na^+)	5–10 ml when required	100 ml = **C**
Asilone® (Berk)	Tablets	dried aluminium hydroxide 500 mg	activated dimethicone 270 mg (low Na^+)	1–2 tablets chewed or sucked when required	20 tabs = **C**
	Gel (viscous suspension) Diluent 5	dried aluminium hydroxide 420 mg, light magnesium oxide 70 mg/5 ml	activated dimethicone 135 mg/5 ml (low Na^+)	5–10 ml when required	100 ml = **C**
	Suspension (=mixture) Diluent 5	active ingredients as for gel	(see above)	5–10 ml when required	100 ml = **C**
Asilone for Infants®	Paediatric Mixture Diluent 2	dried aluminium hydroxide 84 mg, light magnesium oxide 14 mg/5 ml	activated dimethicone 27 mg/5 ml	5 ml when required before or with feeds	100 ml = **C**
Dijex® (Crookes Products)	Tablets (pink)	aluminium hydroxide-magnesium carbonate co-dried gel 400 mg	—	1–2 tablets chewed 2–4 hourly	20 tabs = **A**
	Liquid (=mixture)	aluminium hydroxide mixture 98%, magnesium hydroxide 1.7%	—	5–10 ml, 2–4 hourly	100 ml = **A**
Diloran® (Rona)	Tablets	aluminium hydroxide-magnesium carbonate co-dried gel 85 mg, magnesium oxide 340 mg	activated dimethicone 25 mg	1–2 tablets; CHILD (6–12 years) 1 tablet chewed or sucked when required	20 tabs = **B**
	Suspension (=mixture)	aluminium hydroxide-magnesium carbonate co-dried gel 80 mg, magnesium oxide 320 mg/10 ml	activated dimethicone 25 mg/10 ml	10–20 ml; CHILD 1–5 years 2.5–5 ml, 6–12 years 5–10 ml	100 ml = **B**

Table: Compound Proprietary Antacids *(continued)*

Name and Manufacturer	Presentation Diluent	Antacids	Other Ingredients	Dose	Price
Diovol® (Pharmax)	Tablets (white/ yellow)	aluminium hydroxide-magnesium carbonate co-dried gel 300 mg, magnesium hydroxide 100 mg	dimethicone 25 mg	1–2 tablets chewed or sucked when required	20 tabs = **B**
	Suspension (=mixture) Diluent 3	aluminium hydroxide 200 mg, magnesium hydroxide 200 mg/5 ml	dimethicone 25 mg/5 ml	10–20 ml, when required	100 ml = **B**
Droxalin® (Sterling Health)	Tablets	polyhydroxy-aluminium sodium carbonate 162 mg, magnesium trisilicate 162 mg	—	1–2 tablets chewed when required	20 tabs = **A**
Gastrils® (Jackson)	Pastilles (s/c, green or yellow)	aluminium hydroxide-magnesium carbonate co-dried gel 500 mg	—	1–2 pastilles sucked when required; CHILD 1 pastille 3 times daily	90 g (22) = **B**
Gastrocote® (MCP)	Tablets	dried aluminium hydroxide 80 mg, magnesium trisilicate 40 mg, sodium bicarbonate 70 mg	alginic acid 200 mg	1–3 chewed when required. Not recommended for children under 6 years	20 tabs = **C**
Gaviscon® (R&C)	Tablets	sodium bicarbonate 170 mg, dried aluminium hydroxide 100 mg, magnesium trisilicate 25 mg	alginic acid 500 mg, with sucrose and mannitol. Contains 2 mmol Na^+/tab	1–2 tablets; CHILD 1 tablet chewed when required and followed with liquid	20 tabs = **C**
	Granules in sachets (pale brown)	sodium bicarbonate 177 mg, dried aluminium hydroxide 208 mg, magnesium trisilicate 52 mg/5-g sachet	alginic acid 481 mg, sodium alginate 521 mg/5-g sachet with sucrose. Contains about 5 mmol Na^+/sachet	1 sachet; CHILD ½ sachet chewed when required and followed with liquid	10 sachets = **D**
	Liquid (=mixture) (pink)	sodium bicarbonate 267 mg/10 ml	sodium alginate 500 mg/10 ml, with saccharin. Contains about 6 mmol Na^+/10 ml	10–20 ml; CHILD 5–10 ml when required	100 ml = **C**

Table: Compound Proprietary Antacids *(continued)*

Name and Manufacturer	Presentation Diluent	Antacids	Other Ingredients	Dose	Price
Infant Gaviscon®	Powder in sachets	sodium bicarbonate 340 mg, magnesium trisilicate 50 mg, dried aluminium hydroxide 200 mg/2-g sachet	alginic acid 924 mg/2-g sachet, with colloidal silica and mannitol. Contains 4 mmol Na^+/ sachet	INFANT ½–1 sachet mixed with feeds when required; CHILD 1 sachet in water after meals	10 sachets = **D**
Gelusil® (Warner)	Tablets	dried aluminium hydroxide 250 mg, magnesium trisilicate 500 mg	(low Na^+)	1–2 chewed or sucked when required; CHILD half adult dose	20 tabs = **A**
	Suspension (=mixture) Diluent 4	dried aluminium hydroxide 310 mg, magnesium trisilicate 620 mg/5 ml	—	5–20 ml, with water; CHILD 6–12 years half adult dose when required	100 ml = **B**
Maalox® (Rorer)	Tablets	dried aluminium hydroxide 400 mg, magnesium hydroxide 400 mg	—	1–2 tablets chewed when required	20 tabs = **B**
	Suspension (=mixture) Diluent 2	dried aluminium hydroxide 220 mg, magnesium hydroxide 195 mg/5 ml	(low Na^+)	10–20 ml when required	100 ml = **B**
Maalox Plus®	Tablets (white/ yellow)	dried aluminium hydroxide 200 mg, magnesium hydroxide 200 mg	dimethicone with silica 25 mg	2–4 chewed when required	20 tabs = **C**
	Suspension (=mixture)	dried aluminium hydroxide 220 mg, magnesium hydroxide 195 mg/5 ml	dimethicone with silica 25 mg/5 ml	10–20 ml when required	100 ml = **C**
Polyalk® (Galen)	Tablets	dried aluminium hydroxide 500 mg	activated dimethicone 250 mg	1–2 tablets chewed or sucked when required	20 tabs = **C**
	Suspension (= mixture) and Gel	dried aluminium hydroxide 440 mg, light magnesium oxide 70 mg/5 ml	dimethicone 125 mg/5 ml (low Na^+)	5–10 ml when required	100 ml = **B**
Polycrol® (Nicholas)	Tablets (green/white)	aluminium hydroxide-magnesium carbonate co-dried gel 275 mg, magnesium hydroxide 100 mg	activated dimethicone 25 mg (low Na^+)	1–2 tablets; CHILD 1–5 years ½ tablet, 6–12 years 1 tablet, chewed or sucked when required	20 tabs = **B**
	Gel (=mixture) Diluent 2	aluminium hydroxide mixture 4.75 ml, magnesium hydroxide 100 mg/5 ml	activated dimethicone 25 mg/5 ml (low Na^+)	5–10 ml; CHILD 1–5 years 2.5 ml, 6–12 years 5 ml when required	100 ml = **C**

For all abbreviations and symbols see inside cover. Relative prices: **A** = up to 20p, **B** = 21-50p,

Table: Compound Proprietary Antacids *(continued)*

Name and Manufacturer	Presentation Diluent	Antacids	Other Ingredients	Dose	Price
Polycrol Forte®	Tablets	aluminium hydroxide-magnesium carbonate co-dried gel 275 mg, magnesium hydroxide 100 mg	activated dimethicone 250 mg (low Na^+)	1–2 tablets chewed or sucked when required	20 tabs = **B**
	Gel (=mixture) Diluent 2	aluminium hydroxide mixture 4.75 ml, magnesium hydroxide 100 mg/5 ml	activated dimethicone 125 mg/5 ml (low Na^+)	5–10 ml; CHILD (under 5 years) 2.5 ml, 5–12 years 5 ml when required	100 ml = **C**
Prodexin® (Bencard)	Tablets	aluminium glycinate 900 mg, magnesium carbonate 100 mg	(low Na^+)	1 or more tablets chewed or sucked when required	20 tabs = **B**
Siloxyl® (Concept)	Tablets	dried aluminium hydroxide 500 mg	dimethicone 250 mg	1–2 tablets chewed or sucked when required	20 tabs = **B**
	Suspension (=mixture)	dried aluminium hydroxide 420 mg, light magnesium oxide 70 mg/5 ml	dimethicone 125 mg/5 ml	5–10 ml; CHILD 6–12 years 5 ml when required	100 ml = **B**
Sylopal® (Norton)	Suspension (=mixture)	light magnesium oxide 70 mg, aluminium hydroxide mixture to 5 ml	dimethicone 125 mg/5 ml	5–10 ml when required	100 ml = **B**
Synergel® (Servier)	Gel (=mixture)	aluminium phosphate mixture 55% in 16-ml (20 g) sachets	pectin, agar. contains about 8 mmol Na^+/ 10 ml	1 sachet when required; CHILD 5 ml/ 4.5 kg daily in divided doses	10 sachets = **C**
Topal® (Concept)	Tablets	dried aluminium hydroxide 30 mg, light magnesium carbonate 40 mg	alginic acid 200 mg	1–3 tablets, chewed between meals and at bedtime	20 tabs = **B**

Diluent notes

1. Syrup, life of diluted mixture 14 days
2. Do not dilute
3. Water for preparations, life of diluted mixture 14 days
4. Water for preparations, life of diluted mixture 28 days
5. Purified water, freshly boiled and cooled, life of diluted mixture 14 days

1.1.3 Other antacids

Calcium-containing antacid preparations should be avoided as they may increase gastric acid production. They tend to be constipating and, with prolonged use, may cause hypercalcaemia (milk-alkali syndrome) with headache, nausea, nocturia, irritability, and weakness. Prolonged use may also give rise to alkalosis.

Bismuth antacid preparations have a weak action and they have been implicated in causing encephalopathy.

Surface anaesthetics (**oxethazaine** in Mucaine®) may be included in antacids to relieve the discomfort in oesophagitis but their effectiveness is doubtful and they should be avoided.

Calcium Carbonate Powder, Compound, calcium carbonate 375 mg, light kaolin 125 mg, heavy magnesium carbonate 125 mg, sodium bicarbonate 375 mg. Price 100 g = **A**

Chalk Mixture, Paediatric (see Formulary). Price 100 ml = **A**

Magnesium Carbonate Tablets, Compound, heavy magnesium carbonate 200 mg, light kaolin 60 mg, sodium bicarbonate 120 mg, calcium carbonate 200 mg. Price 20 tabs = **A**

Magnesium Carbonate Powder, Compound, heavy magnesium carbonate 333 mg, light kaolin 83 mg, sodium bicarbonate 250 mg, calcium carbonate 333 mg. Price 100 g = **A**

Bislumina® (MCP)
Suspension (= mixture), bismuth aluminate 750 mg/5 ml. Price 100 ml = **B**

Lac Bismuth® (Philip Harris)
Suspension (= mixture), bismuth carbonate 650 mg/5 ml. Price 100 ml = **B**

Mucaine® (Wyeth)
Suspension (= mixture), aluminium hydroxide mixture 4.75 ml, magnesium hydroxide 100 mg, oxethazaine 10 mg/5 ml. Diluent syrup, life of diluted mixture 14 days. Price 100 ml = **A**

Neutrolactis® (Wander)
Tablets, dried aluminium hydroxide 140 mg, calcium carbonate 280 mg, magnesium trisilicate 200 mg, with milk solids 1.5 g. Price 20 tabs = **B**

Nulacin® (Bencard)
Tablets, calcium carbonate 130 mg, heavy magnesium carbonate 30 mg, heavy magnesium oxide 130 mg, magnesium trisilicate 230 mg, with milk solids, dextrins and maltose. Price 25 tabs = **B**

Roter® (FAIR)
Tablets, pink, bismuth subnitrate 300 mg, frangula 25 mg, magnesium carbonate 400 mg, sodium bicarbonate 200 mg. Price 20 tabs = **B**

Titralac® (Riker)
Tablets, calcium carbonate 420 mg, glycine 180 mg. Price 20 tabs = **A**

1.2 Antispasmodics

Although antispasmodics reduce intestinal spasm they are of value only in the treatment of peptic ulcer, spastic bowel syndrome, and diverticular disease, and in none of these conditions are they of fundamental importance.

For use of antispasmodics in peptic ulcer see below under anticholinergic drugs.

Spastic colon may often respond to reassurance or treatment with a high fibre diet and **bran** supplements. **Mebeverine** has few side-effects and may be of value in colonic spasm. In total ulcerative colitis antispasmodics are potentially dangerous as they encourage the onset of paralysis and toxic megacolon.

The antispasmodics are divided into those with anticholinergic effects, those that have a direct effect on smooth muscle, and metoclopramide.

ANTICHOLINERGICS. The most useful anticholinergic drugs are **dicyclomine** and **propantheline**. Others include ambutonium, atropine, belladonna alkaloids, glycopyrronium, hyoscine, isopropamide, mepenzolate, penthienate, pipenzolate, piperidolate, poldine, and clidinium (in Libraxin®, section 1.2.1). Anticholinergics inhibit parasympathetic innervation and thereby reduce secretion and motility of the stomach and intestine, but effective therapeutic doses are associated with a high incidence of side-effects. Elderly patients are particularly susceptible to glaucoma, urinary retention, difficulty with visual accommodation, and constipation.

In high doses anticholinergics reduce basal and meal-stimulated gastric acid production and although there is little evidence to suggest they heal ulcers they may be useful as a supplement to antacid therapy in peptic ulcers. Their use at night has the justification that side-effects are less objectionable than in the daytime and as they delay gastric emptying this may keep antacids in the stomach for longer and so suppress nocturnal acidity. **Dicyclomine** elixir (Merbentyl®) may be helpful for treating gripe in infants (infantile colic) but dosage should be carefully controlled.

SPASMOLYTICS. Drugs which have a direct effect on smooth muscle but no anticholinergic effect include **alverine** (Spasmonal®), **mebeverine** (Colofac®), and **papaverine.**

Metoclopramide (Maxolon®, Primperan®) differs in action from the anticholinergic drugs. It increases propulsive activity in the stomach and helps to close the lower oesophageal sphincter. It is useful in the treatment of heartburn and of vomiting (see section 4.6), and in radiological procedures. Metoclopramide may give rise to severe extrapyramidal reactions including facial spasms and oculogyric crises. It should therefore be used with caution and is **not** recommended for children.

Peppermint oil is a deflatulent and antispasmodic. It relieves abdominal colic and distension by relaxing the intestinal muscles. Enteric-coated preparations (Colpermin®) are useful as an adjunct in the treatment of spastic colon.

Preparations listed below have been arranged alphabetically according to the antispasmodic drug present in the preparation. Antispasmodic preparations containing antacids are also listed here.

Preparations containing barbiturates, papaverine or other sedative substances are listed separately in section 1.2.1. They should be **avoided** as the sedative component is not usually required but when a sedative is indicated it should be prescribed separately in appropriate dosage (see section 4.1.2): the use of barbiturates for this purpose is **not** justified.

ALVERINE CITRATE

Indications: relief of gastro-intestinal spasm
Side-effects: occasionally hypotension, drowsiness, weakness, headache, and dry mouth
Dose: 60–120 mg 1–3 times daily

Spasmonal® (Norgine)
Tablets, blue, alverine citrate 60 mg. Price 20 tabs = **D**

AMBUTONIUM BROMIDE

Indications: aid in peptic ulcer treatment
Side-effects: mild peripheral anticholinergic effects (see Atropine Sulphate)

Aludrox SA® (Wyeth)
Suspension (=mixture), green, ambutonium bromide 2.5 mg, aluminium hydroxide mixture 4.75 ml, magnesium hydroxide 100 mg/5 ml.

Diluent syrup, life of diluted mixture 14 days. Price 100 ml = **A**
Dose: 5–10 ml 3–4 times daily between meals and at bedtime

ATROPINE SULPHATE

Indications: aid in peptic ulcer treatment
Cautions: in the elderly, in patients with urinary retention, prostatic enlargement, tachycardia, cardiac insufficiency, paralytic ileus, and pyloric stenosis
Contra-indications: glaucoma
Side-effects: peripheral anticholinergic side-effects include dry mouth with difficulty in swallowing and thirst, dilatation of the pupils with loss of accommodation and sensitivity to light, increased intra-ocular pressure, flushing, dry skin, bradycardia followed by tachycardia, palpitations and arrhythmias, difficulty with micturition, and constipation. Drug interactions: see Appendix 1
Dose: *by mouth,* 0.25–2 mg daily in single or divided doses; dosage should be gradually increased to the max. tolerated

Atropine Sulphate Tablets, atropine sulphate 600 micrograms. Price 20 tabs = **A**

BELLADONNA ALKALOIDS

Indications: aid in peptic ulcer and spastic colon treatment
Cautions; Contra-indications; Side-effects: see under Atropine Sulphate

Aluminium Hydroxide and Belladonna Mixture, belladonna alkaloids 300 micrograms/10 ml (see Formulary). Low Na^+. Price 100 ml = **A**
Dose: 5 ml between meals

Belladonna Mixture, Paediatric, belladonna alkaloids 45 micrograms/5 ml (see Formulary). Price 100 ml = **A**
Dose: CHILD: up to 1 year 5 ml, 1–5 years 10 ml half an hour before meals

Magnesium Trisilicate and Belladonna Mixture, belladonna alkaloids 150 micrograms/10 ml (see Formulary). Contains about 6 mmol Na^+/10 ml. Price 200 ml = **B**
Dose: 10–20 ml between meals when necessary

Alka-Donna® (Carlton)
Tablets, belladonna alkaloids 80 micrograms (calc. as hyoscyamine), dried aluminium hydroxide 250 mg, magnesium trisilicate 500 mg. Price 20 tabs = **A**
Dose: 1–2 tablets, sucked 3 times daily before meals
Suspension (=mixture), belladonna alkaloids 60 micrograms (calc. as hyoscyamine), aluminium hydroxide mixture 2.15 ml, magnesium trisilicate 342.5 mg/5 ml. Price 100 ml = **A**
Dose: 5–10 ml 3 times daily between meals

Aluhyde® (Sinclair)
Tablets, scored, belladonna liquid extract 7.8 mg, dried aluminium hydroxide 245 mg, magnesium trisilicate 245 mg. Price 20 tabs = **C**
Dose: 2 tablets 3 times daily before meals

Bellocarb® (Sinclair)
Tablets, beige, scored, belladonna dry extract 10 mg (equivalent to 100 micrograms of hyoscyamine), magnesium carbonate 300 mg, magnesium trisilicate 300 mg. Price 20 tabs = **C**
Dose: 1–2 tablets 4 times daily

Carbellon® (Medo)
Tablets, black, belladonna dry extract 6 mg (equivalent to 60 micrograms hyoscyamine), charcoal 100 mg, magnesium hydroxide 100 mg. Price 20 tabs = **A**
Dose: 2–4 tablets 3–4 times daily; CHILD 1 tablet 3 times daily

Neutradonna® (Nicholas)
Tablets, belladonna alkaloids 48 micrograms (calc. as hyoscyamine), aluminium sodium silicate 650 mg. Price 20 tabs = **B**
Dose: 2–3 tablets, preferably chewed, up to 4 times daily; CHILD 2–5 years ½–1 tablet, 6–12 years 1–1½ tablets
Powder, belladonna alkaloids 75 micrograms (calc. as hyoscyamine), aluminium sodium silicate 989.6 mg/g. Price 25 g = **B**
Dose: 5–10 ml, in liquid, up to 4 times daily after meals; CHILD 2–5 years 2.5 ml, 6–12 years 2.5–5 ml

Peptard® (Riker)
Tablets, hyoscyamine sulphate 200 micrograms. Price 20 tabs = **D**
Dose: 2–3 tablets twice daily; CHILD over 10 years 1–2 tablets

DICYCLOMINE HYDROCHLORIDE

Indications: aid in peptic ulcer and spastic colon treatment; infantile colic
Side-effects: mild peripheral anticholinergic effects (see Atropine Sulphate)
Cautions: caution in infants
Dose: 30–60 mg daily in divided doses; CHILD up to 6 months up to 5 mg 3–4 times daily, 6–24 months 5–10 mg up to 3–4 times daily, 15 minutes before feeds, 2–12 years 10–20 mg 3 times daily

Kolanticon® (Merrell)
Gel (=mixture), dicyclomine hydrochloride 2.5 mg, dried aluminium hydroxide 200 mg, light magnesium oxide 100 mg, dimethicone 20 mg/5 ml. Diluent purified water, freshly boiled and cooled, life of diluted mixture 14 days. Price 125 ml = **B**
Dose: 10–20 ml every 4 hours when required

Kolantyl® (Merrell)
Tablets, dicyclomine hydrochloride 5 mg, dried aluminium hydroxide 240 mg, magnesium hydroxide 144 mg, magnesium trisilicate 90 mg. Price 20 tabs = **B**
Dose: 1–2 tablets chewed 4 hourly when required
Gel (=mixture), dicyclomine hydrochloride 2.5 mg, dried aluminium hydroxide 200 mg, light magnesium oxide 100 mg/5 ml. Diluent purified water, freshly boiled and cooled, life of diluted mixture 14 days. Price 125 ml = **B**
Dose: 10–20 ml 4 hourly when required

Merbentyl® (Merrell)
Tablets, dicyclomine hydrochloride 10 mg. Price 20 tabs = **B**
Syrup (=elixir), red, dicyclomine hydrochloride 10 mg/5 ml. Diluent syrup, life of diluted elixir 14 days. For infants under 6 months dilute with an equal volume of water before use. Price 100 ml = **C**

Ovol® (Pharmax)
Colic drops, yellow, dicyclomine hydrochloride 10 mg, dimethicone 40 mg/ml. Price 15-ml bottle with pipette = **D**
Dose: CHILD 0.5–1 ml before feeds; max. 4 ml daily

GLYCOPYRRONIUM BROMIDE

Indications: aid in peptic ulcer and spastic colon treatment
Side-effects: mild peripheral anticholinergic effects (see under Atropine Sulphate)
Dose: 1–4 mg 2–3 times daily

Robinul® (Robins)
Tablets, pink, scored, glycopyrronium bromide 2 mg. Price 20 tabs = **D**

HYOSCINE BUTYLBROMIDE

Indications: aid in peptic ulcer and spastic colon treatment
Cautions; Contra-indications; Side-effects: see under Atropine Sulphate

Buscopan® (Boehringer Ingelheim)
Tablets, s/c, hyoscine butylbromide 10 mg. Price 20 tabs = **C**
Dose: 20 mg 4 times daily; CHILD 6–12 years, 10 mg 3 times daily
Injection, hyoscine butylbromide 20 mg/ml. Price 1-ml amp = **A**
Dose: by intramuscular or intravenous injection, 20 mg

MEBEVERINE HYDROCHLORIDE

Indications: relief of gastro-intestinal and colonic spasm
Dose: 135 mg 3 times daily before meals

Colofac® (Duphar)
Tablets, s/c, mebeverine hydrochloride 135 mg. Price 20 tabs = **D**

MEPENZOLATE BROMIDE

Indications: relief of gastro-intestinal and colonic spasm
Side-effects: mild peripheral anticholinergic effects (see Atropine Sulphate)
Dose: 25–50 mg 3–4 times daily

Cantil® (MCP)
Tablets, yellow, scored, mepenzolate bromide 25 mg. Price 20 tabs = **C**
Elixir, mepenzolate bromide 12.5 mg/5 ml. Diluent water for preparations, life of diluted elixir 14 days. Price 100 ml = **D**

METOCLOPRAMIDE HYDROCHLORIDE

Indications: digestive disorders, to promote gastric motility and gastric emptying; gastric and duodenal radiological procedures; as an aid in duodenal intubation
Cautions: treatment should begin with a low dose and gradually increase. Avoid doses exceeding 500 micrograms/kg/day. Reduce dose in renal failure. Caution in children. Drug interactions: see Appendix 1
Side-effects: extrapyramidal effects, especially in patients under 15 years of age, rarely drowsiness, constipation
Dose: *by mouth, or by intramuscular or intravenous injection,* up to 10 mg (5 mg in young adults up to 20 years) 3 times daily; CHILD up to 1 year 1 mg twice daily, 1–2 years 1 mg 2–3 times daily, 3–5 years 2 mg 2–3 times daily, 6–14 years 2.5–5 mg 3 times daily
For radiological examinations, as a single dose 5–10 minutes before examination, 10–20 mg; CHILD under 3 years 1 mg, 3–5 years 2 mg, 6–12 years 2.5–5 mg

Metoclopramide Tablets, metoclopramide hydrochloride (anhydrous) 10 mg. Price 20 tabs = **C**
Metoclopramide Elixir, metoclopramide hydrochloride (anhydrous) 5 mg/5 ml. Price 100 ml = **D**
Metoclopramide Injection, metoclopramide hydrochloride (anhydrous) 5 mg/ml. Price 2-ml amp = **A**

Maxolon® (Beecham)
Tablets, scored, metoclopramide hydrochloride (anhydrous) 10 mg. Price 20 tabs = **D**
Syrup (=elixir), yellow, metoclopramide hydrochloride (anhydrous) 5 mg/5 ml. Diluent water for preparations, life of diluted elixir 7 days. Price 100 ml = **D**
Paediatric liquid, yellow, metoclopramide hydrochloride (anhydrous) 1 mg/ml. Price 15 ml with pipette = **D**
Injection, metoclopramide hydrochloride (anhydrous) 5 mg/ml. Price 2-ml amp = **B**

Primperan® (Berk)
Tablets, scored, metoclopramide hydrochloride (anhydrous) 10 mg. Price 20 tabs = **C**
Syrup (=elixir), lime, metoclopramide hydrochloride (anhydrous) 5 mg/5 ml. Diluent syrup, life of diluted elixir 14 days. Price 100 ml = **D**
Injection, metoclopramide hydrochloride (anhydrous) 5 mg/ml. Price 2-ml amp = **A**

PENTHIENATE METHOBROMIDE

Indications: aid in peptic ulcer and spastic colon treatment
Side-effects: mild peripheral anticholinergic effects (see Atropine Sulphate)
Dose: 2.5–10 mg 3 times daily

Monodral® (Sterling Research)
Tablets, yellow, scored, penthienate methobromide 5 mg. Price 20 tabs = **C**

PEPPERMINT OIL

Indications: relief of abdominal colic and distension, particularly in spastic colon

Side-effects: heartburn, local irritation, rarely sensitivity to menthol

Colpermin® (Tillotts)

Capsules, light blue/dark blue, green band, e/c, peppermint oil 0.2 ml. Price 20 caps = **E**

Dose: 1–2 capsules swallowed whole with water 3 times daily before meals usually for 1–2 weeks

PIPENZOLATE BROMIDE

Indications: aid in peptic ulcer and spastic colon treatment

Side-effects: mild peripheral anticholinergic effects (see Atropine Sulphate)

Dose: 5 mg 3 times daily before meals and 5–10 mg at night

Piptal® (MCP)

Tablets, peach, pipenzolate bromide 5 mg. Price 20 tabs = **B**

Piptalin® (MCP)

Elixir, pipenzolate bromide 4 mg, activated dimethicone 40 mg/5 ml. Diluent water for preparations, life of diluted elixir 14 days. Price 100 ml = **D**

Dose: 10 ml 3–4 times daily before meals; CHILD 2.5–5 ml

PIPERIDOLATE HYDROCHLORIDE

Indications: relief of gastro-intestinal spasm

Side-effects: very mild peripheral anticholinergic effects (see Atropine Sulphate)

Dose: 50 mg 4 times daily before meals

Dactil® (MCP)

Tablets, piperidolate hydrochloride 50 mg. Price 20 tabs = **C**

POLDINE METHYLSULPHATE

Indications: aid in peptic ulcer and spastic colon treatment, childhood enuresis

Side-effects: mild peripheral anticholinergic effects (see Atropine Sulphate)

Dose: 2–4 mg every 6 hours, starting with the lower dose; CHILD, for enuresis, 2 mg at night

Nacton® (Bencard)

Tablets, scored, poldine methylsulphate 2 mg. Price 20 tabs = **B**

Tablets forte, orange, scored, poldine methylsulphate 4 mg. Price 20 tabs = **C**

PROPANTHELINE BROMIDE

Indications: aid in peptic ulcer and spastic colon treatment; childhood enuresis; aid in radiological procedures

Cautions: drug interactions, see Appendix 1

Side-effects: mild peripheral anticholinergic effects (see Atropine Sulphate)

Dose: by mouth, 15 mg 3 times daily before meals and 30 mg at night; CHILD, for enuresis, 15–45 mg at night

By intramuscular or intravenous injection, 30 mg every 6 hours when necessary. Rate of intravenous injection should not exceed 6 mg/minute

Propantheline Tablets, s/c, propantheline bromide 15 mg. Price 20 tabs = **A**

Pro-Banthine® (Searle)

Tablets, pink, s/c, propantheline bromide 15 mg. Price 20 tabs = **B**

Injection, powder for reconstitution, propantheline bromide. Price 30-mg vial = **B**

1.2.1 Other antispasmodic preparations

The antispasmodic preparations listed below contain barbiturates, papaverine, or other sedative compounds and their use is **not** recommended for the reasons stated under 1.2 above.

Actonorm® (Wallace Mfg)

Tablets, dried aluminium hydroxide 25 mg, atropine sulphate 50 micrograms, calcium carbonate 109 mg, diastase 5 mg, light kaolin 25 mg, magnesium carbonate 225 mg, magnesium trisilicate 50 mg, pancreatin 5 mg, papaverine hydrochloride 200 micrograms, phenobarbitone 5 mg, thiamine hydrochloride 500 micrograms. Price 20 tabs = **B**

Powder, dried aluminium hydroxide 5%, atropine sulphate 0.01%, calcium carbonate 14.5%, diastase 1%, light kaolin 5%, magnesium carbonate 30%, magnesium trisilicate 5%, pancreatin 1%, papaverine hydrochloride 0.04%, peppermint oil 0.05%, phenobarbitone 1%, sodium bicarbonate 37.3%, thiamine hydrochloride 0.1%. Price 85 g = **D**

Actonorm-Sed® (Wallace Mfg)

Gel (=mixture), dried aluminium hydroxide 220 mg, belladonna tincture 0.15 ml, activated dimethicone 25 mg, magnesium hydroxide 100 mg, peppermint oil 0.00075 ml, phenobarbitone 8 mg/5 ml. Price 100 ml = **C**

Alka-Donna-P® (Carlton)

Tablets, dried aluminium hydroxide 250 mg, belladonna dry extract 8 mg, magnesium trisilicate 500 mg, phenobarbitone 8 mg. Price 20 tabs = **A.**

Mixture, aluminium hydroxide mixture 2.15 ml, belladonna tincture 0.2 ml, magnesium trisilicate 342.5 mg, phenobarbitone 8 mg/5 ml. Price 100 ml = **A**

APP Stomach Powder® (Consolidated)

Powder, aluminium hydroxide mixture 3%, bismuth carbonate 2%, calcium carbonate 37.8%, homatropine methylbromide 0.1%, magnesium carbonate 37%, magnesium trisilicate 19.48%, papaverine hydrochloride 0.1%. Price 100 g = **C**

Tablets, aluminium hydroxide mixture 15 mg, bismuth carbonate 12.5 mg, calcium carbonate 180.5 mg, homatropine methylbromide 1.5 mg, magnesium carbonate 180 mg, magnesium trisilicate 107.5 mg, papaverine hydrochloride 3 mg. Price 20 tabs = **A**

Bellergal® (Sandoz)

Tablets, pinkish brown, s/c, phenobarbitone 20 mg, belladonna alkaloids 100 micrograms, ergotamine tartrate 300 micrograms. Price 20 tabs = **B**

Bellergal Retard® (Sandoz)

Tablets, s/r, coloured, phenobarbitone 40 mg, belladonna alkaloids 200 micrograms, ergotamine tartrate 600 micrograms. Price 20 tabs = **C**

Cantil with Phenobarbitone® (MCP)

Tablets, brown, scored, mepenzolate bromide 25 mg, phenobarbitone 15 mg. Price 20 tabs = **D**

Libraxin® (Roche)
Tablets, green, f/c, chlordiazepoxide 5 mg, clidinium bromide 2.5 mg. Price 20 tabs = **B**

Pro-Banthine with Dartalan® (Searle)
Tablets, peach, compression coated, propantheline bromide 15 mg, thiopropazate hydrochloride 3 mg. Price 20 tabs = **B**

Stelabid® (SK&F)
Tablets, yellow, s/c, isopropamide 5 mg (as iodide), trifluoperazine 1 mg (as hydrochloride). Price 20 tabs = **C**
Tablets forte, yellow, s/c, isopropamide 7.5 mg (as iodide), trifluoperazine 2 mg (as hydrochloride). Price 20 tabs = **D**

1.3 Ulcer-healing drugs

Ulcers may often be treated effectively without drugs by simple measures such as rest in bed, regular meals, and avoidance of smoking. Antacids may be necessary for the relief of pain. **Carbenoxolone** (Biogastrone®, Duogastrone®), **cimetidine** (Tagamet®), **ranitidine** (Zantac®), and tripotassium dicitratobismuthate (De-Nol®), are useful ulcer-healing drugs. Large doses of antacids (see section 1.1.1) may also be effective in healing ulcers. The main problem with all these drugs is the high rate of relapse after treatment is discontinued; surgery may be necessary in such cases.

Tripotassium dicitratobismuthate is a bismuth chelate. It may act to promote healing of gastric and duodenal ulcers by coating the ulcer and so protecting its surface, and it is claimed that healing is longer lasting than with other drugs. Patients should not eat or drink for one hour before and half an hour after each dose.

Carbenoxolone, a synthetic derivative of glycyrrhizic acid (a constituent of liquorice) is more effective in gastric than duodenal ulcer and is better suited to younger rather than older patients because of the nature of its side-effects, which include sodium retention and hypokalaemia and which may aggravate conditions such as oedema, hypertension, cardiac failure, and muscle weakness. It may act by protecting the mucosal barrier from acid–pepsin attack and increasing mucosal mucin production. **Deglycyrrhizinised liquorice** is free from these side-effects but is of doubtful efficacy.

Cimetidine and the recently introduced drug **ranitidine** heal peptic ulcers, particularly duodenal ulcers by producing gastric hypochlorhydria as a result of their H_2-receptor blocking action. They are also used to reduce acid secretion in patients bleeding from erosive gastritis, in severe reflux oesophagitis with ulceration, and in the Zollinger–Ellison syndrome. They should only be used in confirmed ulceration and should **not** be prescribed for non-specific dyspepsia. Abrupt withdrawal of treatment should be avoided. Although rebound hyperacidity does not occur, unexpected perforation or haemorrhage has occurred rarely with cimetidine but not as yet with ranitidine.

Side-effects such as mental confusion and gynaecomastia have been reported with cimetidine. It is important to exclude malignancy before initiating treatment with cimetidine or ranitidine because they may mask the symptoms. It is also thought that long-term hypochlorhydria may be associated with an increased risk of gastric cancer but no hazard has been convincingly demonstrated.

For these reasons cimetidine and ranitidine should be given in single short courses (4 to 6 weeks) and long-term treatments such as prophylactic doses of cimetidine 400 mg or ranitidine 150 mg at night should be avoided unless the circumstances are exceptional. In any case, the relapse rate after discontinuation of long-term treatment is high (80 to 90% of cases) and also about 25% of patients with duodenal ulcer seem resistant to treatment. If relapse occurs then surgery rather than further treatment with cimetidine or ranitidine may be indicated.

BISMUTH CHELATE

Indications: peptic ulceration
Cautions: encephalopathy has been reported with prolonged high dosage; avoid repeated courses
Side-effects: constipation, may blacken faeces

De-Nol® (Brocades)
Liquid (=elixir), red, tripotassium dicitratobismuthate 120 mg/5 ml. Price 100 ml = **E**
Dose: 5 ml, diluted with 15 ml water, 4 times daily, 30 minutes before the 3 main meals and 2 hours after the last meal for at least 28 days

CARBENOXOLONE SODIUM

Indications: gastric ulceration in young patients; also used in duodenal ulceration
Cautions: elderly patients, cardiac disease, hypertension, impaired hepatic and renal function. Potassium supplements and thiazide diuretics may be necessary. Drug interactions: see Appendix 1
Contra-indications: avoid use with spironolactone
Side-effects: sodium and water retention leading to oedema, alkalosis, hypertension, hypokalaemia

Biogastrone® (Winthrop)
Tablets, scored, carbenoxolone sodium 50 mg. Price 20 tabs = **E**
Dose: for gastric ulceration, 2 tablets 3 times daily after meals for 1 week, then 1 tablet 3 times daily until the ulcer is healed (4–6 weeks)

Duogastrone® (Winthrop)
Capsules (for duodenal release), carbenoxolone sodium 50 mg. Price 28 caps = **G**
Dose: for duodenal ulceration, 1 capsule with liquid 4 times daily 15–30 minutes before meals for 6–12 weeks

Pyrogastrone® (Winthrop)
Tablets, carbenoxolone sodium 20 mg, alginic acid 600 mg, dried aluminium hydroxide 240 mg, magnesium trisilicate 60 mg, sodium bicarbonate 210 mg. Price 20 tabs = **E**

Dose: for oesophageal inflammation and ulceration, 1 tablet, chewed, 3 times daily immediately after meals, and 2 at bedtime, for at least 6 weeks

CIMETIDINE

Indications: peptic ulceration; reduction of gastric acid secretion in erosive gastritis, reflux oesophagitis, and Zollinger–Ellison syndrome
Cautions: see notes above. Where possible long-term treatment should be avoided otherwise the patient should be kept under observation. Reduce dosage in impaired renal function. Caution in hepatic impairment. Avoid intravenous injection in high dosage or in cardiovascular impairment (infusion is preferable to minimise risk of arrhythmias). Avoid abrupt withdrawal of treatment. Drug interactions: see Appendix 1
Side-effects: occasional diarrhoea, dizziness, rashes, rarely mental confusion, gynaecomastia, interstitial nephritis
Dose: by mouth, 200 mg, increased to 400 mg if necessary, 3 times daily after meals, and 400 mg at bedtime, for 4–6 weeks; CHILD 20–40 mg/kg daily in divided doses
Maintenance, 400 mg at bedtime *or* 400 mg in the morning and 400 mg at bedtime
By intramuscular or slow intravenous injection, 200 mg every 4–6 hours
By intravenous infusion, 100–150 mg/hour (or 2 mg/kg/hour) for 2 hours, repeated after an interval of 4–6 hours; the average infusion rate should not exceed 75 mg/hour over 24 hours
Max. dose (all routes) 2 g daily in divided doses

▼ Tagamet® (SK&F)
Tablets, green, f/c, cimetidine 200 mg. Price 20 tabs = **E**
Syrup (=elixir), orange, cimetidine 200 mg/5 ml. Diluent syrup, life of diluted elixir 28 days. Price 100 ml = **F**
Injection, cimetidine 100 mg/ml. Price 2-ml amp = **B**

LIQUORICE, DEGLYCYRRHIZINISED

Indications: peptic ulceration

Caved-S® (Tillotts)
Tablets, brown, aluminium hydroxide mixture 100 mg, deglycyrrhizinised liquorice 380 mg, light magnesium carbonate 200 mg, sodium bicarbonate 100 mg. Price 20 tabs = **C**
Rabro® (Sinclair)
Tablets, brown, deglycyrrhizinised liquorice extract 400 mg, calcium carbonate 500 mg, frangula 25 mg, magnesium oxide 100 mg. Price 20 tabs = **C**

RANITIDINE

Indications: see under Cimetidine
Cautions: as for Cimetidine, except drug interactions
Side-effects: as for Cimetidine, except gynaecomastia has not been reported
Dose: by mouth, 150 mg twice daily, increased if necessary to 900 mg daily in divided doses; CHILD 8–12 years up to 150 mg twice daily
Maintenance, 150 mg at bedtime
By slow intravenous injection, 50 mg every 6–8 hours
By intravenous infusion, 25 mg/hour for 2 hours, repeated if necessary after an interval of 6–8 hours

▼ Zantac® (Glaxo)
Tablets, f/c, ranitidine 150 mg (as hydrochloride). Price 20 tabs = **I**
Injection, ranitidine 10 mg (as hydrochloride)/ml. Price 5-ml amp = **C**

1.4 Antidiarrhoeal drugs

1.4.1 Antidiarrhoeal adsorbent mixtures
1.4.2 Antidiarrhoeal drugs which reduce motility
1.4.3 Other antidiarrhoeal preparations

In severe diarrhoea it is important to prevent or treat **fluid and electrolyte depletion**. This is particularly so in infants and in frail or elderly patients, who may become dangerously ill through dehydration alone. See section 9.3.2 for appropriate replacement preparations.

The symptomatic remedies listed below should be used when the diarrhoea is severe or has lasted longer than 24 hours.

When it is necessary to use an antidiarrhoeal agent in children **kaolin mixture**, **paediatric**, should preferably be used and the preparations in section 1.4.2 should be avoided.

Antispasmodics (section 1.2) are occasionally of value in treating abdominal cramps associated with diarrhoea but they should not be used as a primary treatment.

Most cases of diarrhoea are not bacterial in origin but even when a bacterial cause is suspected antibiotics or sulphonamides should be avoided (section 1.4.3).

For treatment of diarrhoea associated with chronic disease see section 1.5; for antibacterial treatment in gastro-intestinal infections see Table 1, section 5.1; for anthelmintic treatment see section 5.5.

1.4.1 Antidiarrhoeal adsorbent mixtures

Mixtures of **chalk** (Paediatric Chalk Mixture, Aromatic Chalk Powder) and **kaolin** (Kaolin Mixture, Paediatric Kaolin Mixture) may be effective in controlling diarrhoea. **Methylcellulose** is used in diarrhoea and is also specially useful in controlling faecal consistency in ileostomy and colostomy.

KAOLIN, LIGHT

Indications: diarrhoea

Kaolin Mixture (see Formulary). Price 200 ml = **B**
Dose: 10–20 ml every 4 hours

Kaolin Mixture, Paediatric (see Formulary). Price 100 ml = **A**
Dose: CHILD up to 1 year 5 ml, 1–5 years 10 ml every 4 hours

Kaopectate® (Upjohn)
Mixture, kaolin 6.18 g/30 ml. Diluent water for preparations, life of diluted mixture 14 days. Price 100 ml = **B**
Dose: 30–120 ml; CHILD 5–60 ml according to age, after each bowel movement

KLN® (Ashe)
Mixture, kaolin 1.15 g/5 ml. Price 100 ml = **B**
Dose: CHILD 6 months–1 year 5 ml, 1–3 years 10 ml, 3–10 years 20 ml every 4 hours

---

CERATONIA

Indications: diarrhoea

Arobon® (Nestlé)
Powder, ceratonia 80%, starch 15%, cocoa 5%. Price 150 g = **C**
Dose: adults and children 20–40 g, in liquid, daily; infants 2–10%, premature infants 1%, added to feeds

---

CHALK

Indications: diarrhoea

Chalk Mixture, Paediatric (see Formulary). Price 100 ml = **A**
Dose: CHILD up to 1 year 5 ml, 1–5 years 10 ml, every 4 hours

Chalk Powder, Aromatic, chalk 250 mg, cardamom seed 30 mg, clove 40 mg, nutmeg 80 mg, cinnamon 100 mg, sucrose 500 mg/g. Price 100 g = **B**
Dose: 0.5–5 g in liquid, every 4 hours

ISPAGHULA HUSK

Indications: diarrhoea (also constipation, section 1.6.1)
Side-effects: flatulence, abdominal distension
Note: for diarrhoea the dose should be taken with a minimum of water

Preparations
Section 1.6.1

METHYLCELLULOSE

Indications: diarrhoea (also ileostomy, colostomy control, and constipation, section 1.6.1)

Preparations
Section 1.6.1

STERCULIA

Indications: diarrhoea (also ileostomy and colostomy control and constipation, section 1.6.1)
Note: for diarrhoea the dose should be taken with a minimum of water

Preparations
Section 1.6.1

1.4.2 Antidiarrhoeal drugs which reduce motility

These are used for the symptomatic relief of diarrhoeas not controlled by adsorbent mixtures. **Codeine, diphenoxylate** (Lomotil®), **loperamide** (Imodium®), **morphine** (Kaolin and Morphine Mixture), and **opium** (Aromatic Chalk with Opium Mixture) are useful agents. There are few side-effects but, except in the case of loperamide, excessive sedation may occur in chronic liver disease and in children. Prolonged use may possibly aggravate spastic bowel syndrome and precipitate the development of diverticular disease. Codeine is preferred to morphine in chronic diarrhoea or mild ulcerative colitis as it is less likely to produce dependence.

CODEINE PHOSPHATE

Indications: diarrhoea
Cautions: ulcerative colitis, spastic bowel syndrome, and hepatic disease; use with caution in children (respiratory depression). Tolerance and dependence may occur with prolonged use. The actions of central nervous depressants are increased. Drug interactions: see Appendix 1
Contra-indications: pseudomembranous colitis, diverticular disease
Side-effects: occasional nausea, dizziness, and sedation; rarely paralytic ileus may occur with prolonged use
Dose: 45–120 mg daily in 3–6 divided doses; CHILD 1–3 mg/kg daily in divided doses

Codeine Phosphate Tablets, codeine phosphate 15 mg, price 20 tabs = **B**; 30 mg, price 20 tabs = **C**; 60 mg, price 20 tabs = **D**

Codeine Phosphate Syrup, codeine phosphate 25 mg/5 ml. Price 100 ml = **C**

Diarrest® (Galen)
Liquid (= elixir), codeine phosphate 5 mg, dicyclomine hydrochloride 2.5 mg, potassium chloride 40 mg, sodium chloride 50 mg, sodium citrate 50 mg/5 ml. For diarrhoea with cramp. Price 100 ml = **D**
Dose: 20 ml; CHILD 4–5 years 5 ml, 6–9 years 10 ml, 10–13 years 15 ml. Doses should be taken with water and given 4 times daily

Kaodene® (Crookes)
Mixture, codeine phosphate 10 mg, light kaolin 3 g/10 ml. Price 250 ml = **C**
Dose: 20 ml 3–4 times daily; CHILD over 5 years 10 ml

DIPHENOXYLATE HYDROCHLORIDE

Indications: diarrhoea
Cautions; Contra-indications: as for Codeine Phosphate (above). Subclinical doses of atropine sulphate are added to formulations to discourage excessive use
Side-effects: as for Codeine Phosphate (above); rarely rashes may also occur. Respiratory depression may occur when excessive doses are given to children
Dose: initially 10 mg, followed by 5 mg every 6 hours until diarrhoea is controlled; CHILD 1–3

years 2.5 mg twice daily, 4–8 years 2.5 mg 3 times daily, 9–12 years 2.5 mg 4 times daily, 13–16 years 5 mg 3 times daily

Lomotil® (Searle)
Tablets, diphenoxylate hydrochloride 2.5 mg, atropine sulphate 25 micrograms. Price 20 tabs = **C**
Liquid (= mixture), red, diphenoxylate hydrochloride 2.5 mg, atropine sulphate 25 micrograms/5 ml. Diluent glycerol, life of diluted elixir 14 days. Price 60 ml = **C**

LOPERAMIDE HYDROCHLORIDE

Indications: diarrhoea
Side-effects: occasional dry mouth, dizziness, headache, gastro-intestinal disturbances, and rashes
Dose: 4 mg initially followed by 2 mg after each loose stool up to a total of 16 mg daily; CHILD 1–3 years 1 mg 2–3 times daily, 4–8 years 1 mg 4 times daily, 9–12 years 2 mg 4 times daily
Chronic diarrhoea, 4–8 mg daily in divided doses initially and then if necessary reduced to a maintenance dose

Imodium® (Janssen)
Capsules, green/grey, loperamide hydrochloride 2 mg. Price 20 caps = **E**
Syrup (= elixir), red, loperamide hydrochloride 1 mg/5 ml. Diluent water for preparations, life of diluted elixir 14 days. Price 100 ml = **E**

MORPHINE HYDROCHLORIDE

Indications: diarrhoea
Cautions; Contra-indications; Side-effects: as for Codeine Phosphate (above). Sedation and the risk of dependence are greater

Kaolin and Morphine Mixture, morphine hydrochloride 916 micrograms/10 ml (see Formulary). Price 200 ml = **A**
Dose: 10 ml every 4 hours

OPIUM

Indications: diarrhoea
Cautions; Contra-indications; Side-effects: as for Codeine Phosphate (above). Sedation and the risk of dependence are greater

Aromatic Chalk with Opium Mixture, morphine 5 mg/10 ml (see Formulary). Price 200 ml = **C**
Dose: 10–20 ml every 4 hours; CHILD up to 1 year 1 ml, 1–5 years 2–5 ml, 6–12 years 5–10 ml

1.4.3 Other antidiarrhoeal preparations

Antibiotic and sulphonamide preparations should be **avoided** for the treatment of diarrhoea even when a bacterial cause is suspected because they may prolong rather than shorten the time taken to control diarrhoea and carrier states. Bacterial resistance to antibiotics may develop and they may cause a bacterial diarrhoea and pseudomembranous colitis. There is no evidence to suggest that antibiotics, sulphonamides, or clioquinol are effective in the prophylaxis of traveller's diarrhoea.

Lactobacillus preparations prevent the growth of putrefying bacteria by acidifying the intestine but there is no evidence that these preparations are beneficial.

Cremostrep® (MSD)
Mixture, kaolin 500 mg, streptomycin 50 mg (as sulphate), succinylsulphathiazole 500 mg/5 ml. Diluent syrup, life of diluted mixture 14 days. Price 100 ml = **C**
Enpac® (Aplin & Barrett)
Powder, Lactobacillus acidophilus cells resistant to various antibiotics. Price 60 g = **D**
Flar® (Consolidated)
Capsules, lactic acid bacilli resistant to antibiotics and sulphonamides 5×10^9 cells, cyanocobalamin 5 micrograms, folic acid 200 micrograms, inositol 20 mg, liver extract from 20 g fresh liver, nicotinamide 20 mg, pyridoxine hydrochloride 500 micrograms, riboflavine 500 micrograms, sodium pantothenate 7.5 mg, thiamine hydrochloride 5 mg. Price 20 caps = **C**
Furoxone® (Eaton)
Suspension (= mixture), furazolidone 25 mg, kaolin 700 mg, pectin 75 mg/5 ml. Price 100 ml = **D**
Guanimycin® (A&H)
Suspension forte (= mixture), dihydrostreptomycin sulphate 250 mg, light kaolin 4·25 g, sulphaguanidine 1·985 g/15 ml when reconstituted. Price 150 ml = **D**
Kaomycin® (Upjohn)
Mixture, light kaolin 1·03 g, neomycin sulphate 53 mg. Diluent water for preparations, life of diluted mixture 14 days. Price 150 ml = **D**
Lomotil with Neomycin® (Searle)
Tablets, scored, atropine sulphate 25 micrograms, diphenoxylate hydrochloride 2·5 mg, neomycin sulphate 250 mg. Price 20 tabs = **E**
Liquid (= elixir), yellow, atropine sulphate 25 micrograms, diphenoxylate hydrochloride 2·5 mg, neomycin sulphate 250 mg/5 ml. Diluent glycerol, life of diluted elixir 14 days. Price 50 ml = **E**
Neo-Sulfazon® (Wallace Mfg)
Mixture, kaolin 750 mg, neomycin sulphate 37·5 mg, pectin 62.5 mg, phthalylsulphathiazole 500 mg/5 ml. Price 75 ml = **C**
Neovax® (Norton)
Mixture, kaolin 6 g, neomycin sulphate 525 mg/30 ml. Price 100 ml = **B**
Sulphamagna® (Wyeth)
Mixture, beige, activated attapulgite 2 g, phthalylsulphathiazole 2 g, streptomycin 200 mg (as sulphate), sulphadiazine 500 mg/30 ml. Price 150 ml = **D**
Unidiarea® (Unigreg)
Capsules, green, activated attapulgite 80 mg, clioquinol 125 mg, neomycin sulphate 200 mg. Price 12 caps = **D**
Uniflor® (Aplin & Barrett)
Tablets, Lactobacillus acidophilus not resistant to antibiotics. Price 20 tabs = **C**

1.5 Treatment of chronic diarrhoeas

When diarrhoea is persistent and the presence of a tumour has been ruled out, the following conditions should be considered. Manipulation of diet or exclusion of certain foods as well as drug treatment is important in the management of such disorders. It is also important to maintain adequate fluid intake (see section 9.2.1.3).

SPASTIC BOWEL SYNDROME. This may require treatment with a high-fibre diet supplemented with bran or other bulk-forming drugs (section 1.6.1) if necessary. In some patients there may be important psychological aggravating factors which respond to reassurance. Antidiarrhoeal drugs such as **loperamide** (Imodium®) may sometimes be necessary but prolonged use may aggravate the condition (section 1.4.2). Antispasmodics such as **mebeverine** (Colofac®), section 1.2, may be necessary.

MALABSORPTION SYNDROME. The most common cause in this country is coeliac disease (intolerance to gluten) and is usually treated with a gluten-free diet (see section 9.3). Pancreatic deficiency states are treated with **pancreatin** supplements (section 1.9.4).

ULCERATIVE COLITIS. Local maintenance treatment with corticosteroid retention enemas for example **prednisolone** enema (section 1.7.2), or with **sulphasalazine** tablets (Salazopyrin®) may be sufficient to control symptoms in localised disease. Extensive disease is also treated with sulphasalazine, which helps to prevent relapses. Treatment may be long-term and dosage requires frequent adjustment; the rate of metabolism of sulphasalazine is genetically determined and side-effects occur frequently. Sulphasalazine enemas and suppositories are generally used only in patients who cannot tolerate the side-effects of oral sulphasalazine. Severe cases may need additional treatment with **oral corticosteroids**. Prednisolone is generally used. In resistant cases immunosuppressants, usually **azathioprine** (Imuran®), can be used. **Sodium cromoglycate** (Nalcrom®) has been used in colitis but results of clinical trials are disappointing.

Laxatives are required to facilitate bowel movement when proctitis is present but a high-fibre diet and bulk-forming drugs such as **methylcellulose** are more useful in adjusting faecal consistency (section 1.6.1).

Symptoms of mild ulcerative colitis may be relieved with antidiarrhoeal drugs such as **codeine** or **loperamide** (Imodium®) but they should be used with caution in severe cases as paralytic ileus and toxic megacolon may be precipitated. For similar reasons antispasmodics should **not** be used in ulcerative colitis.

Cholestyramine (Questran®) is effective in the symptomatic relief of diarrhoea caused by ileal disease, or where the ileum has been resected, and occasionally in post-vagotomy diarrhoea.

See also sections 1.7.2 and 1.7.3 for anti-inflammatory drugs acting on the colon and rectum.

CROHN'S DISEASE. Treatment is similar to that of ulcerative colitis. Oral **sulphasalazine** may relieve symptoms and in certain circumstances oral **corticosteroids** may be used (see section 6.3.2); **corticotrophin** and **tetracosactrin** (see section 6.5.1) are also used. Resistant cases may be treated with **azathioprine**. Antibiotics are not recommended in Crohn's disease except when hospital investigation has revealed definite evidence of the overgrowth of bacteria in the small bowel.

PSEUDOMEMBRANOUS COLITIS. This may develop after antibiotic therapy. Clindamycin and lincomycin have been implicated most frequently but few antibiotics are free of this side-effect. Oral **vancomycin** (see section 5.1.7) or **metronidazole** (see section 5.1.11.1) have been advocated as specific treatment.

DIVERTICULAR DISEASE. This is treated with a high-fibre diet, bran supplements and bulk-forming laxatives. **Antispasmodics** are also of some value (section 1.2). Antibiotics should be used only when the diverticula in the intestinal wall become infected. **Antidiarrhoeal** drugs which slow intestinal motility, for example codeine, diphenoxylate, and loperamide (Imodium®) could possibly exacerbate the symptoms of diverticular disease and are therefore **contra-indicated**.

AZATHIOPRINE

Indications: induction and maintenance of remission in ulcerative colitis and Crohn's disease
Cautions; Side-effects: see section 8.2.1
Dose: 1–3 mg/kg daily

Preparations

See section 8.2.1

CHOLESTYRAMINE

Indications: diarrhoea associated with ileal disease, ileal resection and post-vagotomy diarrhoea.
Cautions: supplements of vitamins A and D may be required during prolonged treatment; absorption of acidic drugs such as warfarin may be impaired. Drug interactions: see Appendix 1
Side-effects: nausea, heartburn, and rashes
Dose: initially 12–24 g daily, in single or divided doses, subsequently adjusted as required

Questran® (Bristol)
Powder, cholestyramine (anhydrous), 4-g sachet. Price 10 sachets = **F**

PREDNISOLONE

Indications: induction and maintenance of remission in ulcerative colitis, and Crohn's disease
Cautions; Contra-indications; Side-effects: see Corticosteroids, section 6.3.3
Dose: *by mouth*, initial dose 40 mg daily, in single or divided doses, until remission occurs, followed by reducing doses
By intravenous injection, for emergency treatment (under hospital supervision only), the equivalent of 20 mg of prednisolone (as prednisolone sodium phosphate) every 8 hours

Preparations
Oral and parenteral, section 6.3.4; rectal, sections 1.7.2 and 1.7.3

SODIUM CROMOGLYCATE

Indications: aid in the treatment of ulcerative colitis (see notes above); food allergy (in conjunction with dietary restriction)
Side-effects: occasional nausea, rashes, and joint pain
Dose: 200 mg 4 times daily before meals; CHILD 2–14 years 100 mg; capsules may be swallowed whole or the contents dissolved in hot water and diluted with cold water before taking

▼ **Nalcrom®** (Fisons)
Capsules, sodium cromoglycate 100 mg. Price 20 caps = **F**

SULPHASALAZINE

Indications: induction and maintenance of remission in ulcerative colitis and Crohn's disease
Cautions: maintain adequate fluid intake to prevent crystalluria; pregnancy; hepatic and renal disease; glucose-6-phosphate dehydrogenase deficiency. Blood counts and urine analysis necessary during prolonged treatment; withdraw treatment if blood dyscrasias or hypersensitivity reactions develop
Contra-indications: salicylate and sulphonamide hypersensitivity
Side-effects: nausea, vomiting, epigastric discomfort, headache, vertigo, tinnitus, rashes, fever, minor haematological abnormalities such as Heinz-body anaemia, reversible neutropenia, folate malabsorption; rarely frank haemolytic anaemias, pancreatitis, agranulocytosis, Stevens–Johnson syndrome, neurotoxicity, photosensitisation, polyarteritis nodosa, allergic myocarditis, pulmonary fibrosis, irreversible azoospermia in men. Urine may be coloured orange
Dose: by mouth, acute attack 1 g 4 times daily until remission occurs (if necessary corticosteroids may also be given), reducing to a maintenance dose of 500 mg 4 times daily; CHILD, acute attack 40–60 mg/kg daily, maintenance dose 20–30 mg/kg daily
By rectum in suppositories, 1–2 g morning and night after defaecation. As an enema, 3 g at bedtime, retained for at least 1 hour

Salazopyrin® (Pharmacia)
Tablets, brown, scored, sulphasalazine 500 mg. Price 20 tabs = **D**
EN-tablets® (= tablets e/c), yellow, f/c, sulphasalazine 500 mg. Price 20 tabs = **D**
Suppositories, brown, sulphasalazine 500 mg. Price 10 suppos = **E**
Retention enema, sulphasalazine 3 g in 100-ml single-dose disposable packs fitted with a nozzle. Price 100 ml = **D**

1.6 Laxatives

Misconceptions about bowel habits have led to excessive laxative use. Abuse may lead to hypokalaemia and an atonic non-functioning colon. Simple constipation is usually relieved by increasing the intake of dietary fibre; in children the introduction of fruit purée may be sufficient. In infants constipation is often remedied by adjustment of the diet, for example by increasing the sugar content of infant feeds based on milk powder.

Laxatives should generally be **avoided** except where straining will exacerbate a condition (such as angina) or increase the risk of rectal bleeding as in haemorrhoids. The use of laxatives is also acceptable in hepatic failure where the administration of **lactulose** (Duphalac®, Gatinar®) may be useful in the treatment of hepatic encephalopathy. Drug-induced constipation may also need treatment with laxatives. The use of laxatives in children is undesirable. It has occasionally resulted in atonic non-functioning colon.

The laxatives that follow have been divided into 4 main groups (sections 1.6.1–4). This simple classification disguises the fact that some laxatives have a complex action. For example **dioctyl sodium sulphosuccinate** (docusate sodium) has been classified as a faecal softener but it also increases intestinal secretions by stimulating adenyl cyclase. This has an important effect on intestinal motility.

The laxatives in section 1.6.6 should preferably be avoided in prescribing.

1.6.1 Bulk-forming drugs

These relieve constipation by increasing faecal mass which stimulates peristalsis. They are useful in the management of patients with colostomy, ileostomy, haemorrhoids, chronic diarrhoea associated with diverticular disease, spastic colon, and ulcerative colitis (section 1.5). Adequate fluid intake must be maintained to avoid intestinal obstruction. Unprocessed **bran**, taken with food, is a most effective bulk-forming preparation. Finely ground bran is less effective than coarsely ground bran but it is less troublesome to take.

Methylcellulose, **ispaghula**, and **sterculia** are useful in patients who cannot tolerate bran. Methylcellulose also acts as a faecal softener.

BRAN (WHEAT)

Indications: constipation caused by inadequate fibre intake, diverticular disease, chronic diarrhoea (section 1.5)
Cautions; Contra-indications; Side-effects: as for Ispaghula Husk (below). Calcium and iron

absorption may be impaired. Avoid in gluten enteropathies and coeliac disease
Dose: 12–24 g or more daily in divided doses

Fybranta® (Norgine)
Tablets, brown, bran 2 g. Price 20 tabs = **B**
Dose: 3–12 tablets daily in divided doses, chewed and swallowed with water

▼ **Proctofibe**® (Roussel)
Tablets, beige, fibrous grain extract 375 mg, fibrous citrus extract 94 mg. Price 20 tabs = **B**
Dose: adults and children over 3 years 4–12 tablets daily in divided doses chewed, swallowed, or dispersed in water

ISPAGHULA HUSK

Indications: constipation caused by inadequate fibre intake, diverticular disease, chronic diarrhoea (section 1.5), haemorrhoids, colostomy control
Cautions: adequate fluid intake should be maintained; caution in ulcerative colitis
Contra-indications: intestinal obstruction and colonic atony
Side-effects: flatulence, abdominal distension, and intestinal obstruction

Fybogel® (R&C)
Granules, buff, effervescent, ispaghula husk 3.5 g/sachet. Contains 6 mmol Na^+/sachet; caution in patients on sodium restricted diet. Price 10 sachets = **C**
Dose: 1 sachet in water twice daily preferably after meals; CHILD ½–1 level 5-ml spoonful

Isogel® (A&H)
Granules, pink, ispaghula husk 90%. Price 100 g = **B**
Dose: constipation, 2 teaspoonsfuls in water once or twice daily, preferably after meals; CHILD 1 teaspoonful
Diarrhoea (section 1.4.1), 1 teaspoonful 3 times daily

Metamucil® (Searle)
Powder, psyllium hydrophilic muciloid (ispaghula husk) 50%. Price 100 g = **D**
Dose: one 5-ml spoonful 1–3 times daily with water

Regulan® (Searle)
Powder, psyllium hydrophilic muciloid (ispaghula husk) 3.6 g/6.4 g sachet. Price 10 sachets = **C**
Dose: 1 sachet in 150 ml water 1–3 times daily

Vi-Siblin® (P-D)
Granules, brown, ispaghula husk 66%. Price 100 g = **D**
Dose: two 5-ml spoonfuls one or more times daily with water

METHYLCELLULOSE

Indications: constipation caused by inadequate fibre intake; diverticular disease, chronic diarrhoea (section 1.5); haemorrhoids, colostomy, and ileostomy control
Cautions; Contra-indications; Side-effects: as for Ispaghula Husk (above)

Methylcellulose Granules, pink, methylcellulose '2500' or '4500' 64%. Price 100 g = **D**
Dose: 1.5–6 g (2.5–10 ml) with water

Celevac® (WBP)
Tablets, pink, methylcellulose '450' 500 mg. Price 20 tabs = **A**
Granules, pink, methylcellulose '450' 64%. Price 100 g = **C**
Dose: 3–6 tablets (5–10 ml granules) twice daily. In constipation the dose should be taken with water. In diarrhoea, ileostomy, and colostomy control, minimise liquid intake for 30 minutes before and after the dose

Cellucon® (Medo)
Tablets, buff, methylcellulose '2500' 500 mg. Price 20 tabs = **A**
Dose: 1–4 tablets, chewed, 3 times daily with water

Cologel® (Lilly)
Mixture, yellow, methylcellulose '450' 900 mg/10 ml. Diluent water for preparations, life of diluted mixture 14 days. Price 100 ml = **B**
Dose: 5–15 ml taken with water preferably after meals 3 times daily initially, reducing to a maintenance dose of 5–15 ml daily

STERCULIA

Indications: constipation caused by inadequate fibre intake; diverticular disease, chronic diarrhoea (section 1.5); haemorrhoids, colostomy and ileostomy control
Cautions; Contra-indications; Side-effects: as for Ispaghula Husk (above)

Inolaxine® (Martindale)
Granules, orange, sterculia 98%. Price 175 g = **E**
Dose: 1–2 heaped teaspoonfuls once or twice daily with water; CHILD half the adult dose

Normacol Antispasmodic® (Norgine)
Granules, orange, coated, sterculia 62%, alverine citrate 0.5% (for the treatment of spastic colon). Price 100 g = **C**
Dose: 1–2 heaped 5-ml spoonfuls once or twice daily after the main meal or at bedtime. CHILD half the adult dose with water

Normacol Special® (Norgine)
Granules, coated, sterculia 62% (for the treatment of diverticular disease, constipation in pregnancy, and colostomy control). Price 100 g = **C**
Dose: in constipation and diverticular disease, as for Normacol Antispasmodic (above)

Normacol X® (Norgine)
Granules, coated, sterculia 62%, 40 g with 2 *tablets*, orange, danthron 200 mg (for bowel evacuation before abdominal radiological procedures); the urine may be coloured red. Price per pack = **B**
Dose: 2 heaped 5-ml spoonfuls of granules after breakfast and 1 tablet at bedtime for 2 days before examination

Normacol Standard (and Sugar-free)—section 1.6.6

1.6.2 Stimulant laxatives

These act by increasing intestinal motility. The most commonly used stimulant laxatives are **bisacodyl**, **danthron**, and standardised **senna** preparations. They often cause abdominal cramp. These preparations should not be used in intestinal obstruction, and prolonged use should be avoided as they can eventually precipitate the onset of an atonic non-functioning colon and hypokalaemia. They should preferably be avoided in children. Other laxatives should be used during pregnancy.

Stimulant laxatives which should be avoided in prescribing are indicated in section 1.6.6.

The anticholinesterases bethanechol, distigmine, neostigmine, and pyridostigmine enhance parasympathetic activity in the gut and increase intestinal motility. They are rarely used for their gastro-intestinal effects but may be needed in cases of paralytic ileus, for example postoperatively. Organic obstruction of the gut must first be excluded and they should be used with caution in bowel anastomosis.

BETHANECHOL CHLORIDE

Indications: see notes above
Cautions; Contra-indications; Side-effects: see under Neostigmine (see section 10.2.1) and notes above
Dose: *by mouth*, 10–30 mg 3–4 times daily

Myotonine Chloride® (Glenwood)
Tablets, pale blue, scored, bethanechol chloride 10 mg. Price 20 tabs = **B**
Tablets, pale blue, scored, bethanechol chloride 25 mg. Price 20 tabs = **C**

BISACODYL

Indications: constipation, bowel evacuation before radiological procedures, endoscopy, and surgery. Tablets act within 6–12 hours; suppositories act within 1 hour (see also section 1.6.5)
Cautions; Contra-indications; Side-effects: see general notes on stimulant laxatives (above). The tablets may cause gastro-intestinal disturbances. The suppositories may cause local irritation
Dose: *by mouth* for constipation, 5–10 mg after meals usually at night. Avoid taking with milk and antacids
By rectum in suppositories for constipation, 10 mg usually in the morning; CHILD 5 mg
Before radiological procedures etc., 10 mg by mouth at bedtime for 2 days before examination and, if necessary, a 10-mg suppository 1 hour before examination. An enema may also be used immediately before the investigation (see section 1.6.5)

Oral preparations
Bisacodyl Tablets, e/c, s/c, bisacodyl 5 mg. Price 20 tabs = **A**

Dulcodos® (Boehringer Ingelheim)
Tablets, e/c, s/c, bisacodyl 5 mg, dioctyl sodium sulphosuccinate 100 mg. Price 20 tabs = **C**
Dose: 2 tablets, usually at bedtime; avoid taking with milk or antacids

Dulcolax® (Boehringer Ingelheim)
Tablets, yellow, e/c, s/c, bisacodyl 5 mg. Price 20 tabs = **A**

Rectal preparations
Section 1.6.5

CASCARA

Indications: constipation. Acts within 6–8 hours
Cautions; Contra-indications; Side-effects: see notes on stimulant laxatives (above). The urine may be coloured red. Caution in nursing mothers

Cascara Tablets, s/c unless otherwise indicated, containing approximately 20 mg of total hydroxyanthracene derivatives of which not less than 40% consists of cascarosides. Price 20 tabs (s/c) = **A**
Dose: 1–2 tablets, usually at bedtime

CASTOR OIL

Indications: constipation; bowel evacuation before radiological procedures, endoscopy, surgery. Acts within 2–8 hours
Cautions: menstruation. See also notes on stimulant laxatives (above)
Contra-indications: intestinal obstruction
Side-effects: nausea, vomiting
Dose: 5–20 ml when required; CHILD up to 1 year 1–5 ml, 1–12 years 5–15 ml, in milk or fruit juice before breakfast or on an empty stomach

Price 100 ml = **B**

DANTHRON

Indications: constipation, bowel evacuation before radiological procedures, endoscopy, and surgery. Acts within 6–12 hours
Cautions; Contra-indications; Side-effects: see notes on stimulant laxatives (above). The urine may be coloured red. Avoid prolonged contact with skin (as in infants with napkins and in incontinent patients) since irritation and excoriation may occur. Caution in nursing mothers
Dose: constipation, 25–75 mg usually at bedtime; CHILD 12.5–25 mg
Before radiological procedures etc, 50–100 mg

Dorbanex® (Riker)
Capsules, yellow, danthron 25 mg, poloxamer '188' 200 mg. Price 20 caps = **C**
Dose: constipation 1–2 capsules; CHILD 1 capsule
Before radiological procedures etc. 2–4 capsules
Liquid (= mixture), orange, danthron 25 mg, poloxamer '188' 200 mg/5 ml. Diluent tragacanth mucilage or syrup, life of diluted elixir 14 days. Price 100 ml = **C**

Dose: constipation, 5–10 ml; CHILD 2.5 ml, usually at bedtime
Liquid forte (= strong mixture), orange, danthron 75 mg, poloxamer '188' 1 g/5 ml. Diluent as above. Price 100 ml = **C**
Dose: constipation, 5 ml usually at bedtime

Normacol-X®—section 1.6.1

Normax® (Bencard)
Capsules, brown, danthron 50 mg, dioctyl sodium sulphosuccinate 60 mg. Price 20 caps = **B**
Dose: 1–3 capsules; CHILD 6–12 years 1 capsule, usually at bedtime

DISTIGMINE BROMIDE

Indications: see notes above
Cautions; Contra-indications; Side-effects: see under Neostigmine (section 10.2.1 and notes above)
Dose: *by mouth*, 5 mg daily half an hour before breakfast
By intramuscular injection, 500 micrograms about 12 hours after surgery, repeated once daily until normal function is restored

Ubretid® (Berk)
Tablets, scored, distigmine bromide 5 mg. Price 20 tabs = **I**
Injection, distigmine bromide 500 micrograms/ml. Price 1-ml amp = **B**

FIG

Indications: mild constipation (also has demulcent properties)

Figs Syrup, Compound, fig 3.2 g, cascara elixir 0.5 ml, compound rhubarb tincture 0.5 ml, senna liquid extract 1 ml/10 ml. Price 100 ml = **B**
Dose: 2.5–10 ml when required

NEOSTIGMINE

Indications: see notes above
Cautions; Contra-indications; Side-effects: see section 10.2.1 and notes above
Dose: *by mouth*, neostigmine bromide 15–30 mg, repeated according to the patient's response; CHILD 2.5–15 mg
By subcutaneous or intramuscular injection, neostigmine methylsulphate 0.5–2.5 mg; CHILD 0.125–1 mg

Preparations
See section 10.2.1

PYRIDOSTIGMINE BROMIDE

Indications; Cautions; Contra-indications; Side-effects: see under Neostigmine
Dose: *by mouth*, 60–240 mg, repeated according to the patient's needs; CHILD 15–60 mg
By subcutaneous or intramuscular injection, 1 to 5 mg; CHILD 0.25–1 mg

Preparations
See section 10.2.1

SENNA

Indications: constipation; bowel evacuation before abdominal radiological procedures, endoscopy, and surgery. Acts in 8–12 hours
Cautions; Contra-indications; Side-effects: see introduction to stimulant laxatives (above). The urine may be coloured red

Agiolax® (M&B)
Granules, brown, tinnevelly senna pods 12.4%, ispaghula seed 54.2%. Price 100 g = **C**
Dose: 1–2 heaped teaspoonfuls with water before breakfast and after supper or every 4–6 hours in resistant cases; CHILD half the adult dose.

Senade® (Andard-Mount)
Tablets, brown, sennosides A and B 13.5 mg (as the calcium salts). Price 20 tabs = **A**
Dose: 1–3 tablets, usually at bedtime; CHILD 1–12 years 1 tablet
Elixir, sennosides A and B 13.5 mg/5 ml (as the calcium salts). Price 100 ml = **C**
Dose: 10 ml, usually at bedtime; CHILD 1–12 years 5 ml

Senokot® (R&C)
Tablets, brown, ≡ sennoside B 7.5 mg. Price 20 tabs = **A**
Dose: 2–4 tablets, usually at bedtime; initial dose should be low then gradually increased; CHILD over 6 years, half adult dose
Granules, brown, sennoside B 14.9 mg/5 ml or 5.5 mg/g (one 5-ml spoonful = 2.7 g). Price 100 g = **C**
Dose: 5–10 ml, usually at bedtime
Syrup (= elixir), brown, ≡ sennoside B 7.5 mg/5 ml. Diluent syrup, life of diluted elixir 14 days. Price 100 ml = **B**
Dose: 10–20 ml, usually at bedtime; CHILD 2–6 years 2.5–5 ml, over 6 years 5–10 ml

X-Prep® (Napp)
Liquid (= mixture), brown, sennosides A and B 142 mg/71 ml (for bowel evacuation before radiological procedures). Price 71-ml bottle = **B**
Dose: 71 ml with a tumblerful of water; CHILD and underweight adult 0·5 ml/kg, repeated after 1 hour

SODIUM PICOSULPHATE

Indications: constipation, bowel evacuation before abdominal radiological procedures, endoscopy, and surgery (acts in 10–14 hours)
Cautions; Contra-indications; Side-effects: see general notes on stimulant laxatives (above)
Dose: 5–15 mg, usually at bedtime; CHILD up to 5 years 2.5 mg, 6–12 years 2.5–5 mg

Laxoberal® (WBP)
Elixir, yellow, sodium picosulphate 5 mg/5 ml. Diluent purified water, freshly boiled and cooled, life of diluted elixir 14 days. Price 100 ml = **C**

Picolax® (Nordic)
Oral powder, sodium picosulphate 10 mg/sachet, with magnesium citrate. For bowel evacuation before radiological procedures, surgery etc. Price 2 sachets = **B**
Dose: 1 sachet in water in the morning and a second in the afternoon of the day preceding investigatory or surgical procedures

1.6.3 Faecal softeners

These act by lubricating the faeces (for example liquid paraffin or poloxamer 188) or they soften faeces by affecting intestinal electrolyte transport (for example dioctyl sodium sulphosuccinate). This may cause sufficient rectal stimulation to promote a bowel action. These drugs are useful in the management of haemorrhoids and anal fissure. See also drugs administered rectally to relieve constipation (section 1.6.5).

DIOCTYL SODIUM SULPHOSUCCINATE

(Docusate Sodium)
Indications: constipation
Dose: 37.5–200 mg; CHILD up to 1 year 12.5 mg, 1–12 years 12.5–100 mg, 2–3 times daily taken with water. Initial doses should be large and gradually reduced

Dioctyl-Medo® (Medo)
Tablets, scored, dioctyl sodium sulphosuccinate 20 mg. Price 20 tabs = **A**
Tablets forte, yellow, s/c, dioctyl sodium sulphosuccinate 100 mg. Price 20 tabs = **B**
Syrup (= elixir), yellow, dioctyl sodium sulphosuccinate 12.5 mg/5 ml (see section 1.6.5 for use as an enema). Diluent syrup, life of diluted elixir 14 days. Price 100 ml = **B**
Elixir concentrate, dioctyl sodium sulphosuccinate 50 mg/5 ml; for dilution before use with 3 parts of orange syrup to make the elixir (see section 1.6.5 for use as an enema). Price 100 ml = **C** (Hosp. only)

LIQUID PARAFFIN

Indications: constipation
Cautions: avoid prolonged use.
Side-effects: anal seepage of paraffin and consequent anal irritation after prolonged use granulomatous reactions caused by absorption of small quantities of liquid paraffin (especially from the emulsion), lipoid pneumonia, and interference with the absorption of fat-soluble vitamins
Dose: 10–30 ml when required

Liquid Paraffin Mixture, liquid paraffin 5 ml/10 ml. Price 100 ml = **A**
Dose: 10–30 ml when required
Liquid Paraffin and Magnesium Hydroxide Mixture—section 1.6.4
Liquid Paraffin and Phenolphthalein Mixture—section 1.6.6

Petrolagar No. 1® (Wyeth)
Mixture, liquid paraffin 7%, light liquid paraffin 18%. Price 100 ml = **A**
Dose: 10 ml morning and night or after meals

1.6.4 Osmotic laxatives

These act by maintaining a volume of fluid in the bowel by osmosis.

Saline purgatives are commonly abused but are satisfactory for occasional use. Adequate fluid intake should be maintained. **Magnesium sulphate** is useful where rapid bowel evacuation is required; a dose taken before breakfast or on an empty stomach and followed by a tumblerful of warm fluid usually causes evacuation within 2 hours. Sodium salts should be avoided as they may give rise to sodium and water retention in susceptible individuals.

Lactulose is a semi-synthetic disaccharide which is not absorbed from the gastro-intestinal tract. It produces an osmotic diarrhoea of low faecal pH, and discourages the proliferation of ammonia-producing organisms. It is also useful in the treatment of hepatic encephalopathy.

LACTULOSE

Indications: constipation, adjunctive treatment of hepatic encephalopathy
Contra-indications: galactosaemia
Side-effects: occasional gastro-intestinal disturbances
Dose: expressed in terms of the elixir containing lactulose 3.35 g/5 ml
Constipation, initially 15–30 ml daily in single or divided doses gradually reduced according to patient's needs; CHILD under 1 year 5 ml, 1–5 years 10 ml, 6–12 years 20 ml daily, gradually reduced
Hepatic encephalopathy, 30–50 ml 3 times daily

Lactulose Elixir, lactulose 3.35 g/5 ml with other ketonic sugars. Price 100 ml = **C**
Duphalac® (Duphar)
Syrup (= elixir), yellow, lactulose 3.35 g/5 ml with other ketonic sugars. Price 100 ml = **C**
Gatinar® (Wander)
Elixir, yellow, lactulose 3.35 g/5 ml with other ketonic sugars. Price 100 ml = **C**

MAGNESIUM CARBONATE

Indications: mild constipation
Cautions: use only occasionally; caution in the elderly and in renal impairment
Contra-indications: intestinal obstruction
Side-effects: eructation due to liberated carbon dioxide
Dose: 2–5 g followed by a tumblerful of water when required

Preparations
Section 1.1.1

MAGNESIUM HYDROXIDE

Indications: mild constipation
Cautions; Contra-indications: as for Magnesium Carbonate (above)
Dose: 2–4 g followed by a tumblerful of water, when required

Liquid Paraffin and Magnesium Hydroxide Mixture, magnesium hydroxide mixture 7.35 ml, liquid paraffin 2.5 ml, chloroform spirit 0.15 ml/10 ml. Price 100 ml = **A**
Dose: 5–20 ml when required

Magnesium Hydroxide Mixture, magnesium oxide (hydrated) about 550 mg/10 ml. Do not store in a cold place. Price 100 ml = **A**
Dose: 25–50 ml when required

MAGNESIUM SULPHATE

Indications: rapid bowel evacuation
Cautions; Contra-indications: as for Magnesium Carbonate (above)
Dose: 5–15 g with water before breakfast or on an empty stomach; CHILD 100–250 mg/kg when required

Magnesium Sulphate Mixture, magnesium sulphate 4 g/10 ml (see Formulary). Price 200 ml = **B**
Dose: 10–20 ml

1.6.5 Rectally administered laxatives

Enemas containing arachis oil or dioctyl sodium sulphosuccinate, and glycerol suppositories lubricate and soften impacted faeces and promote a bowel movement.

Bisacodyl (Dulcolax®), **dioctyl sodium sulphosuccinate** and **phosphate enemas** are useful in bowel clearance before radiological procedures, endoscopy, and surgery.

The use of soft soap enema should be **avoided**, especially in pregnancy as it may inflame the colonic mucosa.

Bisacodyl Suppositories, bisacodyl 10 mg. Price 12 suppos = **C**
Dose: 1 suppository

Glycerol Suppositories, gelatin 140 mg, glycerol 700 mg, purified water to 1 g. Price 12 suppos (all sizes) = **B**
Dose: 1 suppository moistened with water before use. The usual sizes are for *infants* small (1-g mould), *children* medium (2-g mould), *adults* large (4-g mould)

Phosphates Enema Formula B, sodium acid phosphate 12.8 g, sodium phosphate 10.24 g, purified water, freshly boiled and cooled, to 128 ml. Price 128 ml = **B**
Dose: 128 ml

Beogex® (Pharmax)
Adult suppositories, sodium bicarbonate 1.08 g, anhydrous sodium acid phosphate 1.32 g. Price 6 suppos = **B**
Paediatric suppositories, sodium bicarbonate 700 mg, anhydrous sodium acid phosphate 700 mg. Price 6 suppos = **B**
Dose: 1 suppository; CHILD 1 paediatric suppository, inserted 30 minutes before evacuation is required. Moisten with water before use

Dioctyl-Medo® (Medo)—see section 1.6.3 for oral preparations used by rectum
Syrup (= elixir, used also as enema). Price 100 ml = **B**
Dose: by rectum, 15–40 ml; CHILD up to 1 year 5–10 ml, over 1 year 7.5–15 ml
Elixir concentrate, dilute with 3 parts of water for use instead of the elixir, as an enema. Price 100 ml = **C** (Hosp.only)

Dulcolax® (Boehringer Ingelheim)
Suppositories, bisacodyl 10 mg. Price 12 suppos = **B**
Dose: 1 suppository
Paediatric suppositories, bisacodyl 5 mg. Price 12 suppos = **C**
Dose: 1 suppository
Rectal solution (= enema), bisacodyl 2.74 mg/ml. Price 100 ml = **C**
Dose: for bowel evacuation before radiological procedures, endoscopy, and surgery, 2–3 ml; CHILD 1–2 ml
Mixed with barium sulphate enema, 2–5 ml for every 1–3 litres of barium sulphate enema

Fletchers' Arachis Oil Retention Enema® (Pharmax)
Enema, arachis oil in 130-ml single-dose disposable packs. Price 130 ml = **C**
Dose: 130 ml; the enema should be warmed before use

Fletchers' Magnesium Sulphate Retention Enema® (Pharmax)
Enema, magnesium sulphate 50%, in 130-ml single-dose disposable packs. Price 130 ml = **B**
Dose: 130 ml

Fletchers' Phosphate Enema® (Pharmax)
Enema, phosphates enema formula B (see above). Price 128 ml with a standard or long rectal tube = **B**
Dose: 128 ml

Klyx® (Ferring)
Enema, dioctyl sodium sulphosuccinate 0.1%, sorbitol 25% in single-dose disposable packs (with a plastic sleeve). Price 120 and 240 ml (both) = **B**
Dose: 120 or 240 ml; preferably retained for 5 minutes

Micralax® (SK&F)
Enema, sodium citrate 450 mg, sodium alkylsulphoacetate 45 mg, sorbic acid 5 mg in 5-ml single-dose disposable packs. Price 5 ml = **B**
Dose: 5 ml when required

Microlet® (Ayerst)
Enema, sodium citrate 450 mg, sodium lauryl sulphoacetate 45 mg, glycerol 625 mg, with citric acid, potassium sorbate and sorbitol, in 5-ml single-dose disposable packs with nozzle. Price 5 ml = **B**
Dose: 5–10 ml; CHILD up to 3 years 2·5 ml

Relaxit® (Pharmacia)
Enema, sodium citrate 450 mg, sodium lauryl sulphate 75 mg, sorbic acid 5 mg, in a viscous solution in 5-ml single-dose disposable packs fitted with a nozzle. Price 5 ml = **B**
Dose: 5 ml

Veripaque® (Winthrop)
Enema, powder for reconstitution, oxyphenisatin. Price 50-mg vial = **C**
Dose: before diagnostic procedures or surgery, 50 mg in 2 litres of water (or *pro rata*)
Mixed with barium sulphate enema, 50 mg for every 2 litres of barium sulphate enema (or *pro rata*)

1.6.6 Other laxatives

Unstandardised preparations of cascara, frangula, rhubarb, and senna should be **avoided** as their laxative action is unpredictable.

Aloes, colocynth, and jalap should be **avoided** as they have a drastic purgative action.

Phenolphthalein should be **avoided** as it may cause rashes, albuminuria, and haemoglobinuria. Its laxative effects may continue for several days because of enterohepatic recycling.

Liquid Paraffin and Phenolphthalein Mixture, phenolphthalein 30 mg/10 ml in liquid paraffin mixture. Price 100 ml = **A**

Phenolphthalein Tablets, phenolphthalein 125 mg. Price 20 tabs = **A**

Rhubarb Mixture, Compound (see Formulary). Price 100 ml = **A**

Rhubarb and Soda Mixture, Ammoniated (see Formulary). Price 100 ml = **A**

Agarol® (Warner)
Mixture, phenolphthalein 66 mg, liquid paraffin 1.6 ml, agar 10 mg/5 ml. Price 100 ml = **B**

Alophen® (P-D)
Pills, brown, s/c, aloin 15 mg, belladonna dry extract 5 mg, ipecacuanha 4 mg, phenolphthalein 30 mg. Price 20 pills = **A**

Cascara Evacuant® (P-D)
Elixir, 'cascara extract' 2 g/5 ml. Price 125 ml = **C**

Kaylene-Ol® (Dendron)
Mixture, kaolin 7.5%, liquid paraffin 22.5%. Price 100 ml = **B**

Kest® (Berk)
Tablets, magnesium sulphate 300 mg, phenolphthalein 49 mg. Price 20 tabs = **A**

Normacol Standard® (Norgine)
Granules, brown, coated, frangula 8%, sterculia 62%. Price 100 g = **C**

Normacol Standard Sugar-free Formula® (Norgine), as for Normacol Standard (above). Contains no sugar. Price 100 g = **C**

Opobyl® (Bengué)
Pills, aloes 20 mg, bile salts 50 mg, boldo extract 10 mg, euonymus 2 mg, desiccated liver 50 mg, podophyllin 2 mg. Price 20 pills = **B**

Petrolagar No. 2® (Wyeth)
Mixture, phenolphthalein 0.35%, liquid paraffin 7%, light liquid paraffin 18%. Price 100 ml = **A**

Veracolate® (Warner)
Tablets, red, s/c, bile salts 70 mg, capsicum oleoresin 3 mg, 'cascara extract' 65 mg, phenolphthalein 32 mg. Price 20 tabs = **A**

1.7 Rectal and colonic drugs

Pruritus, soreness, and excoriation in the anal and perianal regions, and rectal discharge are common in patients suffering from haemorrhoids, fistulae, and proctitis. They are best treated by careful local toilet, drying and powdering the skin, and adjusting the diet to avoid hard stools. These measures may be supplemented by the application of various bland soothing preparations or preparations containing local anaesthetics (section 1.7.1). Bulk-forming drugs, bran, and high residue diet may be helpful in anal fissure.

When necessary, anti-inflammatory drugs such as sulphasalazine (section 1.5) and corticosteroids (section 1.7.2) are used but it is important to exclude perianal thrush. This is best treated with **nystatin** by mouth and by topical application (see sections 5.2 and 13.10.2).

Glycerol suppositories and phosphates enemas are occasionally used for their local action in severe constipation (section 1.6.5).

1.7.1 Soothing agents

Bland soothing preparations may contain mild astringents such as bismuth subgallate, zinc oxide, and hamamelis. Many proprietary preparations also contain lubricants (such as lauromacrogol 400 and sodium oleate); vasoconstrictors (adrenaline, ephedrine, phenylephrine); or mild antiseptics (chlorothymol, boric acid, Peru balsam, bronopol, and resorcinol). Prolonged application of preparations containing **resorcinol** should be **avoided** because they may interfere with thyroid function. Heparinoids are used to promote the resorption of local oedema and extravasated blood.

Soothing agents such as hamamelis suppositories may give symptomatic relief in haemorrhoids.

Local anaesthetics are used to relieve pain associated with haemorrhoids, anal fissure and pruritus ani. They are added to many proprietary preparations. They should be used only for short periods (no longer than 2 weeks) as they may cause sensitisation of the anal skin.

Lignocaine gel and ointment (see section 15.2) may be useful for application to anal fissures and are best applied on a plastic dilator. This ensures that the ointment comes into contact with the base of the fissure and encourages healing.

Alternative local anaesthetics include amethocaine, cinchocaine, and pramoxine, but they are more irritant.

ADMINISTRATION. Unless otherwise indicated a suppository is usually inserted into the rectum night and morning and after defaecation. Rectal ointments and creams are applied night and morning and after defaecation, externally or by rectum using a rectal nozzle.

Bismuth Subgallate Suppositories, Compound, bismuth subgallate 200 mg, castor oil 60 mg, resorcinol 60 mg, zinc oxide 120 mg, in theobroma oil or other suitable basis. Price 12 suppos = **C**

Hamamelis Suppositories, hamamelis dry extract, usual strength 200 mg in theobroma oil or other suitable basis. Price 12 suppos = **D**

Hamamelis and Zinc Oxide Suppositories. Usual strength hamamelis dry extract 200 mg, zinc oxide 600 mg. Price 12 suppos = **D**

Alcos-Anal® (Norgine)
Ointment, sodium oleate 10%, lauromacrogol '400' 2%, chlorothymol 0.1%. Price 20 g = **D**
Suppositories, sodium oleate 200 mg, lauromacrogol '400' 20 mg, chlorothymol 700 micrograms. Price 10 suppos = **D**

Anodesyn® (Crookes Products)
Ointment, ephedrine hydrochloride 0.25%, lignocaine hydrochloride 0.5%, allantoin 0.5%. Price 25 g = **B**
Prolonged use should be avoided
Suppositories, ephedrine hydrochloride 5.1 mg, lignocaine hydrochloride 10.25 mg, allantoin 10.25 mg, bronopol 4.1 mg. Price 12 suppos = **C**
Prolonged use should be avoided

Anusol® (Warner)
Cream, bismuth oxide 2.14%, Peru balsam 1.8%, zinc oxide 10.75%. Price 23 g = **C**
Ointment, benzyl benzoate 1.25%, bismuth subgallate 2.25%, bismuth oxide 0.87%, zinc oxide 10.75%, Peru balsam 1.87%. Price 25 g = **C**
Suppositories, bismuth oxide 24 mg, bismuth subgallate 59 mg, Peru balsam 49 mg, zinc oxide 296 mg. Price 12 suppos = **C**

Bismodyne® (Loveridge)
Ointment, bismuth subgallate 2%, hexachlorophane 0.5%, lignocaine 0.5%, zinc oxide 7.5%. Price 25 g = **B**
Prolonged use should be avoided
Suppositories, bismuth subgallate 150 mg, hexachlorophane 2.5 mg, lignocaine 10 mg, zinc oxide 120 mg. Price 12 suppos = **B**
Prolonged use should be avoided

Lasonil® (Bayer)
Ointment, hyaluronidase 150 units, heparinoids equivalent to 50 units of heparin/g. Price 14 g = **B**; 40 g = **D**

Nestosyl® (Bengué)
Ointment, benzocaine 2%, butyl aminobenzoate 2%, hexachlorophane 0.1%, resorcinol 2%, zinc oxide 10%. Price 30 g = **B**
Prolonged use should be avoided.

1.7.2 Rectal corticosteroids

Corticosteroids are used to relieve inflammation but should only be used for limited periods and when the presence of infection has been excluded.

Hydrocortisone cream and ointment are useful for treating the perianal regions. Hydrocortisone suppositories and the corticosteroid retention enemas are used to relieve the inflammation of ulcerative colitis and proctitis. Corticosteroid foam preparations such as Colifoam® may be a useful alternative for patients with difficulty in retaining corticosteroid enemas. Oral **sulphasalazine** (section 1.5) may supplement these treatments if necessary.

For compound rectal preparations with corticosteroids see section 1.7.3.

HYDROCORTISONE

Indications: inflammation associated with colitis, proctitis, haemorrhoids, and related conditions
Cautions; Contra-indications; Side-effects: see section 6.3.3. Prolonged use should be avoided. Contra-indicated in untreated infection

Hydrocortisone Cream, hydrocortisone or hydrocortisone acetate 1%—see section 13.4
Apply sparingly 3–4 times daily when required

Hydrocortisone Ointment, hydrocortisone 0.5, 1, or 2.5%—see section 13.4
Apply sparingly 3–4 times daily when required

Hydrocortisone Suppositories, hydrocortisone or hydrocortisone acetate 25 mg in theobroma oil or other suitable basis. Price 6 suppos = **D**
Dose: 1 suppository inserted night and morning and after defaecation

Colifoam® (Stafford-Miller)
Foam in aerosol pack, hydrocortisone acetate 10%. Price 20-g pack = **H**
Dose: initially 1 applicatorful (1.4 g) inserted into the rectum once or twice daily for 2–3 weeks, then once on alternate days

Cortenema® (Bengué)
Retention enema, hydrocortisone (partially solubilised) 100 mg/60 ml. Price 60 ml = **C**
Dose: initially 1 enema at bedtime for 2–3 weeks; then alternate days. The enema should be retained for at least 1 hour

BETAMETHASONE VALERATE

Indications: inflammation of the anus and perianal regions
Cautions; Contra-indications; Side-effects: see section 6.3.3. Prolonged use should be avoided. Contra-indicated in untreated infection

Preparations
See section 1.7.3 for Betnovate® compound rectal preparations and section 13.4 for cream and ointment

PREDNISOLONE

Indications; Cautions; Contra-indications; Side-effects: as for Hydrocortisone (above)

Predenema® (Pharmax)
Retention enema, prednisolone 20 mg (as the sodium metasulphobenzoate salt) in 100-ml single-dose disposable pack fitted with a long or standard tube. Price 100 ml = **C**
Dose: initially 1 enema at bedtime for 2–4 weeks; then on alternate days. The enema should be retained for at least 1 hour

Predsol® (Glaxo)
Retention enema, prednisolone 20 mg (as the sodium phosphate salt) in 100-ml single-dose disposable packs fitted with a nozzle. Price 100 ml = **C**
Dose: initially 1 enema at bedtime for 2–4 weeks then reduced. The enema should be retained for at least 1 hour
Suppositories, prednisolone 5 mg (as the sodium phosphate salt). Price 10 suppos = **D**
Dose: 1 suppository inserted night and morning and after defaecation

1.7.3 Compound preparations with corticosteroids

See section 1.7.2 for discussion of corticosteroids used locally in diseases of the colon and rectum and section 1.7.1 for other ingredients of rectal preparations.

Rectal preparations which contain **antibiotics** should be **avoided** because they are generally ineffective owing to the large bacterial population in the bowel and the development of resistance; hypersensitivity may also occur.

ADMINISTRATION. Unless otherwise indicated a suppository is inserted into the rectum night and morning and after defaecation. Rectal ointments and creams are applied night and morning and after defaecation, externally or by rectum using a rectal nozzle. Prolonged use should be avoided.

Anacal® (Luitpold-Werk)
Ointment, hexachlorophane 0.5%, lauromacrogol '400' 5%, a heparinoid 0.2%, prednisolone 0.15%. Price 30 g = **E**
Apply 1–4 times daily
Suppositories, hexachlorophane 5 mg, lauromacrogol '400' 50 mg, a heparinoid 4 mg, prednisolone 1 mg. Price 10 suppos = **D**

Anugesic-HC® (Warner)
Cream, benzyl benzoate 1.2%, bismuth oxide 0.87%, hydrocortisone acetate 0.5%, Peru balsam 1.8%, pramoxine hydrochloride 1%, resorcinol 0.87%, zinc oxide 12.33%. Price 15 g = **E**

Anugesic-HC® (Warner)
Suppositories, benzyl benzoate 33 mg, bismuth oxide 24 mg, bismuth subgallate 59 mg, hydrocortisone acetate 5 mg, Peru balsam 49 mg, pramoxine hydrochloride 27 mg, zinc oxide 296 mg. Price 12 suppos = **E**

Anusol-HC® (Warner)
Ointment, benzyl benzoate 1.25%, bismuth oxide 0.87%, bismuth subgallate 2.25%, hydrocortisone acetate 0.25%, Peru balsam 1.87%, resorcinol 0.87%, zinc oxide 10.75%. Price 15 g = **E**
Suppositories, benzyl benzoate 33 mg, bismuth oxide 24 mg, bismuth subgallate 59 mg, hydrocortisone acetate 10 mg, Peru balsam 49 mg, resorcinol 24 mg, zinc oxide 296 mg. Price 12 suppos = **D**

Betnovate® (Glaxo)
Rectal ointment, betamethasone valerate 0.05%, lignocaine hydrochloride 2.5%, phenylephrine hydrochloride 0.1%. Price 25 g = **D**
Apply 2–3 times daily until inflammation subsides then once daily, externally or by rectum
Compound suppositories, betamethasone valerate 500 micrograms, lignocaine hydrochloride 40 mg, phenylephrine hydrochloride 2 mg. Price 10 suppos = **D**

Hepacort Plus® (Rona)
Cream, heparin sodium 1000 units/g, hydrocortisone acetate 0.1%. Price 10 g = **C**
Apply 3 times daily
Suppositories, heparin sodium 2000 units, hydrocortisone acetate 2 mg. Price 6 suppos = **C**
Dose: 1 suppository inserted 2–3 times daily

Proctofoam HC® (Stafford-Miller)
Foam in aerosol pack, hydrocortisone acetate 1%, pramoxine hydrochloride 1%. Price 20-g pack (40 applications) = **F**
Insert 1 applicatorful by rectum 2–3 times daily and after defaecation and apply perianally as required

Proctosedyl® (Roussel)
Ointment, aesculin 1%, cinchocaine hydrochloride 0.5%, framycetin sulphate 1%, hydrocortisone 0.5%. Price 15 g = **E**
Suppositories, aesculin 10 mg, cinchocaine hydrochloride 5 mg, framycetin sulphate 10 mg, hydrocortisone 5 mg. Price 12 suppos = **E**

Scheriproct® (Schering)
Ointment, cinchocaine hydrochloride 0.5%, clemizole undecenoate 1%, hexachlorophane 0.5%, prednisolone hexanoate 0.19%. Price 10 g = **D**
In severe cases use 3–4 times daily on first day then once or twice daily, externally or by rectum
Suppositories, cinchocaine hydrochloride 1 mg, clemizole undecenoate 5 mg, hexachlorophane 2.5 mg, prednisolone hexanoate 1.3 mg. Price 12 suppos = **D**
Dose: in severe cases insert 1 suppository 2–3 times daily and then once daily after defaecation

Ultraproct® (Schering)
Ointment, cinchocaine hydrochloride 0.5%, clemizole undecenoate 1%, fluocortolone hexanoate 0.095%, fluocortolone pivalate 0.092%, hexachlorophane 0.5%. Price 10 g = **D**
Apply 3–4 times on the first day then once or twice daily
Suppositories, cinchocaine hydrochloride 1 mg, clemizole undecenoate 5 mg, fluocortolone hexanoate 630 micrograms, fluocortolone pivalate 610 micrograms, hexachlorophane 2.5 mg. Price 12 suppos = **E**
Dose: in severe cases insert 1 suppository 2–3 times daily then once daily after defaecation

Uniroid® (Unigreg)
Ointment, cinchocaine hydrochloride 5 mg, hydrocortisone 5 mg, neomycin sulphate 5 mg, polymyxin B sulphate 6250 units/g. Price 15 g = **D**
Suppositories, cinchocaine hydrochloride 5 mg, hydrocortisone 5 mg, neomycin sulphate 10 mg, polymyxin B sulphate 12500 units. Price 12 suppos = **D**

Xyloproct® (Astra)
Ointment (= cream), aluminium acetate 3.5%, hydrocortisone acetate 0.275%, lignocaine 5%, zinc oxide 18%. Price 15 g = **D**
Apply several times daily

Suppositories, aluminium acetate 50 mg, hydrocortisone acetate 5 mg, lignocaine 60 mg, zinc oxide 400 mg. Price 10 suppos = **D**
Dose: 1 suppository at night and after defaecation

1.7.4 Other rectal preparations

Oily phenol injection is used to inject haemorrhoids but rubber banding has largely replaced injection therapy.

Sulphasalazine enemas and suppositories are available (section 1.5), but are generally not employed except in patients who cannot tolerate the side-effects of oral administration.

BUFEXAMAC

Indications: inflammation associated with haemorrhoids, pruritus ani, and related conditions
Cautions: stinging may occur after application. Occasional hypersensitivity reactions

Parfenac® (Lederle)
Cream, bufexamac 5%. Price 15 g = **C**
Apply sparingly 2–3 times daily

PHENOL

Indications: injection of haemorrhoidal veins
Dose: 0.5–1.5 ml of oily phenol injection into the submucous layer; several injections may be given at different sites

Oily Phenol Injection, phenol 5% in almond oil or other suitable oil. Price 2- and 5-ml amp (both) = **B**; 25-ml vial = **D**

1.8 Stoma care

1.8.1 Local care of stoma
1.8.2 Prescribing for patients with stoma

1.8.1 Local care of stoma

Patients are usually given advice about the use of cleansing agents, protective creams, lotions, deodorants, or sealants whilst in hospital, either by the surgeon or by the health authority stoma care nurses. Voluntary organisations offer help and support to patients with stoma.

Items in the following list are prescribable as drugs without restriction or as borderline substances (see Appendix 3).

Protectives, adhesives, and sealants

Colobase® (Coloplast)
Paste (elastic). Price 50 g = **E**. ACBS: see Appendix 3

Hollister Karaya Paste® (Abbott)
Adhesive paste. Price 126 g = **E**. ACBS: see Appendix 3

Hollister Skin Gel® (Abbott)
Gel. Price 28 g = **E**. ACBS: see Appendix 3

Kerodex Double Seven® (Sterling Industrial)
Barrier cream. Price per tube = **C**. ACBS: see Appendix 3

Orabase® (Squibb)
Ointment (gel), see section 12.3.1

Orahesive® (Squibb)
Powder (adhesive), see section 12.3.1

Translet® (Searle)
Barrier cream. Price 57 g = **D**. ACBS: see Appendix 3

Deodorants

Atmocol® is used as a deodorising spray when emptying the appliance. The other deodorants listed are placed in the appliance.

Atmocol® (Raymed)
Aerosol deodorant. Price 1 unit (400 sprays) = **D**. ACBS: see Appendix 3

Chironair® (Downs)
Deodorant solution. Price 120 ml = **D**. ACBS: see Appendix 3

Dor® (Simpla)
Deodorant solution. Price 7 ml = **C**. ACBS: see Appendix 3

Nilodor® (Loxley)
Deodorant solution. Price (with dropper) 7.5 ml = **D**; 15 ml = **E**. ACBS: see Appendix 3

No-Roma® (Salt)
Deodorant solution. Price 30 ml = **B**; 300 ml = **E**. ACBS: see Appendix 3

Ostobon® (Coloplast)
Deodorant powder. Price 22 g = **D**. ACBS: see Appendix 3

Translet Plus One® (Searle)
Deodorant solution for men. Price 7 ml = **D**. ACBS: see Appendix 3

Translet Plus Two® (Searle)
Deodorant solution for women. Price 7 ml = **D**. ACBS: see Appendix 3

Stomogel® (Raymed)
Deodorant gel. Price 40 g = **C**. ACBS: see Appendix 3

1.8.2. Prescribing for patients with stoma

Enteric-coated and *sustained-release* preparations are **unsuitable**, particularly in patients with ileostomies, as there may not be sufficient release of the active ingredient.

Laxatives. Enemas and washouts should **not** be prescribed for patients with ileostomies as they may cause rapid and severe dehydration.

Colostomy patients may suffer from constipation and whenever possible should be treated by increasing fluid intake or dietary fibre. **Bulk-forming laxatives** (section 1.6.1) should be tried. If they are insufficient, as small a dose as possible of **danthron** or **senna** (section 1.6.2) should be used. Preparations such as **X-Prep**® should be **avoided** when preparing patients for radiological procedures as they may cause severe dehydration with nausea, vomiting, and griping.

Antidiarrhoeals. Intestinal sedatives such as **loperamide**, **codeine phosphate**, or **diphenoxylate** (with atropine) are effective. Bulk-forming drugs (section 1.6.1) may be tried but it is often difficult to adjust the dose appropriately.

Antibiotics should **not** be given for an episode of acute diarrhoea.

Antacids. The tendency to diarrhoea from magnesium salts or constipation from aluminium salts may be increased in these patients.

Diuretics should be used with caution in patients with ileostomies as they may become excessively dehydrated and potassium depletion may easily occur. It is usually advisable to use a **potassium-sparing** diuretic (see section 2.2.3).

Digoxin. Patients with a stoma are particularly susceptible to hypokalaemia whilst on digoxin therapy and potassium supplements may be advisable (see section 9.2.1.1).

Potassium supplements. Liquid formulations are preferred to sustained-release formulations.

Narcotic analgesics (see sections 4.7.1.2 and 4.7.2) may cause troublesome constipation in colostomy patients. When a non-narcotic analgesic is required paracetamol is usually suitable.

Iron preparations may cause loose stools in these patients. If this is troublesome and if iron is definitely indicated one of the intramusuclar iron preparations (see section 9.1.1.2) should be used. Sustained-release preparations should be **avoided** for the reasons given above.

1.9 Drugs affecting intestinal secretions

1.9.1 Drugs acting on the gall bladder

Oral **chenodeoxycholic acid** therapy is used in certain patients to dissolve cholesterol gallstones. It is used when surgery is inadvisable, symptoms are mild, gallbladder function is not impaired, and the stones are small and radiolucent. Since long-term treatment necessitating radiological monitoring is required it should preferably be controlled by hospital clinics. Long-term prophylaxis with chenodeoxycholic acid may be needed even after the stones have disappeared.

Ursodeoxycholic acid (Destolit®) has a similar action to chenodeoxycholic acid. It does not cause diarrhoea, a side-effect that limits the value of chenodeoxycholic acid.

Dehydrocholic acid is used to improve biliary drainage by stimulating the secretion of thin watery bile. It is given after surgery of the biliary tract to flush the common duct and drainage tube and may be useful to wash away small calculi obstructing flow through the common bile duct.

CHENODEOXYCHOLIC ACID

Indications: dissolution of cholesterol gallstones (see above)
Cautions: see above; also pregnancy
Contra-indications: do not use when stones are radio-opaque, in women who may become pregnant, in non-functioning gallbladders, in hepatic damage, and inflammatory diseases of the small intestine and colon
Side-effects: diarrhoea (particularly with high dosage), pruritus
Dose: 10–15 mg/kg daily in divided doses for 3–24 months, depending on size of stone; treatment is continued for 3 months after stones dissolve

▼ **Chendol®** (Weddel)
Capsules, orange/white, chenodeoxycholic acid 125 mg. Price 20 caps = **F**

▼ **Chenofalk®** (Armour)
Capsules, blue, chenodeoxycholic acid 250 mg. Price 20 caps = **F**

DEHYDROCHOLIC ACID

Indications: (improves biliary drainage) biliary tract surgery; to flush away small calculi in the bile duct; to accelerate visualisation and aid elimination of contrast media in the gall bladder
Contra-indications: complete mechanical biliary obstruction and occlusive hepatitis
Dose: 250–750 mg, 3 times daily; not recommended in children.
Cholecystography, 500–750 mg every 4 hours for 12 hours before and after the examination

Dehydrocholic Acid Tablets, dehydrocholic acid 250 mg. Price 50 tabs = **E**

URSODEOXYCHOLIC ACID

Indications; Cautions; Contra-indications: see under Chenodeoxycholic Acid
Side-effects: see under Chenodeoxycholic Acid; diarrhoea may occur less frequently
Dose: 8–10 mg/kg daily divided into 2 doses taken after the evening meal and one other meal; treatment is continued for 3–6 months after stones dissolve

▼ **Destolit®** (Lepetit)
Tablets, scored, ursodeoxycholic acid 150 mg. Price 20 tabs = **G**

1.9.2 Drugs which increase gastric acidity

Acidol-Pepsin® and Muripsin® used in achlorhydria and hypochlorhydria but are of uncertain value. They have replaced dilute hydrochloric acid for these conditions.

Acidol-Pepsin® (Sterling Research)
Tablets, pepsin 97 mg, betaine hydrochloride 388 mg: 1 tablet ≈ 1 ml dilute hydrochloric acid. Price 20 tabs = **B**
Dose: 1–3 tablets crushed and dissolved in water 3 times daily after meals; to be taken through a straw or glass tube

Muripsin® (Norgine)
Tablets, orange, glutamic acid hydrochloride 500 mg, pepsin 35 mg: 1 tablet ≈ 1 ml dilute hydrochloric acid. Price 20 tabs = **C**
Dose: 1–2 tablets with meals

1.9.3 Aprotinin

Aprotinin is a proteolytic enzyme inhibitor used in the treatment of acute pancreatitis. Its value has not been substantiated

Table: Pancreatin Supplements

Preparation and Price	Presentation	Dose	Minimum activity in BP units (approx.) Protease	Amylase	Lipase
Pancreatin BP 1980 Price 100 g = **F**	Powder	2–8 g daily in divided doses	1400/g	24 000/g	20 000/g
Cotazym® (Organon) Price 50 caps = **E**	Capsules, green, to be opened before use	6 capsules daily sprinkled on food or with milk	500	10 000	14 000
Nutrizym® (BDH) Price 50 tabs = **E**	Tablets, s/c, outer core bromelains 50 mg; inner core e/c, pancreatin 400 mg, ox bile 30 mg	1–2 during or after each meal	400	9000	9000
Pancrex® (P&B) Price 100 g = **E**	Granules, e/c	5–10 g 4 times daily before meals swallowed dry or with liquid	300/g	4000/g	5000/g
Pancrex V® (P&B) Price 100 g = **F**	Powder	0.5–2 g 4 times daily before meals swallowed dry or with liquid	1400/g	30 000/g	25 000/g
Price 50 caps = **C**	Capsules, to be opened before use	Up to 1 year 1–2 capsules mixed with feeds. Adults and children over 1 year 2–3 capsules 4 times daily before meals or sprinkled on food	430	9000	8000
Price 50 tabs = **B**	Tablets, e/c, s/c	5–15 tablets 4 times daily before meals	110	1700	1900
Price 50 tabs = **C**	Tablets forte, e/c, s/c	2–6 tablets 4 times daily before meals	330	5000	5600

Notes: Pancreatin BP 1980 is equivalent to Strong Pancreatin Powder BNF 1976–78.
When mixing pancreatin with food or liquid, excessive heat should be avoided.

APROTININ

Indications: prevention of pancreatitis after abdominal surgery, acute pancreatitis; disseminated intravascular coagulation

Side-effects: occasional hypersensitivity reactions

Dose: *by slow intravenous injection*, 500 000 kallidinogenase (kallikrein) inactivator units, then 200 000 units by intravenous infusion every 4 hours

Trasylol® (Bayer)
Injection, aprotinin 20 000 kallidinogenase (kallikrein) inactivator units/ml. Price 5-ml amp = **F**; 10-ml amp = **H**

1.9.4 Pancreatin supplements

Pancreatin preparations may be administered by mouth to compensate for the reduced or absent exocrine secretion in children with cystic fibrosis and in adults following pancreatectomy, total gastrectomy or chronic pancreatitis. They assist the digestion of starch, fat, and protein. As pancreatic enzymes are inactivated by gastric acid, pancreatin supplements are more effective when gastric acid secretion is temporarily inhibited by cimetidine given concurrently.

ENZYME ACTIVITY. For practical purposes, the minimum enzyme activity specified in the *British Pharmacopoeia 1980* for each component is approximately $1\frac{1}{2}$ times the potency originally specified in the *British Pharmacopoeia 1973* and 5 times the minimum potency required by the *British Pharmacopoeia 1968*.

Note. The BP 1980 also includes Pancreatic Extract which has half the potency of Pancreatin.

UNITS. Potencies in the table are expressed in BP units or NF = United States National Formulary, now known as USP units.

One BP unit of protease activity = approximately 62.5 NF (USP) units

One BP unit of lipase activity = approximately 1 NF (USP) unit
One BP unit of amylase activity = approximately 4.15 NF (USP) units
One BP unit of protease, lipase, and amylase activity = approximately 1 FIP unit

PANCREATIN

Indications: see notes above
Cautions: if mixed with liquids or feeds the resulting mixture should not be allowed to stand for longer than 1 hour
Side-effects: it may irritate the skin surrounding the mouth and anus
Dose: 2–8 g of Pancreatin BP daily in divided doses according to the patient's needs; CHILD up to 1 year 500–750 mg with each feed, 1–12 years 0.75–1 g before each meal.
Dosage is adjusted according to the size, number, and consistency of stools so that the patient thrives. It is given immediately before or with the main meals and extra allowance may be needed if snacks are taken between meals

Preparations

The preparations available for replacement therapy are shown in the table. The activity of pancreatin as powder or from capsules is destroyed by the acidity of the stomach. Such preparations are best taken sprinkled over food. **Pancreatin Granules** and **Pancreatin Tablets** are enteric-coated and may be taken before meals. **Cimetidine** (section 1.3) may be given concurrently to reduce gastric acid secretion

1.9.5 Other pancreatin preparations

The following preparations containing pancreatin are claimed to relieve discomfort caused by dietary imbalance. They are of doubtful value.

Combizym® (Luitpold-Werk)
Tablets, yellow, inner layer, pancreatin 220 mg; outer layer amylase, cellulase, hemicellulase, and protease. Price 50 tabs = **D**

Combizym Compositum® (Luitpold-Werk)
Tablets, orange, inner layer, ox bile extract 60 mg, pancreatin 400 mg; outer layer, amylase, cellulase, and protease. Price 50 tabs = **E**

Cotazym B® (Organon)
Tablets, f/c, cellulase, cholic acid 30 mg (as ox bile extract), pancreas powder (lipase 5400 units). Price 50 tabs = **E**

Enzypan® (Norgine)
Tablets, brown, chocolate-coated, inner layer e/c, dried ox bile 60 mg, pancreatin BP 1968 180 mg; outer layer, pepsin 12 mg. Price 50 tabs = **D**

Phazyme® (Stafford-Miller)
Tablets, pink, s/c, outer layer dimethicone with silica 20 mg, inner layer, e/c, dimethicone with silica 40 mg, amylase 2000 USP units, lipase 240 USP units, protease 3000 USP units. Price 20 tabs = **C**

2: Drugs used in the treatment of diseases of the CARDIOVASCULAR SYSTEM

In this chapter, drug treatment is discussed under the following headings:

2.1 Cardiac glycosides

These are used in the treatment of heart failure and supraventricular tachycardias, especially atrial fibrillation. The cardiac stimulant action is probably due to an alteration of the intracellular environment with increased accumulation and availability of calcium ions. The glycosides decrease the rate of conduction through the atrioventricular node and this slows the ventricular response in atrial fibrillation.

Nausea and vomiting are common toxic effects; ventricular extrasystoles, paroxysmal atrial tachycardia with block, and sometimes bradycardia and atrioventricular block also occur. Hypokalaemia predisposes to cardiac toxicity. A serum-digoxin concentration of more than 2 nanograms/ml (2.6 nmol/litre) is likely to cause toxic effects. Cardiac glycosides are not removed by dialysis; heart block may be treated with intravenous atropine, ventricular tachycardia with intravenous phenytoin, and supraventricular arrhythmias with intravenous practolol.

Digoxin (Lanoxin® etc.) is the glycoside of choice. In patients with moderate failure a loading dose is not required and a satisfactory serum concentration can be achieved over a period of about a week using a dose of 125–250 micrograms twice a day which can then be reduced. The final maintenance dose is governed by the clinical response and, in atrial fibrillation, by the ventricular rate, which should not be allowed to fall below 60 beats/minute.

When very rapid control is needed, which is seldom, digoxin may be given intravenously in a digitalising dose of 0.75 to 1.25 mg followed by 250 micrograms intravenously every 4 hours, with electrocardiographic monitoring.

It is often possible to withdraw digoxin without any clinical deterioration once the heart failure has been controlled—clearly desirable in elderly patients; a diuretic may need to be continued.

CHILDREN. The dose is based on body-weight; they require a relatively larger dose of digoxin than adults.

DIGOXIN

Indications: heart failure, supraventricular arrhythmias
Cautions: recent infarction, hypothyroidism; reduce dosage in the elderly and in renal failure; avoid hypokalaemia. Drug interactions: see Appendix 1
Side-effects: nausea, vomiting, arrhythmias, heart block
Dose: by mouth, 250 micrograms twice daily until digitalised, then 125–500 micrograms daily. For rapid digitalisation a dose of 1 mg over 24 hours
By intravenous injection, 0.75–1.25 mg initially, then 250 micrograms every 4 hours, under ECG cover

Digoxin Tablets, digoxin 125 and 250 micrograms. Price 20 tabs (both) = **A**
Diganox Nativelle® (Wilcox)
Tablets, scored, digoxin 250 micrograms. Price 20 tabs = **A**
Lanoxin® (Wellcome)
Tablets, digoxin 125 micrograms. Price 20 tabs = **A**
Tablets, scored, digoxin 250 micrograms. Price 20 tabs = **A**
Injection, digoxin 250 micrograms/ml. Price 2-ml amp = **B**
Lanoxin-PG® (Wellcome)
Tablets, blue, digoxin 62.5 micrograms. Price 20 tabs = **A**
Elixir, yellow, digoxin 50 micrograms/ml. Do not dilute, measure with pipette. Price 60 ml = **E**

DESLANOSIDE

Indications: heart failure, supraventricular arrhythmias
Cautions; Side-effects: see under Digoxin
Dose: by intramuscular or intravenous injection, rapid digitalisation, 0.8–1.6 mg in single or divided doses over 24 hours.

Cedilanid® (Sandoz)
Injection, deslanoside 200 micrograms/ml. Price 2-ml amp = **A**

DIGITOXIN

Indications: heart failure, supraventricular arrhythmias
Cautions; Side-effects: see under Digoxin
Dose: by mouth, 50–200 micrograms daily
By slow intravenous injection, 1–1.5 mg daily in divided doses for 1–2 days

Digitoxin Tablets, digitoxin 100 micrograms. Price 20 tabs = **A**

Digitaline Nativelle® (Wilcox)

Tablets, pink, digitoxin 100 micrograms. Price 20 tabs = **B**

Solution (= elixir), digitoxin 1 mg/ml (5 drops ≈ 100 micrograms). Price 10 ml = **D**

Injection, digitoxin 200 micrograms/ml. Price 1-ml amp = **B**

LANATOSIDE C

Indications: heart failure, supraventricular arrhythmias

Cautions; Side-effects: see under Digoxin

Dose: slow digitalisation 1.5–2 mg daily for 3–5 days; maintenance 0.25–1.5 mg daily

Cedilanid® (Sandoz)

Tablets, scored, lanatoside C 250 micrograms. Price 20 tabs = **B**

MEDIGOXIN

Indications: heart failure, supraventricular arrhythmias

Cautions; Side-effects: see under Digoxin

Dose: *by mouth or by intravenous injection*, 200 micrograms twice daily for 3–5 days, then 200–300 micrograms daily

Lanitop® (Roussel)

Tablets, yellow, scored, medigoxin 100 micrograms. Price 20 tabs = **B**

Injection, medigoxin 100 micrograms/ml. Price 2-ml amp = **A**

OUABAIN

Indications: heart failure, supraventricular arrhythmias

Cautions; Side-effects: see under Digoxin

Dose: *by slow intravenous injection*, 250–500 micrograms, then 100 micrograms every hour *or* digoxin by mouth until digitalised

Ouabaine Arnaud® (Wilcox)

Injection, ouabain 250 micrograms/ml. Price 1-ml amp = **C**

2.2 Diuretics

For potassium supplements, see section 9.2.1.1.

Thiazide diuretics (section 2.2.1) are used to relieve oedema due to heart failure, in which glomerular filtration is reduced, there is increased reabsorption of sodium from the renal tubules, and an increased production of aldosterone contributes to fluid retention.

The more potent **'loop' diuretics** such as frusemide or bumetanide (section 2.2.2) are used in patients with pulmonary oedema due to left ventricular failure and in patients with longstanding heart failure who no longer respond to the thiazide diuretics.

The thiazide diuretics are used in small doses to lower blood pressure, either alone or in combination with other antihypertensive drugs. They reduce peripheral vascular resistance. This antihypertensive effect is not much increased by increasing the dose.

Hypokalaemia may occur with both thiazide and loop diuretics; potassium supplements (see section 9.2.1.1) are usually unnecessary with smaller doses and certainly not when thiazides are used to lower blood pressure. Often the use of potassium-sparing diuretics (section 2.2.3) avoids the need to take potassium supplements. Intermittent diuretic therapy is less likely to induce hypokalaemia than long-continued treatment.

In patients with oedema resistant to treatment, combined use of diuretics which act on different parts of the renal tubule or by antagonising aldosterone may be effective: a thiazide may be combined with a loop diuretic, a potassium-sparing diuretic, or spironolactone (section 2.2.4).

In hepatic failure hypokalaemia caused by diuretics can precipitate encephalopathy.

In late pregnancy thiazide diuretics have been reported to cause neonatal thrombocytopenia.

2.2.1 Thiazides and related diuretics

Thiazides and related compounds act at the beginning of the distal convoluted tubule and are moderately potent diuretics. Side-effects include hypokalaemia, hypochloraemic alkalosis, hyperuricaemia, and hyperglycaemia. Hypokalaemia is dangerous in patients being treated with cardiac glycosides. Less common side-effects include skin rashes and thrombocytopenia. All thiazide diuretics are active by mouth with an onset of action within 1 to 2 hours and duration of 12 to 24 hours.

Small doses of the thiazide diuretics are used long-term to control hypertension—often alone in mild hypertension, but also with other drugs in more severe hypertension. Larger doses, often for only short periods of time, are needed in the treatment of oedema.

Bendrofluazide is the drug of choice in mild or moderate cardiac failure when the patient is not desperately ill and severe pulmonary oedema is not present. This drug is also effective alone in the treatment of mild hypertension and to potentiate other drugs in controlling more severe hypertension. Combined preparations of thiazide diuretics and potassium chloride are available; they may be useful when there is a compliance problem but have no other advantage over bendrofluazide or other thiazide diuretics prescribed in conjunction with potassium supplements (see section 9.2.1.1). Combined preparations and potassium-sparing diuretics should **not** usually be given together.

Chlorthalidone (Hygroton®), a thiazide-related compound, has a longer duration of action than the thiazides and may be given on alternate days to control hypertension.

There are many thiazide and thiazide-related compounds available but none offer any significant advantage over the ones mentioned.

NEWER COMPOUNDS. **Xipamide** (Diurexan®) resembles chlorthalidone structurally, and is more potent than the other thiazides. **Indapamide** (Natrilix®) is chemically related to chlorthalidone; it is claimed to lower blood pressure without causing a diuresis. Neither has been shown to have any advantage over longer-established thiazides.

BENDROFLUAZIDE

Indications: oedema, hypertension, diabetes insipidus (see section 6.5.2)
Cautions: may cause hypokalaemia, aggravates diabetes and gout; renal and hepatic impairment. Drug interactions: see Appendix 1
Contra-indications: renal failure
Side-effects: rashes, thrombocytopenia
Dose: 2.5–10 mg daily

Bendrofluazide Tablets, bendrofluazide 2.5 and 5 mg. Price 20 tabs (both) = **A**

Aprinox® (Boots)
Tablets, scored, bendrofluazide 2.5 and 5 mg. Price 20 tabs (both) = **A**

Berkozide® (Berk)
Tablets, bendrofluazide 2.5 mg. Price 20 tabs = **A**
Tablets, scored, bendrofluazide 5 mg. Price 20 tabs = **A**

Centyl® (Burgess)
Tablets, bendrofluazide 2.5 mg. Price 20 tabs = **B**
Tablets, scored, bendrofluazide 5 mg. Price 20 tabs = **C**

Neo-NaClex® (DF)
Tablets, scored, bendrofluazide 5 mg. Price 20 tabs = **B**

Urizide® (DDSA)
Tablets, bendrofluazide 5 mg. Price 20 tabs = **A**

CHLOROTHIAZIDE

Indications: oedema, hypertension
Cautions; Contra-indications; Side-effects: see under Bendrofluazide
Dose: 0.5–2 g daily

Saluric® (MSD)
Tablets, scored, chlorothiazide 500 mg. Price 20 tabs = **B**

CHLORTHALIDONE

Indications: oedema, hypertension, diabetes insipidus (see section 6.5.2)
Cautions; Contra-indications; Side-effects: see under Bendrofluazide
Dose: 25–100 mg daily *or* 50–200 mg on alternate days

Hygroton® (Geigy)
Tablets, yellow, scored, chlorthalidone 50 mg. Price 20 tabs = **C**
Tablets, scored, chlorthalidone 100 mg. Price 20 tabs = **D**

CLOPAMIDE

Indications: oedema, hypertension
Cautions; Contra-indications; Side-effects: see under Bendrofluazide
Dose: 20–60 mg daily

Brinaldix® (Sandoz)
Tablets, scored, clopamide 20 mg. Price 20 tabs = **D**

CLOREXOLONE

Indications: oedema, hypertension
Cautions; Contra-indications; Side-effects: see under Bendrofluazide
Dose: 10–100 mg daily

Nefrolan® (M&B)
Tablets, scored, clorexolone 10 mg. Price 20 tabs = **B**

CYCLOPENTHIAZIDE

Indications: oedema, hypertension
Cautions; Contra-indications; Side-effects: see under Bendrofluazide
Dose: 0.25–1 mg daily

Navidrex® (Ciba)
Tablets, scored, cyclopenthiazide 500 micrograms. Price 20 tabs = **B**

HYDROCHLOROTHIAZIDE

Indications: oedema, hypertension
Cautions; Contra-indications; Side-effects: see under Bendrofluazide
Dose: 25–200 mg daily

Hydrochlorothiazide Tablets, hydrochlorothiazide 25 mg, price 20 tabs = **B**; 50 mg, price 20 tabs = **C**

Direma® (Dista)
Tablets, hydrochlorothiazide 25 mg. Price 20 tabs = **B**
Tablets, hydrochlorothiazide 50 mg. Price 20 tabs = **C**

Esidrex® (Ciba)
Tablets, scored, hydrochlorothiazide 25 and 50 mg. Price 20 tabs (both) = **C**

HydroSaluric® (MSD)
Tablets, scored, hydrochlorothiazide 25 and 50 mg. Price 20 tabs (both) = **B**

HYDROFLUMETHIAZIDE
Indications: oedema, hypertension
Cautions; Contra-indications; Side-effects: see under Bendrofluazide
Dose: 25–200 mg daily

Hydrenox® (Boots)
Tablets, hydroflumethiazide 50 mg. Price 20 tabs = **A**

INDAPAMIDE
Indications: hypertension
Cautions: severe hepatic or renal impairment
Side-effects: nausea, headache, slight weight loss; diuresis with doses above 2.5 mg daily
Dose: 2.5 mg daily

▼ **Natrilix®** (Servier)
Tablets, pink, s/c, indapamide 2.5 mg. Price 20 tabs = **F**

MEFRUSIDE
Indications: oedema, hypertension
Cautions; Contra-indications; Side-effects: see under Bendrofluazide
Dose: 12.5–100 mg daily

Baycaron® (Bayer)
Tablets, scored, mefruside 25 mg. Price 20 tabs = **D**

METHYCLOTHIAZIDE
Indications: oedema, hypertension
Cautions; Contra-indications; Side-effects: see under Bendrofluazide
Dose: 2.5–10 mg daily

Enduron® (Abbott)
Tablets, pink, scored, methyclothiazide 5 mg. Price 20 tabs = **B**

METOLAZONE
Indications: oedema, hypertension
Cautions; Contra-indications; Side-effects: see under Bendrofluazide
Dose: 5–20 mg daily; max. 80 mg daily

Metenix 5® (Hoechst)
Tablets, blue, metolazone 5 mg. Price 20 tabs = **D**

POLYTHIAZIDE
Indications: oedema, hypertension
Cautions; Contra-indications; Side-effects: see under Bendrofluazide
Dose: 1–4 mg daily

Nephril® (Pfizer)
Tablets, scored, polythiazide 1 mg. Price 20 tabs = **C**

QUINETHAZONE
Indications: oedema, hypertension
Cautions; Contra-indications; Side-effects: see under Bendrofluazide
Dose: 50–100 mg daily

Aquamox® (Lederle)
Tablets, quinethazone 50 mg. Price 20 tabs = **E**

XIPAMIDE
Indications: oedema, hypertension
Cautions; Contra-indications: see under Bendrofluazide
Side-effects: slight gastro-intestinal disturbances; mild dizziness
Dose: 20–40 mg daily

▼ **Diurexan®** (Merck)
Tablets, scored, xipamide 20 mg. Price 20 tabs = **E**

2.2.2 Loop diuretics

These drugs inhibit resorption from the ascending loop of Henle in the renal tubule and are powerful diuretics. Hypokalaemia frequently develops, and care is needed to avoid hypotension. If there is an enlarged prostate, urinary retention may occur and steps should be taken to avoid it.

Frusemide (Lasix® etc.) and **bumetanide** (Burinex®) have similar activity. Oral administration is effective within 1 hour and diuresis is complete within 6 hours, so that the drugs can be given twice daily without interfering with sleep. Given intravenously they act rapidly, the peak effect occurring within 30 minutes. The diuresis is related to the size of dose, and in patients with impaired renal function very large doses may occasionally have to be given. In such doses both drugs can cause deafness and bumetanide can cause myalgia.

Ethacrynic acid (Edecrin®) has a similar onset and duration of action and may be useful in patients who have become refractory to frusemide and bumetanide. Deafness may occur in patients with renal failure, especially when ethacrynic acid is given intravenously.

For the use of potassium supplements with loop diuretics, see section 9.2.1.1.

FRUSEMIDE
Indications: oedema, oliguria due to renal failure
Cautions: causes hypokalaemia and hyponatraemia, aggravates diabetes and gout, liver failure, prostatism. Drug interactions: see Appendix 1
Contra-indications: liver cirrhosis
Side-effects: rashes; tinnitus and deafness in impaired renal function
Dose: *by mouth,* 20–80 mg once or twice daily; up to 2 g daily in oliguria; CHILD 1–3 mg/kg daily
By intramuscular or slow intravenous injection, 20–50 mg; CHILD 0.5–1.5 mg/kg
By intravenous infusion, in oliguria, 0.25–1 g at a rate not exceeding 4 mg/minute

Frusemide Tablets, frusemide 20 mg, price 20 tabs = **C**; 40 mg, price 20 tabs = **B**; 500 mg, price 20 tabs = **I**

Frusemide Injection, frusemide 10 mg/ml. Price 2-ml amp = **B**; 5-ml amp = **C**; 25-ml amp = **D**

Dryptal® (Berk)

Tablets, scored, frusemide 40 mg. Price 20 tabs = **B**

Tablets, yellow, scored, frusemide 500 mg. Price 20 tabs = **I** (Hosp. only)

Injection, frusemide 10 mg/ml. Price 2- and 5-ml amp (both) = **B**; 25-ml amp = **E** (Hosp. only)

Frusetic® (Unimed)

Tablets, scored, frusemide 40 mg. Price 20 tabs = **C**

Frusid® (DDSA)

Tablets, scored, frusemide 40 mg. Price 20 tabs = **B**

Lasix® (Hoechst)

Tablets, scored, frusemide 20 mg. Price 20 tabs = **C**

Tablets, scored, frusemide 40 mg. Price 20 tabs = **D**

Tablets, yellow, scored, frusemide 500 mg. Price 20 tabs = **I** (Hosp. only)

Paediatric liquid (= mixture), frusemide 1 mg/ml when reconstituted with water for preparations. Price 150 ml = **D**

Injection, frusemide 10 mg/ml. Price 2-ml amp = **B**; 5-ml amp = **C**; 25-ml amp = **D**

BUMETANIDE

Indications: oedema, oliguria due to renal failure

Cautions; Contra-indications: see under Frusemide

Side-effects: see under Frusemide, also myalgia

Dose: *by mouth,* 0.5–2 mg once or twice daily; 5 mg in oliguria

By intramuscular or intravenous injection, 0.5–2 mg

By intravenous infusion, 2–5 mg over 30–60 minutes

Burinex® (Leo)

Tablets, yellow, scored, bumetanide 1 mg. Price 20 tabs = **C**

Tablets, scored, bumetanide 5 mg. Price 20 tabs = **G**

Injection, bumetanide 500 micrograms/ml. Price 2-ml amp = **B**; 4-ml amp = **C**; 10-ml amp = **D**

ETHACRYNIC ACID

Indications: oedema, oliguria due to renal failure

Cautions; Contra-indications; Side-effects: see under Frusemide; also pain on injection

Dose: *by mouth,* 25–150 mg daily

By slow intravenous injection or infusion, 50 mg

Edecrin® (MSD)

Tablets, scored, ethacrynic acid 50 mg. Price 20 tabs = **C**

Injection, powder for reconstitution, ethacrynic acid (as sodium salt). Price 50-mg vial = **C**

2.2.3 Potassium-sparing diuretics

Amiloride (Midamor®) and **triamterene** (Dytac®) on their own are weak diuretics. They cause retention of potassium and are therefore used as an alternative to giving potassium supplements with thiazide or loop diuretics. Although it is preferable to prescribe the two types of diuretic separately, the use of fixed combinations of a thiazide with triamterene or amiloride may be justified if compliance is a problem.

AMILORIDE HYDROCHLORIDE

Indications: oedema, potassium conservation with thiazide and loop diuretics

Cautions: diabetes, hepatic cirrhosis. Drug interactions: see Appendix 1

Contra-indications: hyperkalaemia, renal failure

Side-effects: rashes, mental confusion

Dose: 5–20 mg daily

Midamor® (Morson)

Tablets, yellow, amiloride hydrochloride 5 mg. Price 20 tabs = **D**

Moduretic® (MSD)

Tablets, peach, amiloride hydrochloride 5 mg, hydrochlorothiazide 50 mg. Price 20 tabs = **D**

Dose: 1–2, increased if necessary to a max. of 4 tablets daily

---

TRIAMTERENE

Indications: oedema, potassium conservation with thiazide and loop diuretics

Cautions; Contra-indications; Side-effects: see under Amiloride Hydrochloride

Dose: 100–200 mg daily

Dyazide® (SK&F)

Tablets, peach, scored, triamterene 50 mg, hydrochlorothiazide 25 mg. Price 20 tabs = **C**

Dose: 1–3 tablets daily

Dytac® (SK&F)

Capsules, maroon, triamterene 50 mg. Price 20 caps = **D**

Dytide® (SK&F)

Capsules, clear/maroon, triamterene 50 mg, benzthiazide 25 mg. Price 20 caps = **D**

Dose: 1–3 capsules daily

2.2.4 Spironolactone

Spironolactone (Aldactone® etc.) is a weak diuretic but it potentiates thiazide or loop diuretics by antagonising aldosterone. It is of value in the treatment of the oedema of cirrhosis of the liver and occasionally may help in oedema of cardiac failure that is resistant to therapy. Spironolactone promotes the retention of potassium. Potassium supplements must **not** be given with spironolactone.

Spironolactone is also used in Conn's syndrome (primary hyperaldosteronism).

Potassium canrenoate (Spiroctan-M®) has similar uses to spironolactone, but can be given parenterally. It is metabolised to canrenone, which is also a metabolite of spironolactone.

POTASSIUM CANRENOATE

Indications: oedema associated with cardiac dysfunction, secondary aldosteronism, liver failure, nephrotic syndrome

Cautions; Contra-indications: see under Spironolactone; also caution in pregnancy and contra-indicated in hyponatraemia

Side-effects: nausea and vomiting, particularly after high doses; pain and irritation at injection site

Dose: by slow intravenous injection, up to 800 mg daily, in single or divided doses

Spiroctan-M® (MCP)

Injection, potassium canrenoate 10 mg/ml. Price 20-ml amp = **C** (Hosp. only)

SPIRONOLACTONE

Indications: oedema in cirrhosis of the liver, potentiation of thiazide and loop diuretics, Conn's syndrome

Cautions: drug interactions: see Appendix 1

Contra-indications: hyperkalaemia, renal failure

Side-effects: gastro-intestinal disturbances, gynaecomastia

Dose: 100–200 mg daily

Spironolactone Tablets, spironolactone 25 mg. Price 20 tabs = **D**

Aldactide 25® (Searle)

Tablets, buff, f/c, scored, spironolactone 25 mg, hydroflumethiazide 25 mg. Price 20 tabs = **E**
Dose: 1–4 tablets daily

Aldactide 50® (Searle)

Tablets, buff, f/c, scored, spironolactone 50 mg, hydroflumethiazide 50 mg. Price 20 tabs = **F**
Dose: 1–2 tablets daily

Aldactone® (Searle)

Tablets, buff, f/c, scored, spironolactone 25 mg. Price 20 tabs = **D**

Tablets, buff, f/c, spironolactone 100 mg. Price 20 tabs = **G**

Diatensec® (Searle)

Tablets, f/c, spironolactone 50 mg. Price 20 tabs = **E**

Spiroctan® (MCP)

Tablets, blue, spironolactone 25 mg. Price 20 tabs = **D**

Tablets, green, spironolactone 50 mg. Price 20 tabs = **E**

Capsules, green, spironolactone 100 mg. Price 20 caps = **G**

2.2.5 Osmotic diuretics

They are rarely used in heart failure as they may acutely expand the blood volume. **Mannitol** is the most commonly used—in forced diuresis in cases of drug overdose, and in cerebral oedema.

MANNITOL

Indications: cerebral oedema, forced diuresis

Cautions: extravasation causes inflammation and thrombophlebitis

Contra-indications: congestive cardiac failure, pulmonary oedema

Side-effects: chills, fever

Dose: by intravenous infusion, 50–200 g over 24 hours, preceded by a test dose of 200 mg/kg by slow intravenous injection

Mannitol Intravenous Infusion

10% solution. Price 500-ml container = **D**

20% solution. Price 250- and 500-ml containers (both) = **D**

25% solution. Price 50-ml amp = **D**

Osmitrol® (Travenol)

Intravenous infusion, mannitol 10%. Price 500-ml container = **D**

Intravenous infusion, mannitol 15%. Price 500-ml container = **D**

Intravenous infusion, mannitol 20%. Price 500-ml container = **E**

UREA

Indications: cerebral oedema

Cautions: see under Mannitol

Contra-indications: renal failure, hepatic failure, intracerebral haemorrhage

Side-effects: headache, mental confusion

Dose: by intravenous infusion, 40–80 g as a 30% solution in dextrose intravenous infusion 5 or 10%

Ureaphil® (Abbott)

Intravenous infusion, powder for reconstitution, urea. Price 40-g vial = **J**

2.2.6 Mercurial diuretics

They are effective diuretics but are now little used because of their nephrotoxicity. Mersalyl **must** be given by intramuscular injection; intravenous use may cause severe hypotension and sudden death.

MERSALYL

Indications: oedema unresponsive to other diuretics

Cautions: recent myocardial infarction, treatment with cardiac glycosides, frequent extrasystoles

Contra-indications: renal impairment

Side-effects: gastro-intestinal disturbances, allergic reactions

Mersalyl Injection, mersalyl sodium 100 mg and theophylline 50 mg/ml. Price 2-ml amp = **B**
Dose: by deep intramuscular injection, 0.5–2 ml

2.2.7 Carbonic anhydrase inhibitors

Acetazolamide and dichlorphenamide are weak diuretics, and are little used for their diuretic effect, although acetazolamide is being investigated as a prophylactic measure for mountain sickness. They inhibit the formation of aqueous fluid, and are used in glaucoma (see section 11.6).

2.2.8 Combined diuretics and potassium supplements

Many patients on diuretics do not need potassium supplements (see section 9.2.1.1). For many of those who do, the amount of potassium ion in combined preparations may not be enough, and for this reason their use is to be discouraged.

Brinaldix K® (Sandoz)
Tablets, effervescent, clopamide 20 mg, potassium 12 mmol. Price 20 tabs = **D**

Burinex K® (Leo)
Tablets, bumetanide 500 micrograms, potassium 7.7 mmol for sustained release. Price 20 tabs = **C**

Centyl K® (Burgess)
Tablets, green, bendrofluazide 2.5 mg, potassium 7.7 mmol for sustained release. Price 20 tabs = **B**

Diumide-K Continus® (Napp)
Tablets, white/orange, frusemide 40 mg, potassium 8 mmol for sustained release. Price 20 tabs = **D**

Esidrex-K® (Ciba)
Tablets, hydrochlorothiazide 12.5 mg, potassium 8.1 mmol for sustained release. Price 20 tabs = **B**

Hygroton-K® (Geigy)
Tablets, red, s/c, chlorthalidone 25 mg, potassium 6.7 mmol for sustained release. Price 20 tabs = **B**

Lasikal® (Hoechst)
Tablets, white/yellow, f/c, frusemide 20 mg, potassium 10 mmol for sustained release. Price 20 tabs = **D**

Lasix + K® (Hoechst)
Tablets, scored, frusemide 40 mg, with *tablets,* s/r, yellow, potassium chloride (potassium 10 mmol). Price 30 + 60 tabs = **F**

Navidrex-K® (Ciba)
Tablets, yellow, s/c, cyclopenthiazide 250 micrograms, potassium 8.1 mmol for sustained release. Price 20 tabs = **B**

Neo-NaClex-K® (DF)
Tablets, pink/white, f/c, bendrofluazide 2.5 mg, potassium 8.4 mmol for sustained release. Price 20 tabs = **B**

2.3 Anti-arrhythmic drugs

2.3.1 Treatment of individual arrhythmias

Management of an arrhythmia, apart from the treatment of associated heart failure, requires precise diagnosis of the type of arrhythmia, and electrocardiography is essential.

Atrial fibrillation. The ventricular rate can be controlled by digoxin (section 2.1).

Ectopic beats. If spontaneous with a normal heart, these rarely require treatment beyond reassurance. If they are particularly troublesome, oral procainamide or quinidine is satisfactory.

Atrial flutter. This can often be converted to atrial fibrillation by digoxin. The ventricular rate can then be controlled by digoxin, or reversion to sinus rhythm by d.c. shock may be attempted. There is some evidence that calcium antagonists may be effective.

Atrial paroxysmal tachycardia. About half the patients may revert spontaneously or can be returned to sinus rhythm by reflex vagal stimulation, achieved by pressure over one carotid sinus or over the eyeballs. If this fails full digitalisation or d.c. shock may be effective; propranolol offers an alternative.

Acute arrhythmias after myocardial infarction. It is best to do nothing in patients with a paroxysmal tachycardia or rapid irregularity of the pulse until an ECG record is obtainable. If the condition of the patient is such that death due to the arrhythmia seems imminent, 100 mg of lignocaine should be given intravenously. Bradycardia, particularly if complicated by hypotension, should be treated by atropine sulphate 1 mg intravenously.

Ventricular paroxysmal tachycardia. In an emergency with a severely ill patient reversion is best achieved by d.c. shock. Alternatively, lignocaine (section 2.3.3) is at present the preferred drug. Propranolol (section 2.4) can be given by intravenous injection, preceded by atropine sulphate.

2.3.2 Drugs used in supraventricular tachycardias

Digoxin (section 2.1) by mouth is the treatment of choice in slowing ventricular response in cases of atrial fibrillation and atrial flutter. Intravenous digoxin is occasionally required if the ventricular rate needs rapid control.

Beta-adrenoceptor blocking drugs (section 2.4) prolong atrioventricular nodal conduction and may be used in conjunction with digoxin to control the ventricular response, especially in patients with thyrotoxicosis. Beta-adrenoceptor blocking drugs are also useful in the management of atrioventricular nodal reciprocating tachycardias but care should be taken to avoid reducing cardiac output or precipitating bronchospasm in susceptible patients.

Verapamil (Cordilox®) is the best treatment for atrioventricular, nodal, and Wolff-Parkinson-White reciprocating tachycardias, and atrial flutter; an initial intravenous dose is followed by oral treatment. Hypotension may occur with larger doses. Verapamil should not be injected for 8 hours after giving a beta-adrenoceptor blocking drug because of the risk of causing hypotension and asystole due to prolongation of atrioventricular node conduction time. However, when verapamil injection has been given first, an interval of 30 minutes before giving a beta-adrenoceptor blocking drug is sufficient. (For use in angina see section 2.6.1.)

Amiodarone (Cordarone X®) is used in the treatment of the Wolff-Parkinson-White syndrome. It is also used in supraventricular, nodal, and ventricular tachycardia, atrial flutter and fibrillation, and ventricular fibrillation when other drugs cannot be used. Amiodarone has a long half-life and need only be given once daily when therapeutic blood concentrations have been established. Most patients develop corneal microdeposits; these rarely interfere with vision and are reversible on withdrawal of treatment. Amiodarone contains iodine which can be released and cause disorders of thyroid function (both hypothyroidism and hyperthyroidism have been reported).

Quinidine (section 2.3.3) is useful in supraventricular tachycardia to suppress atrial ectopic activity which may precede these arrhythmias.

In cases of paroxysmal atrial tachycardia with block, digitalis toxicity should be suspected, especially if the patient is hypokalaemic. Apart from stopping administration of the cardiac glycoside and giving potassium supplements, phenytoin or practolol given intravenously may be useful in controlling the tachycardia.

AMIODARONE HYDROCHLORIDE

Indications: see notes above
Cautions: heart failure; interferes with thyroid function tests. Drug interactions: see Appendix 1
Contra-indications: sinus bradycardia, atrioventricular block, thyroid dysfunction
Side-effects: corneal microdeposits, peripheral neuropathy, tremor, photosensitisation and rarely skin discoloration; hypothyroidism, hyperthyroidism
Dose: 200 mg 3 times daily for at least 1 week; maintenance, 200 mg daily

▼ Cordarone X® (Labaz)
Tablets, scored, amiodarone hydrochloride 200 mg. Price 20 tabs = **G**

ATROPINE SULPHATE

Indications: bradycardia after myocardial infarction, bradycardia caused by beta-adrenoceptor blocking drugs
Cautions: glaucoma, paralytic ileus, enlarged prostate. Drug interactions: see Appendix 1
Side-effects: dry mouth, confusion, tachycardia
Dose: by intravenous injection, 0.3–1 mg. Max. 3 mg in 24 hours

Atropine Sulphate Injection
400 micrograms/ml. Price 1-ml amp = **B**
600 micrograms/ml. Price 1-ml amp = **A**; 25-ml vial = **C**
800 micrograms/ml. Price 1-ml amp = **B**
1 mg/ml. Price 1-ml amp = **B**
1.2 mg/ml. Price 0.5-ml amp = **A**
1.25 mg/ml. Price 1-ml amp = **B**

VERAPAMIL HYDROCHLORIDE

Indications: supraventricular arrhythmias, angina pectoris
Cautions: do not give within 8 hours of a beta-adrenoceptor blocking drug
Contra-indications: bradycardia, heart block, heart failure
Side-effects: nausea, vomiting; hypotension, bradycardia, and asystole after intravenous administration
Dose: by mouth, arrhythmias, 40–120 mg 3 times daily; angina, 80–120 mg 3 times daily
By slow intravenous injection, 5 mg, repeated after 5–10 minutes if necessary
By intravenous infusion, 5–10 mg over 1 hour; max. 100 mg in 24 hours

Cordilox® (Abbott)
Tablets, yellow, f/c, verapamil hydrochloride 40 mg. Price 20 tabs = **C**
Tablets, yellow, f/c, verapamil hydrochloride 80 mg. Price 20 tabs = **E**
Tablets, 'Cordilox-120', yellow, f/c, verapamil hydrochloride 120 mg. Price 20 tabs = **E**
Injection, verapamil hydrochloride 2.5 mg/ml. Price 2-ml amp = **C**

2.3.3 Drugs used in ventricular arrhythmias

Lignocaine is the treatment of choice to suppress ventricular extrasystoles and ventricular tachycardia following an acute myocardial infarction. Its effectiveness in preventing ventricular fibrillation after an acute infarct is controversial but apparent ineffectiveness may be due to inadequate plasma concentrations. An intravenous bolus given over 2 minutes is followed immediately by an infusion, the rate being adjusted according to the clinical response. Lignocaine infusion should be continued for 36 hours and care should be taken in patients with cardiac or hepatic failure; doses may need to be reduced to avoid central nervous system depression or convulsions.

Tocainide (Tonocard®) is an analogue of lignocaine with similar activity, and can be given by mouth or intravenous injection.

If lignocaine is ineffective **mexiletine** (Mexitil®), which has a similar action, can be given as a slow intravenous injection followed by infusion at a decreasing rate until the arrhythmia is controlled. Adverse cardiovascular and central nervous system effects may limit the dose which can be tolerated.

Other drugs that may be given by slow intravenous injection to control arrhythmias include **procainamide** (Pronestyl®), which should be used cautiously if lignocaine has already been given, as the cumulative negative inotropic effect may severely depress the myocardium; **disopyramide** (Norpace®, Rythmodan®) and **practolol** (Eraldin®), both of which may impair cardiac contractility; and **phenytoin** (Epanutin®), which is particularly useful in digitalis-induced arrhythmias.

Bretylium (Bretylate®) has been given by intramuscular injection, but can cause severe hypotension.

Once the arrhythmia has been controlled, treatment by mouth is introduced, but all available drugs have disadvantages. Nausea and vomiting associated with mexiletine may prevent an effective dose being given; prolonged use of procainamide can cause a syndrome resembling lupus erythematosus; disopyramide has an anticholinergic effect which limits its use in patients with glaucoma or urinary retention; and quinidine can cause hypersensitivity reactions and gastro-intestinal upsets. Amiodarone (section 2.3.2) is also used.

BRETYLIUM TOSYLATE

Indications: ventricular arrhythmias resistant to other treatment
Cautions: do not give noradrenaline or other sympathomimetic amines
Side-effects: hypotension, nausea
Dose: *by intramuscular injection,* 5 mg/kg repeated after 6–8 hours if necessary

Bretylate® (Wellcome)
Injection, bretylium tosylate 50 mg/ml. Price 2-ml amp = **E**

DISOPYRAMIDE

Indications: ventricular arrhythmias, especially after myocardial infarction
Cautions: renal failure, glaucoma. Drug interactions: see Appendix 1
Side-effects: myocardial depression, hypotension, atrioventricular block; anticholinergic effects include dry mouth, blurred vision, urinary retention
Dose: *by mouth,* 100 mg every 6 hours
By slow intravenous injection, 2 mg/kg to a max. of 150 mg, with ECG monitoring; maintenance, 400 micrograms/kg/hour *by intravenous infusion*

Disopyramide Capsules, disopyramide 100 mg, price 20 caps = **D**; 150 mg, price 20 caps = **E**
Disopyramide Phosphate Capsules, disopyramide 100 and 150 mg (as phosphate). Price 20 caps (both) = **D**
Dirythmin SA® (Astra)
Durules® (= tablets, s/r), f/c, disopyramide 150 mg (as phosphate). Price 20 tabs = **E**
Dose: 300 mg every 12 hours
Norpace® (Searle)
Capsules, orange/white, disopyramide 100 mg (as phosphate). Price 20 caps = **D**
Capsules, orange/brown, disopyramide 150 mg (as phosphate). Price 20 caps = **D**
Injection, disopyramide 20 mg (as phosphate)/ml. Price 5-ml amp = **C**; 7.5 ml amp = **D**
Rythmodan® (Roussel)
Capsules, green/yellow, disopyramide 100 mg. Price 20 caps = **D**
Capsules, disopyramide 150 mg. Price 20 caps = **E**
Injection, disopyramide 10 mg (as phosphate)/ml. Price 5-ml amp = **C**; 10- and 15-ml amp (both) = **D**
Rythmodan Retard® (Roussel)
Tablets, s/r, scored, f/c, disopyramide 250 mg (as phosphate). Price 20 tabs = **F**
Dose: 250–375 mg every 12 hours

LIGNOCAINE HYDROCHLORIDE

Indications: ventricular arrhythmias, especially after myocardial infarction
Cautions: lower doses in congestive cardiac failure and hepatic failure. Drug interactions: see Appendix 1
Contra-indications: complete heart block; supraventricular tachycardias
Side-effects: confusion, convulsions
Dose: *by intravenous injection,* 50–100 mg as a bolus, repeated after 5 minutes if necessary; maintenance, 1–4 mg/minute by intravenous infusion

Lignocaine 0.1% in Dextrose Injection, lignocaine hydrochloride 1 mg/ml in dextrose intravenous infusion. Price 500-ml container = **D**; 1-litre container = **D**
Lignocaine 0.2% in Dextrose Injection, lignocaine hydrochloride 2 mg/ml in dextrose intravenous infusion. Price 500-ml container = **D**; 1-litre container = **D**
Lidothesin® (Pharm. Mfg Co.)
Injection 5%, lignocaine hydrochloride 50 mg/ml. To be diluted before use. Price 10-ml amp = **A**
Xylocard® (Astra)
Injection 100 mg, lignocaine hydrochloride (anhydrous) 20 mg/ml. Price 5-ml syringe = **D**
Intravenous infusion, lignocaine hydrochloride (anhydrous) 200 mg/ml. To be diluted before use. Price 5-ml syringe (1 g) = **D**; 10-ml syringe (2 g) = **E**

MEXILETINE HYDROCHLORIDE

Indications: ventricular arrhythmias, especially after myocardial infarction
Cautions: drug interactions: see Appendix 1
Contra-indications: bradycardia, heart block
Side-effects: bradycardia, hypotension, confusion, dysarthria, nystagmus, tremor
Dose: *by mouth,* 200 mg 3–4 times daily
By intravenous injection, 100–250 mg over 5–10 minutes, followed by *infusion* of 250 mg as a 0.1% solution over 1 hour, 125 mg/hour for 2 hours, then 500 micrograms/minute

Mexitil® (Boehringer Ingelheim)
Capsules, purple/red, mexiletine hydrochloride 50 mg. Price 20 caps = **C**
Capsules, red, mexiletine hydrochloride 200 mg. Price 20 caps = **E**
Injection, mexiletine hydrochloride 25 mg/ml. Price 10-ml amp = **D**

PHENYTOIN SODIUM

Indications: ventricular arrhythmias, especially those caused by cardiac glycosides (for use in epilepsy, see section 4.8.1)
Cautions: do not give with lignocaine hydrochloride
Contra-indications: supraventricular tachycardias, heart block
Side-effects: bradycardia, hypotension, asystole, confusion
Dose: *by intravenous injection,* 250 mg at a rate not exceeding 50 mg/minute. Repeat after 10 minutes if necessary

Epanutin Ready Mixed Parenteral® (P-D)
Injection, phenytoin sodium 50 mg/ml. Price 5-ml amp = **E**

PRACTOLOL

Indications: supraventricular tachycardias; ventricular arrhythmias, especially after myocardial infarction
Cautions: chronic obstructive airways disease; do not give with digitalis; for cautions with verapamil see notes (section 2.3.2)
Side-effects: bradycardia, hypotension, heart failure, bronchospasm
Dose: by slow intravenous injection, 5 mg, repeated after 5 minutes if required

Eraldin® (ICI)
Injection, practolol 2 mg/ml. Price 5-ml amp = **B** (Hosp. only)

PROCAINAMIDE HYDROCHLORIDE

Indications: ventricular arrhythmias, especially after myocardial infarction
Cautions: renal impairment, asthma, myasthenia gravis
Contra-indications: heart block, heart failure, hypotension
Side-effects: nausea, diarrhoea, rashes, fever, myocardial depression, heart failure, lupus erythematosus-like syndrome, agranulocytosis after prolonged treatment
Dose: by mouth, 250–500 mg every 4 hours
By slow intravenous injection, 25–50 mg/minute with ECG monitoring, until arrhythmia is controlled. Max. dose 1 g
Maintenance, 0.25–2 mg/minute *by intravenous infusion*

Procainamide Durules® (Astra)
Tablets, s/r, yellow, procainamide hydrochloride 500 mg. Price 20 tabs = **D**
Dose: 1–1·5 g every 8 hours

Pronestyl® (Squibb)
Tablets, scored, procainamide hydrochloride 250 mg. Price 20 tabs = **C**
Injection, procainamide hydrochloride 100 mg/ml. Price 10-ml vial = **C**

QUINIDINE

Indications: prevention of supraventricular tachycardias, ventricular arrhythmias
Cautions: 200-mg test dose to detect hypersensitivity reactions. Drug interactions: see Appendix 1
Contra-indications: heart block
Side-effects: see under Procainamide Hydrochloride; also ventricular arrhythmias, thrombocytopenia, haemolytic anaemia
Dose: by mouth, quinidine sulphate 200–400 mg 3–4 times daily
Note: quinidine sulphate 200 mg ≡ quinidine bisulphate 250 mg

Quinidine Sulphate Tablets, quinidine sulphate 200 and 300 mg. Price 20 tabs (both) = **D**

Kiditard® (Delandale)
Capsules, s/r, blue, quinidine bisulphate 250 mg. Price 20 caps = **D**
Dose: 500 mg every 12 hours, adjusted as required

Kinidin Durules® (Astra)
Tablets, s/r, f/c, quinidine bisulphate 250 mg. Price 20 tabs = **E**
Dose: 500 mg every 12 hours, adjusted as required

Quinicardine® (Wilcox)
Tablets, scored, quinidine sulphate 200 mg. Price 20 tabs = **F**

TOCAINIDE HYDROCHLORIDE

Indications: ventricular arrhythmias, especially after myocardial infarction
Cautions: severe hepatic or renal impairment, uncompensated heart failure, pregnancy (toxicity in *animal* studies). Drug interactions: see Appendix 1
Contra-indications: atrioventricular block
Side-effects: CNS effects including tremor, dizziness, convulsions, paraesthesia; gastro-intestinal effects including nausea and vomiting; bradycardia and hypotension after injection; rash and fever; rarely lupus erythematosus-like syndrome, fibrosing alveolitis, agranulocytosis, transient neutropenia
Dose: chronic arrhythmias, *by mouth,* 1.2 g daily in 2–3 divided doses; max. 2.4 g daily
Acute treatment, *by slow intravenous injection or infusion,* 500–750 mg over 15–20 minutes, followed immediately by 600–800 mg by mouth
Maintenance, *by mouth,* 1.2 g daily, in 2–3 divided doses

▼ **Tonocard®** (Astra)
Tablets, yellow, f/c, tocainide hydrochloride 400 mg. Price 20 tabs = **F**
Tablets, yellow, f/c, tocainide hydrochloride 600 mg. Price 20 tabs = **F**
Injection, tocainide hydrochloride 50 mg/ml. Price 15-ml vial = **G**

2.4 Beta-adrenoceptor blocking drugs

The beta-adrenoceptor blocking drugs or 'beta-blockers' are used in the treatment of hypertension, angina, supraventricular arrhythmias, and thyrotoxicosis. They block the response of beta-adrenoceptors in the heart and other sites to sympathetic stimuli. They slow the heart and reduce its liability to arrhythmias. Unfortunately in a few patients the deprivation of sympathetic stimuli to the heart muscle may induce myocardial depression and precipitate heart failure. They should not be given to patients with atrioventricular block as they decrease conduction in the atrioventricular node and bundle of His.

It is unfortunate too that the direct effects of beta-blockers in peripheral blood vessels may exacerbate Raynaud's phenomenon and intermittent claudication. In diabetics, effects on glycogenolysis may cause a fall of blood sugar to unacceptable levels, and in some patients effects on bronchial smooth muscle may cause severe bronchospasm.

Some of the drugs such as **propranolol** (Inderal®), **oxprenolol** (Trasicor®), and **pindolol** (Visken®) cause vivid dreams and hallucinations, but usually only in large doses.

Practolol (Eraldin®) is now used only for the emergency control of certain arrhythmias (section 2.3.3). It was withdrawn from general use after it was shown to cause the oculo-mucocutaneous syndrome, including conjunctival scarring, corneal opacity, psoriasiform rash, and peritoneal fibrosis. This is probably a delayed immunological reaction. Isolated cases of peritoneal fibrosis have been reported in association with acebutolol, atenolol, metoprolol, oxprenolol, pindolol, propranolol, and sotalol.

There are differences between these drugs. **Acebutolol** (Sectral®), **atenolol** (Tenormin®), and **metoprolol** (Betaloc®, Lopresor®) are relatively cardioselective and therefore slightly less likely to cause bronchospasm, peripheral vasoconstriction, or hypoglycaemia. Acebutolol, oxprenolol, and pindolol have some intrinsic sympathomimetic activity as well as their blocking activity and they are, therefore, less likely to cause bradycardia and reduction in cardiac output than the others; this property makes them less effective in controlling thyrotoxicosis.

Labetalol (Trandate®) combines alpha- and beta-adrenoceptor blocking activity; alpha blockade in peripheral arteries lowers peripheral resistance, and helps to reduce blood pressure.

HYPERTENSION

Beta-blockers are effective antihypertensive drugs but their mode of action in lowering blood pressure remains contentious, and it seems likely that several distinct mechanisms may contribute to their hypotensive effect. Both resting and exercising cardiac output are reduced by beta-blockers after acute administration; baroceptor reflex sensitivity is altered, and (with some beta-blockers) plasma-renin activity is reduced. A further contributory effect may be that beta-blockers have a direct central effect on hypothalamic control of the sympathetic nervous system.

The major advantage of these drugs in lowering blood pressure is their relative freedom from side-effects such as postural hypotension and failure of ejaculation. There is currently little good clinical evidence that any one beta-blocker is a more effective antihypertensive than any other.

Beta-blockers can be given either separately or in combination with diuretics or with antihypertensive drugs of other classes. Further, they need only be given once or twice daily to control blood pressure. Slow-release formulations of several beta-blockers are currently being compared with conventional formulations.

The effective dose range of beta-blockers in hypertension is probably smaller than originally believed; doses of above 400 mg of propranolol or oxprenolol confer little additional hypotensive effect and will only cause additional adverse reactions. Start with a small daily dose and build up the dosage gradually leaving at least 5 days between each increment.

In hypertension due to **phaeochromocytoma** it is essential to use both alpha-blocking drugs (section 2.5.4) and beta-blocking drugs. Giving only a beta-blocking drug may lead to very severe hypertension.

ANGINA AND MYOCARDIAL INFARCTION

Many reports have now shown that regular administration of beta-blockers improves exercise tolerance in most patients with angina. This effect is caused by their ability to reduce cardiac work. The dose should be increased until the symptoms are controlled: usually control is accompanied by some slowing of the pulse. As in hypertension there is no good evidence as to the superiority of any one drug, although the occasional patient will respond better to one beta-blocker than another. In patients with asthma and angina, the beta-blocker of choice would be one with cardioselective properties.

Sudden withdrawal of these drugs may cause an exacerbation of angina in patients with severe coronary disease.

ARRHYTHMIAS

Beta-blockers will control cardiac arrhythmias due either to excessive catecholamine liberation or to increased sensitivity to catecholamines. Situations in which such arrhythmias may occur include anaesthesia with drugs such as halothane and surgery for patients with phaeochromocytoma (after pre-operative therapy with an alpha-adrenoceptor blocking drug—beta-blockers should **never** be used alone in phaeochromocytoma).

Beta-blockers will also control supraventricular tachycardia following myocardial infarction. There is little to choose between beta-blockers in the long-term prophylaxis of cardiac arrhythmias except when they are due to thyrotoxicosis, when perhaps those with intrinsic sympathomimetic activity are less effective.

If a cardiac arrhythmia is life-threatening and beta-blockers are to be administered, they can be given intravenously. **Practolol** is still the favoured drug but is only available as an injection for hospital use.

THYROTOXICOSIS

Beta-blockers that do not have intrinsic sympathomimetic activity are used in pre-operative preparation for thyroidectomy. Doses of 40–

200 mg of propranolol 6-hourly can render a patient clinically euthyroid within 4 days, although the routine tests of increased thyroid function remain unaltered. Further, the gland is less vascular and firmer at operation, making surgery easier.

In hyperthyroid crisis, administration of up to 5 mg of propranolol, initially by slow intravenous injection, will result in rapid improvement of symptoms and signs.

Propranolol has also been used as an adjunct to radioactive iodine treatment instead of conventional antithyroid drugs. One of its advantages is that it permits laboratory assessment of radioiodine therapy since laboratory tests of thyroid function are not altered by beta-blockers. In addition beta-blockers are useful in neonatal thyrotoxicosis and in supraventricular arrhythmias due to hyperthyroidism. Presumably all beta-blockers will manifest an antithyroid action, but those without intrinsic sympathomimetic activity, for example **propranolol** and **sotalol**, appear preferable. Most experience has been gained with propranolol.

PSYCHIATRIC ILLNESS

Beta-blockers have been used to treat neurotic anxiety and acute psychotic states. Probably patients whose symptoms are palpitations, tremor, and tachycardia respond best.

PROPRANOLOL HYDROCHLORIDE

Indications: hypertension, angina, arrhythmias, thyrotoxicosis
Cautions: avoid abrupt withdrawal. Drug interactions: see Appendix 1
Contra-indications: asthma, heart failure, peripheral vascular disease, late pregnancy
Side-effects: bradycardia, heart failure, bronchospasm, peripheral vasoconstriction
Dose: by mouth, daily in divided doses, hypertension, 160–320 mg; angina, 120–320 mg; arrhythmias, 30–160 mg; thyrotoxicosis, 30–160 mg
By intravenous injection, 0.5–1 mg over 1 minute, preceded by atropine sulphate 1–2 mg

Propranolol Tablets, propranolol hydrochloride 10 mg, price 20 tabs = **B**; 40 mg and 80 mg, price 20 tabs (both) = **C**; 160 mg, price 20 tabs = **D**

Angilol® (DDSA)
Tablets, pink, f/c, propranolol hydrochloride 10 mg. Price 20 tabs = **B**
Tablets, pink, f/c, propranolol hydrochloride 40 mg. Price 20 tabs = **C**
Tablets, pink, f/c, propranolol hydrochloride 80 mg. Price 20 tabs = **D**
Tablets, pink, f/c, propranolol hydrochloride 160 mg. Price 20 tabs = **D**

Apsolol® (APS)
Tablets, pink, f/c, scored, propranolol hydrochloride 10 mg. Price 20 tabs = **B**
Tablets, pink, f/c, scored, propranolol hydrochloride 40 mg. Price 20 tabs = **C**
Tablets, pink, f/c, scored, propranolol hydrochloride 80 mg. Price 20 tabs = **C**
Tablets, pink, f/c, scored, propranolol hydrochloride 160 mg. Price 20 tabs = **E**

Berkolol® (Berk)
Tablets, pink, f/c, scored, propranolol hydrochloride 10 mg. Price 20 tabs = **B**
Tablets, pink, f/c, scored, propranolol hydrochloride 40 mg. Price 20 tabs = **C**
Tablets, pink, f/c, scored, propranolol hydrochloride 80 mg. Price 20 tabs = **C**
Tablets, pink, f/c, scored, propranolol hydrochloride 160 mg. Price 20 tabs = **D**

Inderal® (ICI)
Tablets, pink, f/c, propranolol hydrochloride 10 mg. Price 20 tabs = **B**
Tablets, pink, f/c, propranolol hydrochloride 40 mg. Price 20 tabs = **C**
Tablets, pink, f/c, propranolol hydrochloride 80 mg. Price 20 tabs = **D**
Tablets, pink, f/c, propranolol hydrochloride 160 mg. Price 20 tabs = **E**
Injection, propranolol hydrochloride 1 mg/ml. Price 1-ml amp = **B**

Inderal-LA® (ICI)
Capsules, s/r, lavender/pink, propranolol hydrochloride 160 mg. Price 28 caps = **H**
Dose: 160 mg daily

ACEBUTOLOL

Indications: hypertension, angina, arrhythmias
Cautions; Contra-indications; Side-effects: see under Propranolol Hydrochloride
Dose: by mouth, daily in divided doses, hypertension, 400–800 mg; angina, 400–800 mg; arrhythmias, 300–600 mg
By intravenous injection, 5–25 mg over 3–5 minutes

Sectral® (M&B)
Capsules, buff/white, acebutolol 100 mg (as hydrochloride). Price 20 caps = **D**
Capsules, buff/pink, acebutolol 200 mg (as hydrochloride). Price 20 caps = **E**
Tablets, f/c, acebutolol 400 mg (as hydrochloride). Price 28 tabs = **H**
Injection, acebutolol 5 mg (as hydrochloride)/ml. Price 5-ml amp = **C**

ATENOLOL

Indications: hypertension, angina
Cautions; Contra-indications; Side-effects: see under Propranolol Hydrochloride; reduce dose in renal failure
Dose: hypertension, 100 mg daily; angina, 100 mg daily in 1 or 2 doses

Tenormin® (Stuart)
Tablets, orange, f/c, scored, atenolol 100 mg. Price 28 tabs = **H**

Tenormin LS® (Stuart)
Tablets, f/c, atenolol 50 mg. Price 20 tabs = **F**

LABETALOL HYDROCHLORIDE

Indications: hypertension; controlled hypotension in surgery

Cautions: heart block, heart failure; avoid abrupt withdrawal; interferes with laboratory tests for catecholamines. Drug interactions: see Appendix 1

Side-effects: postural hypotension, tiredness, weakness, headache, rashes, scalp tingling

Dose: by mouth, initially 100 mg 2–3 times daily after food, increased after 1 or 2 weeks; max. 2.4 g daily

By intravenous injection, 50 mg over 1 minute, repeated after 5 minutes if necessary; max. 200 mg

By intravenous infusion, 2 mg/minute to a max. of 200 mg

▼ **Trandate®** (A&H)

Tablets, orange, f/c, labetalol hydrochloride 100 mg. Price 20 tabs = **D**

Tablets, orange, f/c, labetalol hydrochloride 200 mg. Price 20 tabs = **E**

Tablets, orange, f/c, labetalol hydrochloride 400 mg. Price 20 tabs = **F**

Injection, labetalol hydrochloride 5 mg/ml. Price 20-ml amp = **E**

METOPROLOL TARTRATE

Indications: hypertension, angina, arrhythmias (including arrhythmias during anaesthesia), thyrotoxicosis

Cautions; Contra-indications; Side-effects: see under Propranolol Hydrochloride

Dose: by mouth, hypertension, 100–400 mg daily in 1 or 2 doses; angina, 50–100 mg 2 or 3 times daily; arrhythmias, 50 mg 2–3 times daily; thyrotoxicosis, 50 mg 4 times daily

By intravenous injection, up to 5 mg at rate 1–2 mg/minute, repeated after 5 minutes if necessary

In surgery, 2–4 mg *by slow intravenous injection* at induction or to control arrhythmias developing during anaesthesia; 2-mg doses may be repeated to a max. of 10 mg

Metoprolol Tartrate Tablets, metoprolol tartrate 50 mg, price 20 tabs = **C**; 100 mg, price 20 tabs = **D**

Betaloc® (Astra)

Tablets, scored, metoprolol tartrate 50 mg. Price 20 tabs = **C**

Tablets, scored, metoprolol tartrate 100 mg. Price 20 tabs = **D**

Injection, metoprolol tartrate 1 mg/ml. Price 5-ml amp = **B**

Betaloc-SA® (Astra)

Durules (= tablets, s/r), metoprolol tartrate 200 mg. Price 20 tabs = **G**

Dose: 200–400 mg daily

Lopresor® (Geigy)

Tablets, pink, f/c, scored, metoprolol tartrate 50 mg. Price 20 tabs = **C**

Tablets, blue, f/c, scored, metoprolol tartrate 100 mg. Price 20 tabs = **D**

Injection, metoprolol tartrate 1 mg/ml. Price 5-ml amp = **A** (Hosp. only)

Lopresor SR® (Geigy)

Tablets, s/r, yellow, f/c, metoprolol tartrate 200 mg. Price 28 tabs = **H**

Dose: 200–400 mg daily

NADOLOL

Indications: hypertension, angina

Cautions; Contra-indications; Side-effects: see under Propranolol Hydrochloride; reduce dose in renal failure

Dose: hypertension, 80 mg daily, increased at weekly intervals; angina, 40 mg daily, increased at weekly intervals. Max. 240 mg daily

▼ **Corgard®** (Squibb)

Tablets, nadolol 40 mg. Price 20 tabs = **E**

Tablets, scored, nadolol 80 mg. Price 20 tabs = **F**

OXPRENOLOL HYDROCHLORIDE

Indications: hypertension, angina, arrhythmias, thyrotoxicosis

Cautions; Contra-indications; Side-effects: see under Propranolol Hydrochloride

Dose: by mouth, daily in divided doses, hypertension 160–320 mg; angina, 120–480 mg; arrhythmias, 60–240 mg; thyrotoxicosis, 40–120 mg

By slow intravenous injection, 1–2 mg, repeated after 10–20 minutes if required

Oxprenolol Tablets, f/c, oxprenolol hydrochloride 20 mg, price 20 tabs = **C**; 40 mg, price 20 tabs = **C**; 80 mg, price 20 tabs = **D**; 160 mg, price 20 tabs = **E**

Apsolox® (APS)

Tablets, f/c, oxprenolol hydrochloride 20 mg. Price 20 tabs = **C**

Tablets, f/c, oxprenolol hydrochloride 40 mg. Price 20 tabs = **D**

Tablets, yellow, f/c, oxprenolol hydrochloride 80 mg. Price 20 tabs = **D**

Tablets, orange, f/c, oxprenolol hydrochloride 160 mg. Price 20 tabs = **E**

Slow-Trasicor® (Ciba)

Tablets, s/r, f/c, oxprenolol hydrochloride 160 mg. Price 28 tabs = **H**

Dose: 160–480 mg daily

Trasicor® (Ciba)

Tablets, f/c, oxprenolol hydrochloride 20 mg. Price 20 tabs = **C**

Tablets, f/c, scored, oxprenolol hydrochloride 40 mg. Price 20 tabs = **D**

Tablets, yellow, f/c, oxprenolol hydrochloride 80 mg. Price 20 tabs = **D**

Tablets, orange, f/c, oxprenolol hydrochloride 160 mg. Price 20 tabs = **F**

Injection, powder for reconstitution, oxprenolol hydrochloride. Price 2-mg amp = **B**

PINDOLOL

Indications: hypertension, angina

Cautions; Contra-indications; Side-effects: see under Propranolol Hydrochloride; reduce dose in renal failure
Dose: daily in divided doses, hypertension, 10–45 mg; angina, 7.5–15 mg

Visken® (Sandoz)
Tablets, scored, pindolol 5 mg. Price 20 tabs = **E**
Tablets, scored, pindolol 15 mg. Price 20 tabs = **G**

PRACTOLOL
Section 2.3.3

SOTALOL HYDROCHLORIDE
Indications: hypertension, angina, arrhythmias, thyrotoxicosis
Cautions; Contra-indications; Side-effects: see under Propranolol Hydrochloride; reduce dose in renal failure
Dose: by mouth, daily in divided doses, hypertension, 200–480 mg; angina, 160–480 mg; arrhythmias, 120–240 mg; thyrotoxicosis, 120–240 mg
By slow intravenous injection, 10–20 mg, repeated if necessary

Sotalol Hydrochloride Tablets, sotalol hydrochloride 80 mg. Price 20 tabs = **B**
Beta-Cardone® (DF)
Tablets, green, scored, sotalol hydrochloride 40 mg. Price 20 tabs = **C**
Tablets, red, scored, sotalol hydrochloride 80 mg. Price 20 tabs = **D**
Tablets, scored, sotalol hydrochloride 200 mg. Price 28 tabs = **F**
Injection, sotalol hydrochloride 2 mg/ml. Price 5-ml amp = **C**
Sotacor® (Bristol)
Tablets, pink, scored, sotalol hydrochloride 80 mg. Price 20 tabs = **B**
Tablets, blue, scored, sotalol hydrochloride 160 mg. Price 14 tabs = **D**
Injection, sotalol hydrochloride 2 mg/ml. Price 5-ml amp = **B**

TIMOLOL MALEATE
Indications: hypertension, angina, prophylaxis after acute myocardial infarction
Cautions; Contra-indications; Side-effects: see under Propranolol Hydrochloride
Dose: daily in divided doses, hypertension, 15–45 mg; angina, 15–45 mg, prophylaxis after infarction, 10–20 mg

Timolol Maleate Tablets, timolol maleate 10 mg. Price 20 tabs = **D**
▼ **Betim®** (Burgess)
Tablets, scored, timolol maleate 10 mg. Price 20 tabs = **D**
Blocadren® (MSD)
Tablets, blue, scored, timolol maleate 10 mg. Price 20 tabs = **D**

COMPOUND PREPARATIONS

When both a diuretic and a beta-adrenoceptor blocking drug are required to control hypertension, they should be prescribed separately so that the dosage of the components can be adjusted independently; fixed combinations should only be used when compliance is a problem.

Co-Betaloc® (Astra) *tablets,* scored, metoprolol tartrate 100 mg, hydrochlorothiazide 12.5 mg. Price 20 tabs = **F**
Inderetic® (ICI) *capsules,* propranolol hydrochloride 80 mg, bendrofluazide 2.5 mg. Price 20 caps = **E**
▼ **Lopresoretic®** (Geigy) *tablets,* f/c, scored, metoprolol tartrate 100 mg, chlorthalidone 12.5 mg. Price 28 tabs = **F**
▼ **Moducren®** (Morson) *tablets,* blue, scored, timolol maleate 10 mg, amiloride hydrochloride 2.5 mg, hydrochlorothiazide 25 mg. Price 28 tabs = **G**
▼ **Prestim®** (Leo) *tablets,* scored, timolol maleate 10 mg, bendrofluazide 2.5 mg. Price 20 tabs = **E**
▼ **Sotazide®** (Bristol) *tablets,* blue, scored, sotalol hydrochloride 160 mg, hydrochlorothiazide 25 mg. Price 28 tabs = **H**
Tenoretic® (Stuart) *tablets,* f/c, scored, atenolol 100 mg, chlorthalidone 25 mg. Price 28 tabs = **H**
▼ **Trasidrex®** (Ciba) *tablets,* red, s/c, oxprenolol hydrochloride 160 mg for sustained release, cyclopenthiazide 250 micrograms. Price 28 tabs = **H**
▼ **Viskaldix®** (Sandoz) *tablets,* scored, pindolol 10 mg, clopamide 5 mg. Price 28 tabs = **H**

2.5 Antihypertensive drugs

Antihypertensive therapy has improved the outlook of the patient with high blood pressure by decreasing the incidence of stroke, heart failure, and renal failure, but there is little convincing evidence that it has reduced the number of patients suffering myocardial infarction. In starting treatment, the practitioner should have definite goals in mind, both in terms of levels of blood pressure to reach and end-organ function to preserve. Periodic assessment of how far these goals have been achieved forms the basis of good antihypertensive management.

Malignant (or accelerated) hypertension and established persistent hypertension are two situations where lowering of blood pressure is mandatory.

Malignant hypertension is characterised by high levels of pressure accompanied by papilloedema, retinal haemorrhage, or soft exudates. The immediate aim of treatment is to avert vascular catastrophe such as stroke or myocardial infarction and thus the blood pressure should be lowered as rapidly as possible and subsequently maintained within acceptable limits.

Rapid reduction of blood pressure can be achieved *within minutes* by intravenous administration of diazoxide, hydralazine, sodium nitroprusside, or labetalol, or *within hours* by oral treatment with methyldopa, bethanidine, or labetalol. These treatments must be followed by long-term oral treatment as for established persistent hypertension.

Established persistent hypertension is characterised by blood pressure persistently above 105 mmHg (14 kPa) diastolic. The aim of treatment is to reverse or prevent end-organ damage.

The practitioner has the choice of using one or more of the following classes of drugs:

thiazide diuretics—section 2.2.1
beta-adrenoceptor blocking drugs—section 2.4
vasodilator antihypertensive drugs—2.5.1
centrally-acting antihypertensive drugs—2.5.2
adrenergic neurone blocking drugs—2.5.3

The **thiazides** or **beta-adrenoceptor blocking drugs** alone may be adequate to control mild hypertension and are widely used for this purpose, but in moderate or severe hypertension a combination of drugs is usually needed.

If more than one drug is to be used they should be selected from different classes, so that they have different modes of action. It is illogical to combine two drugs from the same class. Knowledge of the class to which a drug belongs is important in understanding and predicting side-effects and warning the patient of them. The practitioner need only familiarise himself with one drug from each class, and this will enable him to treat the majority of his hypertensive patients.

Three other situations where long-term antihypertensive therapy is frequently used but for which the evidence is less convincing are mild hypertension, disparately elevated systolic pressure, and hypertension in the elderly.

Mild hypertension is characterised by diastolic blood pressures between 90 and 105 mmHg (12–14 kPa). The normal lability of blood pressure frequently causes problems in deciding whether to treat these patients or not, and current opinion is divided on the need for long-term therapy.

Five useful stratagems for treatment are:

1. Diuretics—any thiazide diuretic (for example bendrofluazide 5 mg/day) is acceptable (section 2.2.1) and potassium supplements are seldom necessary. Potassium-sparing diuretics (spironolactone, amiloride, or triamterene) are **not** indicated for routine antihypertensive treatment.
2. Beta-adrenoceptor blocking drugs (section 2.4) are all antihypertensive and there is no proven evidence of the superiority of any one member of this class.
3. Low doses of potent antihypertensive drugs, such as vasodilators, centrally-acting drugs, or adrenergic neurone blockers may be suitable. In low doses, side-effects are minimal and if necessary the dose may be increased to cope with altered circumstances. This contrasts with diuretics, which have a poor dose-response relationship.
4. Drug combinations are sometimes used, but these are probably to be avoided in the interests of keeping treatment uncomplicated.
5. Non-drug methods such as weight loss will lower blood pressure if significant and sustained. Cigarette smoking should be discontinued or drastically reduced. The place of meditation and yoga as antihypertensive therapy remains controversial.

Disparately elevated systolic pressure, with relatively normal diastolic pressures. The case for treatment here rests on the assumption that end-organ damage is caused by an elevation of the mean blood pressure which has both systolic and diastolic components.

Hypertension in the elderly has treatment goals different from those in the young, but treatment is justified if one can avert disabling complications such as stroke, without inducing unacceptable side-effects. Elderly hypertensive patients who have already had a stroke are still frequently worthwhile candidates for antihypertensive therapy.

2.5.1 Vasodilator antihypertensive drugs

These are potent drugs, especially when used in combination with beta-adrenoceptor blocking drugs or thiazides. **Prazosin** (Hypovase®) does not cause tachycardia, unlike the other vasodilators. **Diazoxide** (Eudemine®) is markedly diabetogenic and is not used by mouth in hypertension, but is given by intravenous injection in the emergency treatment of severe hypertension. **Hydralazine** (Apresoline®) is given by injection to control severe hypertension; given by mouth it is effective in the long-term management of hypertension, usually combined with a beta-blocker which reduces tachycardia. **Sodium nitroprusside** (Nipride®) is given by intravenous infusion to control severe hypertensive crises.

Minoxidil (Loniten®) should be reserved for the treatment of severe hypertension resistant to other drugs. Vasodilatation is accompanied by increased cardiac output and tachycardia, which is controlled by giving a beta-adrenoceptor blocking drug such as propranolol 80–160 mg daily. Minoxidil also causes marked fluid retention, and a diuretic **must** be given; thiazides are usually adequate in patients with normal renal function, but a loop diuretic should be used in patients with impaired renal function or who gain weight. Hirsutism is a troublesome side-effect in women, and may require use of a depilatory preparation.

DIAZOXIDE

Indications: hypertensive crisis, (for use in hypoglycaemia, see section 6.1.4)
Cautions: ischaemic heart disease, pregnancy, labour, impaired renal function
Side-effects: tachycardia, hyperglycaemia, fluid retention
Dose: by rapid intravenous injection, 300 mg, repeated up to 3 times in 24 hours

Eudemine® (A&H)
Injection, diazoxide 15 mg/ml. Price 20-ml amp = **E**

HYDRALAZINE HYDROCHLORIDE

Indications: moderate to severe hypertension, in addition to a beta-adrenoceptor blocking drug or diuretic; hypertensive crisis
Cautions: avoid in early pregnancy. Drug interactions: see Appendix 1
Side-effects: postural hypotension, tachycardia, fluid retention, nausea, and vomiting; systemic lupus erythematosus-like syndrome after long-term therapy with more than 200 mg daily
Dose: by mouth, 25 mg twice daily, increased to a max. of 100 mg twice daily
By slow intravenous injection or infusion, 20–40 mg, repeated if necessary

Apresoline® (Ciba)
Tablets, yellow, scored, hydralazine hydrochloride 25 mg. Price 20 tabs = **B**
Tablets, violet, s/c, hydralazine hydrochloride 50 mg. Price 20 tabs = **C**
Injection, powder for reconstitution, hydralazine hydrochloride. Price 20-mg amp = **B**

MINOXIDIL

Indications: severe hypertension, in addition to a diuretic and a beta-adrenoceptor blocking drug
Cautions: avoid oedema, may aggravate heart failure and angina, lower doses in dialysis patients
Contra-indications: phaeochromocytoma
Side-effects: gastro-intestinal disturbances, weight gain, peripheral oedema, tachycardia, hypertrichosis, breast tenderness
Dose: initially 5 mg daily, in 1–2 doses, increased by 5–10 mg every 3 or more days; max. usually 50 mg

▼ **Loniten®** (Upjohn)
Tablets, scored, minoxidil 2.5 mg. Price 20 tabs = **D**
Tablets, scored, minoxidil 5 mg. Price 20 tabs = **E**
Tablets, scored, minoxidil 10 mg. Price 20 tabs = **F**

PRAZOSIN HYDROCHLORIDE

Indications: hypertension; congestive heart failure
Cautions: first dose may cause loss of consciousness for up to 1 hour; lower dose in renal failure. Avoid abrupt withdrawal. Drug interactions: see Appendix 1
Side-effects: postural hypotension, drowsiness, weakness
Dose: hypertension, 500 micrograms 2–3 times daily, the initial dose being given with the evening meal; increased to a max. of 20 mg daily
Heart failure, 500 micrograms initially, then 1 mg 3–4 times daily; maintenance 4–20 mg daily

Hypovase® (Pfizer)
Tablets, prazosin hydrochloride 500 micrograms. Price 20 tabs = **C**
Tablets, orange, scored, prazosin hydrochloride 1 mg. Price 20 tabs = **D**
Tablets, scored, prazosin hydrochloride 2 mg. Price 20 tabs = **D**
Tablets, scored, prazosin hydrochloride 5 mg. Price 20 tabs = **F**
Treatment pack, 8 tablets, prazosin hydrochloride 500 micrograms; 32 orange tablets, prazosin hydrochloride 1 mg. Price per pack = **E**

SODIUM NITROPRUSSIDE

Indications: hypertensive crisis; controlled hypotension in surgery; acute or chronic heart failure
Cautions: hypothyroidism, severe renal impairment
Contra-indications: hepatic failure; vitamin B_{12} deficiency; Leber's optic atrophy; compensatory hypertension
Side-effects: headache, dizziness, nausea, and vomiting; palpitations and retrosternal pain—reduce infusion rate
Dose: hypertensive crisis, *by intravenous infusion,* 0.5–1.5 microgram/kg/minute initially, then adjusted; usual range 0.5–8 micrograms/kg/minute
Heart failure, *by intravenous infusion,* initially 10–15 micrograms/minute, increased every 5–10 minutes as necessary; usual range 10–200 micrograms/minute

▼ **Nipride®** (Roche)
Infusion, powder for reconstitution, sodium nitroprusside. Price 50-mg amp (with diluent) = **F** (Hosp. only)

2.5.2 Centrally-acting antihypertensive drugs

Fewer patients are being started on centrally-acting antihypertensives, as vasodilators and beta-adrenoceptor blocking drugs are now preferred. This group includes **methyldopa** (Aldomet®) which is usually given with a diuretic, and **clonidine** (Catapres®). Clonidine reduces both supine and erect blood pressure with little postural hypotension, but sudden withdrawal may cause a hypertensive crisis, a danger if a patient omits a few doses.

Rauwolfia and **reserpine** derivatives are generally ineffective by mouth and cause an unacceptably high incidence of depression.

CLONIDINE HYDROCHLORIDE

Indications: moderate to severe hypertension (for use in migraine, see section 4.7.4.2)
Cautions: must be withdrawn gradually to avoid hypertensive crisis. Drug interactions: see Appendix 1
Contra-indications: history of depression
Side-effects: dry mouth, sedation, depression, fluid retention, bradycardia, Raynaud's phenomenon
Dose: *by mouth,* 50–100 micrograms 3 times daily, increased every 3rd day; max. daily dose usually 1.2 mg
By slow intravenous injection, 150–300 micrograms

Catapres® (Boehringer Ingelheim)
Tablets, scored, clonidine hydrochloride 100 micrograms. Price 20 tabs = **D**
Tablets, scored, clonidine hydrochloride 300 micrograms. Price 20 tabs = **F**
Perlongets® (= capsules s/r), red/yellow, clonidine hydrochloride 250 micrograms. Price 14 caps = **F**
Dose: 250–750 micrograms daily
Injection, clonidine hydrochloride 150 micrograms/ml. Price 1-ml amp = **B**

METHYLDOPA

Indications: moderate to severe hypertension, in conjunction with a diuretic; hypertensive crisis
Cautions: positive direct Coombs' test in 20% of patients (may affect blood cross-matching); interference with laboratory tests; blood counts and liver-function tests advised. Drug interactions: see Appendix 1
Contra-indications: history of depression, active liver disease, phaeochromocytoma
Side-effects: dry mouth, sedation, depression, drowsiness, diarrhoea, fluid retention, failure of ejaculation, liver damage, haemolytic anaemia, systemic lupus erythematosus-like syndrome
Dose: *by mouth,* 250 mg 3 times daily, gradually increased; max. daily dose 3 g
By intravenous infusion, methyldopate hydrochloride 250–500 mg, repeated after 6 hours if required

Methyldopa Tablets, f/c, methyldopa (anhydrous) 125 mg, price 20 tabs = **B**; 250 mg, price 20 tabs = **C**; 500 mg, price 20 tabs = **D**

Aldomet® (MSD)
Tablets, yellow, f/c, methyldopa (anhydrous) 125 and 250 mg. Price 20 tabs (both) = **C**
Tablets, yellow, f/c, methyldopa (anhydrous) 500 mg. Price 20 tabs = **D**
Injection, methyldopate hydrochloride 50 mg/ml. Price 5-ml amp = **E**

Dopamet® (Berk)
Tablets, yellow, f/c, methyldopa (anhydrous) 125 mg. Price 20 tabs = **B**
Tablets, yellow, f/c, methyldopa (anhydrous) 250 mg. Price 20 tabs = **C**
Tablets, yellow, f/c, methyldopa (anhydrous) 500 mg. Price 20 tabs = **D**

Hydromet® (MSD)
Tablets, pink, f/c, methyldopa, hydrochlorothiazide Price 20 tabs = **D**

Medomet® (DDSA)
Capsules, yellow, methyldopa (anhydrous) 250 mg. Price 20 caps = **C**
Capsules, yellow, methyldopa (anhydrous) 500 mg. Price 20 caps = **C**
Tablets, yellow, f/c, methyldopa (anhydrous) 250 mg. Price 20 tabs = **C**
Tablets, yellow, f/c, methyldopa (anhydrous) 500 mg. Price 20 tabs = **D**

RESERPINE AND RAUWOLFIA ALKALOIDS

Indications: hypertension
Cautions: drug interactions: see Appendix 1
Contra-indications: history of depression, phaeochromocytoma, peptic ulcer, Parkinson's disease
Side-effects: dry mouth, nasal congestion, sedation, depression, postural hypotension, bradycardia, fluid retention

Reserpine Tablets, reserpine 100 and 250 micrograms. Price 20 tabs (both) = **A**

Abicol® (Boots)
Tablets, pink, scored, reserpine 150 micrograms, bendrofluazide 2.5 mg. Price 20 tabs = **A**

Decaserpyl® (Roussel)
Tablets, scored, methoserpidine 5 mg. Price 20 tabs = **D**.
Tablets, pink, scored, methoserpidine 10 mg. Price 20 tabs = **E**

Decaserpyl Plus® (Roussel)
Tablets, scored, methoserpidine 10 mg, benzthiazide 20 mg. Price 20 tabs = **E**

Enduronyl® (Abbott)
Tablets, yellow, scored, deserpidine 250 micrograms, methyclothiazide 5 mg. Price 20 tabs = **C.**
Tablets forte, grey, scored, deserpidine 500 micrograms, methyclothiazide 5 mg. Price 20 tabs = **C**

Harmonyl® (Abbott)
Tablets, pink, scored, deserpidine 250 micrograms. Price 20 tabs = **B**

Hypercal® (Carlton)
Tablets, rauwolfia alkaloids 2 mg. Price 20 tabs = **A**

Raudixin® (Squibb)
Tablets, orange, s/c, rauwolfia serpentina 50 mg. Price 20 tabs = **B**

Rautrax® (Squibb)
Tablets, red, s/c, rauwolfia serpentina 50 mg, hydroflumethiazide 50 mg, potassium chloride 625 mg (8.4 mmol K^+). Price 20 tabs = **D**

Rauwiloid® (Riker)
Tablets, cream, alseroxylon 2 mg. Price 20 tabs = **B**

Serpasil® (Ciba)
Tablets, blue, reserpine 100 micrograms. Price 20 tabs = A.
Tablets, blue, scored, reserpine 250 micrograms. Price 20 tabs = **A**

Serpasil-Esidrex® (Ciba)
Tablets, scored, reserpine 150 micrograms, hydrochlorothiazide 10 mg. Price 20 tabs = **B**

Serpasil-Esidrex-K® (Ciba)
Tablets, blue, s/c, reserpine 150 micrograms, hydrochlorothiazide 10 mg, potassium chloride 600 mg (8.1 mmol K^+). Price 20 tabs = **B**

2.5.3 Adrenergic neurone blocking drugs

These drugs prevent the release of noradrenaline from postganglionic adrenergic neurones. Guanethidine (Ismelin®) also depletes the nerve endings of noradrenaline. In many patients their value is limited by their failure to control supine blood pressure without causing an unacceptable degree of postural hypotension. Their action is potentiated by diuretics.

BETHANIDINE SULPHATE

Indications: moderate to severe hypertension, in conjunction with a diuretic or beta-adrenoceptor blocking drug
Cautions; Contra-indications; Side-effects: see under Guanethidine Monosulphate (except diarrhoea)
Dose: 10 mg 3 times daily, increased by 5 mg every 2 days; max. daily dose 200 mg

Esbatal® (Calmic)
Tablets, peach, scored, bethanidine sulphate 10 mg. Price 20 tabs = **C**
Tablets, peach, scored, bethanidine sulphate 50 mg. Price 20 tabs = **G**

DEBRISOQUINE

Indications: moderate to severe hypertension, in conjunction with a diuretic or beta-adrenoceptor blocking drug
Cautions; Contra-indications; Side-effects: see under Guanethidine Monosulphate (except diarrhoea)
Dose: 10 mg 1–2 times daily, increased by 10 mg every 3 days; max. daily dose usually 120 mg

Declinax® (Roche)
Tablets, scored, debrisoquine 10 mg (as sulphate). Price 20 tabs = **C**
Tablets, blue, scored, debrisoquine 20 mg (as sulphate). Price 20 tabs = **C**

GUANETHIDINE MONOSULPHATE

Indications: moderate to severe hypertension, in conjunction with a diuretic or beta-adrenoceptor blocking drug
Cautions: postural hypotension may cause falls in elderly patients. Drug interactions: see Appendix 1
Contra-indications: phaeochromocytoma, renal failure
Side-effects: postural hypotension, failure of ejaculation, fluid retention, nasal congestion, diarrhoea
Dose: by mouth, 10–20 mg daily, increased by 10 mg every 5–7 days; max. daily dose usually 75 mg
By intramuscular injection, 10–20 mg

Ismelin® (Ciba)
Tablets, guanethidine monosulphate 10 mg. Price 20 tabs = **B**
Tablets, pink, guanethidine monosulphate 25 mg. Price 20 tabs = **D**
Injection, guanethidine monosulphate 10 mg/ml. Price 1-ml amp = **B**

GUANOCLOR SULPHATE

Indications: moderate to severe hypertension, in conjunction with a diuretic
Cautions; Contra-indications; Side-effects: see under Guanethidine Monosulphate
Dose: 5 mg twice daily, increased by 10 mg daily at weekly intervals

Vatensol® (Pfizer)
Tablets, mauve, scored, guanoclor sulphate 10 mg. Price 20 tabs = **C**
Tablets, mauve, scored, guanoclor sulphate 40 mg. Price 20 tabs = **E**

GUANOXAN SULPHATE

Indications: moderate to severe hypertension, in conjunction with a diuretic
Cautions; Contra-indications; Side-effects: see under Guanethidine Monosulphate
Dose: see under Guanoclor Sulphate

Envacar® (Pfizer)
Tablets, yellow, scored, guanoxan sulphate 10 mg. Price 20 tabs = **D**
Tablets, yellow, scored, guanoxan sulphate 40 mg. Price 20 tabs = **G**

2.5.4 Alpha-adrenergic blocking drugs

Phenoxybenzamine (Dibenyline®) and **phentolamine** (Rogitine®) are not used in the routine management of hypertension as they cause reflex tachycardia and an unacceptable degree of orthostatic hypotension. Their main use is in phaeochromocytoma, given before and during surgery to control paroxysmal hypertension or for long-term therapy if the tumour is inoperable. They are also used to control hypertensive crises precipitated by clonidine withdrawal, and by reactions between monoamine-oxidase inhibitors and foods containing pressor amines.

Indoramin (Baratol®) is used in the treatment of hypertension, usually in combination with a diuretic or beta-adrenoceptor blocking drug.

INDORAMIN

Indications: hypertension, usually in conjunction with a diuretic or a beta-adrenoceptor blocking drug
Cautions: patient's ability to drive or operate machinery may be impaired; control incipient heart failure with diuretics and digoxin; hepatic or renal impairment; Parkinson's disease
Contra-indications: established heart failure; patients being treated with monoamine-oxidase inhibitors

Side-effects: sedation; weight gain, dizziness, failure of ejaculation, dry mouth, nasal congestion occur less frequently
Dose: initially 25 mg twice daily, increased by 25–50 mg at intervals of 2 weeks; max. daily dose 200 mg

▼ Baratol® (Wyeth)
Tablets, blue, f/c, indoramin 25 mg (as hydrochloride). Price 20 tabs = **E**
Tablets, green, scored, f/c, indoramin 50 mg (as hydrochloride). Price 20 tabs = **F**

PHENOXYBENZAMINE HYDROCHLORIDE

Indications: hypertension due to phaeochromocytoma, Raynaud's disease
Contra-indications: renal impairment
Side-effects: marked tachycardia and postural hypotension
Dose: *by mouth,* phaeochromocytoma, 20–30 mg at night, increased by 10–20 mg every 4 days; maintenance dose usually 40–100 mg twice daily
Raynaud's disease, 10 mg at night increased by 10 mg every 4 days; maintenance 30–60 mg daily divided into 2 doses

Dibenyline® (SK&F)
Capsules, red, phenoxybenzamine hydrochloride 10 mg. Price 20 caps = **E**
Injection, phenoxybenzamine hydrochloride 50 mg/ml. To be diluted before use. 2-ml amp (Hosp. only)

PHENTOLAMINE MESYLATE

Indications: hypertensive crises due to phaeochromocytoma, clonidine withdrawal, reaction between monoamine-oxidase inhibitors and foods containing pressor amines; acute left ventricular failure
Side-effects: see under Phenoxybenzamine Hydrochloride; also flushing
Dose: *by intravenous injection,* 5–10 mg repeated as necessary
By intravenous infusion, 5–60 mg over 10–30 minutes at a rate of 0.1–2 mg/minute

Rogitine® (Ciba)
Injection, phentolamine mesylate 10 mg/ml. Price 1-ml amp = **B**; 5-ml amp = **D**

2.5.5 Angiotensin-converting enzyme inhibitors

Captopril (Capoten®) inhibits the conversion of angiotensin I to angiotensin II; it is used in the treatment of severe hypertension refractory to other treatment. A thiazide (or loop diuretic in patients with impaired renal function) may also be required. The principle adverse effects of captopril are rashes and loss of taste; proteinuria may also occur.

CAPTOPRIL

Indications: severe hypertension resistant to other treatment
Cautions: first dose may cause marked hypotension within 3 hours in patients taking diuretics, on a low-sodium diet, or on dialysis (may recur with next 1 or 2 doses); renal impairment. Drug interactions: see Appendix 1
Side-effects: loss of taste, stomatosis, abdominal pain, rashes, hypotension (see Cautions), proteinuria, agranulocytosis, neutropenia, hyperkalaemia
Dose: initially 25 mg 3 times daily, increased to 50 mg after 2 weeks if necessary; a diuretic should be added before further increase in captopril dose; max. 450 mg daily

▼ Capoten® (Squibb)
Tablets, captopril 25 mg. Price 20 tabs = **F**
Tablets, scored, captopril 50 mg. Price 20 tabs = **H**
Tablets, scored, captopril 100 mg. Price 20 tabs = **I**

2.5.6 Ganglion-blocking drugs

Mecamylamine (Inversine®) and trimetaphan (Arfonad®) are now seldom used because of their anticholinergic side-effects.

MECAMYLAMINE HYDROCHLORIDE

Indications: moderate to severe hypertension if other drugs are ineffective
Cautions: impaired renal function, cardiovascular disease
Contra-indications: glaucoma, pyloric stenosis
Side-effects: postural hypotension, drowsiness, dry mouth, impotence, paralytic ileus
Dose: 2.5 mg twice daily, increased by 2.5 mg every 2 days; maintenance dose 20–30 mg daily

Inversine® (MSD)
Tablets, yellow, scored, mecamylamine hydrochloride 2.5 mg. Price 20 tabs = **A**
Tablets, scored, mecamylamine hydrochloride 10 mg. Price 20 tabs = **B**

TRIMETAPHAN CAMSYLATE

Indications: controlled hypotension in surgery
Cautions; Contra-indications; Side-effects: see under Mecamylamine Hydrochloride
Dose: *by intravenous infusion,* 3–4 mg/minute initially

Arfonad® (Roche)
Injection, trimetaphan camsylate 50 mg/ml. Price 5-ml amp = **E**

2.5.7 Other antihypertensive drugs

Pargyline is a monoamine-oxidase inhibitor and because dietary restrictions are necessary it is now used only in resistant hypertension when other drugs have proved ineffective.

Veratrum alkaloids have a very low therapeutic index and should no longer be used in the treatment of hypertension.

There is no justification for the use of barbiturates in the treatment of hypertension.

Hypercal-B® (Carlton)
Tablets, rauwolfia alkaloids 2 mg, amylobarbitone 15 mg. Price 20 tabs = **A**

Seominal® (Winthrop)
Tablets, yellow, scored, reserpine 200 micrograms, phenobarbitone 10 mg, theobromine 325 mg. Price 20 tabs = **E**

Theominal® (Winthrop)
Tablets, phenobarbitone 30 mg, theobromine 300 mg. Price 20 tabs = **C**

PARGYLINE HYDROCHLORIDE

Indications: refractory hypertension
Cautions: impaired liver and renal function. MAOI—see section 4.3.2. Drug interactions: see Appendix 1
Contra-indications: phaeochromocytoma, hyperthyroidism, schizophrenia
Side-effects: postural hypotension, oedema, nausea, vomiting, dry mouth, impotence, headache, insomnia, nightmares
Dose: 25 mg daily, increased by 10 mg at weekly intervals; maintenance usually 25–50 mg daily

Eutonyl® (Abbott)
Tablets, orange, f/c, pargyline hydrochloride 25 mg. Price 20 tabs = **D**

VERATRUM ALKALOIDS

Alkavervir
Indications: see notes above
Cautions: drug interactions: see Appendix 1
Contra-indications: cardiovascular disease, phaeochromocytoma
Side-effects: postural hypotension, bradycardia, arrhythmias, nausea, vomiting, epigastric pain, shallow respiration

Rauwiloid + Veriloid® (Riker)
Tablets, brown, alkavervir 3 mg, alseroxylon 1 mg. Price 20 tabs = **D**

Thiaver® (Riker)
Tablets, blue, scored, alkavervir 4 mg, epithiazide 4 mg. Price 20 tabs = **D**

Veriloid® (Riker)
Tablets, yellow, scored, alkavervir 2 mg. Price 20 tabs = **D**

2.6 Vasodilators

2.6.1 Vasodilators used in angina pectoris
2.6.2 Vasodilators used in heart failure
2.6.3 Peripheral vasodilators
2.6.4 Cerebral vasodilators

For the use of vasodilators in hypertension, see section 2.5.1.

2.6.1 Vasodilators used in angina pectoris

A short-acting nitrite or nitrate is usually the first drug used; **glyceryl trinitrate** is one of the most effective drugs for providing symptomatic relief. Taken sublingually its onset of action is rapid but its effect lasts only for 20–30 minutes. It does not appreciably dilate diseased coronary vessels but, by causing a reduction in venous return and therefore ventricular stroke output, systolic pressure falls and left ventricular work decreases. However, in severe angina frequent administration of glyceryl trinitrate may be necessary and side-effects such as flushing, headache, and postural hypotension may limit therapy.

Isosorbide dinitrate is active sublingually and also after oral administration. The value of long-acting nitrates such as **pentaerythritol tetranitrate** in the treatment of angina is still strongly debated since nitrates are metabolised rapidly in the liver, so that little active drug reaches the systemic circulation. The activity of isosorbide dinitrate may depend on the production of active metabolites.

Glyceryl trinitrate injection (Tridil®) or isosorbide dinitrate injection (Cedocard IV®, Isoket®) may be tried when the sublingual form is ineffective in patients with chest pain due to myocardial infarction or severe ischaemia.

Verapamil (section 2.3.2) has been used for the treatment of angina. It interferes with the inward displacement of calcium ions across cardiac cell membranes (and thereby inhibits excitation-contraction coupling), decreases cardiac contractility, decreases oxygen requirements of the heart, and does not block beta-adrenoceptors. Its effectiveness in the treatment of angina is still a matter of debate. It may precipitate heart failure and cause hypotension at high doses and should not be used in conjunction with beta-adrenoceptor blocking drugs.

Perhexiline maleate (Pexid®) has been shown to reduce the frequency and severity of anginal attacks when compared with placebo, and it does not appear to precipitate heart failure or airways obstruction. It reduces exercise-induced tachycardia but has no effect on the resting heart-rate, unlike beta-adrenoceptor blocking drugs. Serious side-effects, usually associated with long-term treatment, include peripheral neuropathy, raised intracranial pressure, and liver damage; perhexiline should not be prescribed unless patients can be regularly monitored.

Nifedipine (Adalat®) is a more potent peripheral and coronary vasodilator than verapamil and does not have anti-arrhythmic activity. It increases coronary blood flow and decreases myocardial oxygen consumption in *animals.* Like verapamil and the beta-adrenoceptor blocking drugs it has a negative inotropic effect. Minor side-effects associated with vasodilatation such as flushing and headaches, and gastro-intestinal intolerance have been reported.

Lidoflazine (Clinium®) is a long-acting coronary vasodilator and also inhibits the influx of calcium ions across cardiac cell membranes. Increased exercise tolerance develops gradually over several weeks.

Dipyridamole (section 2.9) is also used in the treatment of angina.

GLYCERYL TRINITRATE

Indications: prophylaxis and treatment of angina; congestive heart failure
Side-effects: throbbing headache, flushing, dizziness, postural hypotension, tachycardia
Dose: *sublingually,* 0.5–1 mg, repeated as required
By mouth, 2.6–6.4 mg as sustained-release tablets, 2–3 times daily
By intravenous infusion, 10–200 micrograms/minute

Glyceryl Trinitrate Tablets, glyceryl trinitrate 300, 500, and 600 micrograms. Price 20 tabs (all) = **A**

Natirose® (Wilcox) *tablets,* pink, s/c, glyceryl trinitrate, ethylmorphine hydrochloride, hyoscyamine hydrobromide. Price 20 tabs = **C**

Nitrocontin Continus® (Napp)
Tablets, s/r, pink, glyceryl trinitrate 2.6 mg. Price 20 tabs = **B**
Tablets, s/r, pink, glyceryl trinitrate 6.4 mg. Price 20 tabs = **C**

Percutol® (R&C)
Ointment, glyceryl trinitrate 2%. Price 30 g = **F**
Dose: prophylaxis of angina pectoris, 8–32 mg (½–2 inches of ointment extruded from nozzle of tube) 3–4 hourly

Sustac® (Pharmax)
Tablets, s/r, pink, glyceryl trinitrate 2.6 mg. Price 20 tabs = **C**
Tablets, s/r, pink, glyceryl trinitrate 6.4 mg. Price 20 tabs = **D**
Tablets, s/r, pink, glyceryl trinitrate 10 mg. Price 20 tabs = **D**
Dose: severe angina, 10 mg 3 times daily

▼ **Tridil®** (American Hospital Supply)
Injection, glyceryl trinitrate 500 micrograms/ml. To be diluted before use. Price 10-ml amp = **G**
Injection, glyceryl trinitrate 5 mg/ml. To be diluted before use. Price 10-ml amp = **J**
Infusion apparatus should be of glass or suitable polyethylene, but not PVC

ISOSORBIDE DINITRATE

Indications: prophylaxis and treatment of angina; congestive heart failure
Side-effects: see under Glyceryl Trinitrate
Dose: *sublingually,* 5–10 mg
By mouth, daily in divided doses, angina 40–120 mg, congestive heart failure 40–160 mg
By intravenous infusion, 2–7 mg/hour

Isosorbide Dinitrate Tablets, isosorbide dinitrate 10 mg. Price 20 tabs = **B**

Cedocard® (Tillotts)
Tablets, scored, isosorbide dinitrate 5 mg. Price 20 tabs = **B**

Cedocard-20® (Tillotts)
Tablets, blue, scored, isosorbide dinitrate 20 mg. Price 20 tabs = **C**

Cedocard Retard® (Tillots)
Tablets, s/r, yellow, scored, isosorbide dinitrate 20 mg. Price 20 tabs = **D**
Dose: 20 mg every 12 hours

▼ **Cedocard IV®** (Tillotts)
Injection, isosorbide dinitrate 1 mg/ml. To be diluted before use. Price 10-ml amp = **G**
Glass or polythene infusion apparatus is preferable; loss of potency will occur if PVC apparatus is used

Isoket® (Sanol Schwarz)
Injection, isosorbide dinitrate 1 mg/ml. To be diluted before use. Price 10-ml amp = **G**
Glass or polythene infusion apparatus is preferable; loss of potency will occur if PVC apparatus is used

Isoket Retard® (Sanol Schwarz)
Tablets, s/r, yellow, scored, isosorbide dinitrate 20 mg. Price 20 tabs = **D**
Dose: prophylaxis, 20 mg every 12 hours; treatment of anginal attack, 10 mg chewed and dissolved in the mouth

Isordil® (Ayerst)
Tablets (sublingual), pink, isosorbide dinitrate 5 mg. Price 20 tabs = **B**
Tablets, scored, isosorbide dinitrate 10 mg. Price 20 tabs = **B**
Tablets, pale yellow, scored, isosorbide dinitrate 30 mg. Price 20 tabs = **C**
Tembids®(= capsules s/r), blue/clear, isosorbide dinitrate 40 mg. Price 20 caps = **D**
Dose: 40 mg 2–3 times daily

Soni-Slo® (Rona)
Capsules, s/r, pink/clear, enclosing white/yellow pellets, isosorbide dinitrate 20 mg. Price 20 caps = **D**
Dose: 20 mg every 8–12 hours

Sorbitrate® (Stuart)
Tablets (chewable), green, scored, isosorbide dinitrate 5 mg. Price 20 tabs = **B**
Tablets, yellow, scored, isosorbide dinitrate 10 mg. Price 20 tabs = **B**
Tablets, blue, scored, isosorbide dinitrate 20 mg. Price 20 tabs = **B**

Vascardin® (Nicholas)
Tablets, scored, isosorbide dinitrate 10 mg. Price 20 tabs = **B**

LIDOFLAZINE

Indications: prophylaxis of angina
Contra-indications: pregnancy
Side-effects: gastro-intestinal disturbances, dizziness, tinnitus, headaches
Dose: 1st week, 120 mg once daily; 2nd week, 120 mg twice daily; 3rd and subsequent weeks, 120 mg 3 times daily

▼ **Clinium®** (Janssen)
Tablets, lidoflazine 120 mg. Price 20 tabs = **E**

NIFEDIPINE

Indications: prophylaxis and treatment of angina
Cautions: withdraw the drug if ischaemic pain occurs or existing pain worsens shortly after initiating treatment
Contra-indications: women of childbearing age
Side-effects: see under Glyceryl Trinitrate
Dose: 10–20 mg 3 times daily; in elderly patients, initially 5 mg 3 times daily; for immediate effect bite into capsule and retain liquid in mouth

Adalat® (Bayer)
Capsules, orange, nifedipine 5 mg. Price 20 caps = **D**
Capsules, orange, nifedipine 10 mg. Price 20 caps = **E**

PENTAERYTHRITOL TETRANITRATE

Indications: prophylaxis of angina; congestive heart failure
Side-effects: see under Glyceryl Trinitrate
Dose: 20–60 mg 3–4 times daily

Cardiacap® (Consolidated)
Capsules, s/r, blue/yellow, pentaerythritol tetranitrate 30 mg. Price 20 caps = **C**
Dose: 30 mg every 12 hours
Mycardol® (Winthrop)
Tablets, scored, pentaerythritol tetranitrate 30 mg. Price 20 tabs = **B**
Pentoxylon® (Riker) *tablets,* brown, pentaerythritol tetranitrate, alseroxylon. Price 20 tabs = **B**
Peritrate® (Warner)
Tablets, green, pentaerythritol tetranitrate 10 mg. Price 20 tabs = **A**
Peritrate SA® (Warner)
Tablets, s/r, green, pentaerythritol tetranitrate 80 mg. Price 20 tabs = **B**
Dose: 80 mg every 12 hours

PERHEXILINE MALEATE

Indications: prophylaxis of angina, when not controlled by nitrates or beta-adrenoceptor blocking drugs
Cautions: regular determination of weight, blood glucose, and liver function required during treatment; also check for symptoms of peripheral neuropathy
Contra-indications: severe liver and renal disease
Side-effects: postural hypotension, headache, dizziness, flushing; on prolonged treatment, changes in liver-function tests, peripheral neuropathy, raised intracranial pressure, hypoglycaemia, marked weight loss
Dose: 100 mg twice daily; max. 400 mg daily

Pexid® (Merrell)
Tablets, scored, perhexiline maleate 100 mg. Price 20 tabs = **E**

PRENYLAMINE LACTATE

Indications: prophylaxis of angina
Cautions: drug interactions: see Appendix 1
Contra-indications: severe hepatic or renal impairment, cardiac conduction defects, severe uncompensated heart failure
Side-effects: nausea, vomiting, diarrhoea, myocardial depression, ventricular tachycardia (in hypokalaemia)
Dose: 60 mg 3 times daily, increased to 300 mg daily if response is inadequate after 14 days; reduce to lowest effective dose after 3 weeks

Synadrin® (Hoechst)
Tablets, pink, s/c, prenylamine 60 mg (as lactate). Price 20 tabs = **D**

2.6.2 Vasodilators used in heart failure

Until recently, treatment of heart failure was restricted to restoring contractility with cardiac glycosides and relieving congestion with diuretics. Cardiac glycosides have been shown to have limited inotropic potential in long-term treatment and it now appears that vasodilators may produce improvement in cardiac performance comparable with that achieved by the most potent inotropic drugs.

Vasodilators act in heart failure by one of two methods: by arteriolar dilatation which reduces both peripheral vascular resistance and left ventricular pressure at systole and results in improved cardiac output, or by venous dilatation which results in a dilatation of capacitance vessels, an increase of venous pooling, and diminution of venous return to the heart thus decreasing left ventricular and diastolic pressure. Symptoms of heart failure are therefore relieved. Three groups of drugs should be considered—nitrates (glyceryl trinitrate, isosorbide dinitrate, pentaerythritol tetranitrate) which act predominantly by venous dilatation; hydralazine which acts predominantly by arteriolar dilatation; and phentolamine, prazosin, and sodium nitroprusside which produce both arteriolar and venous dilatation. Combinations of drugs with different effects can be tried.

Glyceryl trinitrate and other nitrates—section 2.6.1
Hydralazine hydrochloride—section 2.5.1
Phentolamine mesylate—section 2.5.4
Prazosin hydrochloride—section 2.5.1
Sodium nitroprusside—section 2.5.1

2.6.3 Peripheral vasodilators

Most serious peripheral disorders are now known to be due to occlusion of vessels, either by spasm or sclerotic plaques; use of vasodilators tends to dilate healthy, but not diseased, vessels and may even decrease blood flow in ischaemic areas.

BAMETHAN SULPHATE

Indications: Raynaud's disease, poor peripheral circulation

Cautions: angina
Contra-indications: recent myocardial infarction
Side-effects: postural hypotension, tachycardia, flushing
Dose: 25 mg 4 times daily

Vasculit® (Boehringer Ingelheim)
Tablets, bamethan sulphate 12.5 mg. Price 20 tabs = **B**

CINNARIZINE

Indications: peripheral vascular disease, Raynaud's disease
Cautions; Side-effects: see under Cyclizine (section 4.6); also hypersensitivity reactions, caution in hypotension
Dose: initially, 75 mg 3 times daily; maintenance, 75 mg 2–3 times daily

Stugeron Forte® (Janssen)
Capsules, orange/yellow, cinnarizine 75 mg. Price 20 caps = **F**
Stugeron: see section 4.6

NICOTINIC ACID DERIVATIVES

Indications: peripheral vascular disease (for the use of nicotinic acid and derivatives in hyperlipidaemia, see section 2.12)
Cautions: diabetes
Side-effects: flushing, dizziness, nausea, vomiting, hypotension
Dose: inositol nicotinate, 1.5–4 g daily; nicofuranose, 500 mg 3 times daily; nicotinyl alcohol (as tartrate), 25–50 mg 4 times daily *or* 150–300 mg twice daily in sustained-release form

Amisyn® (Armour)
Tablets, nicotinamide 50 mg, acetomenaphthone 10 mg. Price 20 tabs = **B**
Bradilan® (Napp)
Tablets, e/c and s/c, nicofuranose 250 mg. Price 20 tabs = **D**
Hexopal® (Winthrop)
Tablets, scored, inositol nicotinate 500 mg. Price 20 tabs = **E**
Tablets forte, scored, inositol nicotinate 750 mg. Price 20 tabs = **E**
Dose: 1.5–3 g daily
Suspension (= mixture), inositol nicotinate 1 g/5 ml. Diluent syrup, life of diluted mixture 14 days. Price 100 ml = **F**
Pernivit® (DF)
Tablets, pink, s/c, nicotinic acid 25 mg, acetomenaphthone 7 mg. Price 20 tabs = **A**
Ronicol® (Roche)
Tablets, scored, nicotinyl alcohol 25 mg (as tartrate). Price 20 tabs = **B**
Timespan® (= tablets s/r), red, s/c, nicotinyl alcohol 150 mg (as tartrate). Price 20 tabs = **D**

OXPENTIFYLLINE

Indications: peripheral vascular disease
Cautions: hypotension
Side-effects: nausea, dizziness, flushing
Dose: *by mouth,* 200 mg 3 times daily, reducing to 100 mg
By slow intravenous injection or infusion, 100 mg; max. 400 mg daily

Trental® (Hoechst)
Tablets, pink, s/c, oxpentifylline 100 mg. Price 20 tabs = **D**
Tablets, s/r, pink, s/c, oxpentifylline 400 mg. Price 20 tabs = **E**
Dose: 400 mg 2–3 times daily
Injection, oxpentifylline 20 mg/ml. Price 5-ml amp = **C**

THYMOXAMINE

Indications: Raynaud's disease, peripheral vascular disease, vascular spasm
Cautions: coronary artery disease, diabetes
Side-effects: nausea, diarrhoea, flushing, headache, dizziness
Dose: *by mouth,* 40 mg 4 times daily
By intravenous injection, 100 micrograms/kg 4 times daily
By intravenous infusion, 30 mg every 6 hours
By intra-arterial injection, 5 mg

Opilon® (Warner)
Tablets, yellow, scored, thymoxamine 40 mg (as hydrochloride). Price 20 tabs = **E**
Injection, thymoxamine 5 mg (as hydrochloride)/ml. Price 1-ml amp = **B**
Injection forte, thymoxamine 15 mg (as hydrochloride)/ml. Price 2-ml amp = **C**

TOLAZOLINE HYDROCHLORIDE

Indications: peripheral vascular disease
Cautions; Contra-indications; Side-effects: see under Bamethan Sulphate; also contra-indicated in peptic ulcer
Dose: 12.5 mg 1–2 times daily, increased to max. of 50 mg 4 times daily

Priscol® (Ciba)
Tablets, scored, tolazoline hydrochloride 25 mg. Price 20 tabs = **A**

OTHER PREPARATIONS USED IN PERIPHERAL VASCULAR DISEASE

Rutosides (Paroven®) are not vasodilators and are not generally regarded as effective preparations as capillary sealants or for the treatment of cramps.

Depropanex® (MSD)
Injection, deproteinated pancreatic extract. Price 10-ml vial = **D**
Paroven® (Zyma)
Capsules, yellow, oxerutins 250 mg. Price 20 caps = **E**

2.6.4 Cerebral vasodilators

These drugs are claimed to improve mental function. Some improvements in performance of psychological tests have been reported but the drugs have not been shown clinically to be of much benefit in senile dementia.

CO-DERGOCRINE MESYLATE
Indications: adjunct in the management of senile dementia
Cautions: severe bradycardia
Side-effects: nausea, vomiting, flushing, rashes, nasal congestion, postural hypotension in hypertensive patients
Dose: 4.5 mg daily in single or divided doses

Hydergine® (Sandoz)
Tablets, scored, co-dergocrine mesylate 1.5 mg. Price 20 tabs = **E**
Tablets, co-dergocrine mesylate 4.5 mg. Price 28 tabs = **I**

CYCLANDELATE
Indications: peripheral vascular disease; adjunct in the management of senile dementia
Contra-indications: recent myocardial infarction
Side-effects: nausea, flushing, dizziness with high doses
Dose: 1.2–1.6 g daily in divided doses

Cyclobral® (Norgine)
Capsules, pink/brown, cyclandelate 400 mg. Price 20 caps = **D**
Cyclospasmol® (Brocades)
Capsules, pink/grey, cyclandelate 400 mg. Price 20 caps = **D**
Tablets, pink, s/c, cyclandelate 400 mg. Price 20 tabs = **D**
Suspension (= mixture), cyclandelate 400 mg /5 ml when reconstituted with freshly boiled and cooled purified water. Diluent syrup, life of diluted mixture 14 days. Price 100 ml = **E**

ISOXSUPRINE HYDROCHLORIDE
Indications: cerebral and peripheral vascular disease
Contra-indications: recent arterial haemorrhage
Side-effects: flushing, tachycardia, palpitations, nausea, vomiting
Dose: by mouth, 20 mg 4 times daily *or* 40 mg (in sustained-release form) every 12 hours
By intramuscular injection, 5–10 mg 3–4 times daily
By intravenous infusion, 100–400 micrograms/minute

Defencin CP® (Bristol)
Capsules, s/r, pink/red, isoxsuprine hydrochloride (as resinate) 40 mg. Price 28 caps = **F**
Duvadilan® (Duphar)
Tablets, pink, scored, isoxsuprine hydrochloride 20 mg. Price 20 tabs = **C**
Injection, isoxsuprine hydrochloride 5 mg/ml. Price 2-ml amp = **B**; 10-ml amp = **D**
Duvadilan Retard® (Duphar)
Capsules, s/r, red/white, isoxsuprine hydrochloride (as resinate) 40 mg. Price 28 caps = **F**

NAFTIDROFURYL OXALATE
Indications: cerebral and peripheral vascular disease
Contra-indications: parenteral administration in atrioventricular block
Side-effects: nausea, epigastric pain
Dose: by mouth, 100–200 mg 3 times daily
By intravenous or intra-arterial infusion, 200 mg over at least 90 minutes, twice daily

Praxilene® (Lipha)
Capsules, pink, naftidrofuryl oxalate 100 mg. Price 20 caps = **E**
Injection forte, naftidrofuryl oxalate 20 mg/ml. Price 10-ml amp = **D**

2.7 Sympathomimetics

Xanthine derivatives such as aminophylline are also used as cardiac stimulants, particularly in congestive heart failure. For details of preparations, see section 3.1.3.

2.7.1 Sympathomimetics with inotropic activity

The cardiac stimulants **dobutamine** (Dobutrex®) and **dopamine** (Intropin®) act on sympathetic receptors in cardiac muscle, and increase contractility with little effect on rate; they are used in cardiogenic shock.

Prenalterol (Hyprenan®, Varbian®) has similar cardiac stimulant activity but has a more selective action on $beta_1$ receptors, so may also be used to reverse the cardiac effects of beta-adrenoceptor blocking drugs.

Isoprenaline also acts on sympathetic receptors and increases both heart rate and contractility; it may prevent Stokes-Adams attacks, but insertion of a pacemaker is preferable.

DOBUTAMINE HYDROCHLORIDE
Indications: inotropic support in infarction or cardiac surgery
Cautions: low dose in acute myocardial shock
Side-effects: tachycardia and increase in blood pressure indicate overdosage
Dose: by intravenous infusion, 2.5–10 micrograms/kg/minute, adjusted according to response

▼ **Dobutrex®** (Lilly)
Injection, powder for reconstitution, dobutamine hydrochloride. Price 250-mg vial = **H**

DOPAMINE HYDROCHLORIDE
Indications: cardiogenic shock in infarction or cardiac surgery
Cautions: correct hypovolaemia; extravasation at infusion site may cause necrosis. Drug interactions: see Appendix 1

Contra-indications: tachyarrhythmia, phaeochromocytoma
Side-effects: nausea and vomiting, peripheral vasoconstriction, hypotension, hypertension, tachycardia
Dose: by intravenous infusion, 5–20 micrograms/kg/minute initially, increased if necessary

Intropin® (American Hospital Supply)
Injection, dopamine hydrochloride 40 mg/ml. To be diluted before use. Price 5-ml amp or syringe = **F**
Injection, dopamine hydrochloride 160 mg/ml. To be diluted before use. Price 5-ml amp = **J**

ISOPRENALINE HYDROCHLORIDE

Indications: heart block, severe bradycardia
Cautions: ischaemic heart disease, diabetes, hyperthyroidism
Side-effects: tachycardia, arrhythmias, hypotension, sweating, tremor, headache
Dose: by mouth, 30 mg every 8 hours, then increased; max. daily dose usually 750 mg
By intravenous infusion, 0.5–10 micrograms/minute

Isuprel® (Winthrop)
Injection, isoprenaline hydrochloride 200 micrograms/ml. Price 1-ml amp = **E**; 5-ml amp = **G**

Saventrine® (Pharmax)
Tablets, s/r, isoprenaline hydrochloride 30 mg. Price 20 tabs = **D**

Saventrine IV® (Pharmax)
Injection, isoprenaline hydrochloride 1 mg/ml. Price 2-ml amp = **B**

PRENALTEROL HYDROCHLORIDE

Indications: inotropic support in infarction, cardiac surgery or shock; reversal of the cardiac effect of beta-blockers
Cautions: correct hypovolaemia; angina pectoris and recent myocardial infarction, obstructive subvalvular cardiomyopathy, diabetes, hypokalaemia, pregnancy (toxicity in *animal* studies)
Contra-indications: serious ventricular arrhythmias
Side-effects: palpitations, nervousness; isolated ventricular ectopic beats, increase in attack rate in patients with angina pectoris, excessive increase in blood pressure or heart rate (may be counteracted by intravenous injection of beta-blocker)
Dose: inotropic support, *by intravenous infusion,* 500 micrograms/minute, adjusted according to response; max. total dose 20 mg.
Reversal of beta-blockade, *by intravenous injection,* 2–5 mg over 5 minutes, repeated if necessary to a max. of 20 mg

▼ **Hyprenan®** (Astra)
Injection, prenalterol hydrochloride 1 mg/ml. Price 5-ml amp = **H**

▼ **Varbian®** (Ciba)
Injection, prenalterol hydrochloride 1 mg/ml. Price 5-ml amp = **H**

2.7.2 Sympathomimetics causing vasoconstriction

Vasoconstrictors raise blood pressure transiently by constricting peripheral vessels. They are sometimes used as an emergency method of elevating blood pressure while preparations are being made for more effective therapy such as transfusion. They may also be used in general and spinal anaesthesia to control blood pressure.

The danger of vasoconstrictors is that although they raise blood pressure they do so at the expense of perfusion of vital organs such as the kidney. Further, in many patients with shock the peripheral resistance is already high, and to raise it further is unhelpful. Thus the use of vasoconstrictors in the treatment of shock is to be generally **deprecated**. The use of volume expanders such as blood or plasma, or the inotropic agents dopamine, dobutamine, or isoprenaline is more appropriate (section 2.7.1). Treatment of the underlying condition with, for example antibiotics in septic shock, is obviously important, and, in addition high doses of corticosteroids may be helpful.

METARAMINOL

Indications: acute hypotension
Cautions: extravasation at injection site may cause necrosis. Drug interactions: see Appendix 1
Contra-indications: myocardial infarction, pregnancy
Side-effects: tachycardia, arrhythmia, reduced renal blood flow
Dose: by subcutaneous or intramuscular injection, 2–10 mg
By intravenous infusion, 15–100 mg

Aramine® (MSD)
Injection, metaraminol 10 mg (as tartrate)/ml. Price 1-ml amp = **B**; 10-ml vial = **D**

METHOXAMINE HYDROCHLORIDE

Indications: hypotension in anaesthesia
Cautions: hyperthyroidism. Drug interactions: see Appendix 1
Contra-indications: severe coronary or cardiovascular disease
Side-effects: headache, hypertension, bradycardia
Dose: by intramuscular injection, 5–20 mg
By slow intravenous injection, 5–10 mg

Vasoxine® (Calmic)
Injection, methoxamine hydrochloride 20 mg/ml. Price 1-ml amp = **B**

NORADRENALINE ACID TARTRATE

Indications: acute hypotension, cardiac arrest
Cautions; Contra-indications: see under Metaraminol Tartrate
Side-effects: headache, palpitations, bradycardia
Dose: by intravenous infusion, 8–12 micrograms/minute, adjusted as required
By rapid intravenous or intracardiac injection, 100–150 micrograms
Note: noradrenaline acid tartrate 2 mg ≡ noradrenaline 1 mg

Levophed® (Winthrop)
Injection, noradrenaline acid tartrate 2 mg/ml. Price 2-ml amp = **B**; 4-ml amp = **C**
Special injection, noradrenaline acid tartrate 200 micrograms/ml. Price 2-ml amp = **B**

OXEDRINE TARTRATE

Indications: hypotension
Cautions; Contra-indications; Side-effects: see under Phenylephrine Hydrochloride

Sympatol® (Lewis)
Liquid (oral), oxedrine tartrate 10%. Price 20 ml = **C**; 100 ml = **F**
Dose: 20–30 drops 3 times daily
Injection, oxedrine tartrate 60 mg/ml. Price 1-ml amp = **A**
Dose: by subcutaneous, intramuscular, or intravenous injection, 60–120 mg every 1–2 hours

PHENYLEPHRINE HYDROCHLORIDE

Indications: acute hypotension
Cautions; Contra-indications: see under Metaraminol Tartrate; also contra-indicated in severe hypertension and hyperthyroidism
Side-effects: hypertension with headache, palpitations, vomiting; tachycardia or reflex bradycardia; tingling and coolness of skin
Dose: by subcutaneous or intramuscular injection, 5 mg
By slow intravenous injection, 100–500 micrograms
By intravenous infusion, 5–20 mg

Phenylephrine Injection 1%, phenylephrine hydrochloride 10 mg/ml. Price 1-ml amp = **B**

2.8 Anticoagulants and Protamine

The main use of anticoagulants is to prevent thrombus formation or the extension of an existing thrombus in the slower-moving venous side of the circulation, where the thrombus consists of a fibrin web enmeshed with platelets and red cells. Anticoagulants are therefore widely used in the prevention and treatment of deep-vein thrombosis in the legs.

Anticoagulants are of less use in preventing thrombus formation in arteries, for in faster-flowing vessels thrombi are composed mainly of platelets with little fibrin. Anticoagulants are used to prevent thrombi forming on prosthetic heart valves. Any success anticoagulants have had in reducing mortality after myocardial infarction is probably due to the decreased incidence of deep-vein thrombosis in recumbent patients.

2.8.1 Parenteral anticoagulants

Heparin is given to initiate anticoagulation and is rapidly effective. As its effects are short-lived it is best given by continuous infusion; if given by intermittent intravenous injection, the interval between doses must not exceed 6 hours. Oral anticoagulants are started at the same time, and the heparin infusion withdrawn after 3 days.

If oral anticoagulants cannot be given and heparin is continued, its dose is adjusted after determination of the whole blood clotting time or partial thromboplastin time.

If haemorrhage occurs it is usually sufficient to withdraw heparin, but if rapid reversal of the effects of heparin is required, protamine sulphate is a specific antidote (section 2.8.3).

For the prophylaxis of thrombosis in patients undergoing heart surgery or renal dialysis full therapeutic doses of heparin are given for the duration of the procedure. Low-dose heparin by subcutaneous injection is used to prevent post-operative deep-vein thrombosis and pulmonary embolism. Laboratory monitoring is not required with this regimen.

Ancrod (Arvin®) has been shown to be as effective as heparin in the resolution of deep-vein thromboses, but some patients develop resistance. The initial infusion must be given slowly, as there is a risk of massive intravascular formation of unstable fibrin. The response can be monitored by observing clot size after blood has been allowed to stand for about 2 hours, the aim being to predict a dose that produces a 2–3 mm clot. Alternatively, plasma-fibrinogen concentrations can be measured directly.

The major complication is haemorrhage. Since it takes 12–24 hours to reach haemostatic fibrinogen concentrations after administration has ceased it may be necessary to give ancrod antivenom (0.2-ml test dose subcutaneously followed by 0.8 ml intramuscularly, and 30 minutes later 1 ml intravenously). Anaphylaxis may occur and adrenaline and hydrocortisone should be available. As an alternative to antiserum, reconstituted freeze-dried fibrinogen may be given. Subcutaneous injection of ancrod has been used for prophylaxis in patients likely to develop deep-vein thrombosis.

HEPARIN

Indications: deep-vein thrombosis, disseminated intravascular coagulation, prevention of post-operative thrombosis

Contra-indications: haemophilia and other haemorrhagic disorders, peptic ulcer, cerebral aneurysm, severe hypertension, severe liver disease, bacterial endocarditis
Side-effects: haemorrhage, thrombocytopenia, hypersensitivity reactions; osteoporosis after prolonged use
Dose: *by intravenous injection,* loading dose of 5000 units followed by continuous *infusion* of 40 000 units over 24 hours *or* 10 000 units by *intravenous injection* every 6 hours
By subcutaneous injection, 5000 units before surgery, then every 12 hours until patient is ambulant

Heparin Injection (heparin sodium)
1000 units/ml. Price 5-ml amp = **C**; 5-ml vial = **B**
5000 units/ml. Price 5-ml amp or vial = **D**
25 000 units/ml. Price 0.2-ml amp = **B**
Heparin Injection (heparin calcium)
25 000 units/ml (subcutaneous). Price 0.2-ml amp = **B**; 0.2-ml syringe = **C**
Calciparine® (Labaz)
Injection (subcutaneous), heparin calcium 25 000 units/ml. Price 0.2-ml syringe = **C**
Heparin Retard® (Boots)
Injection (intramuscular or subcutaneous), heparin sodium 10 000 units/ml. Price 2-ml amp = **E**
Hep-Rinse® (Leo)
Injection, heparin sodium 100 units/ml. Price 2-ml amp = **B**
Dose: to maintain patency of catheters, cannulae, etc., 200 units flushed through every 4–8 hours. Not for therapeutic use
Hepsal® (Weddel)
Solution (sterile), heparin sodium 10 units/ml. Price 5-ml amp = **A**
Dose: to maintain patency of catheters, cannulae, etc., 50 units flushed through every 4 hours. Not for systemic administration
Minihep® (Leo)
Injection (subcutaneous), heparin sodium 25 000 units/ml. Price 0.2-ml amp = **B**
Minihep Calcium® (Leo)
Injection (subcutaneous), heparin calcium 25 000 units/ml. Price 0.2-ml amp = **B**
Uniparin® (Weddel)
Injection (subcutaneous), heparin sodium 25 000 units/ml. Price 0.2-ml syringe = **C**

ANCROD

Indications: deep-vein thrombosis, prevention of postoperative thrombosis
Cautions; Contra-indications; Side-effects: see under Heparin; resistance may develop
Dose: *by intravenous infusion,* 2 units/kg over 6–12 hours, then *by infusion or slow intravenous injection,* 2 units/kg every 12 hours

Arvin® (Berk)
Injection, ancrod 70 units/ml. Price 1-ml amp = **I** (Hosp. only)

2.8.2 Oral anticoagulants

They antagonise the effects of vitamin K, and take 36–48 hours for the anticoagulant effect to develop; if an immediate effect is required, heparin must be given concomitantly. The dose of oral anticoagulants is adjusted to prolong the prothrombin time to 2–3 times normal values. The prothrombin time should be measured daily from the 4th day of treatment, at weekly intervals once a steady dose has been established, then monthly.

The main indication for oral anticoagulant therapy is deep-vein thrombosis. Patients with poorly controlled atrial fibrillation who are at risk of embolisation should also be treated, as should patients with heart valve prostheses, to prevent emboli developing on the valves; antiplatelet drugs may also be useful in these patients.

Oral anticoagulants should not be used in cerebral thrombosis or peripheral arterial occlusion, but may be of value in patients with transient brain ischaemic attacks whether due to carotid or vertebrobasilar arterial disease; if these patients also have severe hypertension anticoagulants are contra-indicated, and antiplatelet drugs are an alternative (section 2.9).

Warfarin and other coumarins are the drugs of choice, as they are less likely to cause sensitivity reactions than phenindione.

The main adverse effect of all oral anticoagulants is haemorrhage; if this is mild, omission of several doses may be all that is required. If it is more serious, blood transfusion or phytomenadione (vitamin K_1) is required; the dose is 10–20 mg given intravenously, but will take up to 12 hours to act and will prevent oral anticoagulants from acting for several days or even weeks (see section 9.6.6).

Minor bleeding is usually shown as bruising, haematuria, or melaena, while massive bleeding may occur into viscera, muscles, or brain, when it is likely to be fatal. Placental and foetal haemorrhage may also occur.

Haemorrhage is more likely in patients with liver disease, and those who are taking other drugs such as phenylbutazone, aspirin, or clofibrate. Patients taking a fixed dose of warfarin and a microsomal enzyme-inducing agent such as phenobarbitone are at risk of haemorrhage if the barbiturate is withdrawn and the anticoagulant dose maintained.

Oral anticoagulants are weakly teratogenic and should not be given in the first trimester of pregnancy. Also, since they cross the placenta, they should not be given in the last few weeks of pregnancy. The elderly are more sensitive to the effects of oral anticoagulants and the starting dose should be lower and great attention paid to subsequent monitoring.

Anticoagulant treatment cards must be carried by patients, and cards are available from:
DHSS Store
No. 2 Site
Manchester Rd

Heywood
Lancs OL10 2PZ
In Scotland the cards are available from:
SHHD (Div IIID)
Room 9
St. Andrew's House
Edinburgh EH1 3DE

WARFARIN SODIUM

Indications: deep-vein thrombosis, transient brain ischaemic attacks, prophylaxis with prosthetic heart valves
Cautions: hepatic or renal disease, recent surgery. Drug interactions: see Appendix 1
Contra-indications: first trimester and last weeks of pregnancy, peptic ulcer, severe hypertension, bacterial endocarditis
Side-effects: haemorrhage
Dose: 10 mg daily for 3 days; maintenance usually 3–10 mg daily

Marevan® (DF)
Tablets, brown, scored, warfarin sodium 1 mg. Price 20 tabs = **A**
Tablets, blue, scored, warfarin sodium 3 mg. Price 20 tabs = **A**
Tablets, pink, scored, warfarin sodium 5 mg. Price 20 tabs = **A**
Warfarin WBP (WBP)
Tablets, brown, scored, warfarin sodium 1 mg. Price 20 tabs = **A**
Tablets, blue, scored, warfarin sodium 3 mg. Price 20 tabs = **A**
Tablets, pink, scored, warfarin sodium 5 mg. Price 20 tabs = **A**

NICOUMALONE

Indications: deep-vein thrombosis, transient brain ischaemic attacks, prophylaxis with prosthetic heart valves
Cautions; Contra-indications; Side-effects: see under Warfarin Sodium
Dose: 8–16 mg on 1st day; 4–12 mg on 2nd day; maintenance dose usually 1–6 mg daily

Sinthrome® (Geigy)
Tablets, pink, nicoumalone 1 mg. Price 20 tabs = **A**
Tablets, scored, nicoumalone 4 mg. Price 20 tabs = **B**

PHENINDIONE

Indications: deep-vein thrombosis
Cautions; Contra-indications; Side-effects: see under Warfarin Sodium; also hypersensitivity reactions including rashes, fever, leucopenia, agranulocytosis, diarrhoea, renal and hepatic damage; urine coloured pink
Dose: 200 mg on 1st day; 100 mg on 2nd day; maintenance dose usually 50–150 mg daily

Dindevan® (DF)
Tablets, phenindione 10 mg. Price 20 tabs = **A**
Tablets, green, phenindione 25 mg. Price 20 tabs = **A**
Tablets, phenindione 50 mg. Price 20 tabs = **B**

2.8.3 Protamine sulphate

Although protamine sulphate is used to counteract overdosage with heparin, if used in excess protamine has an anticoagulant effect.

PROTAMINE SULPHATE

Indications: neutralisation of the anticoagulant effect of heparin
Cautions: overdose of protamine sulphate has an anticoagulant effect
Side-effects: flushing, hypotension, bradycardia
Dose: by slow intravenous injection, 1 mg neutralises 100 units heparin when given within 15 minutes; if a longer time has elapsed, less protamine is required as heparin is rapidly excreted; max. dose 50 mg

Protamine Sulphate Injection, protamine sulphate 10 mg/ml. Price 5-ml amp = **B**

2.9 Antiplatelet drugs

By decreasing platelet adhesiveness, these drugs may inhibit thrombus formation on the arterial side of the circulation, where thrombi are formed by platelet aggregation and anticoagulants have little effect. Antiplatelet drugs have little effect in venous thromboembolism.

Dipyridamole (Persantin®) is used with anticoagulants to prevent thrombus formation on prosthetic valves, and its use in diabetic retinopathy is under investigation. **Aspirin** (section 10.1.1.1) and **sulphinpyrazone** (Anturan®) are under investigation for prophylactic use in coronary disease including infarction, and transient brain ischaemic attacks, but appropriate dosage has not been established.

DIPYRIDAMOLE

Indications: thromboembolism, angina
Cautions: may exacerbate migraine, hypotension. Drug interactions: see Appendix 1
Side-effects: nausea, diarrhoea, throbbing headache, hypotension
Dose: angina, *by mouth,* 50 mg 3 times daily
By slow intravenous injection, 10–20 mg 2–3 times daily
Thromboembolism, *by mouth,* 100–200 mg 3–4 times daily before food

Persantin® (Boehringer Ingelheim)
Tablets, orange, s/c, dipyridamole 25 mg. Price 20 tabs = **C**
Tablets, s/c, dipyridamole 100 mg. Price 20 tabs = **E**
Injection, dipyridamole 5 mg/ml. Price 2-ml amp = **A**

SULPHINPYRAZONE

Indications: prophylaxis after myocardial infarction (for use in gout, see section 10.1.4)
Cautions; Contra-indications; Side-effects: see section 10.1.4
Dose: 200 mg 4 times daily with food, starting 1 month after infarction

▼ **Anturan**® (Geigy)
Tablets, yellow, s/c, sulphinpyrazone 200 mg. Price 28 tabs = **E**

2.10 Fibrinolytic drugs

These activate plasminogen to form plasmin, which degrades fibrin and so breaks up thrombi. **Streptokinase** is used in the treatment of life-threatening venous thrombosis, and in pulmonary embolism. Treatment must be started rapidly, within an hour of the event, and controlled by measurement of the thrombin clotting time. Corticosteroids or antihistamines may be required to control allergic reactions.

Urokinase is currently used for thrombolysis in the eye and in arteriovenous shunts; its use in pulmonary embolism is under study. It has the advantage of being non-antigenic.

STREPTOKINASE

Indications: venous thrombosis, pulmonary embolism
Cautions: atrial fibrillation, recovery from streptococcal infection
Contra-indications: recent haemorrhage, coagulation defects, severe hypertension, streptococcal infections, surgery in previous 72 hours, menstruation, first 18 weeks of pregnancy
Side-effects: allergic reactions, fever, rashes, haemorrhage (if due to overdose, can give tranexamic acid)
Dose: *by intravenous infusion,* 250 000–600 000 units over 30 minutes, then 100 000 units every hour for up to 1 week

Kabikinase® (KabiVitrum)
Injection, powder for reconstitution, streptokinase 100 000 units, price per vial = **H**; 250 000 and 600 000 units, price per vial (both) = **J**

Streptase® (Hoechst)
Injection, powder for reconstitution, streptokinase 100 000 units, price per vial = **G**; 250 000 and 750 000 units, price per vial (both) = **J**

UROKINASE

Indications: thrombosed arteriovenous shunts; thrombolysis in the eye
Contra-indications: recent haemorrhage, surgery in previous 72 hours, pregnancy
Side-effects: haemorrhage (if due to overdose, give aminocaproic acid), fever
Dose: *by instillation into arteriovenous shunt,* 5000–37 500 International units in 2–3 ml sodium chloride intravenous infusion
Intra-ocular administration, 5000–37 500 International units in 2 ml sodium chloride intravenous infusion
Note: 1.5 International units ≈ 1 Ploug unit

▼ **Abbokinase**® (Abbott)
Injection, powder for reconstitution, urokinase 250 000 International units. Price per vial = **J**
Dose: in pulmonary embolism, by intravenous infusion, 4400 units/kg over 10 minutes, then 4400 units/kg/hour for 12 hours

Ukidan (Serono)
Injection, powder for reconstitution, urokinase 5000 International units, price per vial = **G**; 25 000 International units, price per vial = **J**

Urokinase (Leo)
Injection, powder for reconstitution, urokinase 7500 International units (5000 Ploug units), price per amp = **I**; 37 500 International units (25 000 Ploug units) and 150 000 International units (100 000 Ploug units), price per amp (both) = **J**

2.11 Antifibrinolytic drugs

Fibrin stabilisation can be encouraged by the administration of **aminocaproic acid** (Epsikapron®) or **tranexamic acid** (Cyklokapron®), which inhibit plasminogen activation and interfere with fibrinolysis. They may be useful when haemorrhage cannot be staunched, for example in prostatectomy, dental extraction in haemophiliacs, or menorrhagia associated with intra-uterine contraceptive devices.

Ethamsylate (Dicynene®) has similar uses but its mode of action is unknown.

Aprotinin (section 1.9.3) is used in disseminated intravascular coagulation.

AMINOCAPROIC ACID

Indications: haemorrhage after surgery, particularly prostatectomy, menorrhagia
Cautions: lower dose in renal impairment, haemophilia
Contra-indications: history of thromboembolic disease, early pregnancy
Side-effects: nausea, diarrhoea, dizziness
Dose: 3 g 4–6 times daily

Epsikapron® (KabiVitrum)
Powder, effervescent, aminocaproic acid 3 g in sachet. Price 10 sachets = **E**
Syrup (= mixture), aminocaproic acid 1.5 g/5 ml. Price 100 ml = **E**

ETHAMSYLATE

Indications: haemorrhage from small blood vessels
Side-effects: nausea, headache, rashes
Dose: *by mouth,* 500 mg 4 times daily

By intramuscular or intravenous injection, 0.75–1 g

Dicynene® (Delandale)
Tablets, ethamsylate 250 mg. Price 20 tabs = **D**
Tablets, ethamsylate 500 mg. Price 20 tabs = **F**
Injection, ethamsylate 125 mg/ml. Price 2-ml amp = **C**
Injection, ethamsylate 500 mg/ml. Price 2-ml syringe = **E**

TRANEXAMIC ACID

Indications: see under Aminocaproic Acid; also streptokinase overdose
Cautions; Contra-indications; Side-effects: see under Aminocaproic Acid
Dose: *by mouth,* 1 g 3–4 times daily
By slow intravenous injection, 1–2 g 3 times daily

Cyklokapron® (KabiVitrum)
Tablets, tranexamic acid 500 mg. Price 20 tabs = **F**
Injection, tranexamic acid 100 mg/ml. Price 5-ml amp = **D**

2.12 Drugs used in the treatment of hyperlipidaemia

Five categories of hyperlipidaemia are recognised, the most common being Type II, familial hypercholesterolaemia in which cholesterol binds to lipoprotein and elevates the concentration of low-density lipoproteins (LDL), and Type IV, in which concentrations of serum triglycerides and thus very-low-density lipoproteins (VLDL) are elevated.

Any drug treatment given must be combined with a strict dietary regimen. Young patients with severe hyperlipidaemia who already have ischaemic heart disease or have a family history of vascular disease seem most likely to benefit.

Clofibrate (Atromid-S®) inhibits cholesterol formation in the liver and reduces binding of triglycerides to lipoproteins. It is used in the treatment of both Type II and Type IV hyperlipidaemia, but may increase the incidence of gallstones.

Cholestyramine (Questran®) and **colestipol** (Colestid®) are ion-exchange resins which bind cholesterol and prevent its reabsorption from the gut; they are used in Type II hyperlipidaemia.

Dextrothyroxine (Choloxin®) lowers the blood cholesterol concentration so is used in Type II hyperlipidaemia, but may cause tachycardia and, in patients with ischaemic heart disease, angina.

Probucol (Lurselle®) lowers serum concentrations of cholesterol by increasing the excretion of bile acids; absorption of cholesterol may also be decreased.

Nicotinic acid and **nicofuranose** (Bradilan®) reduce both cholesterol and triglyceride concentrations, so are used in Type II hyperlipidaemia, but effective doses cause flushing and postural hypotension.

BEZAFIBRATE

Indications: hypercholesterolaemia and hyperlipidaemia
Cautions: reduced dose in moderate renal impairment. Drug interactions: see Appendix 1
Contra-indications: severe renal or hepatic impairment, primary biliary cirrhosis, nephrotic syndrome, pregnancy
Side-effects: abdominal discomfort; rarely myositis-like syndrome, hypersensitivity
Dose: 600 mg daily; may be reduced to 400 mg daily in hypertriglyceridaemia

Bezalip® (MCP)
Tablets, f/c, bezafibrate 200 mg. Price 20 tabs = **E**

CHOLESTYRAMINE

Indications: hypercholesterolaemia, Type II hyperlipidaemia
Cautions: supplements of fat-soluble vitamins required with high doses. Drug interactions: see Appendix 1
Contra-indications: complete biliary obstruction
Side-effects: nausea, constipation, heartburn, rashes
Dose: 12–16 g daily in liquid, in divided doses; up to 36 g may be required

Questran® (Bristol)
Powder, sachets, cholestyramine (anhydrous) 4 g. Price 10 sachets = **F**

CLOFIBRATE

Indications: hyperlipidaemia, especially Type IV
Cautions: impaired liver or kidney function, low serum-albumin concentrations. Drug interactions: see Appendix 1
Contra-indications: pregnancy
Side-effects: nausea, diarrhoea, myalgia
Dose: 1.5–2 g daily in divided doses after meals

Atromid-S® (ICI)
Capsules, red, clofibrate 500 mg. Price 20 caps = **C**

COLESTIPOL HYDROCHLORIDE

Indications: hypercholesterolaemia, Type II hyperlipidaemia
Cautions; Contra-indications; Side-effects: see under Cholestyramine
Dose: 15–20 g daily in liquid, in 2–4 divided doses

▼ **Colestid®** (Upjohn)
Granules, yellow, colestipol hydrochloride. Price 10 × 5-g sachets = **F**; 250-g bottle = **J**

DEXTROTHYROXINE SODIUM

Indications: hypercholesterolaemia, Type II hyperlipidaemia
Cautions: ischaemic heart disease. Drug interactions: see Appendix 1
Contra-indications: severe kidney or liver disease

Side-effects: tachycardia, angina in patients with ischaemic heart disease
Dose: 1–2 mg daily, increased by 1–2 mg at monthly intervals; max. dose 8 mg daily

Choloxin® (Travenol)
Tablets, yellow, scored, dextrothyroxine sodium 2 mg. Price 20 tabs = **G**

NICOTINIC ACID AND DERIVATIVES
Indications: hyperlipidaemia, especially Type II (for use in peripheral vascular disease, see section 2.6.3)
Cautions; Side-effects: see section 2.6.3
Dose: nicotinic acid, 1–2 g 3 times daily; nicofuranose, 0.5–1 g 3 times daily

Nicotinic Acid Tablets, nicotinic acid 25, 50, and 100 mg. Price 20 tabs (all) = **A**
Bradilan® (Napp)
Tablets, e/c and s/c, nicofuranose 250 mg. Price 20 tabs = **D**

PROBUCOL
Indications: hypercholesterolaemia
Cautions: in women of childbearing age; avoid pregnancy during and for 6 months after stopping treatment
Contra-indications: pregnancy
Side-effects: nausea, vomiting, flatulence, diarrhoea, abdominal pain; rarely angioneurotic oedema, hypersensitivity reactions
Dose: 500 mg twice daily

▼ **Lurselle®** (Lepetit)
Tablets, probucol 250 mg. Price 20 tabs = **E**

2.13 Local sclerosants

Ethanolamine oleate and sodium tetradecyl sulphate are used in sclerotherapy of varicose veins, and phenol is used in thrombosed haemorrhoids (see section 1.7.4).

ETHANOLAMINE OLEATE
Indications: sclerotherapy of varicose veins
Cautions: extravasation may cause necrosis of tissues
Contra-indications: inability to walk, acute phlebitis, oral contraceptive use, obese legs
Side-effects: allergic reactions

Ethanolamine Oleate Injection, ethanolamine oleate 5%. Price 2- and 5-ml amp (both) = **B**
Dose: by intravenous injection, 2–5 ml divided between 3–4 sites; repeated at weekly intervals

---

SODIUM TETRADECYL SULPHATE
Indications: sclerotherapy of varicose veins
Cautions; Contra-indications; Side-effects: see under Ethanolamine Oleate

STD® (STD Pharmaceutical)
Injection, sodium tetradecyl sulphate 3%. Price 1-ml amp = **B**; 30-ml vial = **F**
Dose: by intravenous injection, 0.5–1 ml at up to 4 sites; repeated after 2 weeks if necessary

3: Drugs used in the treatment of diseases of the RESPIRATORY SYSTEM

In this chapter, drug treatment is described under the following headings:

The treatment of upper respiratory tract infections leading to exacerbation of chronic bronchitis and pneumonia is indicated in section 5.1 (table 1) and the treatment of tuberculosis is indicated in section 5.1.9.

3.1 Bronchodilators

3.1.1 Adrenoceptor stimulants (sympathomimetics)

Most mild or moderate attacks of asthma respond rapidly to *aerosol* administration of a selective beta$_2$-adrenoceptor stimulant. **Salbutamol** (Ventolin®) and **terbutaline** (Bricanyl®) are available in a wide range of formulations and can be given by aerosol inhalation, by mouth, or intravenously (see below—severe asthma). **Fenoterol** (Berotec®) and **rimiterol** (Pulmadil®) are available as aerosol inhalations and **isoetharine** (Numotac®) as tablets. **Reproterol** (Bronchodil®) is a new drug available as an aerosol inhalation and tablets. These selective beta$_2$-adrenoceptor stimulants are preferable to the non-selective drugs adrenaline, ephedrine, isoprenaline, methoxyphenamine, and pseudoephedrine and the partly selective orciprenaline which also stimulate the heart rate.

All bronchodilator aerosols act for about 3–5 hours after inhalation (rimiterol less than the others). Patients should be advised that if they fail to obtain their usual degree of symptomatic relief they should seek medical advice. In such circumstances a short course of corticosteroid therapy by mouth will usually be required to bring the asthma under control (see section 6.3.4).

Aerosol inhalations provide relief more rapidly than *tablets* and are generally preferable to preparations of beta$_2$-adrenoceptor stimulants given systemically since the higher doses usually required by mouth may result in tremor or nervous tension. Oral preparations are often used in children but many can use an inhaler successfully if taught and supervised by parents, provided they understand that it should not be used excessively. Some adrenoceptor stimulants are available both as pressurised aerosol inhalations and as insufflation cartridges. A decision on which form is the more suitable should be made for each patient.

In severe bronchospasm or status asthmaticus, beta$_2$-adrenoceptor stimulants such as salbutamol or terbutaline may be given intravenously and this is usually preferable to intravenous aminophylline. Alternatively, large doses may be administered as an aqueous aerosol inhaled from a nebuliser or delivered by intermittent positive-pressure ventilation through a tightly-fitting mask. However, the treatment of patients with severe asthma is safer in hospital, where oxygen therapy and resuscitation facilities are immediately available.

In many instances the dose or frequency of administration of beta$_2$-adrenoceptor stimulants can be reduced by use in conjunction with corticosteroid aerosol inhalations (which are normally preferable to the systemic use of corticosteroids) or by use of sodium cromoglycate (section 3.3).

EMERGENCY TREATMENT. *Severe asthma* can be fatal and must be treated promptly and energetically. It is characterised by persistent dyspnoea poorly relieved by bronchodilators, restlessness, exhaustion, a high pulse rate (usually over 110/minute), and a very low peak expiratory flow. The respiration is so shallow that wheezing may be absent. Such patients should be given salbutamol or terbutaline by subcutaneous or intravenous injection, or aminophylline by slow intravenous injection. They must also be given a large dose of a corticosteroid—adults 200 mg of hydrocortisone (as sodium phosphate or succinate) intravenously or 40 mg of prednisolone orally, children half these doses (see also section 3.2).

The further treatment of these patients is safer in hospital where oxygen therapy and resuscitation facilities are immediately available. Treatment should never be delayed for investigations, patients should never be sedated, and the possibility of a pneumothorax should also be remembered.

3.1.1.1 SELECTIVE BETA$_2$-ADRENOCEPTOR STIMULANTS

SALBUTAMOL

Indications: bronchospasm, status asthmaticus
Cautions: hyperthyroidism, ischaemic heart disease. Caution in intravenous administration to diabetics

Side-effects: tachycardia, tremor, headache, dizziness; seldom troublesome when given by aerosol inhalation

Dose: *by mouth,* 3–4 times daily, 2–4 mg; CHILD 2–5 years 1–2 mg, 6–12 years 2 mg

By subcutaneous or intramuscular injection, 500 micrograms every 4 hours

By slow intravenous injection, 250 micrograms, repeated if necessary

By continuous intravenous infusion, 3–20 micrograms/minute

By aerosol inhalation, 100–200 micrograms (1–2 puffs) 3–4 times daily (every 4 hours in severe bronchospasm); CHILD 100 micrograms (1 puff) 3–4 times daily

By inhalation of powder (insufflation cartridges), 200–400 micrograms 3–4 times daily (every 4 hours in severe bronchospasm); CHILD 200 micrograms 3–4 times daily

By inhalation of nebulised solution (respirator solution), 2 ml of a 0.5% solution (over a period of 3 minutes) 4 times daily, or 1–2 mg per hour as a solution containing 0.005–0.01%. (50–100 micrograms/ml)

Oral preparations

Ventolin® (A&H)

Tablets, pink, salbutamol 2 mg (as sulphate). Price 20 tabs = **B**

Tablets, pink, salbutamol 4 mg (as sulphate). Price 20 tabs = **C**

Spandets® (= tablets s/r), pink/white, salbutamol 8 mg (as sulphate). Price 20 tabs = **D**

Dose: 8 mg twice daily, increased if necessary to a max. of 32 mg daily; CHILD over 12 years 8 mg twice daily

Syrup (=elixir), red, salbutamol 2 mg (as sulphate)/5 ml. Diluent syrup (without preservative), life of diluted elixir 14 days. Price 100 ml = **C**

Parenteral preparations

Ventolin® (A&H)

Injection, salbutamol 50 micrograms (as sulphate)/ml. Price 5-ml amp = **C**

Injection, salbutamol 500 micrograms (as sulphate)/ml. Price 1-ml amp = **B**

Solution for intravenous infusion, salbutamol 1 mg (as sulphate)/ml. Price 5-ml amp = **F**

Inhalation preparations

Ventolin® (A&H)

Inhaler (= aerosol inhalation), salbutamol 100 micrograms/metered inhalation, 200-dose unit. Price (complete unit) = **E**

Advise patients not to exceed prescribed dose and to follow manufacturer's directions

Rotacaps® (= insufflation cartridges), light blue/clear, salbutamol 200 micrograms (as sulphate). Price 20 cartridges = **D**

Rotacaps® (= insufflation cartridges), dark blue/clear, salbutamol 400 micrograms (as sulphate). Price 20 cartridges = **D**

Rotahaler® (for use with Rotacaps). Price per unit = **C**

Respirator solution (for use with a nebuliser or ventilator), salbutamol 0.5% (5 mg/ml, as sulphate). Price 20 ml = **F**

TERBUTALINE SULPHATE

Indications; Cautions; Side-effects: see under Salbutamol

Dose: *by mouth,* 5 mg 2–3 times daily; CHILD 2–5 years 0.75–1.5 mg 3 times daily, 6–12 years 2.5 mg 2–3 times daily

By subcutaneous, intramuscular, or slow intravenous injection, 250–500 micrograms 2–4 times daily; CHILD 2–15 years 10 micrograms/kg to a max. of 300 micrograms

By continuous intravenous infusion, 1.5–5 micrograms/minute for 8–10 hours; reduce dose for children

By aerosol inhalation, 250–500 micrograms (1–2 puffs) 3–4 times daily (every 4 hours in severe bronchospasm); CHILD 250 micrograms (1 puff) 3–4 times daily

By inhalation of nebulised solution (respirator solution), 2–5 mg increasing if necessary to 10 mg

Bricanyl® (Astra)

Tablets, scored, terbutaline sulphate 5 mg. Price 20 tabs = **C**

Syrup (= elixir), terbutaline sulphate 1.5 mg/5 ml. Diluent water, life of diluted elixir 14 days. Price 100 ml = **C**

Injection, terbutaline sulphate 500 micrograms/ml. Price 1-ml amp = **A**

Inhaler (= aerosol inhalation), terbutaline sulphate 250 micrograms/metered inhalation, 400-dose unit. Price (complete unit) = **G**

Advise patients not to exceed prescribed dose and to follow manufacturer's directions

Spacer inhaler (= aerosol inhalation), terbutaline sulphate 250 micrograms/metered inhalation in 'spacer' unit (extended mouthpiece device), 400-dose unit. Price (complete unit) = **H**

Advise patients as above

Respirator solution (for use with a nebuliser or ventilator), terbutaline sulphate 10 mg/ml. rice 10 ml = **C**

Bricanyl SA® (Astra)

Tablets, s/r, terbutaline sulphate 7.5 mg. Price 20 tabs = **D**

Dose: 7.5 mg twice daily.

FENOTEROL HYDROBROMIDE

Indications: bronchospasm

Cautions; Side-effects: see under Salbutamol

Dose: *by aerosol inhalation,* 180–360 micrograms (1–2 puffs) 3–4 times daily (every 4 hours in severe bronchospasm); CHILD 180 micrograms (1 puff) 3–4 times daily

▼ **Berotec®** (WBP)

Inhaler (= aerosol inhalation), fenoterol hydrobromide 180 micrograms/metered inhalation, 200-dose unit. Price (complete unit) = **E**

Advise patients not to exceed prescribed dose and to follow manufacturer's directions

ISOETHARINE HYDROCHLORIDE

Indications: bronchospasm
Cautions; Side-effects: see under Salbutamol
Dose: 10–20 mg 3–4 times daily

Numotac® (Riker)
Tablets, s/r, isoetharine hydrochloride 10 mg. Price 20 tabs = **C**

REPROTEROL HYDROCHLORIDE

Indications: bronchospasm
Cautions; Side-effects: see under Salbutamol
Dose: by mouth, 20 mg 3 times daily, reduced to 10 mg 3 times daily if side-effects occur; CHILD 6–12 years 10 mg 3 times daily
By aerosol inhalation, 0.5–1 mg (1–2 puffs) 3–4 times daily, max. 1 mg (2 puffs) every 3 hours; CHILD 6–12 years 500 micrograms (1 puff) 3 times daily, max. 500 micrograms (1 puff) every 3 hours

▼ Bronchodil® (Keymer)
Tablets, scored, reproterol hydrochloride 20 mg. Price 20 tabs = **C**
Aerosol inhalation, reproterol hydrochloride 500 micrograms/metered inhalation, 400-dose unit. Price (complete unit) = **G**
Advise patients not to exceed prescribed dose and to follow manufacturer's directions

RIMITEROL HYDROBROMIDE

Indications: bronchospasm
Cautions; Side-effects: see under Salbutamol
Dose: by aerosol inhalation, 200–600 micrograms (1–3 puffs) 3–4 times daily as required; the dose should not be repeated within 30 minutes and not more than 8 times in 24 hours

Pulmadil® (Riker)
Inhaler (= aerosol inhalation), rimiterol hydrobromide 200 micrograms/metered inhalation, 300-dose unit. Price (complete unit) = **G**
Advise patients not to exceed prescribed dose and to follow manufacturer's directions
Auto (= aerosol inhalation), rimiterol hydrobromide 200 micrograms/metered inhalation, 300-dose cartridge in breath-actuated unit. Price (complete unit) = **H**; replacement cartridge = **G**
Advise patients as above

3.1.1.2 NON-SELECTIVE ADRENOCEPTOR STIMULANTS

These preparations are now regarded as less suitable and less safe as bronchodilators than the selective beta$_2$-adrenoceptor stimulants, as they are more likely to cause cardiac irregularities and other side-effects (section 3.4).

Adrenaline is used by injection in the emergency treatment of acute allergic and anaphylactic reactions.

ADRENALINE

Indications: bronchospasm, emergency treatment of acute anaphylaxis
Cautions: hyperthyroidism, diabetes, ischaemic heart disease, ventricular excitability induced by cyclopropane, digitalis, halothane, mercurial diuretics, quinidine, or tricyclic antidepressants. Not to be given intravenously because of increased risk of cardiac irregularities. Drug interactions: see Appendix 1
Side-effects: anxiety, tremor, tachycardia, cardiac arrhythmias; seldom troublesome when given by aerosol inhalation
Dose: bronchospasm, as a single dose, *by subcutaneous or intramuscular injection,* 200–500 micrograms
By aerosol inhalation, adrenaline acid tartrate 280–560 micrograms (1–2 puffs) up to 3–4 times daily
By inhalation of nebulised solution, adrenaline 200–500 micrograms
Acute anaphylaxis, *by subcutaneous or intramuscular injection,* 0.5–1 mg

Adrenaline Injection, adrenaline 1 in 1000 (adrenaline acid tartrate 1.8 mg/ml). Price 0.5- and 1-ml amp (both) = **A**

Adrenaline Solution, adrenaline 1 in 1000 (adrenaline acid tartrate 1.8 mg/ml). For use with nebuliser. Price 25- and 28-ml (both) = **B**; 100 ml = **D**

Adrenaline and Atropine Spray, Compound—see section 3.1.4

Medihaler-Epi® (Riker) *aerosol inhalation,* adrenaline acid tartrate 280 micrograms/metered inhalation, 400-dose unit. Price (complete unit) = **E**. Advise patients not to exceed prescribed dose and to follow manufacturer's directions

EPHEDRINE HYDROCHLORIDE

Indications: bronchospasm
Cautions: ischaemic heart disease, hypertension, hyperthyroidism, prostatism. Drug interactions: see Appendix 1
Side-effects: tremor, tachycardia, insomnia, urinary retention
Dose: 3 times daily, 15–60 mg; CHILD 3 times daily, up to 1 year 7.5 mg, 1–5 years 15 mg, 6–12 years 30 mg

Ephedrine Hydrochloride Tablets, ephedrine hydrochloride 15, 30, and 60 mg. Price 20 tabs (all) = **A**

Ephedrine Elixir, yellow, ephedrine hydrochloride 15 mg/5 ml. Diluent syrup, life of diluted elixir 14 days. Price 100 ml = **B**

ISOPRENALINE SULPHATE

Indications: bronchospasm
Cautions: diabetes, ischaemic heart disease, hyperthyroidism
Side-effects: tremor, tachycardia

Dose: by mouth, sublingually, 10–20 mg 3 times daily, increased if necessary to 40 mg
By aerosol inhalation, 160–240 micrograms (2–3 puffs of iso-autohaler or medihaler-iso), or up to 1.2 mg (3 puffs of medihaler-isoforte); the dose should not be repeated within 30 minutes and not more than 8 times in 24 hours
By inhalation of a spray containing 1%, 1 ml

Aleudrin® (Lewis)
Tablets, scored (sublingual), isoprenaline sulphate 20 mg. Price 20 tabs = **B**.
Solution (= spray), isoprenaline sulphate 1%. Price 10 ml = **B**
Iso-Autohaler® (Riker)
Aerosol inhalation, isoprenaline sulphate 80 micrograms/metered inhalation, 400-dose vial in breath-actuated unit. Price (complete unit) = **G**; 400-dose refill vial = **E**. Advise patients not to exceed prescribed dose and to follow manufacturer's directions
Medihaler-Iso® (Riker)
Aerosol inhalation, isoprenaline sulphate 80 micrograms/metered inhalation, 400-dose vial. Price (complete unit) = **E**. Advise patients as above.
Medihaler-Iso Forte® (Riker)
Aerosol inhalation, isoprenaline sulphate 400 micrograms/metered inhalation, 400-dose vial. Price (complete unit) = **F**. Advise patients as above

METHOXYPHENAMINE HYDROCHLORIDE

Indications; bronchospasm
Cautions; Side-effects: see under Isoprenaline Sulphate
Dose: 50–100 mg every 3–4 hours; CHILD 25–50 mg every 4–6 hours

Orthoxine Hydrochloride® (Upjohn) *tablets,* scored, methoxyphenamine hydrochloride 100 mg. Price 20 tabs = **C**

ORCIPRENALINE SULPHATE

Indications: bronchospasm
Cautions; Side-effects: see under Isoprenaline Sulphate
Dose: *by mouth,* 20 mg 4 times daily; CHILD up to 1 year 5–10 mg 3 times daily, 1–5 years 5–10 mg 4 times daily, 6–12 years 40–60 mg daily in divided doses
By deep intramuscular injection, 500 micrograms, repeated if necessary after 30 minutes; CHILD up to 5 years 250 micrograms
By aerosol inhalation, 670–1340 micrograms (1–2 puffs) up to 6 times daily; CHILD up to 6 years 670 micrograms (1 puff) up to 4 times daily, 6–12 years 670–1340 micrograms (1–2 puffs) up to 4 times daily
By inhalation of nebulised solution (inhalant solution), up to 1 minute with 5% solution 5–10 times daily

Alupent® (Boehringer Ingelheim)
Tablets, scored, orciprenaline sulphate 20 mg. Price 20 tabs = **C**.
Syrup (= elixir), orciprenaline sulphate 10 mg/5 ml. Diluents syrup or sorbitol solution, life of diluted elixir 14 days. Price 100 ml = **C**.
Injection, orciprenaline sulphate 500 micrograms/ml. Price 1-ml amp = **A**.
Metered aerosol (= aerosol inhalation), orciprenaline sulphate 670 micrograms/metered inhalation, 300-dose vial with mouthpiece. Price complete unit (15 ml) = **F**; 300-dose refill vial (15 ml) = **E**. Advise patients not to exceed prescribed dose and to follow manufacturer's directions.
Inhalant solution (for use with nebuliser or ventilator), orciprenaline sulphate 5%. Price 7.5 ml = **C**

3.1.2 Anticholinergic bronchodilators

Atropine-like substances have been used for many years in bronchial asthma, but unpleasant side-effects limit their usefulness. However, the new drug **ipratropium** (Atrovent®) may have a more potent bronchodilator action than the beta$_2$-adrenoceptor stimulants in patients with airways obstruction caused by chronic bronchitis. Unlike other anticholinergic drugs it has been shown not to affect sputum viscosity and mucociliary clearance of sputum. Its onset of action is slow, beginning 30 to 60 minutes after administration and lasting 3–4 hours.

IPRATROPIUM BROMIDE

Indications: bronchospasm in chronic bronchitis, especially when bronchial secretion or patient's intolerance to sympathomimetic drugs is increased
Cautions: glaucoma; prostatic hypertrophy
Side-effects: dry mouth
Dose: *by aerosol inhalation,* 18–36 micrograms (1–2 puffs) 3–4 times daily; CHILD up to 5 years 18 micrograms (1 puff), 6–12 years 18–36 micrograms (1–2 puffs) 3 times daily

▼ **Atrovent®** (Boehringer Ingelheim)
Aerosol inhalation, ipratropium bromide 18 micrograms/metered inhalation, 200-dose unit. Price (complete unit) = **F**
Advise patient not to exceed prescribed dose and to follow manufacturer's directions

3.1.3 Xanthine bronchodilators

The use of **aminophylline** injection intravenously is of established value in the treatment of severe attacks of asthma and is still preferred by many physicians to the intravenous injection of beta$_2$-adrenoceptor stimulants (section 3.1.1.1). However, the latter are probably equally effective and the tremor they are liable to produce may be less disturbing than the vomiting often caused by aminophylline.

There has recently been a revival of interest in oral xanthine derivatives, particularly the newer longer-acting preparations of **aminophylline** and **theophylline** such as Nuelin SA®, Phyllocontin Continus®, Slo-Phyllin®, Theocontin Continus®, and Theograd®. Only occasionally are they more effective than sympathomimetic drugs. However, the sustained-release preparations have the advantage of producing adequate blood concentrations for up to 12 hours, allowing twice-daily dosage and overnight control.

ACEPIFYLLINE

Indications: see under Aminophylline

Cautions; Side-effects: see under Aminophylline; less liable to cause nausea and gastro-intestinal disturbances; intramuscular injection is less painful

Dose: by mouth, 0.5–1 g 3 times daily; CHILD, 3–4 times daily, up to 1 year 62.5 mg, 1–5 years 125 mg, 6–12 years 250 mg

By intramuscular injection, 0.5–2 g daily

By slow intravenous injection, 0.5–1 g when required

By rectum in suppositories, 0.5–1.5 g daily; CHILD 1–5 years 200 mg daily, 6–12 years 300 mg daily

Etophylate® (Delandale)

Tablets, acepifylline 250 mg. Price 20 tabs = **B**

Tablets forte, scored, acepifylline 500 mg. Price 20 tabs = **C**

Syrup (= elixir), yellow, acepifylline 125 mg/5 ml. Diluent syrup, life of diluted elixir 14 days. Price 100 ml = **C**

Syrup forte (= strong elixir), orange, acepifylline 500 mg/5 ml. Diluent as above. Price 100 ml = **D**

Injection, acepifylline 250 mg/ml. Price 2-ml amp = **B**

Suppositories, acepifylline 500 mg. Price 12 suppos = **C**

Suppositories, paediatric, acepifylline 100 mg. Price 12 suppos = **C**

AMINOPHYLLINE

Indications: bronchospasm, status asthmaticus, left ventricular failure

Cautions: liver disease, epilepsy, lactation

Side-effects: tachycardia, palpitations, nausea, gastro-intestinal disturbances, cardiac arrhythmias, and convulsions especially if given rapidly by intravenous injection; use of suppositories for more than a few days may cause proctitis; intramuscular injection is painful (this route is therefore not used)

Dose: by mouth, preferably after meals, 100–300 mg, repeated as necessary; CHILD up to 1 year 10–25 mg, 1–5 years 25–50 mg, 6–12 years 50–100 mg

By slow intravenous injection over a period of at least 10–15 minutes, 250–500 mg; CHILD 5 mg/kg

By rectum in suppositories, 360 mg once or twice daily; CHILD, once or twice daily, up to 1 year 12.5–25 mg, 1–5 years 50–100 mg, 6–12 years 100–200 mg

Aminophylline Tablets, aminophylline 100 mg. Price 20 tabs = **A**

Aminophylline Injection, aminophylline 25 mg/ml. Price 10-ml amp = **B**

Aminophylline 250 mg/ml. Price 2-ml amp = **A**

Aminophylline Suppositories, aminophylline usual strengths 50, 100, 150, 180, and 360 mg. Price 12 suppos 50, 100, 150, and 180 mg = **D**; 360 mg = **C**

Cardophylin® (Fisons)

Tablets, aminophylline 100 mg. Price 20 tabs = **B**

Phyllocontin Continus® (Napp)

Tablets, s/r, yellow, f/c, aminophylline 225 mg. Price 20 tabs = **D**

Dose: 225 mg, increased if necessary to 450 mg twice daily

Tablets, paediatric, s/r, pale orange, aminophylline 100 mg. Price 20 tabs = **C**

Dose: CHILD, twice daily, 4–8 years 100 mg, 9–13 years 100–200 mg

Theodrox® (Riker)

Tablets, aminophylline 195 mg, dried aluminium hydroxide gel 260 mg. Price 20 tabs = **B**

CHOLINE THEOPHYLLINATE

Indications: bronchospasm

Cautions; Side-effects: see under Aminophylline

Dose: by mouth, 100–400 mg 2–4 times daily; CHILD, 3 times daily, 3–5 years 62.5–125 mg, 6–12 years 100 mg

Choledyl® (Warner)

Tablets, pink, compression coated, choline theophyllinate 100 mg. Price 20 tabs = **B**

Tablets, yellow, compression coated, choline theophyllinate 200 mg. Price 20 tabs = **B**

Syrup (= elixir), yellow, choline theophyllinate 62.5 mg/5 ml. Diluent syrup (without preservative), life of diluted elixir 14 days. Price 100 ml = **C**

DIPROPHYLLINE

Indications: see under Aminophylline

Cautions; Side-effects: see under Aminophylline but less liable to cause nausea and gastro-intestinal disturbances; intramuscular injection is less painful

Dose: by mouth, 3–4 times daily, 200–400 mg; CHILD, 3–4 times daily, up to 1 year 10–50 mg, 1–5 years 50–100 mg, 6–12 years 100–200 mg

By intramuscular or slow intravenous injection, up to 3 times daily, 500 mg; CHILD, up to 1 year 5 mg/kg body-weight, 1–5 years 50–100 mg, 6–12 years 100–200 mg

By rectum in suppositories, 400 mg once or twice daily

Silbephylline® (Berk)

Tablets, scored, diprophylline 200 mg. Price 20 tabs = **B**

Syrup (= elixir), red, diprophylline 100 mg/5 ml. Diluent syrup, life of diluted elixir 14 days. Price 100 ml = **C**

Injection, diprophylline 250 mg/ml. Price 2-ml amp = **B**

Suppositories, diprophylline 400 mg. Price 10 suppos = **D**

ETAMIPHYLLINE CAMSYLATE

Indications: see under Aminophylline
Cautions; Side-effects: see under Aminophylline but less liable to cause nausea and gastro-intestinal disturbances; intramuscular injection is less painful
Dose: by mouth, 100–300 mg 3–4 times daily; CHILD, 1–5 years 100 mg, 6–12 years 100–200 mg
By intramuscular injection, 700 mg 3–4 times daily; CHILD, as a 3.5% solution, up to 1 year 10–25 mg, 1–5 years 25–50 mg, 6–12 years 50–100 mg
By slow intravenous injection, as a 3.5% solution, 350 mg, repeated as required; CHILD, doses as for intramuscular route
By rectum in suppositories, 500 mg once or twice daily; CHILD 1–5 years 50–100 mg, 6–12 years 100–200 mg

Millophyline® (Martindale)
Tablets, red, s/c, etamiphylline camsylate 100 mg. Price 20 tabs = **B**
Injection, etamiphylline camsylate 140 mg/ml (14%). Price 5-ml amp = **B**. When necessary dilute with water for injections
Suppositories, adult, etamiphylline camsylate 500 mg. Price 10 suppos = **D**
Suppositories, paediatric, etamiphylline camsylate 200 mg. Price 10 suppos = **D**

PROXYPHYLLINE

Indications: bronchospasm
Cautions; Side-effects: see under Aminophylline but less liable to cause nausea and gastro-intestinal disturbances
Dose: by mouth, 300 mg 3 times daily and 600 mg at night
By rectum in suppositories, 500 mg once or twice daily

Thean® (Astra)
Tablets, scored, proxyphylline 300 mg. Price 20 tabs = **B**
Suppositories, proxyphylline 500 mg. Price 20 suppos = **D**

THEOPHYLLINE

Indications: bronchospasm
Cautions; Side-effects: see under Aminophylline
Dose: by mouth, 60–200 mg 3–4 times daily; CHILD, 3–4 times daily, up to 2 years 4–5 mg/kg body-weight, 2–6 years 60–90 mg, 7–12 years 62.5–125 mg
By rectum in suppositories, 300–600 mg daily

Monotheamin® (Lilly)
Capsules, pink, theophylline monoethanolamine 200 mg. Price 20 caps = **C**
Dose: 400–800 mg daily in divided doses

Nuelin® (Riker)
Tablets, theophylline 125 mg. Price 20 tabs = **C**
Liquid (= elixir), theophylline 60 mg (as sodium glycinate) /5 ml. Diluent syrup, life of diluted elixir 14 days. Price 100 ml = **C**

Nuelin SA® (Riker)
Tablets, s/r, theophylline 175 mg. Price 20 tabs = **C**
Dose: 175–350 mg twice daily; CHILD over 6 years 175 mg twice daily

Nuelin SA 250® (Riker)
Tablets, s/r, scored, theophylline 250 mg. Price 20 tabs = **D**
Dose: 250–500 mg twice daily; CHILD over 6 years half adult dose

Slo-Phyllin® (Rona)
Gyrocaps® (= capsules s/r), white/clear, enclosing white pellets, theophylline 60 mg. Price 20 caps = **C**
Gyrocaps® (= capsules s/r), brown/clear, enclosing brown and white pellets, theophylline 125 mg. Price 20 caps = **C**
Gyrocaps® (= capsules s/r), blue/clear, enclosing blue and white pellets, theophylline 250 mg. Price 20 caps = **D**
Dose: 250–500 mg twice daily; CHILD 2–6 years 60–120 mg, 7–12 years 125–250 mg twice daily

Theocontin Continus® (Napp)
Tablets, s/r, theophylline 200 mg. Price 20 tabs = **D**
Dose: 200–400 mg twice daily

Theograd® (Abbott)
Tablets, s/r, f/c, theophylline 350 mg. Price 20 tabs = **B**
Dose: 350 mg twice daily

Theosol® (Martindale)
Suppositories, theophylline 300 mg. Price 12 suppos = **C**

3.1.4 Other bronchodilator preparations

There is no advantage in using compound preparations compared with simple preparations of adrenoreceptor stimulants, xanthines etc.

Solutions of adrenaline deteriorate rapidly on exposure to air.

Adrenaline and Atropine Spray, Compound, adrenaline acid tartrate 0.8%, atropine methonitrate 0.1%, papaverine hydrochloride 0.8%. Price 100 ml = **E**. For use in hand spray

Amesec® (Lilly)
Capsules, blue/orange, aminophylline 130 mg, ephedrine hydrochloride 25 mg. Price 20 caps = **B**

Asmapax® (Nicholas)
Tablets, buff, scored, ephedrine resinate ≡ ephedrine hydrochloride 50 mg, theophylline 65 mg. Price 20 tabs = **C**

Asma-Vydrin® (Lewis)
Spray, adrenaline 0.55%, atropine methonitrate 0.14%, chlorbutol 0.5%, papaverine hydrochloride 0.85%. Price 30 ml = **C**

Bronchilator® (Sterling Research)
Aerosol inhalation, isoetharine mesylate 350 micrograms, phenylephrine hydrochloride 70 micrograms, thenyldiamine hydrochloride 28 micrograms/metered dose. Price 250-dose unit = **G**; refill = **F**

Bronchotone® (Rorer)
Liquid (= mixture), damson-coloured, belladonna tincture 0.52 ml, caffeine 86.5 mg, ephedrine hydrochloride 22.89 mg, sodium iodide 57.04 mg, sodium salicylate 91.85 mg/5 ml. Price 100 ml = **C**

Brontina® (Brocades)
Tablets, scored, deptropine citrate 1 mg. Price 20 tabs = **A**
Dose: 1 mg night and morning

Brontisol® (Brocades)
Aerosol inhalation, deptropine citrate 100 micrograms, isoprenaline hydrochloride 150 micrograms/metered dose. Price 300-dose unit = **D**

Brovon® (Napp)
Inhalant spray, adrenaline 0.5%, atropine methonitrate 0.14%, chlorbutol 0.5%, papaverine hydrochloride 0.88%. Price 20-ml bottle = **C**; 50-ml bottle = **D**; midget inhaler = **D**; reservoir and closure = **D**; rubber bulb = **B**

Brovon, Pressurised: see Pressurised Brovon (below)

CAM Bronchial Antispasmodic Syrup® (Rybar)
Mixture, green, butethamate citrate 4 mg, ephedrine hydrochloride 4 mg/5 ml. Diluent syrup or water for preparations, life of diluted mixture 14 days. Price 150 ml = **C**

Duo-Autohaler® (Riker)
Aerosol inhalation, isoprenaline hydrochloride 160 micrograms, phenylephrine bitartrate 240 micrograms/metered inhalation, 400-dose unit. Price (complete unit) = **G**; refill = **F**

Eumydrin® (Winthrop)
Oral solution, atropine methonitrate 0.6% in 90% alcohol. Dropper provides approximately 200 micrograms of atropine methonitrate/drop. Price 15-ml dropper bottle = **D**
Note: store in a cool place, tightly closed to prevent concentration by evaporation
Dose: CHILD, every 4 hours, up to 6 months 2–4 drops, 6 months–2 years 3–6 drops, 3–5 years 4–8 drops

Labophylline® (LAB)
Tablets, lysine 74 mg, theophylline 100 mg. Price 20 tabs = **B**

Medihaler-Duo® (Riker)
Aerosol inhalation, isoprenaline hydrochloride 160 micrograms, phenylephrine bitartrate 240 micrograms/metered inhalation, 400-dose unit. Price (complete unit) = **F**

Nethaprin Dospan® (Merrell)
Tablets, s/r, scored, bufylline 180 mg, doxylamine succinate 25 mg, etafedrine hydrochloride 50 mg, phenylephrine hydrochloride 25 mg. Price 20 tabs = **D**

Pressurised Brovon® (Napp)
Aerosol inhalation, adrenaline 0.5%, atropine methonitrate 0.1%. Price 17 ml (complete unit) = **E**

Pressurised Iso-Brovon (PIB)® (Napp)
Aerosol inhalation, atropine methonitrate 50 micrograms isoprenaline hydrochloride 180 micrograms/metered inhalation. Price 17 ml (complete unit) = **E**

Pressurised Iso-Brovon Plus (PIB Plus)® (Napp)
Aerosol inhalation, atropine methonitrate 50 micrograms, isoprenaline hydrochloride 500 micrograms/metered inhalation. Price 17 ml (complete unit) = **E**

Rybarvin® (Rybar)
Spray, adrenaline 0.4%, atropine methonitrate 0.1%, benzocaine 0.08%, papaverine hydrochloride 0.08%, in saline vehicle. Price 28 ml = **D**

Silbe® (Berk)
Inhalant (= spray), adrenaline acid tartrate 1%, atropine methonitrate 0.125%, chlorbutol 1%, hyoscine hydrobromide 0.05%, papaverine hydrochloride 0.95%. Price 25 ml = **C**

Taumasthman® (Wallace Mfg)
Tablets, atropine sulphate 300 micrograms, caffeine 50 mg, ephedrine hydrochloride 10 mg, phenazone 100 mg, theophylline 100 mg. Price 20 tabs = **B**

Tedral® (Warner)
Tablets, ephedrine hydrochloride 24 mg, theophylline 120 mg. Price 20 tabs = **A**
Suspension (= mixture), yellow, ephedrine hydrochloride 12 mg, theophylline 65 mg/5 ml. Diluent syrup, life of diluted mixture 28 days. Price 100 ml = **C**

Tedral SA® (Warner)
Tablets, s/r, coloured, ephedrine hydrochloride 48 mg, theophylline 180 mg. Price 20 tabs = **B**

COMPOUND BRONCHODILATORS WITH SEDATIVES

Preparations of this type, especially those containing barbiturates, should be **avoided**.

Expansyl® (SK&F)
Spansules® (= capsules s/r), black/clear, enclosing blue, green, and white pellets, diphenylpyraline hydrochloride 5 mg, ephedrine sulphate 50 mg, trifluoperazine 2 mg (as hydrochloride). Price 20 caps = **D**

Franol® (Winthrop)
Tablets, ephedrine hydrochloride 11 mg, phenobarbitone 8 mg, theophylline 120 mg. Price 20 tabs = **B**

Franol Plus® (Winthrop)
Tablets, ephedrine sulphate 15 mg, phenobarbitone 8 mg, theophylline 120 mg, thenyldiamine hydrochloride 10 mg. Price 20 tabs = **C**

Franol Expect® (Winthrop)
Elixir, red, ephedrine 4.75 mg, guaiphenesin 25 mg, phenobarbitone 4 mg, theophylline 60 mg/5 ml. Price 100 ml = **C**

Lotussin® (Searle)
Linctus, amber, dextromethorphan hydrobromide 6.25 mg, diphenhydramine hydrochloride 5 mg, ephedrine hydrochloride 7.5 mg, guaiphenesin 50 mg/5 ml. Diluent syrup, life of diluted linctus 14 days. Price 100 ml = **C**

Phyldrox® (Carlton)
Tablets, ephedrine hydrochloride 12 mg, phenobarbitone 8 mg, theophylline 128 mg. Price 20 tabs = **A**
Tablets, e/c, ingredients as above. Price 20 tabs = **A**

3.2 Corticosteroids

The action of these substances on the bronchi is not fully understood. They probably give relief by reducing the inflammatory reaction in bronchial walls but they may also modify allergic reactions. The aerosol inhalation preparations introduced in recent years have the great advantage that the side-effects associated with the systemic use of these drugs are much reduced.

If patients on regular treatment with a corticosteroid aerosol inhalation have even a mild degree of bronchospasm they should inhale a bronchodilator (such as salbutamol, section 3.1.1.1) about 10 minutes before each dose of corticosteroid to ensure that the maximum amount of the second drug enters the bronchi.

Patients with severe bronchospasm should be treated with high doses of **prednisolone** by mouth; in an emergency 200 mg of **hydrocortisone** (as sodium succinate) should be given by intravenous injection (see section 6.3.4) and may be repeated every 4 hours, until it is possible to use corticosteroids by mouth. The initial injection may not take effect for 4 to 8 hours and the patient should be carefully observed during this latent period for further signs of deterioration. Slow intravenous infusion is ineffective.

It is often possible to replace administration of corticosteroids by mouth with aerosol inhalation but this is best done when the asthma is well controlled.

BECLOMETHASONE DIPROPIONATE

Indications: bronchospasm, especially in asthma not controlled by bronchodilators

Side-effects: hoarseness; candidiasis of mouth, usually only with large doses (responds to antifungals such as amphotericin lozenges, see section 12.3.2, without discontinuation of therapy)

Dose: by aerosol inhalation, 100 micrograms (2 puffs) 3–4 times daily; CHILD 50 micrograms (1 puff) 2–4 times daily, reduced to the minimum effective dose

By inhalation of powder (insufflation cartridges), 200 micrograms 3–4 times daily; CHILD 100 micrograms 2–4 times daily

Becotide® (A&H)

Inhaler (= aerosol inhalation), beclomethasone dipropionate 50 micrograms/metered inhalation, 200-dose unit. Price (complete unit) = **G**
Advise patient not to exceed prescribed dose and to follow manufacturer's directions

Rotacaps® (= insufflation cartridges), buff/clear, beclomethasone dipropionate 100 micrograms. Price 20 cartridges = **D**

Rotacaps® (= insufflation cartridges), brown/clear, beclomethasone dipropionate 200 micrograms. Price 20 cartridges = **E**

Rotahaler® (for use with Rotacaps). Price per unit = **C**

BETAMETHASONE VALERATE

Indications; Side-effects: see under Beclomethasone Dipropionate (above)

Dose: by aerosol inhalation, 200 micrograms (2 puffs) 3–4 times daily; CHILD 100 micrograms (1 puff) 2–3 times daily, reduced to the minimum effective dose

Bextasol® (Glaxo)

Inhaler (= aerosol inhalation), betamethasone valerate 100 micrograms/metered inhalation, 200-dose unit. Price (complete unit) = **G**
Advise patient not to exceed prescribed dose and to follow manufacturer's directions

HYDROCORTISONE ACETATE

Indications; Side-effects: see under Beclomethasone Dipropionate (above)

Dose: by inhalation of powder (insufflation cartridges), initially 30–45 mg daily; maintenance 7.5–15 mg daily

Pabracort® (P&B)

Insufflation cartridges, hydrocortisone acetate 15 mg. For use with Pabryn® insufflator. Price 10 cartridges = **C**; with insufflator = **D**

3.3 Prophylaxis of asthma

Sodium cromoglycate (Intal®) has the property of stabilising cell membranes and preventing the release of pharmacological mediators of bronchospasm. In patients whose asthma has an allergic basis, and in some patients in whom an allergic basis does not seem to be present, continued use of this drug can reduce the incidence of asthmatic attacks. The prophylactic effect takes some time to develop and so the drug is of no value in the treatment of acute attacks.

There is no advantage in using sodium cromoglycate in combination with isoprenaline, unless the patient finds that inhalation of sodium cromoglycate alone produces bronchospasm or causes a dry, sore throat; in such cases the best procedure is to use a bronchodilator inhalation such as salbutamol or terbutaline a few minutes before a sodium cromoglycate inhalation is given.

Use of sodium cromoglycate may allow a reduction in the dose of corticosteroids or bronchodilators required by the patient. He must be instructed to take the drug regularly whether or not symptoms are present, and it is important to ensure that he understands this.

Ketotifen (Zaditen®) is a newer drug with an action resembling that of sodium cromoglycate but the drug has not been studied for sufficient time to permit a reliable evaluation. It is given by mouth and, while this may be an advantage to patients who find inhalation difficult, ketotifen may have to be given for 4 weeks or more to achieve full prophylaxis. In addition, ketotifen has the properties of an antihistamine and as such may cause drowsiness.

SODIUM CROMOGLYCATE

Indications: prophylaxis of asthma

Side-effects: transient bronchospasm and throat irritation due to inhalation of powder (see also notes above)

Dose: by aerosol inhalation, 2 mg (2 puffs) 4 times daily, increased in severe cases or during periods of risk to 6–8 times daily

By inhalation of powder (insufflation cartridges) 20 mg 4 times daily, increased in severe cases to 8 times daily

By inhalation of nebulised solution 10 mg up to 6 times daily

Intal® (Fisons)

Inhaler (=aerosol inhalation), sodium cromoglycate 1 mg/metered inhalation. 200-dose unit. Price (complete unit) = **I**

Spincaps® (=insufflation cartridges), yellow/clear, sodium cromoglycate 20 mg. Price 20 cartridges = **E**

Spinhaler insufflator® (for use with insufflation cartridges). Price per unit = **D**

Nebuliser solution, sodium cromoglycate 10 mg/ml. Price 2-ml amp = **A**. For use with power-operated nebuliser

Intal Compound® (Fisons)

Spincaps® (=insufflation cartridges), orange/clear, isoprenaline sulphate 100 micrograms, sodium cromoglycate 20 mg. Price 20 cartridges = **D**

KETOTIFEN

Indications: prophylaxis of asthma

Cautions: may affect ability to drive or operate machinery and increase effects of alcohol; previous anti-asthmatic treatment should be continued for a minimum of 2 weeks after initiation of ketotifen treatment

Side-effects: dry mouth, sedation

Dose: 1–2 mg twice daily with meals; initial treatment in readily sedated patients 1 mg at night

▼ **Zaditen**® (Wander)

Capsules, ketotifen 1 mg (as hydrogen fumarate). Price 20 caps = **E**

Tablets, scored, ketotifen 1 mg (as hydrogen fumarate). Price 20 tabs = **E**

3.4 Allergic disorders

Drugs affecting allergic disorders of the upper respiratory tract are discussed under the following headings:

3.4.1 Antihistamines
3.4.2 Hyposensitisation
3.4.3 Allergic emergencies

For the treatment of asthma see sections 3.1.1 and 3.2. For the treatment of hay fever by nasal application of corticosteroids and prophylaxis with sodium cromoglycate see section 12.2. For eye preparations see section 11.4. For the treatment of allergic skin conditions with topical corticosteroid preparations see section 13.4.

Depot **corticosteroid** preparations such as those containing methylprednisolone acetate and triamcinolone acetonide (see section 6.3.4), administered by intramuscular injection every 2 to 4 weeks, are highly effective in the treatment of nasal allergy, but as they are apt to cause impairment of pituitary-adrenal function they should be reserved for very severe cases.

3.4.1 Antihistamines

There is no evidence that any antihistamine is superior to another but they differ in duration of action and incidence of the main side-effects, drowsiness and anticholinergic effects.

Most antihistamines are relatively short-acting, but some, such as promethazine hydrochloride, are active for up to 12 hours. All are of potential value in the treatment of nasal allergy (hay fever), particularly of the seasonal type but have the serious disadvantage of causing drowsiness in most patients who take them regularly. This can be dangerous in certain circumstances as, for example, when the patient is driving a motor vehicle or operating machinery.

Antihistamines are of some value in preventing urticaria and in treating allergic rashes (section 13.3), hay fever, vasomotor rhinitis, pruritus, allergic reactions associated with bites and stings, and drug allergy.

Antihistamines are of no value whatever in the treatment of bronchial asthma, but Type III hypersensitivity reactions, such as allergic alveolitis and serum sickness, respond to corticosteroids.

Several antihistamines are described in other chapters (see Index).

AZATADINE MALEATE

Indications: nasal allergy, urticaria

Cautions; Side-effects: see under Promethazine Hydrochloride

Dose: 1 mg twice daily; CHILD 6–12 years 0.5–1 mg twice daily

▼ **Optimine**® (Kirby-Warrick)

Tablets, scored, azatadine maleate 1 mg. Price 20 tabs = **C**

Syrup (= elixir), orange, azatadine maleate 500 micrograms/5 ml. Price 120 ml = **C**

BROMPHENIRAMINE MALEATE

Indications: nasal allergy, urticaria

Cautions; Side-effects: see under Promethazine Hydrochloride

Dose: 4–8 mg 3–4 times daily; CHILD up to 3 years up to 100 micrograms/kg daily in divided doses, 3–5 years 2 mg 4 times daily, 6–12 years 2–4 mg 3–4 times daily

Dimotane® (Robins)

Tablets, peach, scored, brompheniramine maleate 4 mg. Price 20 tabs = **B**

Elixir, yellow/green, brompheniramine maleate 2 mg/5 ml. Diluent syrup, life of diluted elixir 14 days. Price 100 ml = **C**

Dimotane LA® (Robins)

Tablets, s/r, peach, s/c, brompheniramine maleate 12 mg. Price 20 tabs = **C**

Dose: 12–24 mg twice daily; CHILD 6–12 years 12 mg at bedtime, increased if necessary to 12 mg twice daily

CHLORPHENIRAMINE MALEATE

Indications: nasal allergy, urticaria, emergency treatment of anaphylactic reactions

Cautions; Side-effects: see under Promethazine Hydrochloride

Dose: by mouth, 4 mg 3–4 times daily; CHILD, daily in divided doses, up to 1 year 3 mg, 1–5 years 6 mg, 6–12 years 6–12 mg

Allergic emergencies, *by subcutaneous, intramuscular, or slow intravenous injection,* 10–20 mg to a max. of 40 mg in 24 hours

Chlorpheniramine Tablets, chlorpheniramine maleate 4 mg. Price 20 tabs = **A**

Piriton® (A&H)

Tablets, yellow, chlorpheniramine maleate 4 mg. Price 20 tabs = **A**

Duolets® (= tablets s/r), yellow, s/c, chlorpheniramine maleate 8 mg. Price 20 tabs = **B**

Dose: 8 mg 3 times daily; CHILD over 12 years 8 mg daily

Spandets® (= tablets s/r), yellow/white, chlorpheniramine maleate 12 mg. Price 20 tabs = **C**

Dose: 12 mg 2–3 times daily; CHILD over 12 years 12 mg daily

Syrup (= elixir), chlorpheniramine maleate 2 mg/5 ml. Diluent syrup (without preservative), life of diluted elixir 14 days. Price 150 ml = **B**
Injection, chlorpheniramine maleate 10 mg/ml. Price 1-ml amp = **A**

CLEMASTINE

Indications: nasal allergy, urticaria
Cautions; Side-effects: see under Promethazine Hydrochloride
Dose: 1 mg twice daily; CHILD up to 12 years 0.5–1 mg twice daily

Tavegil® (Wander)
Tablets, scored, clemastine 1 mg (as hydrogen fumarate). Price 20 tabs = **C**
Elixir, clemastine 500 micrograms (as hydrogen fumarate)/5 ml. Diluent syrup or water for preparations, life of diluted elixir 14 days. Price 100 ml = **B**

CYPROHEPTADINE HYDROCHLORIDE

Indications: nasal allergy, urticaria, stimulation of appetite
Cautions: see under Promethazine Hydrochloride
Side-effects: see under Promethazine Hydrochloride; also may inhibit lactation
Dose: allergy, 4–20 mg daily in divided doses; CHILD up to 1 year 1.5–3 mg, 1–5 years 6 mg, 6–12 years 12 mg, daily in divided doses
Stimulation of appetite, as above, but in single or divided doses

Periactin® (MSD)
Tablets, scored, cyproheptadine hydrochloride 4 mg. Price 20 tabs = **B**
Syrup (= elixir), yellow, cyproheptadine hydrochloride 2 mg/5 ml. Diluent syrup (without preservative), life of diluted elixir 14 days. Price 100 ml = **C**

DIMETHINDENE MALEATE

Indications: nasal allergy, urticaria
Cautions; Side-effects: see under Promethazine Hydrochloride

Fenostil Retard® (Zyma)
Tablets, s/r, dimethindene maleate 2.5 mg. Price 20 tabs = **C**
Dose: 2.5 mg twice daily

DIMETHOTHIAZINE

Indications: nasal allergy, urticaria
Cautions; Side-effects: see under Promethazine Hydrochloride
Dose: 20–40 mg 3 times daily; CHILD 6–12 years 10–20 mg twice daily

Banistyl® (M&B)
Tablets, scored, dimethothiazine 20 mg (as mesylate). Price 20 tabs = **C**

DIPHENHYDRAMINE HYDROCHLORIDE

Indications: nasal allergy, urticaria
Cautions; Side-effects: see under Promethazine Hydrochloride
Dose: 50–200 mg daily in divided doses; CHILD 6–12 years 25–50 mg 3–4 times daily

Benadryl® (P-D)
Capsules, pink/clear, diphenhydramine hydrochloride 25 mg. Price 20 caps = **A**

DIPHENYLPYRALINE HYDROCHLORIDE

Indications: nasal allergy, urticaria
Cautions; Side-effects: see under Promethazine Hydrochloride

Histryl® (SK&F)
Spansules®(=capsules s/r), pink/clear, enclosing pink and white pellets, diphenylpyraline hydrochloride 5 mg. Price 20 caps = **C**
Dose: 5–10 mg twice daily
Paediatric Spansules® (=capsules s/r), pink/clear, enclosing pink and white pellets, diphenylpyraline hydrochloride 2.5 mg. Price 20 caps = **B**
Dose: CHILD over 7 years 2.5 mg twice daily

Lergoban® (Riker)
Tablets, s/r, diphenylpyraline hydrochloride 5 mg. Price 20 tabs = **C**
Dose: 5–10 mg twice daily; CHILD over 10 years 5 mg twice daily

MEBHYDROLIN

Indications: nasal allergy, urticaria
Cautions; Side-effects: see under Promethazine Hydrochloride
Dose: 100–300 mg daily in divided doses; CHILD, daily in divided doses, up to 2 years 50–100 mg, 2–5 years 50–150 mg, 6–12 years 100–200 mg

Fabahistin® (Bayer)
Tablets, orange, s/c, mebhydrolin 50 mg. Price 20 tabs = **B**
Suspension (=mixture), orange, mebhydrolin 50 mg (as napadisylate)/5 ml. Diluents tragacanth mucilage for few days storage, *or* methyl hydroxybenzoate 0.07% and sodium carboxymethylcellulose 0.5% in water for preparations for longer storage. Price 100 ml = **C**

MEPYRAMINE MALEATE

Indications: nasal allergy, urticaria
Cautions; Side-effects: see under Promethazine Hydrochloride
Dose: *by mouth,* 100 mg 3 times daily increased if necessary to a max. of 1 g daily

Anthisan® (M&B)
Tablets, green, s/c, mepyramine maleate 50 mg. Price 20 tabs = **B**
Tablets, green, s/c, mepyramine maleate 100 mg. Price 20 tabs = **B**

MEQUITAZINE

Indications: nasal allergy, urticaria
Cautions; Side-effects: see under Promethazine Hydrochloride
Dose: 5 mg twice daily

Primalan® (S&N Pharm.)
Tablets, mequitazine 5 mg. Price 20 tabs = **D**

PHENINDAMINE TARTRATE

Indications: nasal allergy, urticaria
Cautions; Side-effects: see under Promethazine Hydrochloride
Dose: 25–50 mg up to 4 times daily; CHILD 6–12 years half adult dose

Thephorin® (Roche)
Tablets, yellow, s/c, phenindamine tartrate 25 mg. Price 20 tabs = **A**

PHENIRAMINE MALEATE

Indications: nasal allergy, urticaria
Cautions; Side-effects: see under Promethazine Hydrochloride

Daneral-SA® (Hoechst)
Tablets, s/r, pink, s/c, pheniramine maleate 75 mg. Price 20 tabs = **D**
Dose: 75–150 mg at night or 75 mg night and morning

PROMETHAZINE HYDROCHLORIDE

Indications: nasal allergy, urticaria, emergency treatment of anaphylactic reactions; for use in premedication see section 15.1.4.2; sedation see section 4.1.1
Cautions: may impair ability to drive or operate machinery and increase the effects of alcohol. Caution in epilepsy, protatism, glaucoma. Drug interactions: see Appendix 1
Side-effects: drowsiness, urinary retention, dryness of mouth, gastro-intestinal disturbances
Dose: by mouth, 20–50 mg daily in single or divided doses; CHILD up to 1 year 5–10 mg, 1–5 years 5–20 mg, 6–10 years 20–25 mg daily
By deep intramuscular injection, up to 50 mg; CHILD half the oral dose

Phenergan® (M&B)
Tablets, blue, s/c, promethazine hydrochloride 10 mg. Price 20 tabs = **A**
Tablets, blue, s/c, promethazine hydrochloride 25 mg. Price 20 tabs = **B**
Elixir, orange, promethazine hydrochloride 5 mg/5 ml. Diluent syrup, life of diluted elixir 14 days. Price 100 ml = **B**
Injection, promethazine hydrochloride 25 mg /ml. Price 1-ml amp = **A**; 2-ml amp = **B**

TRIMEPRAZINE TARTRATE

Indications: symptomatic relief of allergy, particularly pruritus
Cautions; Side-effects: see under Promethazine Hydrochloride
Dose: 10–40 mg daily in divided doses; CHILD 7.5–25 mg daily in 3 or 4 divided doses

Preparations
See section 15.1.4.2

TRIPROLIDINE HYDROCHLORIDE

Indications: nasal allergy, urticaria
Cautions; Side-effects: see under Promethazine Hydrochloride
Dose: 5–15 mg daily in divided doses; CHILD, 3 times daily, up to 1 year 1 mg, 1–5 years 2 mg, 6–12 years 3 mg

Actidil® (Wellcome)
Tablets, scored, triprolidine hydrochloride 2.5 mg. Price 20 tabs = **C**
Elixir, orange, triprolidine hydrochloride 2 mg /5 ml. Diluent syrup, life of diluted elixir 14 days. Price 100 ml = **C**
Pro-Actidil® (Wellcome)
Tablets, s/r, white/blue/pink, triprolidine hydrochloride 10 mg. Price 20 tabs = **E**
Dose: 10 mg daily increased to 20 mg daily when necessary; CHILD over 10 years 10 mg daily

3.4.2 Hyposensitisation

Specific hyposensitisation with extracts of common allergens, such as grass pollen or the house dust mite, *Dermatophagoides pteronyssinus,* is claimed to be of value in some atopic patients with allergic rhinitis (hay fever) and bronchial asthma, but since the majority of these patients are also sensitive to a wide range of other allergens, hyposensitisation with an extract of a single allergen is in most cases no more than partially effective.

If, however, it is decided to undertake specific hyposensitisation, the only extracts likely to be of value are those of grass pollen and house dust mite. Courses for hay fever should usually begin in January so that they are completed before exposure to pollen.

Hyposensitisation with a mixture of several allergens is **not** recommended, because allergens combined in a single solution have unpredictable effects which may include dangerous reactions. The safest and most convenient preparations to use are probably the precipitated or adsorbed preparations.

Allergic reactions may occur during specific hyposensitisation, especially in small children. The patient should be kept under observation for at least 20 minutes (small children 1 hour) after the injection. Subcutaneous adrenaline should be given as soon as symptoms appear and repeated until they subside.

Freeze-dried wasp and bee venoms are available for the diagnosis and treatment of allergy to wasp or bee strings. Skin testing must be done with careful attention to instructions and is not without risk of precipitating severe reactions.

ALLERGEN EXTRACT VACCINES

Sterile aqueous solutions (**sol**), alum-precipitated extracts of aqueous pyridine solutions (**ape**), aluminium-adsorbed extracts (**aae**), or tyrosine-adsorbed extracts (**tae**) are available in treatment sets of graded strengths. Each set usually contains 3 vials graded so that if the strength of the first is *x*, the others are of strengths 10*x* and 100*x*. Additional vials for maintenance treatment at the highest strength are also available

Indications: hypersensitivity to one or more common allergens (see notes above)

Contra-indications: pregnancy

Side-effects: allergic reactions, especially in small children

Dose: by subcutaneous injection, a volume appropriate to the needs of the patient initially, followed by further doses at suitable intervals, gradually increasing the amount of allergen; additional doses are administered if necessary to maintain reduced sensitivity

Note: PNU = protein nitrogen unit; BU = biological unit equivalent to one thousandth 'histamine-equivalent-prick'

Pollen allergy (hay fever) preparations

Alavac-P® (Bencard)

Injection, ape, prepared from 12 varieties of common grass pollen, set of 3 × 5-ml vials containing 250, 2500, and 25 000 Noon units/ml. Price (complete set) = **J**

Allpyral-G® (Dome)

Injection, ape, prepared from 5 varieties of common grasses, set of 3 × 5-ml vials containing 100, 1000, and 10 000 PNU/ml. Price (complete set) = **J**

Norisen Grass® (Merck)

Injection, aae, prepared from 6 varieties of grass, set of 3 × 4.5-ml vials containing 100, 1000, and 10 000 PNU/ml. Price (complete set) = **J**

Pollinex® (Bencard)

Injection, tae, prepared from 12 varieties of common grasses, set of 3 × pre-filled syringes containing 300, 800 and 2000 Noon units/0.5 ml. Price (complete set) = **J**

Spectralgen Single Species® (Pharmacia)

Injection, powder for reconstitution as sol or aae with normal serum albumin or depot diluent (as specified), prepared from anyone of 7 types of common grass or tree pollen, set of 4 vials containing 100, 1000, 10000, and 100000 BU/ml. Price (complete set with diluent) = **J**

Injection, for maintenance, vial containing 10000 or 100000 BU/ml (as specified). Price with diluent = **J**

Spectralgen 4 Grass Mix® (Pharmacia)

Injection, powder for reconstitution as sol or aae with normal serum albumin or depot diluent (as specified), prepared from 4 varieties of common grass pollen, set of 4 vials containing 100, 1000, 10000, and 100000 BU/ml. Price (complete set with diluent) = **J**

Injection, for maintenance, vial containing 10000 or 100000 BU/ml (as specified). Price with diluent = **J**

Spectralgen 3 Tree Mix® (Pharmacia)

Injection, powder for reconstitution as sol or aae with normal serum albumin or depot diluent (as specified), prepared from 3 varieties of common tree pollen, set of 4 vials containing 100, 1000, 10000, and 100000 BU/ml. Price (complete set with diluent) = **J**

Injection, for maintenance, vial containing 10000 or 100000 BU/ml (as specified). Price with diluent = **J**

House dust mite allergy preparations

Allpyral D. pteronyssinus® (Dome)

Injection, ape, prepared from *D. pteronyssinus,* preparation form as for Allpyral-G except that highest strength vial contains 4000 PNU/ml. Price (complete set) = **J**

Injection, content as above at 4000 PNU/ml strength, 3 × 2-ml vial for maintenance therapy. Price (complete set) = **J**

Allpyral-Mite Fortified House Dust® (Dome)

Injection, ape, prepared from house dust mite (*Dermatophagoides* spp.), fortified, preparation form as for Allpyral-G. Price (complete set) = **J**

Injection, content as above for maintenance, 10-ml vial only, preparation form as for Allpyral-G. Price per vial = **J**

Migen® (Bencard)

Injection, tae, prepared from *D. pteronyssinus,* set of 6 pre-filled syringes containing 4, 10, 25, 60, 150, and 400 Noon units/0.5 ml. Price per set = **J**

Injection, content as above, for maintenance of reduced sensitivity, set of 6 pre-filled syringes containing 400 Noon units/0.5 ml. Price (complete set) = **J**

Specific allergy preparations

Alavac-S® (Bencard)

Injection, ape, prepared from the specific allergens to which patient is hypersensitive, up to a maximum of 7 allergens in any one vaccine. Set of 3 × 5-ml vials in graded doses for different sensitivities. No. 1 and no. 2 vial are 1 in 100 and 1 in 10 dilutions of no. 3 vial. Price (complete set) = **J**

Allpyral-specific® (Dome)

Injection, ape, prepared from the specific allergens to which patient is hypersensitive (*D. pteronyssinus* vaccines, see above), preparation form as for Allpyral-G (above). Price (complete set) = **J**

Injection, specific allergens for maintenance, preparation form as above. Price per vial = **J**

Norisen® (Merck)

Injection, aae, prepared from the specific allergens to which patient is hypersensitive. If allergens include stinging insects, extracts of these cannot be mixed with extracts of other materials. Set of 3 × 4.5-ml vials containing 100, 1000, and 10 000 PNU/ml. For extremely sensitive patients, a 10 PNU/ml vial can also be supplied. Price (complete set) = **J**

Injection, content as above at highest strength, 10-ml vial for maintenance of reduced sensitivity. Price per vial = **J**

SDV® (Bencard)

Injection, sol, specific allergens to which patient is hypersensitive, max. 8 allergens per vaccine. Various strengths, set of 3 × 10-ml vials with 2 of the vials being respectively $\frac{1}{64}$th and $\frac{1}{8}$th the strength of the third. Price (complete set) = **J**

Wasp and bee venom allergy preparations

▼ **Pharmalgen**® (Pharmacia)

Injection, powder for reconstitution, freeze-dried bee venom 100 micrograms. Price 4 vials (with diluent) = **J**

Injection, powder for reconstitution, freeze-dried wasp venom 100 micrograms. Price 4 vials (with diluent) = **J**

Diluent (for further dilution). Price 10 vials of 4.5 ml = **H**

3.4.3 Allergic emergencies

Allergic emergencies include anaphylactic shock and angioneurotic oedema.

Anaphylactic shock is usually precipitated by injections of antisera, some vaccines, and antibiotics, or by insect stings. It is one of the most immediate emergencies in medicine. Adrenaline injection, 0.5 to 1 ml (equivalent to 0.5 to 1 mg of adrenaline), section 3.1.1.2, should be given by intramuscular or subcutaneous injection; several times the usual dose can be given if the patient is unconscious.

Angioneurotic oedema is dangerous when it affects respiration. When this is threatened, **corticosteroids** should be given by mouth or by injection according to the urgency (see section 6.3.4). When obstruction is present **adrenaline** should be injected as above and an intravenous corticosteroid should be given. An injection of **antihistamine** may also be given (if available). Other measures may be necessary, for example maintenance of blood pressure or tracheal intubation.

3.5 Respiratory stimulants

Analeptic drugs have a limited but useful place in the treatment of ventilatory failure in patients with chronic obstructive airways disease. They are effective only when given by intravenous injection or infusion. Respiratory stimulants should be given only under expert supervision in hospital, except in dire emergency and are best combined with active physiotherapy. There is no significant evidence that long-term use is of any value in chronic respiratory failure.

A dose of 4 to 8 ml of **nikethamide** injection given as a bolus injection will usually arouse a patient with carbon dioxide narcosis and it may then be possible, with low-concentration oxygen therapy, supervised coughing, and antibacterial treatment, to avoid recourse to tracheal intubation and artificial ventilation.

Maintenance treatment with a respiratory stimulant may, however, be required in patients who cannot tolerate even a 24% inspired oxygen concentration without becoming drowsy or comatose, and in whom artificial ventilation is contra-indicated by a long history of intolerable respiratory disability.

In these patients the choice lies between regular bolus injections of small doses of nikethamide into the tubing of an intravenous drip, and the continuous intravenous infusion of **doxapram** (Dopram®). Both these forms of treatment must be monitored by frequent arterial blood gas studies and pH measurements to ensure correct dosage. Nikethamide is much less expensive than doxapram and although the latter, being given by continuous infusion, has theoretical advantages, it only occasionally proves effective when treatment with nikethamide has failed. Doxapram is used postoperatively in anaesthetic practice (see section 15.1.7). Overdosage with either drug produces convulsions. **Ethamivan** (Clairvan®) has properties similar to those of nikethamide.

In an asphyxiated newborn infant, clearing the airway is the first essential. Valuable time may be wasted by giving stimulant drugs, but if they are used at all a drop of nikethamide should be placed on the tongue.

NIKETHAMIDE

Indications: acute respiratory failure

Contra-indications: respiratory failure due to neurological disease or drug overdose; status asthmaticus, coronary artery disease, thyrotoxicosis

Side-effects: nausea, restlessness, convulsions

Dose: *by slow intravenous injection,* 0.5–2 g repeated at intervals of 15–30 minutes as necessary

Nikethamide Injection, nikethamide 250 mg/ml. Price 2- and 5-ml amp (both) = **B**

DOXAPRAM HYDROCHLORIDE

Indications: see under Nikethamide

Cautions: cardiovascular disease

Contra-indications: see under Nikethamide

Side-effects: see under Nikethamide; also dizziness, perineal warmth, rarely cough, laryngospasm, bronchospasm, dyspnoea, cardiac arrhythmias

Dose: *by intravenous infusion,* 1–4 mg per minute according to patient's response

Dopram® (Robins)

Injection, doxapram hydrochloride 20 mg/ml. Price 5-ml amp = **D**

Intravenous infusion, doxapram hydrochloride 2 mg/ml. Price 500-ml bottle = **J**

ETHAMIVAN

Indications; Contra-indications; Side-effects: see under Nikethamide

Dose: *by mouth,* PREMATURE INFANTS 12.5 mg (0.25 ml of a 5% solution), FULL-TERM INFANTS 25 mg (0.5 ml of a 5% solution)

By intravenous injection, in barbiturate poisoning, 5–10 ml of a 5% solution

Clairvan® (Sinclair)

Oral solution, ethamivan 50 mg/ml (5%). Price 5-ml dropper bottle = **G**

Injection, ethamivan 50 mg/ml (5%). Price 2-ml amp = **C**

PRETHCAMIDE
(Cropropamide with Crotethamide)

Indications: respiratory insufficiency in chronic bronchitis

Cautions: epilepsy

Side-effects: headache, paraesthesias, restlessness, muscular twitching, tremors, dyspnoea, flushing

Dose: 400 mg 3–4 times daily

Micoren® (Geigy)

Capsules, red, prethcamide 400 mg. Price 20 caps = **D**

3.6 Oxygen

Oxygen should be regarded as a drug and prescribed as such, since the administration of an inappropriate inspired concentration of the gas may have serious or even lethal effects.

In some conditions, such as pneumonia, pulmonary oedema, pulmonary thrombo-embolism, and fibrosing alveolitis, a high inspired oxygen concentration is both essential and safe.

In chronic obstructive airways disease, however, the inspired oxygen concentration should **not** exceed 28%, higher concentrations may cause hypoventilation and progressive carbon dioxide retention. Indeed in some patients even a concentration exceeding 24% may cause hypoventilation and in these patients a variable performance mask (Edinburgh or MC) is needed with the oxygen flow rate adjusted appropriately in accordance with the instructions supplied with the mask.

In severe acute asthma the P_aCO_2 is subnormal initially because of hyperventilation but may later rise steeply, especially in children. If facilities for arterial blood gas studies are not immediately available, the safest policy is probably to compromise by using a Ventimask while the patient is being moved to hospital.

In the domiciliary service, cylinders equipped with an oxygen flowmeter with 'medium' (2 litres/minute) and 'high' (4 litres/minute) setting are available and a constant performance mask such as Mix-O-Mask 28% or Ventimask MkII 28%, or a variable-performance mask such as Edinburgh Mask or MC Mask is supplied. If any other type of equipment is required for domiciliary use, it must be supplied and serviced through the hospital service.

It is seldom possible, because of difficulty in providing a sufficient supply of cylinders, to give effective continuous oxygen therapy in the home, but many patients with severe dyspnoea seem to obtain symptomatic relief from exercise-induced respiratory distress by inhaling oxygen in the correct concentration for short periods.

3.7 Mucolytics

Mucolytics reduce the tenacity of sputum and thereby facilitate expectoration. Those given by mouth include **bromhexine** (Bisolvon®), **carbocisteine** (Mucodyne®), and **methylcysteine** (Visclair®); **acetylcysteine** (Airbron®) and **tyloxapol** (Alevaire®) are administered by inhalation. Although these drugs reduce the viscosity of mucoid sputum, few chronic bronchitics or chronic asthmatic patients seem to derive symptomatic benefit from them. Inhalation of steam or an aerosol of water is probably more effective for liquefying sputum. This treatment followed by postural drainage is good 'expectorant' therapy for patients with bronchiectasis and for some chronic bronchitics.

INHALATIONAL MUCOLYTICS

ACETYLCYSTEINE

Indications: to facilitate expectoration

Side-effects: bronchospasm, nausea, occasionally chills

Dose: *by inhalation of a nebulised solution,* 2–5 ml of a 20% solution through a mask or face-piece every 6–8 hours; may also be given *by direct instillation* into trachea or nebulised into a tent

Airbron® (DF)

Spray, acetylcysteine 200 mg/ml (20%). Price 2-ml amp = **B**; 10-ml vial = **E**

Note. Apparatus must be of glass or suitable plastic, not metal or rubber

DEOXYRIBONUCLEASE

See section 10.3.1

TYLOXAPOL

Indications: to facilitate expectoration

Dose: *by inhalation of a nebulised solution,* 6–20 ml of a 0.125% solution over a period of 24 hours

Alevaire® (Winthrop)

Spray, tyloxapol 0.125%. Price 60 ml = **F**

Note. Brass or copper apparatus should not be used

ORAL AND PARENTERAL MUCOLYTICS

BROMHEXINE HYDROCHLORIDE

Indications: to facilitate expectoration
Cautions: gastric ulceration
Side-effects: gastro-intestinal irritation, transient increased transaminase level
Dose: by mouth, 8–16 mg 4 times daily; CHILD up to 1 year 2 mg twice daily, 1–5 years 4 mg twice daily, 6–12 years 4 mg 4 times daily
By slow intravenous injection, intravenous infusion, or intramuscular injection, 8–24 mg daily

Bisolvon® (Boehringer Ingelheim)
Tablets, yellow, bromhexine hydrochloride 8 mg. Price 20 tabs = **D**
Elixir, yellow, bromhexine hydrochloride 4 mg/5 ml. Diluent sorbitol solution or water for preparations, life of diluted elixir 14 days. Price 100 ml = **C**
Injection, bromhexine hydrochloride 2 mg/ml. Price 2-ml amp = **B**

CARBOCISTEINE

Indications: to facilitate expectoration
Side-effects: occasional gastro-intestinal irritation
Dose: 750 mg 3 times daily initially, then 375 mg 4 times daily; CHILD 1–5 years 62.5–125 mg 4 times daily, 6–12 years 250 mg 3 times daily

Mucodyne® (Berk)
Capsules, yellow, carbocisteine 375 mg. Price 20 caps = **E**
Syrup (=elixir), amber-coloured, carbocisteine 250 mg/5 ml. Diluent syrup, life of diluted elixir 14 days. Price 100 ml = **E**
Paediatric syrup (= elixir), carbocisteine 125 mg/5 ml. Price 100 ml = **D**

Mucolex® (Warner)
Syrup (= elixir), red, carbocisteine 250 mg/5 ml. Price 100 ml = **D**

METHYLCYSTEINE HYDROCHLORIDE

Indications: to facilitate expectoration
Dose: 200 mg 3–4 times daily reduced to 200 mg twice daily after 6 weeks

Visclair® (Sinclair)
Tablets, yellow, e/c, methylcysteine hydrochloride 100 mg. Price 20 tabs = **E**

3.8 Inhalations

Inhalations containing volatile substances such as eucalyptus oil are traditionally used and although the vapour may contain little of the additive it encourages deliberate inspiration of warm moist air which is often comforting in bronchitis. Inhalations are also used for the relief of nasal obstruction in acute rhinitis or sinusitis.

Menthol and Benzoin Inhalation, menthol 2%, in benzoin inhalation (see Formulary). Price 50 ml = **B**
Directions for use: add one teaspoonful to a pint of hot, not boiling, water and inhale the vapour

Menthol and Eucalyptus Inhalation, (see Formulary). Price 50 ml = **A**
Directions for use: as above

Karvol® (Crookes Products)
Inhalation capsules, menthol 35.9 mg, with chlorbutol, cinnamon oil, pine oil, terpineol, and thymol. Price 20 caps = **B**
Directions for use: inhale vapour from contents of 1 capsule expressed into handkerchief or a pint of hot water

3.9 Antitussives

3.9.1 Cough suppressants

Diamorphine and **methadone** (Physeptone®) are effective cough suppressants and, when administered as linctuses, may control distressing cough in patients with terminal lung cancer. In other circumstances these drugs are contra-indicated because of the dangers of inducing sputum retention, ventilatory failure, and narcotic dependence.

Less potent but also less addictive drugs including **codeine, isoaminile citrate** (Dimyril®), **morphine, noscapine, and pholcodine** are commonly prescribed, sometimes in conjunction with other ingredients (section 3.9.2), for the suppression of cough in patients with acute bronchitis, pneumonia, chronic bronchitis, and bronchiectasis. In the first two conditions such treatment is seldom necessary if antibacterial therapy is started promptly. In the latter two, cough suppression is undesirable, except perhaps when sleep is constantly disturbed by a dry cough. However, those drugs which can safely be prescribed are seldom sufficiently potent to be effective and all are liable to cause intractable constipation. In short, the drawbacks are not outweighed by the benefits of such prescribing.

CODEINE PHOSPHATE

Indications: dry or painful cough
Cautions: asthma; see also notes above
Side-effects: constipation, in large doses respiratory depression

Codeine Linctus, codeine phosphate 15 mg/5 ml. Diluent syrup, life of diluted linctus 14 days. Price 100 ml = **B**
Dose: 5 ml 3–4 times daily

Codeine Linctus, Diabetic, codeine phosphate 15 mg/5 ml. Diluent chloroform water, life of diluted linctus 14 days. Price 100 ml = **B**

Codeine Linctus, Paediatric, codeine phosphate 3 mg/5 ml (see Formulary). Price 100 ml = **A**
Dose: CHILD up to 1 year 5 ml, 1–5 years 10 ml

DEXTROMETHORPHAN HYDROBROMIDE

Indications: dry or painful cough
Cautions: see notes above
Side-effects: see under Codeine Phosphate

Cosylan® (P-D)
Syrup (=elixir), dextromethorphan hydrobromide 13.5 mg/5 ml. Diluent syrup, life of diluted elixir 14 days. Price 100 ml = **B**
Dose: 5–10 ml 3–4 times daily

DIAMORPHINE HYDROCHLORIDE

Indications: dry or painful cough in terminal disease
Cautions; Contra-indications; Side-effects: see under Codeine Phosphate and notes above
Dose: 1.5–6 mg

CD Diamorphine Linctus, diamorphine hydrochloride 3 mg/5 ml (see Formulary). Price 100 ml = **C**

ISOAMINILE CITRATE

Indications: dry or painful cough
Cautions: see notes above
Side-effects: constipation
Dose: 40 mg 3–5 times daily; CHILD, 20–40 mg 3–5 times daily

Dimyril® (Fisons)
Linctus, red, isoaminile citrate 40 mg/5 ml. Diluent syrup, life of diluted linctus 14 days. Price 150 ml = **D**

METHADONE HYDROCHLORIDE

Indications: dry or painful cough in terminal disease
Cautions; Contra-indications; Side-effects: see under Codeine Phosphate and notes above
Dose: 1–2 mg 3–4 times daily; CHILD, 4 times daily, 5–10 years 250 micrograms, 11–14 years 500 micrograms

CD Methadone Linctus, yellow, methadone hydrochloride 2 mg/5 ml. Diluent syrup, life of diluted linctus 14 days. Price 100 ml = **B**
CD Physeptone® (Wellcome)
Linctus, brown, methadone hydrochloride 2 mg/5 ml. Diluent syrup, life of diluted linctus 14 days. Price 100 ml = **C**

NOSCAPINE

Indications: dry or painful cough
Cautions: see notes above
Dose: 15–30 mg 3–4 times daily; CHILD, 4 times daily, up to 1 year 1 mg, 2–5 years 2–5 mg, 6–12 years 6–12 mg

Noscapine Linctus, yellow, noscapine 15 mg/5 ml. Diluent syrup, life of diluted linctus 14 days. Price 100 ml = **B**

PHOLCODINE

Indications: dry or painful cough
Cautions: see notes above
Dose: 10 mg up to 6 times daily; CHILD 5 mg up to 6 times daily

Pholcodine Linctus, orange, pholcodine 5 mg/5 ml. Diluent syrup. Price 100 ml = **B**
Pholcodine Linctus, Strong, orange, pholcodine 10 mg/5 ml. Diluent syrup. Price 100 ml = **B**
Dia-tuss® (Rona)
Syrup (=linctus), diabetic, orange, pholcodine 10 mg/5 ml. Diluent sorbitol solution, life of diluted linctus 14 days. Price 100 ml = **C**
Sancos® (Sandoz)
Syrup (=linctus), pholcodine 5 mg/5 ml. Diluent syrup, life of diluted linctus 14 days. Price 100 ml = **B**
Triopaed® (Wander)
Linctus, pholcodine 4 mg/5 ml. Diluent syrup, life of diluted linctus 14 days. Price 100 ml = **B**

3.9.2 Expectorants, demulcents, and compound preparations

EXPECTORANTS. There is no evidence that any drug given by mouth, by inhalation, or by injection has a specific action in promoting expectoration of bronchial secretions by stimulation or augmentation of the cough reflex. The retching and vomiting which can be provoked by gastric irritants, such as ammonium chloride, ipecacuanha, and squill, can certainly expel mucus from the air passages at the same time, particularly in children, but the assumption that 'subemetic' doses of these and other drugs promote expectoration is a myth. There is thus no scientific basis for prescribing these drugs although a harmless expectorant mixture may have a useful role as a placebo. It is irrational to prescribe an expectorant in conjunction with a cough suppressant, antihistamine, or bronchodilator drug.

DEMULCENTS. Some patients have the impression that the demulcent effect of a linctus containing syrup or glycerol relieves a dry irritating cough and preparations such as **simple linctus** and the corresponding paediatric preparation certainly have the advantage of being harmless and inexpensive.

COMPOUND PREPARATIONS. There is no advantage in prescribing a preparation containing several ingredients that have similar therapeutic properties, or in which each ingredient has a different action.

Combinations such as expectorant and cough suppressant, sympathomimetic and sedative, and any or all of these with other types of drug such as antihistamines are to be **deprecated.** If particular components are needed they should be prescribed separately and dosage adjusted independently.

Ammonia and Ipecacuanha Mixture, ammonium bicarbonate, ipecacuanha tincture (see Formulary). Price 100 ml = **A**

Ammonium Chloride Mixture, ammonium chloride 1 g/10 ml (see Formulary). Price 100 ml = **A**
Dose: 10 to 20 ml 3–4 times daily

Ammonium Chloride and Morphine Mixture, ammonium bicarbonate, ammonium chloride, chloroform and morphine tincture (see Formulary). Price 100 ml = **A**

Ipecacuanha and Morphine Mixture, ipecacuanha tincture, chloroform and morphine tincture (see Formulary). Price 100 ml = **A**

Simple Linctus, citric acid monohydrate 125 mg/5 ml (see Formulary). Price 100 ml = **A**
Dose: 5 ml 3–4 times daily

Simple Linctus, Paediatric, citric acid monohydrate 31.25 mg/5 ml (see Formulary). Price 100 ml = **A**
Dose: CHILD, 5–10 ml 3–4 times daily

Squill Linctus, Opiate, squill oxymel, camphorated opium tincture, tolu syrup (see Formulary). Price 100 ml = **A**

Squill Linctus, Opiate, Paediatric, as above diluted (see Formulary). Price 100 ml = **B**

Squill Pastilles, Opiate, squill liquid extract 0.03 ml, concentrated camphorated opium tincture 0.075 ml. Price 20 pastilles = **B**

Tolu Linctus, Compound, Paediatric, citric acid monohydrate 30 mg/5 ml. Price 100 ml = **B**
Dose: CHILD, 5–10 ml

Actifed® (Wellcome)
Compound linctus, red, codeine phosphate 10 mg, pseudoephedrine hydrochloride 30 mg, triprolidine hydrochloride 1.25 mg/5 ml. Diluent syrup, life of diluted linctus 14 days. Price 100 ml = **C**
Syrup (= elixir), yellow, pseudoephedrine hydrochloride 30 mg, triprolidine hydrochloride 1.25 mg/5 ml. Diluent syrup, life of diluted elixir 14 days. Price 100 ml = **C**

Actifed Expectorant® (Wellcome)
Elixir, orange, guaiphenesin 100 mg, pseudoephedrine hydrochloride 30 mg, triprolidine hydrochloride 1.25 mg/5 ml. Price 100 ml = **C**

Alupent Expectorant® (Boehringer Ingelheim)
Tablets, scored, bromhexine hydrochloride 8 mg, orciprenaline sulphate 20 mg. Price 20 tabs = **D**
Mixture, bromhexine hydrochloride 4 mg, orciprenaline sulphate 10 mg/5 ml. Diluents sorbitol solution or syrup, life of diluted mixture 14 days. Price 100 ml = **D**

Benafed® (P-D)
Linctus, orange-red, ammonium chloride 125 mg, dextromethorphan hydrobromide 15 mg, diphenhydramine hydrochloride 12.5 mg, menthol 1 mg, pseudoephedrine hydrochloride 30 mg, sodium citrate 57 mg/5 ml. Diluent syrup, life of diluted linctus 14 days. Price 100 ml = **C**

Benylin Expectorant® (P-D)
Syrup (=elixir), red, ammonium chloride 135 mg, diphenhydramine hydrochloride 14 mg, menthol 1.1 mg, sodium citrate 57 mg/5 ml. Diluent syrup, life of diluted elixir 14 days. Price 100 ml = **B**

Benylin Paediatric® (P-D)
Syrup (=elixir), red, diphenhydramine hydrochloride 7 mg, menthol 0.55 mg, sodium citrate 28.5 mg/5 ml. Diluent syrup, life of diluted elixir 14 days. Price 100 ml = **B**

Benylin with Codeine® (P-D)
Syrup (=elixir), red, codeine phosphate 5.7 mg, diphenhydramine hydrochloride 14 mg, menthol 1.1 mg, sodium citrate 57 mg/5 ml. Diluent syrup, life of diluted elixir 14 days. Price 100 ml = **C**

Bricanyl Compound® (Astra)
Tablets, guaiphenesin 100 mg, terbutaline sulphate 2.5 mg. Price 20 tabs = **C**

Bricanyl Expectorant® (Astra)
Elixir, guaiphenesin 66.5 mg, terbutaline sulphate 1.5 mg/5 ml. Diluent water for preparations, life of diluted elixir 14 days. Price 100 ml = **C**

Copholco® (Rorer)
Linctus, brown, cineole 0.0026 ml, menthol 1.41 mg, pholcodine 5.63 mg, terpin hydrate 2.82 ml/5 ml. Price 100 ml = **B**

Copholcoids® (Rorer)
Pastilles, black, cineole 0.004 ml, menthol 2 mg, pholcodine 4 mg, terpin hydrate 16 mg. Price 50 g = **C**

Davenol® (Wyeth)
Linctus, orange, carbinoxamine maleate 2 mg, ephedrine hydrochloride 7 mg, pholcodine 4 mg/5 ml. Diluent syrup, life of diluted linctus 15 days. Price 100 ml = **B**

Dimotane Expectorant® (Robins)
Elixir, pink, brompheniramine maleate 2 mg, guaiphenesin 100 mg, phenylephrine hydrochloride 5 mg, phenylpropanolamine hydrochloride 5 mg/5 ml. Diluent syrup, life of diluted elixir 14 days. Price 100 ml = **B**

Dimotane Expectorant DC® (Robins)
Elixir, pink, brompheniramine maleate 2 mg, guaiphenesin 100 mg, hydrocodone acid tartrate 1.8 mg, phenylephrine hydrochloride 5 mg, phenylpropanolamine hydrochloride 5 mg/5 ml. Diluent syrup, life of diluted elixir 14 days. Price 100 ml = **C**

Dimotane with Codeine® (Robins)
Elixir, pink, brompheniramine maleate 2 mg, codeine phosphate 10 mg, guaiphenesin 100 mg, phenylephrine hydrochloride 5 mg, phenylpropanolamine hydrochloride 5 mg/5 ml. Diluent syrup, life of diluted elixir 14 days. Price 100 ml = **C**

Dimotane with Codeine Paediatric® (Robins)
Elixir, pink, brompheniramine maleate 1 mg, codeine phosphate 3 mg, guaiphenesin 50 mg, phenylephrine hydrochloride 2.5 mg, phenylpropanolamine hydrochloride 2.5 mg/5 ml. Diluent syrup, life of diluted elixir 14 days. Price 100 ml = **C**

Expulin® (Galen)
Linctus, chlorpheniramine maleate 2 mg, ephedrine hydrochloride 8 mg, pholcodine 5 mg/5 ml. Price 100 ml = **C**

Extil Compound® (DF)
Linctus, reddish-pink, carbinoxamine maleate 6 mg, noscapine 25 mg, pseudoephedrine 49.2 mg/10 ml. Price 100 ml = **C**

Exyphen® (Norton)
Elixir, red, brompheniramine maleate 2 mg, guaiphenesin 120 mg, phenylephrine hydrochloride 4.75 mg, phenylpropanolamine hydrochloride 5 mg/5 ml. Price 100 ml = **B**

Falcodyl® (Norton)
Linctus, ephedrine hydrochloride 4 mg, pholcodine 4 mg/5 ml. Price 100 ml = **B**

Flavelix® (Pharmax)
Elixir, yellow, ammonium chloride 90 mg, ephedrine hydrochloride 10 mg, mepyramine maleate 12.5 mg, sodium citrate 40 mg/5 ml. Diluent syrup, life of diluted elixir 14 days. Price 100 ml = **B**

Franolyn Expect® (WinPharm)
Elixir, ephedrine 4.75 mg, guaiphenesin 25 mg, theophylline 60 mg/5 ml. Price 110 ml = **C**

Guanor Expectorant® (RP Drugs)
Mixture, ammonium chloride 135 mg, diphenhydramine hydrochloride 14 mg, menthol 1.1 mg. sodium citrate 57 mg/5 ml. Price 100 ml = **A**

Guanor Paediatric® (RP Drugs)
Mixture, diphenhydramine hydrochloride 7 mg, menthol

550 micrograms, sodium citrate 28.5 mg/5 ml. Price 100 ml = **B**

Histalix® (Wallace Mfg)
Mixture, ammonium chloride 135 mg, diphenhydramine hydrochloride 14 mg, menthol 1.1 mg, sodium citrate 57 mg/5 ml. Price 150 ml = **C**

Iodo-Ephedrine® (Philip Harris)
Mixture, caffeine 90 mg, ephedrine hydrochloride 8 mg, glycerol 0.9 ml, sodium iodide 90 mg/5 ml in decoction of coffee. Price 100 ml = **B**

Linctifed Expectorant® (Wellcome)
Syrup (=elixir), orange, codeine phosphate 7.5 mg, guaiphenesin 100 mg, pseudoephedrine hydrochloride 20 mg, triprolidine hydrochloride 1.25 mg/5 ml. Diluent syrup, life of diluted elixir 14 days. Price 100 ml = **C**

Linctifed Expectorant Paediatric® (Wellcome)
Syrup (=elixir), red, codeine phosphate 3 mg, guaiphenesin 50 mg, pseudoephedrine hydrochloride 12 mg, triprolidine hydrochloride 600 micrograms/5 ml. Diluent syrup, life of diluted elixir 14 days. Price 100 ml = **C**

Muflin® (Concept)
Syrup (=elixir), red, citric acid 20 mg, dextromethorphan hydrobromide 10 mg, pheniramine maleate 7.5 mg, sodium citrate 130 mg/5 ml. Diluent syrup, life of diluted elixir 14 days. Price 100 ml = **B**

Nethaprin Expectorant® (Merrell)
Syrup (=elixir), orange, bufylline 60 mg, doxylamine succinate 6 mg, etafedrine hydrochloride 20 mg, guaiphenesin 100 mg/5 ml. Price 100 ml = **C**

Noradran® (Norma)
Syrup (=elixir), diphenhydramine hydrochloride 5 mg, diprophylline 50 mg, ephedrine hydrochloride 7.5 mg, guaiphenesin 25 mg/5ml. Price 100 ml = **B**

Organidin® (WBP)
Elixir, yellow, iodinated glycerol 60 mg/5 ml. Diluent glycerol and water for preparations equal parts, life of diluted elixir 14 days. Price 100 ml = **D**

Orthoxicol® (Upjohn)
Syrup (=elixir), red, codeine phosphate 10.95 mg, methoxyphenamine hydrochloride 16·9 mg, sodium citrate 325 mg/5 ml. Diluent syrup, life of diluted elixir 14 days. Price 100 ml = **C**

Pavacol-D® (WBP)
Mixture, brown, papaverine hydrochloride 1 mg, pholcodine 5 mg/5 ml, suitable for diabetics. Diluent sorbitol solution, life of diluted mixture 14 days. Price 100 ml = **C**

Phenergan Compound Expectorant® (M&B)
Linctus, straw coloured, citric acid 65 mg, ipecacuanha liquid extract 0.01 ml, potassium guaiacolsulphonate 45 mg, promethazine hydrochloride 5 mg/5 ml. Diluent syrup, life of diluted linctus 14 days. Price 100 ml = **B**

Phensedyl® (M&B)
Linctus, orange, codeine phosphate 9 mg, ephedrine hydrochloride 7.2 mg, promethazine hydrochloride 3.6 mg/5 ml. Diluent syrup, life of diluted linctus 14 days. Price 100 ml = **B**

Pholcolix® (Warner)
Syrup (=elixir), paracetamol 150 mg, phenylpropanolamine hydrochloride 12.5 mg, pholcodine 5 mg/5 ml. Diluent syrup, life of diluted elixir 14 days. Price 100 ml = **D**

Pholcomed® (Medo)
Linctus, red, papaverine hydrochloride 1.25 mg, pholcodine 5 mg/5 ml. Diluent syrup, life of diluted linctus 14 days. Price 150 ml = **B**
Pastilles, red, papaverine hydrochloride 1 mg, pholcodine 4 mg. Price 20 pastilles = **C**

Pholcomed Diabetic® (Medo)
Linctus, red, ingredients as for Pholcomed but without sugar. Diluent water for preparations, life of diluted linctus 14 days. Price 150 ml = **C**

Pholcomed Expectorant® (Medo)
Syrup (= elixir), guaiphenesin 62.5 mg, methylephedrine hydrochloride 625 micrograms/5 ml. Price 100 ml = **B**. This preparation was previously known as Pulmodrine Expectorant

Pholcomed Forte® (Medo)
Linctus, red, papaverine hydrochloride 5 mg, pholcodine 19 mg/5 ml. Diluent syrup, life of diluted linctus 14 days. Price 100 ml = **C**

Pholcomed Forte Diabetic® (Medo)
Linctus, red, ingredients as for Pholcomed Forte but without sugar. Diluent water for preparations, life of diluted linctus 14 days. Price 100 ml = **C**

Pholtex® (Riker)
Mixture, s/r, orange, phenyltoloxamine 10 mg, pholcodine 15 mg/5 ml, as resin complexes, sugar-free. Diluent syrup or tragacanth mucilage, life of diluted mixture 14 days. Price 100 ml = **C**

Rinurel® (Warner)
Linctus, yellow, paracetamol 150 mg, phenylpropanolamine hydrochloride 12.5 mg, phenyltoloxamine citrate 11 mg, pholcodine 5 mg/5 ml. Diluent syrup, life of diluted linctus 28 days. Price 100 ml = **C**

Robitussin® (Robins)
Liquid (=elixir), red, guaiphenesin 100 mg/5 ml. Diluent syrup, life of diluted elixir 14 days. Price 100 ml = **B**

Robitussin AC® (Robins)
Elixir, amber coloured, codeine phosphate 10 mg, guaiphenesin 100 mg, pheniramine maleate 7.5 mg/5 ml. Diluent syrup, life of diluted elixir 14 days. Price 100 ml = **C**

Rubelix® (Pharmax)
Elixir, red, ephedrine hydrochloride 6 mg, pholcodine 4 mg/5 ml. Diluent syrup, life of diluted elixir 14 days. Price 150 ml = **B**

Sancos Co® (Sandoz)
Syrup (=elixir), chlorpheniramine maleate 2 mg, glycerol 600 mg, pholcodine 5 mg, pseudoephedrine hydrochloride 20 mg/5 ml. Diluent syrup, life of diluted elixir 14 days. Price 100 ml = **B**

Sedatussin® (Lilly)
Syrup (=elixir), orange-brown, cephaëline hydrochloride 350 micrograms, menthol 1.43 mg, sodium benzoate 43.8 mg, squill syrup 0.5 ml, tolu syrup 0.25 ml/5 ml. Diluent syrup, life of diluted elixir 14 days. Price 100 ml = **B**

Sudafed Expectorant® (Calmic)
Syrup (=elixir), red, guaiphenesin 100 mg, pseudoephedrine hydrochloride 30 mg/5 ml. Price 100 ml = **C**

Syrtussar® (Armour)
Syrup (=elixir), red, dextromethorphan hydrobromide 10 mg, pheniramine maleate 7.5 mg/5 ml. Diluent syrup, life of diluted elixir 14 days. Price 150 ml = **C**

Tancolin® (Ashe)
Linctus (paediatric), ascorbic acid 12.35 mg, citric acid 45.85 mg, dextromethorphan hydrobromide 2.62 mg, glycerol 655 mg, methyl hydroxybenzoate 5.9 mg, sodium citrate 99.56 mg, theophylline 15 mg/5 ml. Price 100 ml = **B**

Tedral Expectorant® (Warner)
Elixir, diprophylline 100 mg, ephedrine hydrochloride 10 mg, guaiphenesin 50 mg/5 ml. Price 200 ml = **D**

Tercoda® (Sinclair)
Elixir, yellow, cineole 0.02 ml, codeine phosphate 8 mg, menthol 4 mg, peppermint oil 0.01 ml, pumilio pine oil 0.02 ml, terpin hydrate 8 mg/5 ml. Price 100 ml = **C**

Terpalin® (Norton)
Mixture, cineole 0.002 ml, codeine phosphate 13 mg, menthol 1.5 mg, terpin hydrate 6.5 mg/5 ml. Price 100 ml = **C**

Terpoin® (Hough)
Elixir, yellow, cineole 4.15 mg, codeine phosphate

18.3 mg, guaiphenesin 50 mg, menthol 18.3 mg, terpin hydrate 9.15 mg/5 ml. Price 100 ml = **C**

Tixylix® (M&B)
Linctus, red, phenylpropanolamine hydrochloride 5 mg, pholcodine 1.5 mg (as citrate), promethazine hydrochloride 1.5 mg/5 ml. Diluent syrup, life of diluted linctus 14 days. Price 100 ml = **B**

Totolin® (Galen)
Elixir (paediatric), red, guaiphenesin 30 mg, phenylpropanolamine hydrochloride 7.5 mg/5 ml. Price 100 ml = **B**

Triocos® (Wander)
Syrup (=elixir), chlorpheniramine maleate 5 mg, glycerol 600 mg, pholcodine 5 mg, menthol 80 micrograms, pseudoephedrine hydrochloride 20 mg/5 ml. Diluent syrup, life of diluted elixir 14 days. Price 100 ml = **B**

Triotussic® (Wander)
Suspension (=mixture), orange, mepyramine maleate 6.25 mg, noscapine 20 mg, paracetamol 160 mg, pheniramine maleate 6.25 mg, phenylpropanolamine hydrochloride 12.5 mg, terpin hydrate 90 mg/5 ml. Diluent syrup, life of diluted mixture 14 days. Price 100 ml = **C**

Tussifans® (Norton)
Mixture, anise oil 0.0015 ml, belladona liquid extract 0.007 ml, ipecacuanha liquid extract 0.013 ml, potassium citrate 250 mg, squill syrup 0.3 ml, tolu syrup 0.4 ml/5 ml. Price 100 ml = **A**

Valledrine® (M&B)
Linctus, brown, ephedrine hydrochloride 7.5 mg, pholcodine 4 mg (as citrate), trimeprazine tartrate 2.5 mg/5 ml. Diluent syrup, life of diluted linctus 14 days. Price 100 ml = **B**

Vallex® (M&B)
Linctus, brown, citric acid 65 mg, guaiphenesin 25 mg, ipecacuanha liquid extract 0.015 ml, menthol 1.2 mg, phenylpropanolamine hydrochloride 10 mg, sodium citrate 200 mg, trimeprazine tartrate 2.5 mg/5 ml. Diluent syrup, life of diluted linctus 14 days. Price 100 ml = **B**

3.10 Oral nasal decongestants

These preparations are of doubtful value but unlike the preparations for local application (see section 12.2.2) they do not give rise to rebound nasal congestion. They contain sympathomimetics, and should therefore be avoided in patients with hypertension, hyperthyroidism, or diabetes, and in patients taking monoamine-oxidase inhibitors. Many of the preparations also contain antihistamines which may cause drowsiness and affect ability to drive or operate machinery.

Ephedrine Preparations
Section 3.1.1.2

Actifed® (Wellcome)
Tablets, scored, pseudoephedrine hydrochloride 60 mg, triprolidine hydrochloride 2.5 mg. Price 20 tabs = **C**

Benylin Decongestant® (P-D)
Syrup (= elixir), yellow, diphenhydramine hydrochloride 14 mg, menthol 1.1 mg, pseudoephedrine hydrochloride 10 mg, sodium citrate 57 mg/5 ml. Price 100 ml = **C**

Co-Pyronil® (Lilly)
Capsules, cyclopentamine hydrochloride 12.5 mg, pyrrobutamine phosphate 15 mg. Price 20 caps = **C**

Dimotapp® (Robins)
Elixir, red-brown, brompheniramine maleate 4 mg, phenylephrine hydrochloride 5 mg, phenylpropanolamine hydrochloride 5 mg/5 ml. Diluent syrup, life of diluted elixir 14 days. Price 100 ml = **C**
Elixir, paediatric, red-brown, brompheniramine maleate 1 mg, phenylephrine hydrochloride 2.5 mg, phenylpropanolamine hydrochloride 2.5 mg/5 ml. Price 100 ml = **C**

Dimotapp LA® (Robins)
Tablets, s/r, brown, s/c, brompheniramine maleate 12 mg, phenyleprine hydrochloride 15 mg, phenylpropanolamine hydrochloride 15 mg. Price 20 tabs = **C**

Dimotapp P® (Robins)
Tablets, brompheniramine maleate 2 mg, paracetamol 325 mg, phenylephrine hydrochloride 5 mg, phenylpropanolamine hydrochloride 5 mg. Price 20 tabs = **D**

Emprazil® (Wellcome)
Tablets, orange/white, asprin 300 mg, caffeine 30 mg, pseudoephedrine hydrochloride 20 mg. Price 12 tabs = **B**

Eskornade® (SK&F)
Spansules® (= capsules s/r), grey/clear, enclosing red, grey, and white pellets, isopropamide 2.5 mg (as iodide), diphenylpyraline hydrochloride 5 mg, phenylpropanolamine hydrochloride 50 mg. Price 20 caps = **C**
Syrup (= elixir), green, diphenylpyraline hydrochloride 1.5 mg, isopropamide 750 micrograms (as iodide), phenylpropanolamine hydrochloride 15 mg/5 ml. Diluent syrup, life of diluted elixir 14 days. Price 150 ml = **D**

Haymine® (Pharmax)
Tablets, s/r, yellow, chlorpheniramine maleate 10 mg, ephedrine hydrochloride 15 mg. Price 30 tabs = **D**

Orthoxine®
Section 3.1.1.2

Paragesic® (Sandoz)
Tablets, effervescent, yellow, caffeine 10 mg, paracetamol 500 mg, pseudoephedrine hydrochloride 20 mg. Price 20 tabs = **C**

Rinurel® (Warner)
Tablets, pink, scored, paracetamol 300 mg, phenylpropanolamine hydrochloride 25 mg, phenyltoloxamine citrate 22 mg. Price 20 tabs = **B**

Rinurel SA® (Warner)
Tablets, s/r, pink, scored, paracetamol 600 mg, phenylpropanolamine hydrochloride 100 mg, phenyltoloaxime citrate 66 mg. Price 20 tabs = **C**

Sudafed® (Calmic)
Tablets, pseudoephedrine hydrochloride 60 mg. Price 20 tabs = **C**
Elixir, pink, pseudoephedrine hydrochloride 30 mg/5 ml. Diluent syrup, life of diluted elixir 14 days. Price 100 ml = **C**

Triogesic® (Wander)
Tablets, pink, scored, paracetamol 500 mg, phenylpropanolamine hydrochloride 12.5 mg. Price 20 tabs = **B**
Elixir, red, paracetamol 125 mg, phenylpropanolamine hydrochloride 3 mg/5 ml. Diluents syrup or water for preparations, life of diluted elixir 14 days. Price 100 ml = **B**

Triominic® (Wander)
Tablets, yellow, mepyramine maleate 25 mg, pheniramine maleate 25 mg, phenylpropanolamine hydrochloride 50 mg. Price 20 tabs = **B**
Syrup (= elixir), orange, mepyramine maleate 6.25 mg, pheniramine maleate 6.25 mg, phenylpropanolamine hydrochloride 12.5 mg/5 ml. Diluents syrup or water for preparations, life of diluted elixir 14 days. Price 100 ml = **B**

Uniflu Plus Gregovite C® (Unigreg)
Tablets, composite pack of pairs of tablets: Uniflu *tablets*, mauve, s/c, caffeine 30 mg, codeine phosphate 10 mg, diphenhydramine hydrochloride 15 mg, paracetamol 500 mg, phenylephrine hydrochloride 10 mg; Gregovite C *tablets,* yellow, ascorbic acid 300 mg. Price 12 of each tab = **C**

4: Drugs acting on the CENTRAL NERVOUS SYSTEM

In this chapter, drug treatments are discussed under the following headings:

4.1 Hypnotics, sedatives, and anxiolytics

Most anxiolytics will induce sleep when given in large doses at night and most hypnotics will sedate when given in divided doses during the day. Prescribing of these drugs is widespread but dependence (either physical or psychological) and tolerance to their effects can occur, notably with the barbiturates, but also, after prolonged use, with the benzodiazepines. This may lead to difficulty in withdrawing the drug after the patient has been taking it regularly for more than a few weeks. A withdrawal syndrome (section 4.1.2) may occur if drug treatment is terminated too abruptly. Hypnotics, sedatives, and anxiolytics should therefore not be prescribed indiscriminately and are generally reserved for short courses to alleviate acute conditions after the causal factors have been established.

The increasing trend towards prescribing more than one of these drugs for the same indication is **not** recommended. It may constitute a hazard and there is no evidence that side-effects are minimised.

The **benzodiazepines** are the most common class of drugs used as hypnotics, sedatives, and anxiolytics. They tend to have a hypnotic action in high dosage and an anxiolytic action in low dosage. They have replaced the barbiturates (section 4.1.3).

The advantages of the benzodiazepines over the barbiturates are that side-effects are less frequent and psychological and physical dependence less likely to occur; benzodiazepines are also much less dangerous in overdosage and are less likely to interact with other drugs because they do not induce liver microsomal enzymes.

Drugs in this section have been divided into the following subsections:

4.1.1 Hypnotics and sedatives

A drug which acts as a hypnotic in a high dose will act as a sedative in a low dose. Hypnotics should **not** be prescribed indiscriminately and routine prescribing, especially in hospitals, is undesirable though commonplace.

Ideally, hypnotics should be reserved for short courses of treatment in the acutely distressed. In any case tolerance to their effects develops within 3 to 14 days of continuous use.

The prescribing of hypnotics to children, except for occasional use such as for night terrors and somnambulism, is not justified. Hypnotics should also be avoided in the elderly who are at risk of becoming ataxic and confused and so liable to fall and injure themselves.

A major drawback of using hypnotics over prolonged periods is that they may cause rebound insomnia and precipitate a withdrawal syndrome (section 4.1.2) when the drug is discontinued.

Where prolonged administration cannot be avoided hypnotics should be discontinued as soon as possible and the patient should be warned that sleep may be disturbed for a few days before normal rhythm is re-established; broken sleep with vivid dreams and increased REM (rapid eye movement) may persist for several weeks. This must represent a mild form of dependence even if clinical doses are used.

Before a hypnotic is prescribed the cause of the insomnia should be established and, where possible, the underlying factors should be treated. However, it should be noted that some patients have unrealistic sleep expectations.

Chronic insomnia is commonly caused by prolonged use of hypnotics or alcohol; daytime catnapping; physical causes such as pain, cough, pruritus, and dyspnoea; or psychiatric causes such as anxiety, depression, and alcoholism. Sleep disturbance is very common in depressive illness and early wakening is often a useful pointer. The psychiatric complaint should therefore be treated, adapting the drug regimen to alleviate insomnia. For example, in the treatment of depressive illness, amitriptyline, given at night, will also help to promote sleep.

The benzodiazepines are used as hypnotics (see below) and anxiolytics (section 4.1.2). **Nitrazepam** (Mogadon® etc.) and **flurazepam** (Dalmane®) have a prolonged action which may give rise to residual effects on the following day and with repeated dosage tend to be cumulative. **Lormetazepam** (Noctamid®), **temazepam** (Euhypnos®, Normison®) and **triazolam** (Halcion®) act for a shorter time and have little or no hangover effect but are inappropriate for use in patients with early wakening. Benzodiazepine anxiolytics such as **diazepam** (Valium® etc.) and **clorazepate dipotassium** (Tranxene®) (section 4.1.2) given as a single dose at night may also be used as hypnotics.

Chlormethiazole (Heminevrin®) may be a useful hypnotic for elderly patients because of its freedom from hangover but, as with all hypnotics, routine administration is undesirable. Dependence occurs occasionally. It is used in the treatment of acute withdrawal symptoms in alcoholics but to minimise the risk of dependence administration should be limited to 9 days under hospital supervision. The **benzodiazepines** of section 4.1.2 and less commonly, antipsychotic drugs (section 4.2.1) are also used in the treatment of alcohol withdrawal.

Promethazine (Phenergan®) and **trimeprazine** (Vallergan®) are popular for use in children.

The use of **paraldehyde** as a hypnotic or sedative is obsolete.

Barbiturates and related drugs (section 4.1.3) should be **avoided. Alcohol** is a poor hypnotic as its diuretic action interferes with sleep during the latter part of the night. With chronic use, alcohol disturbs sleep patterns and causes insomnia.

CHLORAL HYDRATE

Indications: insomnia, sedation in the elderly

Cautions; Side-effects: see under Nitrazepam; doses are taken well diluted to minimise gastro-intestinal disturbances. Rashes may occur. Contact with skin and mucous membranes should be avoided. Drug interactions: see Appendix 1

Contra-indications: severe cardiac disease, gastritis, marked hepatic or renal dysfunction

Dose: insomnia, 0.5–2 g; CHILD 30–50 mg/kg up to a max. single dose of 1 g
Sedation, 250 mg 3 times daily

Chloral Mixture, chloral hydrate 500 mg/5 ml (see Formulary). Price 100 ml = **A**
Dose: insomnia, 5–20 ml; CHILD 1–5 years 2.5–5 ml, 6–12 years 5–10 ml, taken well diluted with water 15–30 minutes before bedtime

Chloral Elixir, Paediatric, chloral hydrate 200 mg/5 ml (see Formulary). Price 100 ml = **B**
Dose: up to 1 year 5 ml, well diluted with water

Noctec® (Squibb)
Capsules, red, chloral hydrate 500 mg. Price 20 caps = **B**

CHLORMETHIAZOLE EDISYLATE

Indications: relief of insomnia, agitation in elderly patients, acute alcohol withdrawal

Cautions: see under Nitrazepam, but hangover is less pronounced, doses less cumulative and fewer precautions are required in neuromuscular disease, in pregnancy, and in nursing mothers or elderly patients. Special precautions for intravenous infusion; see also section 4.8.2

Side-effects: sneezing, conjunctival irritation, headache, gastro-intestinal disturbances; rarely, confusion. On intravenous infusion in high doses, cardiovascular and respiratory depression and localised thrombophlebitis

Dose: *by mouth,* insomnia, 2 capsules at bedtime
Sedation, 1 capsule 3 times daily
Alcohol withdrawal, adjusted according to the response, 3 capsules every 6 hours for 2 days, reducing to 2 capsules every 6 hours for 3 days, then to 1 capsule every 6 hours for 4 days
Note: for an equivalent therapeutic effect: 1 capsule (192 mg chlormethiazole base) ≡ 5 ml elixir (250 mg/5 ml chlormethiazole edisylate)
By intravenous infusion, acute alcohol withdrawal, 40–100 ml (320–800 mg) initially as 0.8% solution at a rate of about 60 drops (4 ml)/minute, adjusted according to the response

Heminevrin® (Astra)
Capsules, yellow, chlormethiazole base 192 mg in arachis oil. Price 20 caps = **D**
Syrup (= elixir), chlormethiazole edisylate 250 mg/5 ml. Diluent water for preparations, life of diluted elixir 14 days. Price 100 ml = **C**
Intravenous infusion 0.8%, chlormethiazole edisylate 8 mg/ml. Price 500-ml bottle = **F**

DICHLORALPHENAZONE

Indications: insomnia

Cautions; Contra-indications; Side-effects: see under Chloral Hydrate (above) but fewer gastro-intestinal disturbances. Also contra-indicated in acute intermittent porphyria. Drug interactions: see Appendix 1

Dose: insomnia, 1.3–1.95 g (2–3 tablets); CHILD up to 1 year 112.5–225 mg (2.5–5 ml elixir), 1–5 years 225–450 mg (5–10 ml elixir), 6–12 years 450–900 mg (10–20 ml elixir) taken well diluted with water 20 minutes before bedtime

Welldorm® (S&N Pharm.)
Tablets, purple, f/c, dichloralphenazone 650 mg. Price 30 tabs = **C**
Elixir, red, dichloralphenazone 225 mg/5 ml. Diluent syrup, life of diluted elixir 14 days. Price 150 ml = **D**

FLURAZEPAM

Indications: insomnia where daytime sedation is acceptable

Cautions; Side-effects: see under Nitrazepam

Dose: 15–30 mg half an hour before bedtime

Dalmane® (Roche)
Capsules, grey/yellow, flurazepam 15 mg (as hydrochloride). Price 20 caps = **C**
Capsules, black/grey, flurazepam 30 mg (as hydrochloride). Price 20 caps = **D**

LORMETAZEPAM

Indications: insomnia (useful in the elderly)

Cautions; Side-effects: see under Nitrazepam but hangover is uncommon; doses less cumulative. Less appropriate in patients with early wakening

Dose: 1 mg (elderly patients 500 micrograms) at bedtime

▼ **Noctamid®** (Schering)
Tablets, scored, lormetazepam 500 micrograms. Price 20 tabs = **C**
Tablets, scored, lormetazepam 1 mg. Price 20 tabs = **D**

NITRAZEPAM

Indications: insomnia
Cautions: hangover may affect a patient's ability to drive or operate machinery and increase the effects of alcohol, avoid prolonged use and abrupt withdrawal thereafter. Caution in neuromuscular disease, respiratory disease, pregnancy, nursing mothers; reduce dosage in elderly and debilitated patients, liver disease, renal impairment. Drug interactions: see Appendix 1
Side-effects: hangover with drowsiness, dizziness, ataxia (particularly in the elderly); occasionally confusion, dry mouth, hypersensitivity reactions. Prolonged use may give rise to cumulation, tolerance, rebound insomnia, and dependence
Dose: 5–10 mg, 30 minutes before bedtime; CHILD 2.5–5 mg

Nitrazepam Capsules, nitrazepam 5 mg. Price 20 caps = **B**
Nitrazepam Tablets, nitrazepam 5 mg. Price 20 tabs = **B**
Mogadon® (Roche)
Capsules, purple/black, nitrazepam 5 mg. Price 20 caps = **B**
Tablets, scored, nitrazepam 5 mg. Price 20 tabs = **B**
Nitrados® (Berk)
Tablets, scored, nitrazepam 5 mg. Price 20 tabs = **B**
Remnos® (DDSA)
Tablets, scored, nitrazepam 5 mg. Price 20 tabs = **B**
Tablets, yellow, scored, nitrazepam 10 mg. Price 20 tabs = **B**
Somnite® (Norgine)
Tablets, scored, nitrazepam 5 mg. Price 20 tabs = **B**
Surem® (Galen)
Capsules, mauve/grey, nitrazepam 5 mg. Price 20 caps = **B**
Unisomnia® (Unigreg)
Tablets, scored, nitrazepam 5 mg. Price 20 tabs = **B**

PROMETHAZINE HYDROCHLORIDE

Indications: sedation
Cautions; Side-effects: see under Promethazine Hydrochloride (section 3.4.1)
Dose: 20–50 mg; CHILD up to 1 year 5–10 mg, 1–5 years 15–20 mg, 6–10 years 20–25 mg, at bedtime or, for daytime sedation, once or twice daily using the lower dose

Preparations
See section 3.4.1

TEMAZEPAM

Indications: insomnia (useful in the elderly)
Cautions; Side-effects: see under Nitrazepam, but except at high dosage hangover is uncommon and doses less cumulative. Inappropriate in patients with early wakening
Dose: 10–30 mg, increasing in severe insomnia to 60 mg, 30 minutes before bedtime

Temazepam Capsules, temazepam 10 mg, price 20 caps = **C**; 20 mg, price 20 caps = **D**
▼ **Euhypnos®** (Farmitalia Carlo Erba)
Capsules, green, temazepam 10 mg. Price 20 caps = **C**
▼ **Euhypnos Forte®** (Farmitalia Carlo Erba)
Capsules, green, temazepam 20 mg. Price 20 caps = **D**
▼ **Normison®** (Wyeth)
Capsules, yellow, temazepam 10 mg. Price 20 caps = **C**
Capsules, yellow, temazepam 20 mg. Price 20 caps = **D**

TRIAZOLAM

Indications: insomnia (useful in the elderly)
Cautions; Side-effects: see under Nitrazepam, but hangover is uncommon and doses less cumulative. Inappropriate in patients with early wakening. Psychological disturbances have been reported
Dose: 125–250 micrograms 15–30 minutes before bedtime

▼ **Halcion®** (Upjohn)
Tablets, lavender, scored, triazolam 125 micrograms. Price 20 tabs = **C**
Tablets, blue, scored, triazolam 250 micrograms. Price 20 tabs = **D**

TRICLOFOS SODIUM

Indications: insomnia
Cautions; Contra-indications; Side-effects: see under Chloral Hydrate, but gastro-intestinal disturbances are less common and it is not irritant to skin and mucous membranes
Dose: insomnia, 1–2 g 30 minutes before bedtime; CHILD up to 1 year 100–250 mg, 1–5 years 250–500 mg, 6–12 years 0.5–1 g

Triclofos Elixir, triclofos sodium 500 mg/5 ml. Price 100 ml = **D**

TRIMEPRAZINE TARTRATE

Indications: sedation
Cautions; Side-effects: see under Trimeprazine Tartrate (section 15.1.4.2)
Dose: CHILD 3–6 years 15–60 mg, 7–12 years 60–90 mg, daily in divided doses

Preparations
See section 15.1.4.2

4.1.2 Anxiolytics

Benzodiazepine anxiolytics are generally effective in alleviating definite anxiety states and they are widely prescribed. Although there is a tendency to prescribe these drugs to almost anyone with stress-related symptoms, unhappiness, or minor physical disease, their use in many situations is unjustified. They should be limited to patients whose anxiety is clearly handicapping, as when it interferes with their work, leisure, or family relationships. In children anxiolytic treatment should be used only to relieve acute anxiety (with insomnia) caused by fear.

Anxiolytic treatment should be limited to short periods because tolerance to its effects develops within four months of continuous use and because of the danger of insidious development of dependence and subsequent difficulty in withdrawing the drug. Addiction is particularly likely in patients with a history of alcoholism or drug abuse and in patients with marked personality disorders. Withdrawal of the drug following either high dosage or long-term administration should be gradual as abrupt withdrawal may produce confusion, toxic psychosis, convulsions, or a condition resembling delirium tremens. In milder cases, symptoms may be similar to the original complaint and encourage further prescribing.

Anxiolytics, particularly the benzodiazepines, have been termed 'minor tranquillisers'. This term is misleading because not only do they differ markedly from the antipsychotic drugs ('major tranquillisers') but their use is by no means minor. Antipsychotics, in low doses, are also sometimes used in severe anxiety for their sedative action (section 4.2.1).

Benzodiazepines are the most important anxiolytics. They include chlordiazepoxide (Librium® etc.), clorazepate (Tranxene®), diazepam (Valium® etc.), lorazepam (Ativan®), medazepam (Nobrium®), and oxazepam (Serenid-D®, Serenid Forte®). **Diazepam, chlordiazepoxide, medazepam,** and **clorazepate** are the most appropriate drugs for relieving chronic anxiety as they have a long half-life and consequently a sustained anxiolytic action. Shorter-acting compounds such as **oxazepam** and **lorazepam** may be more appropriate in acute anxiety or for relieving phobic panic attacks; they may be preferred in patients with hepatic impairment.

Clobazam (Frisium®) is a newly introduced benzodiazepine anxiolytic and is claimed to produce less psychomotor impairment. **Diazepam** or **lorazepam**, by intravenous injection or by mouth, may have a place in the control of severe panic attacks. The intravenous route is the most rapid but the procedure is not without risk (section 4.8.2) and should be used only when alternative measures have failed. The intramuscular route has no advantage over the oral route.

Benzodiazepines are also used in the treatment of alcohol withdrawal, beginning with a large dose which is gradually reduced.

Of the other anxiolytics, benzoctamine (Tacitin®) and meprobamate are **less effective** than the benzodiazepines. Meprobamate is also more hazardous in overdosage and is liable to induce dependence.

Barbiturates and related drugs should not be used as anxiolytics (section 4.1.3).

Propranolol (see section 2.4) is often very effective in alleviating the palpitations, diarrhoea, and tremor which accompany anxiety and apprehension. Oxprenolol may also be used.

DIAZEPAM

Indications: anxiety, insomnia, adjunctive treatment of acute alcohol withdrawal

Cautions: may affect a patient's ability to drive or operate machinery and increase the effects of alcohol, avoid prolonged use and abrupt withdrawal thereafter. Caution in neuromuscular disease, closed-angle glaucoma, respiratory disease, late pregnancy, nursing mothers; reduce dosage in elderly and debilitated patients, liver disease, renal impairment. Special precautions are necessary when diazepam is given by intravenous injection (section 4.8.2). Drug interactions: see Appendix 1

Side-effects: drowsiness, dizziness, ataxia (particularly in the elderly); occasionally confusion, dry mouth, hypersensitivity reactions; respiratory depression; on intravenous injection, pain, thrombophlebitis

Dose: by mouth, anxiety, 2 mg 3 times daily increased in severe anxiety to 15–30 mg daily in divided doses; CHILD 1–5 mg daily in divided doses

Insomnia, 5–30 mg at bedtime

By intramuscular or slow intravenous injection, (at a rate of not more than 5 mg/minute) for severe anxiety, control of acute panic attacks, and acute alcohol withdrawal, 10 mg, repeated if necessary after 4 hours

By intravenous infusion—section 4.8.2

By rectum in suppositories, 5–10 mg; max. 60 mg daily in divided doses

Diazepam Capsules, diazepam 2 and 5 mg. Price 20 caps (both) = **A**

Diazepam Tablets, diazepam 2 mg, price 20 tabs = **A;** 5 mg, price 20 tabs = **A;** 10 mg, price 20 tabs = **A**

Diazepam Elixir, diazepam 2 mg/5 ml. Diluent syrup or sorbitol solution, life of diluted elixir 14 days. Price 100 ml = **D**

Atensine® (Berk)

Tablets, scored, diazepam 2 mg. Price 20 tabs = **A**

Tablets, yellow, scored, diazepam 5 mg. Price 20 tabs = **A**

Tablets, blue, scored, diazepam 10 mg. Price 20 tabs = **B**

Diazemuls® (KabiVitrum)

Injection (emulsion), diazepam 5 mg/ml. For intravenous injection or infusion. Price 2-ml amp = **B**

Evacalm® (Unimed)
Tablets, scored, diazepam 2 mg. Price 20 tabs = **A**
Tablets, yellow, scored, diazepam 5 mg. Price 20 tabs = **A**

Sedapam® (DF)
Tablets, scored, diazepam 2 mg. Price 20 tabs = **A**
Tablets, yellow, scored, diazepam 5 mg. Price 20 tabs = **A**

Solis® (Galen)
Capsules, violet/turquoise, diazepam 2 mg. Price 20 caps = **A**
Capsules, violet/mauve, diazepam 5 mg. Price 20 caps = **A**

Tensium® (DDSA)
Tablets, scored, diazepam 2 mg. Price 20 tabs = **A**
Tablets, yellow, scored, diazepam 5 mg. Price 20 tabs = **A**
Tablets, blue, scored, diazepam 10 mg. Price 20 tabs = **B**

Valium® (Roche)
Capsules, blue/white, diazepam 2 mg. Price 20 caps = **A**
Capsules, blue/yellow, diazepam 5 mg. Price 20 caps = **B**
Tablets, scored, diazepam 2 mg. Price 20 tabs = **A**
Tablets, yellow, scored, diazepam 5 mg. Price 20 tabs = **B**
Tablets, blue, scored, diazepam 10 mg. Price 20 tabs = **B**
Syrup(=elixir), pink, diazepam 2 mg/5 ml. Diluent syrup or sorbitol solution, life of diluted elixir 14 days. Price 100 ml = **D**
Injection, diazepam 5 mg/ml. Do not dilute (except for intravenous infusion). Price 2- and 4-ml amp (both) = **B**
Suppositories, diazepam 5 mg. Price 5 suppos = **C**
Suppositories, diazepam 10 mg. Price 5 suppos = **C**

BENZOCTAMINE HYDROCHLORIDE

Indications: anxiety (see notes above)
Cautions; Side-effects: see under Diazepam. Dry mouth occurs more frequently
Dose: 10–20 mg 3 times daily

Tacitin® (Ciba)
Tablets, f/c, scored, benzoctamine hydrochloride 10 mg. Price 20 tabs = **C**

CHLORDIAZEPOXIDE

Indications: anxiety, insomnia, acute alcohol withdrawal
Cautions; Side-effects: see under Diazepam
Dose: *by mouth,* anxiety, 10 mg 3 times daily increased in severe anxiety to 100 mg daily in divided doses; reduce in elderly and debilitated patients; CHILD 5–20 mg daily in divided doses Insomnia, 25 mg at bedtime
By intramuscular injection, control of acute panic attacks and acute alcohol withdrawal, 50–100 mg, followed, if necessary, by 25–100 mg 3–4 times daily
Note: chlordiazepoxide and its hydrochloride are used interchangeably

Chlordiazepoxide Capsules, chlordiazepoxide hydrochloride 5 and 10 mg. Price 20 caps (both) = **A**

Librium® (Roche)
Capsules, green/yellow, chlordiazepoxide hydrochloride 5 mg. Price 20 caps = **B**
Capsules, green/black, chlordiazepoxide hydrochloride 10 mg. Price 20 caps = **B**
Tablets, yellowish green, s/c, chlordiazepoxide 5 mg. Price 20 tabs = **B**
Tablets, pale green, s/c, chlordiazepoxide 10 mg. Price 20 tabs = **B**
Tablets, dark green, s/c, chlordiazepoxide 25 mg. Price 20 tabs = **B**
Injection, powder for reconstitution, chlordiazepoxide (as hydrochloride). Price 100-mg amp (with solvent) = **C**

Tropium® (DDSA)
Capsules, yellow/black, chlordiazepoxide hydrochoride 5 mg. Price 20 caps = **A**
Capsules, green/white, chlordiazepoxide hydrochloride 10 mg. Price 20 caps = **A**
Tablets, green, s/c, chlordiazepoxide hydrochloride 5 mg. Price 20 tabs = **A**
Tablets, green, s/c, chlordiazepoxide hydrochloride 10 mg. Price 20 tabs = **A**
Tablets, green, s/c, chlordiazepoxide hydrochloride 25 mg. Price 20 tabs = **B**

CHLORMEZANONE

Indications: anxiety
Cautions; Side-effects: see under Diazepam
Dose: 200 mg 3 times daily *or* 400 mg at bedtime; max. 800 mg daily

Trancopal® (Sterling Research)
Tablets, yellow, chlormezanone 200 mg. Price 20 tabs = **D**

CLOBAZAM

Indications: anxiety
Cautions; Side-effects: see under Diazepam
Dose: 10 mg 3 times daily, increased in severe anxiety (in hospitalised patients) to a max. of 60 mg daily in divided doses, reduce frequency of dosage in elderly and debilitated patients to twice daily; CHILD, half the adult dose

▼ **Frisium**® (Hoechst)
Capsules, blue, clobazam 10 mg. Price 20 caps = **D**

CLORAZEPATE DIPOTASSIUM

Indications: anxiety, insomnia, adjunctive treatment of acute alcohol withdrawal
Cautions; Side-effects: see under Diazepam
Dose: 15 mg, usually at bedtime

Tranxene® (Boehringer Ingelheim)
Capsules, pink/grey, clorazepate dipotassium 15 mg. Price 20 caps = **D**

HYDROXYZINE HYDROCHLORIDE

Indications: anxiety, adjunctive treatment in stress-related urticaria and dermatoses
Cautions; Side-effects: see under Diazepam
Dose: 25 mg 3–4 times daily, increased in severe anxiety to 400 mg daily in divided doses; CHILD 2–3 mg/kg daily in divided doses

Atarax® (Pfizer)
Tablets, orange, s/c, hydroxyzine hydrochloride 10 mg. Price 20 tabs = **C**
Tablets, green, s/c, hydroxyzine hydrochloride 25 mg. Price 20 tabs = **D**
Syrup (= elixir), hydroxyzine hydrochloride 10 mg/5 ml. Diluent syrup, life of diluted elixir 14 days. Price 150 ml = **D**

KETAZOLAM

Indications: anxiety
Cautions; Side-effects: see under Diazepam
Dose: initially 30 mg at bedtime, adjusted according to the response to 15–60 mg daily

▼ **Anxon®** (Beecham)
Capsules, dark pink/light pink, ketazolam 15 mg. Price 20 caps = **D**
Capsules, dark pink/light pink, ketazolam 30 mg. Price 20 caps = **E**

LORAZEPAM

Indications: anxiety, insomnia
Cautions; Side-effects: see under Diazepam. It is less cumulative and excessive drowsiness is therefore less likely
Dose: *by mouth,* anxiety, 1–4 mg, increased to 10 mg in severe anxiety, daily in divided doses
Insomnia, 1–4 mg at bedtime
By slow intramuscular or slow intravenous injection, for the control of acute panic attacks, 25–30 micrograms/kg every 6 hours if necessary

Ativan® (Wyeth)
Tablets, blue, scored, lorazepam 1 mg. Price 20 tabs = **B**
Tablets, yellow, scored, lorazepam 2.5 mg. Price 20 tabs = **C**
▼ *Injection,* lorazepam 4 mg/ml. Price 1-ml amp = **B.** For intramuscular injection it should be diluted with an equal volume of water for injections or sodium chloride intravenous infusion 0.9%

MEDAZEPAM

Indications: anxiety, insomnia, adjunctive treatment of acute alcohol withdrawal
Cautions; Side-effects: see under Diazepam. It is less cumulative and excessive drowsiness is therefore less likely
Dose: anxiety, 5 mg 2–3 times daily, increased in severe anxiety to a max. of 40 mg daily in divided doses; CHILD 1–1.5 mg/kg daily to a max. of 40 mg
Insomnia, 10–15 mg at bedtime

Nobrium® (Roche)
Capsules, red/white, medazepam 5 mg. Price 20 caps = **B**
Capsules, red/black, medazepam 10 mg. Price 20 caps = **B**

MEPROBAMATE

Indications: anxiety, particularly with muscle spasm
Cautions: see under Diazepam, but the risk of dependence is higher; avoid in acute intermittent porphyria. Caution in epilepsy, abrupt withdrawal may precipitate convulsions
Side-effects: see under Diazepam, but the incidence is greater and drowsiness is the most common side-effect. Also gastro-intestinal disturbances, paraesthesia, weakness, CNS effects which include headache, paradoxical excitement, disturbances of vision; rarely agranulocytosis and rashes
Dose: 400 mg 3 times daily, increased when necessary to a max. of 2.4 g daily in divided doses

Meprobamate Tablets, meprobamate 400 mg. Price 20 tabs = **B**
Equanil® (Wyeth)
Tablets, meprobamate 200 mg. Price 20 tabs = **A**
Tablets, scored, meprobamate 400 mg. Price 20 tabs = **A**
Meprate® (DDSA)
Tablets, meprobamate 400 mg. Price 20 tabs = **A**
Miltown® (Pharmax)
Tablets, scored, meprobamate 400 mg. Price 20 tabs = **B**
Tenavoid® (Burgess)
Tablets, orange, meprobamate 200 mg, bendrofluazide 3 mg. Price 24 tabs = **D**

OXAZEPAM

Indications: anxiety, adjunctive treatment of acute alcohol withdrawal
Cautions; Side-effects: see under Diazepam; drowsiness is the most common side-effect
Dose: anxiety, 15–30 mg 3 to 4 times daily, increased in severe anxiety to a max. of 60 mg 3 times daily

Serenid-D® (Wyeth)
Tablets, oxazepam 10 mg. Price 20 tabs = **B**
Tablets, oxazepam 15 mg. Price 20 tabs = **B**
Serenid-Forte® (Wyeth)
Capsules, red/green, oxazepam 30 mg. Price 20 caps = **B**

PROPRANOLOL HYDROCHLORIDE

Indications: relief of somatic symptoms of anxiety
Cautions; Contra-indications; Side-effects: see section 2.4
Dose: 80–160 mg daily in divided doses

Preparations
See section 2.4

4.1.3 Barbiturates and similar hypnotics and sedatives

The benzodiazepines have supplanted the barbiturates for most purposes as hypnotics, sedatives, and anxiolytics because the barbiturates are more hazardous in use.

The intermediate-acting **barbiturates** and **methyprylone** (Noludar®), given orally, may still have a place in the treatment of severe intractable insomnia, but they should be avoided in the elderly. This group includes amylobarbitone, butobarbitone, cyclobarbitone, heptabarbitone, pentobarbitone, and quinalbarbitone. Some of the long-acting barbiturates, for example phenobarbitone, are of value in epilepsy but their use as sedatives is unjustified. The very short-acting barbiturates are of value in anaesthesia (see section 15.1.1).

Glutethimide (Doriden®) is similar in nature to the barbiturates and its use is likewise not recommended.

AMYLOBARBITONE

Indications: severe intractable insomnia
Cautions: avoid use where possible. Dependence and tolerance readily occur. Abrupt withdrawal may precipitate a serious withdrawal syndrome (rebound insomnia, anxiety, tremor, dizziness, nausea, fits, and delirium). Repeated doses are cumulative and may lead to excessive sedation; may affect ability to drive or operate machinery and increase the effects of alcohol. Caution in respiratory disease, renal disease, hepatic impairment, pregnancy, breast feeding, elderly and debilitated patients. Drug interactions: see Appendix 1
Contra-indications: insomnia caused by pain; porphyria
Side-effects: hangover with drowsiness, dizziness, ataxia, respiratory depression, headache, particularly with the elderly. Also paradoxical excitement and confusion, occasionally precedes sleep
Dose: 100–200 mg 30 minutes before bedtime

Amytal® (Lilly)
Tablets, amylobarbitone 15, 30, 50, and 100 mg. Price 20 tabs (all) = **A**
Tablets, scored, amylobarbitone 200 mg. Price 20 tabs = **B**

AMYLOBARBITONE SODIUM

Indications; Cautions; Contra-indications; Side-effects: see under Amylobarbitone
Dose: 100–200 mg 15–30 minutes before bedtime

Sodium Amytal® (Lilly)
Pulvules® (= capsules), blue, amylobarbitone sodium 60 mg. Price 20 caps = **A**
Pulvules® (= capsules), blue, amylobarbitone sodium 200 mg. Price 20 caps = **B**
Tablets, amylobarbitone sodium 60 mg. Price 20 tabs = **A**
Tablets, amylobarbitone sodium 200 mg. Price 20 tabs = **B**
Injection, powder for reconstitution, amylobarbitone sodium 250 mg and 500 mg. Price per amp (both) = **D**

Tuinal® (Lilly)
Pulvules® (= capsules), orange/blue, amylobarbitone sodium 50 mg, quinalbarbitone sodium 50 mg. Price 20 caps = **B**
Dose: 1–2 capsules 15–30 minutes before bedtime

BUTOBARBITONE

Indications; Cautions; Contra-indications; Side-effects: see under Amylobarbitone
Dose: 100–200 mg 30 minutes before bedtime

Soneryl® (M&B)
Tablets, pink, scored, butobarbitone 100 mg. Price 20 tabs = **A**

CYCLOBARBITONE CALCIUM

Indications; Cautions; Contra-indications; Side-effects: see under Amylobarbitone
Dose: 200–400 mg 30 minutes before bedtime

Cyclobarbitone Tablets, cyclobarbitone calcium 200 mg. Price 20 tabs = **B**

Evidorm® (Winthrop)
Tablets, scored, cyclobarbitone calcium 100 mg, hexobarbitone 250 mg. Price 20 tabs = **D**
Dose: 1–2 tablets 15–30 minutes before bedtime

Phanodorm® (Winthrop)
Tablets, cyclobarbitone calcium 200 mg. Price 20 tabs = **C**

GLUTETHIMIDE

Indications: insomnia (see notes above)
Cautions; Contra-indications; Side-effects: see under Amylobarbitone. Also rashes and gastro-intestinal disturbances may occur
Dose: 250–500 mg 20 minutes before bedtime

Doriden® (Ciba)
Tablets, scored, glutethimide 250 mg. Price 20 tabs = **A**

HEPTABARBITONE

Indications; Cautions; Contra-indications; Side-effects: see under Amylobarbitone
Dose: 200–400 mg 30 minutes before bedtime

Medomin® (Geigy)
Tablets, scored, heptabarbitone 200 mg. Price 20 tabs = **B**

METHYPRYLONE

Indications; Cautions; Contra-indications; Side-effects: see under Amylobarbitone, but side-effects occur less frequently. Rashes and gastro-intestinal disturbances may occur
Dose: 200–400 mg 15 minutes before bedtime

Noludar® (Roche)
Tablets, scored, methyprylone 200 mg. Price 20 tabs = **C**

PENTOBARBITONE SODIUM
Indications; Cautions; Contra-indications; Side-effects: see under Amylobarbitone
Dose: 100–200 mg 30 minutes before bedtime

Nembutal® (Abbott)
Capsules, yellow, pentobarbitone sodium 100 mg. Price 20 caps = **A**

PHENOBARBITONE
Cautions; Contra-indications; Side-effects: see section 4.8.1. The use of phenobarbitone to relieve tension is not justified. Compound preparations containing phenobarbitone as a sedative are found in various chapters

QUINALBARBITONE SODIUM
Indications; Cautions; Contra-indications; Side-effects: see under Amylobarbitone
Dose: 100–200 mg 30 minutes before bedtime

Seconal Sodium® (Lilly)
Pulvules® (= capsules), orange, quinalbarbitone sodium 50 and 100 mg. Price 20 caps (both) = **B**

4.2 Drugs used in psychoses and related disorders

These consist of several groups of chemically related compounds. The most important antipsychotic drugs are the phenothiazine derivatives, the thioxanthenes, the butyrophenones, and pimozide (section 4.2.1). Some of these compounds are given as long-acting depot injections which are described in section 4.2.2.

Lithium salts (section 4.2.3) are used in manic depressive illnesses.

4.2.1 Antipsychotic drugs

Antipsychotic drugs are also known as 'neuroleptics' and (misleadingly) as 'major tranquillisers'. Antipsychotic drugs generally tranquillise without impairing consciousness and without causing paradoxical excitement but they should not be regarded merely as tranquillisers. For conditions such as schizophrenia the tranquillising effect is of secondary importance.

In the short-term they are used to quieten disturbed patients whatever the underlying psychopathology, which may be brain damage, mania, toxic delirium, agitated depression, or acute behavioural disturbance.

They are used to alleviate severe anxiety but this also should be a short-term treatment. In patients with anxiety and depression, caution is necessary as the symptoms of depression may be masked.

TREATMENT OF SCHIZOPHRENIA. The main use of antipsychotic drugs is in the treatment of schizophrenia where they relieve florid psychotic symptoms such as thought disorder, hallucinations, and delusions and prevent relapse. They are usually less effective in apathetic withdrawn patients.

Sometimes they appear to have an activating influence. For example, large doses of chlorpromazine may restore the acutely ill schizophrenic to normal activity and social behaviour where previously he was withdrawn or even mute and akinetic. Patients with acute schizophrenia generally respond better than those with chronic symptoms.

Long-term treatment of patients with a definite diagnosis of schizophrenia may be necessary even after their first episode of illness in order to prevent the manifest illness from becoming chronic. Withdrawal of drug treatment requires careful surveillance because the patient who appears well on medication may suffer a disastrous relapse if treatment is withdrawn inappropriately. In addition the need for continuation of treatment may not become immediately evident because relapse is often delayed for several weeks after cessation of treatment.

Antipsychotic drugs are considered to act by interfering with dopaminergic transmission in the brain by blocking dopamine receptors and may give rise to the extrapyramidal effects described below, and also to hyperprolactinaemia. The antipsychotic drugs also affect to varying degrees cholinergic, alpha-adrenergic, histaminergic, and tryptaminergic receptors.

SIDE-EFFECTS OF ANTIPSYCHOTICS. The most troublesome side-effects of antipsychotic drugs are extrapyramidal symptoms. They are caused most frequently by fluphenazine, haloperidol, and the depot preparations. They are easy to recognise but cannot be accurately predicted because they depend partly on the dose and partly on the type of drug, and on patient idiosyncrasy. They consist of dystonia (abnormal face and body movements) which may appear after only a few doses, akathisia which may resemble an exacerbation of the condition being treated, and a parkinsonism-like syndrome which usually takes longer to develop.

These symptoms remit if the drug is withdrawn. Parkinsonian effects may be suppressed by the administration of **anticholinergic** drugs (section 4.9.2), but routine administration of such drugs is **not** justified as not all patients are affected and because tardive dyskinesia is worsened by them. Tardive dyskinesia is of particular concern because it may be irreversible on withdrawing therapy and treatment may be ineffective. It occurs fairly frequently in patients on long-term therapy and with high dosage, and the treatment of such patients must be carefully and regularly reviewed. Tardive dyskinesia may also occur occasionally after short-term treatment with low dosage.

Hypotension and interference with temperature regulation are dose-related side-effects and are liable to cause dangerous falls and hypothermia in the elderly.

SELECTION OF ANTIPSYCHOTIC DRUGS. The various antipsychotic drugs differ somewhat in predominant actions and side-effects. Selection is influenced by whether a more or less sedating secondary psychotropic effect is required and the patient's susceptibility to extrapyramidal side-effects. The differences between the antipsychotic drugs are less important than the great variability in patient response, and tolerance to these secondary effects usually develops. The increasing trend towards prescribing more than one antipsychotic for the same indication is **not** recommended. It may constitute a hazard and there is no significant evidence that side-effects are minimised.

In the paragraphs below specific antipsychotic drugs are discussed first and a classification then follows.

Chlorpromazine (Largactil® etc.) remains widely used. It has a marked sedating effect and is particularly useful for treating violent patients without causing stupor. Agitated states in the elderly can be controlled without confusion, a dose of 25 mg usually being adequate.

Flupenthixol (Depixol®) and **pimozide** (Orap®) are less sedating than chlorpromazine. Pimozide is regarded by many psychiatrists as the current drug of choice in schizophrenia particularly for apathetic withdrawn patients.

Fluphenazine, haloperidol, and **trifluoperazine** are also of value but their use is limited by the high incidence of extrapyramidal symptoms. **Haloperidol** may be preferred for the rapid control of hyperactive psychotic states.

Thioridazine (Melleril®) is popular for treating the elderly as there is a reduced incidence of extrapyramidal symptoms.

Promazine (Sparine®) is not sufficiently active to be used as an antipsychotic drug but may be of value in elderly patients with minor psychiatric problems.

Paraldehyde is **not** now used for the treatment of psychoses.

DEPOT PREPARATIONS. For maintenance therapy, **long-acting depot injections** of antipsychotic drugs are used because they are more convenient than oral preparations and ensure better patient compliance. However, they may give rise to a higher incidence of extrapyramidal reactions than oral preparations. Patients should first be given a small test-dose as undesirable effects are prolonged. They are administered by intramuscular injection at intervals of 1 to 4 weeks.

Fluphenazine or **clopenthixol** may be suitable for the treatment of excited or agitated patients. **Flupenthixol** can cause over-excitement in such patients but there is no clear-cut division in the usage of these drugs. In children fluphenazine is generally used as experience with the other depot preparations is limited. **Fluspirilene** (Redeptin®) has a shorter duration of action than the depot injections. The incidence of extrapyramidal reactions is similar for all these drugs. The depot preparations are described in section 4.2.2.

OTHER USES. Antipsychotic drugs are also used for many other purposes. **Chlorpromazine** and **prochlorperazine** are effective drugs for the relief of nausea, vomiting (section 4.6), and hiccups. They are used in anaesthetic practice for premedication and in neuroleptanalgesia (section 15.1.4.2). They can also be used to produce hypothermia and in terminal disease to promote calm. **Benperidol** is used in deviant and antisocial sexual behaviour but its value is not established.

CLASSIFICATION OF ANTIPSYCHOTICS. The **phenothiazine** derivatives can be divided into 3 main groups.

Group 1: chlorpromazine and promazine, characterised by pronounced sedative effects and moderate anticholinergic and extrapyramidal side-effects.

Group 2: pericyazine and thioridazine, characterised by moderate sedative effects, marked anticholinergic effects, but fewer extrapyramidal side-effects than groups 1 or 3.

Group 3: fluphenazine, perphenazine, prochlorperazine, thiethylperazine, thiopropazate, and trifluoperazine, characterised by fewer sedative effects, fewer anticholinergic effects than groups 1 or 2, but pronounced extrapyramidal side-effects.

Drugs of other chemical groups tend to resemble the phenothiazines of *group 3*. They include the **butyrophenones** (benperidol, droperidol, and haloperidol); **diphenylbutylpiperidines** (fluspirilene and pimozide); **thioxanthenes** (chlorprothixene, clopenthixol, and flupenthixol); and **oxypertine.**

CHLORPROMAZINE HYDROCHLORIDE

Indications: schizophrenia and related psychoses, tranquillisation and emergency control in behavioural disturbances, short-term adjunctive treatment of severe anxiety, terminal disease, intractable hiccup

Cautions: cardiovascular disease, respiratory disease, phaeochromocytoma, parkinsonism, epilepsy, pregnancy, renal and hepatic impairment, past history of jaundice, leucopenia; reduce dose in elderly and debilitated patients. Avoid drugs such as phenylbutazone that depress leucopoiesis. Initially, sedation may affect the ability to drive or operate machinery and increase the effects of alcohol. For prolonged use examinations for eye defects and abnormal skin pigmentation are required and abrupt discontinuation of therapy should be avoided. Patients should remain supine for 30 minutes after intramuscular injection. Drug interactions: see Appendix 1

Contra-indications: poisoning caused by CNS depressants; bone-marrow depression

Side-effects: extrapyramidal symptoms (reversed by dose reduction or anticholinergic drugs) and, on prolonged administration, occasionally tardive dyskinesia; hypothermia (occasionally pyrexia), drowsiness, apathy, pallor, nightmares, insomnia, depression, and, more rarely, agitation. Anticholinergic symptoms such as dry mouth, constipation, difficulty with micturition, and blurred vision; cardiovascular symptoms such as hypotension and cardiac arrhythmias; endocrine effects such as menstrual disturbances, galactorrhoea, and weight gain; sensitivity reactions such as agranulocytosis, leucopenia, leucocytosis, and haemolytic anaemia, photosensitisation, contact sensitisation, rashes, and jaundice. With prolonged high dosage, corneal and lens opacities and purplish pigmentation of the skin, cornea, conjunctiva, and retina. Intramuscular injection may be painful and may give rise to nodule formation

Dose: *by mouth,* psychoses and severe anxiety, initially 25 mg 3 times daily (may be doubled in bedpatients), adjusted according to the response, to 1 g daily or more in psychoses; CHILD up to 5 years 0.5–1 mg/kg daily, 6–12 years ⅓–½ adult dose

By intramuscular injection, (for relief of acute symptoms), 25–50 mg every 6–8 hours; CHILD, as dose by mouth

By rectum in suppositories, up to 400 mg chlorpromazine daily in divided doses

Intractable hiccup, *by mouth or by intramuscular injection,* 25–50 mg 3–4 times daily

Note: for equivalent therapeutic effect 100 mg chlorpromazine base given *rectally* as a suppository ≡ 20–25 mg chlorpromazine hydrochloride *by intramuscular injection* ≡ 40–50 mg of chlorpromazine base or hydrochloride *by mouth*

Chlorpromazine Tablets, s/c, chlorpromazine hydrochloride 25 and 50 mg, price 20 tabs (both) = **A**; 100 mg, price 20 tabs = **B**

Chlorpromazine Elixir, chlorpromazine hydrochloride 25 mg/5 ml. Price 100 ml = **A**

Chloractil® (DDSA)

Tablets, s/c, chlorpromazine hydrochloride 25 and 50 mg, price 20 tabs (both) = **A**; 100 mg, price 20 tabs = **B**

Dozine® (RP Drugs)

Syrup (= elixir), brown, chlorpromazine hydrochloride 25 mg/5 ml. Diluent sorbitol solution, life of diluted elixir 14 days. Price 100 ml = **A** (Hosp. only)

Largactil® (M&B)

Tablets, s/c, chlorpromazine hydrochloride 10 mg. Price 20 tabs = **A;** 25 mg, price 20 tabs = **A;** 50 mg, price 20 tabs = **B;** 100 mg, price 20 tabs = **C**

Syrup (= elixir), brown, chlorpromazine hydrochloride 25 mg/5 ml. Diluent syrup (without preservative), life of diluted elixir 14 days. Price 100 ml = **A**

Suspension forte (= strong mixture), orange, chlorpromazine hydrochloride 100 mg (as embonate)/5 ml. Diluent syrup (without preservative), life of diluted mixture 14 days. Price 100 ml = **C**

Injection, chlorpromazine hydrochloride 10 mg/ml. Price 5-ml amp = **B**

Injection, chlorpromazine hydrochloride 25 mg/ml. Price 1- and 2-ml amp (both) = **A**

Suppositories, chlorpromazine 100 mg. Price 5 suppos = **C**

BENPERIDOL

Indications: see notes above

Cautions; Contra-indications; Side-effects: see under Haloperidol. Special caution in liver disease

Dose: initially 0.25–1.5 mg daily in divided doses, adjusted according to the response

Anquil® (Janssen)

Tablets, benperidol 250 micrograms. Price 20 tabs = **E**

CHLORPROTHIXENE

Indications: schizophrenia and related psychoses, tranquillisation in behavioural disturbances, short-term adjunctive treatment of severe anxiety

Cautions; Contra-indications; Side-effects: see under Chlorpromazine Hydrochloride. Possibly less effective than chlorpromazine but extrapyramidal symptoms are much less frequent and anticholinergic side-effects are more frequent

Dose: psychoses, up to 400 mg (in elderly patients up to 150 mg) daily in divided doses, adjusted according to the response

Severe anxiety, 30–45 mg daily in divided doses, adjusted according to the response; CHILD up to 6 years, 1–2 mg/kg daily in divided doses, over 6 years 15 mg 3–4 times daily

Taractan® (Roche)

Tablets, pink, s/c, chlorprothixene 15 mg. Price 20 tabs = **B**

Tablets, brown, s/c, chlorprothixene 50 mg. Price 20 tabs = **D**

DROPERIDOL

Indications: tranquillisation and emergency control in psychoses, particularly mania, and in behavioural disturbances

Cautions; Contra-indications; Side-effects: see under Haloperidol. Contra-indicated in severe depression; special caution in liver disease

Dose: *by mouth,* 5–20 mg every 4–8 hours; CHILD, 200–600 micrograms/kg

By intramuscular injection, up to 10 mg every 4–6 hours; CHILD, as dose by mouth
By intravenous injection, 5–15 mg; CHILD 200–300 micrograms/kg

Droleptan® (Janssen)
Tablets, yellow, scored, droperidol 10 mg. Price 20 tabs = **F**
Oral liquid (= elixir), droperidol 1 mg/ml. Do not dilute. Price 100 ml (with graduated cap) = **E**
Injection, droperidol 5 mg/ml. Price 2-ml amp = **C**

FLUPENTHIXOL DIHYDROCHLORIDE

Indications: schizophrenia and related psychoses, particularly with apathy and withdrawal but not mania or psychomotor hyperactivity; short-term adjunctive treatment of severe anxiety
Cautions; Contra-indications; Side-effects: see under Chlorpromazine Hydrochloride but less sedating; extrapyramidal symptoms are more frequent (25% of patients) and tardive dyskinesia also occurs. Oral administration may cause restlessness and insomnia. Avoid in children, senile confusional states, excitable and overactive patients
Dose: flupenthixol, initially 3–9 mg twice daily adjusted according to the response; max. 18 mg daily

Depixol® (Lundbeck)
Tablets, yellow. s/c, flupenthixol 3 mg (as dihydrochloride). Price 20 tabs = **E**
For Depixol® depot injections (flupenthixol decanoate) see section 4.2.2

FLUPHENAZINE HYDROCHLORIDE

Indications: schizophrenia and related psychoses, tranquillisation in behavioural disturbances, short-term adjunctive treatment of severe anxiety
Cautions; Contra-indications; Side-effects: see under Chlorpromazine Hydrochloride, but less sedating and fewer anticholinergic or hypotensive symptoms. Extrapyramidal symptoms, particularly dystonic reactions and akathisia, are more frequent, especially in elderly patients. Occasionally tardive dyskinesia also occurs. Caution when used in depression
Dose: psychoses, initially adults and children 2.5–10 mg daily as a single dose, adjusted according to the response to a max. of 20 mg daily
Severe anxiety, initially 1–2 mg daily in divided doses, increased as necessary to 4 mg; CHILD 0.25–1 mg daily in divided doses, adjusted according to the response

Moditen® (Squibb)
Tablets, pink, s/c, fluphenazine hydrochloride 1 mg. Price 20 tabs = **C**
Tablets, yellow, s/c, fluphenazine hydrochloride 2.5 mg. Price 20 tabs = **D**
Tablets, s/c, fluphenazine hydrochloride 5 mg. Price 20 tabs = **D**
For Modecate® and Moditen Enanthate® depot injections see section 4.2.2

HALOPERIDOL

Indications: schizophrenia and related psychoses, particularly mania; tranquillisation and emergency control in behavioural disturbances; short-term adjunctive treatment of severe anxiety
Cautions; Contra-indications; Side-effects: see under Chlorpromazine Hydrochloride but less sedating, and fewer anticholinergic or hypotensive symptoms. Extrapyramidal symptoms, particularly dystonic reactions and akathisia are more frequent especially in thyrotoxic patients. Occasionally tardive dyskinesia also occurs. Rarely, alterations in liver function, gastro-intestinal disturbances, and weight loss. Caution in depression. Avoid in basal ganglia disease. Drug interactions: see Appendix 1
Dose: *by mouth*, psychoses, initially 0.5–5 mg 2–3 times daily adjusted according to the response; max. 200 mg daily; usual maintenance dose 5–10 mg daily; CHILD initially 50–150 micrograms/kg daily divided into 2 doses, adjusted according to response; usual maintenance dose 50 micrograms/kg daily divided into 2 doses
Severe anxiety, adults 500 micrograms twice daily
By intramuscular or intravenous injection, (for relief of acute symptoms) 10 mg (increasing to 30 mg for emergency control) every 6 hours. CHILD, as dose by mouth

Haloperidol Tablets, haloperidol 1.5 mg, price 20 tabs = **B**; 5 mg, price 20 tabs = **D**; 10 mg, price 20 tabs = **E**; 20 mg, price 20 tabs = **G**
Haldol® (Janssen)
Tablets, yellow, scored, haloperidol 1.5 mg. Price 20 tabs = **B**
Tablets, blue, scored, haloperidol 5 mg. Price 20 tabs = **D**
Tablets, yellow, scored, haloperidol 10 mg. Price 20 tabs = **E**
Tablets, scored, haloperidol 20 mg. Price 20 tabs = **G**
Oral liquid (= elixir), haloperidol 2 mg/ml. Diluent purified water, freshly boiled and cooled, life of diluted elixir 14 days. Price 100 ml (with pipette) = **F**
Oral liquid concentrate (= concentrated elixir), haloperidol 10 mg/ml. Diluent purified water, freshly boiled and cooled, life of diluted concentrate 14 days. Alternatively, purified water, freshly boiled and cooled, containing 0.05% of methyl hydroxybenzoate and 0.005% of propyl hydroxybenzoate, life of diluted concentrate 2 months. Price 10 ml = **E**

Injection, haloperidol 5 mg/ml. Price 1-ml amp = **B**; 2-ml amp = **C**

Serenace® (Searle)

Capsules, green, haloperidol 500 micrograms. Price 20 caps = **B**

Tablets, scored, haloperidol 1.5 mg. Price 20 tabs = **C**

Tablets, pink, scored, haloperidol 5 mg. Price 20 tabs = **D**

Tablets, pale pink, scored, haloperidol 10 mg. Price 20 tabs = **E**

Tablets, dark pink, scored, haloperidol 20 mg. Price 20 tabs = **G**

Oral liquid (= elixir), haloperidol 2 mg/ml. Diluent purified water, freshly boiled and cooled, life of diluted elixir 14 days (2 months for dilutions containing more than 50% of the elixir). Price 100 ml = **F**

Injection, haloperidol 5 mg/ml. Price 1-ml amp = **B**

Injection, haloperidol 10 mg/ml. Price 2-ml amp = **C**

OXYPERTINE

Indications: schizophrenia and related psychoses, particularly with apathy and withdrawal, also suitable in mania and psychomotor hyperactivity; tranquillisation in behavioural disturbances; short-term adjunctive treatment of severe anxiety

Cautions; Side-effects: see under Chlorpromazine Hydrochloride, but extrapyramidal symptoms may occur less frequently. With low doses agitation and hyperactivity occur and with high doses sedation. Occasionally gastro-intestinal disturbances, photophobia, and rashes may occur. Drug interactions: see Appendix 1

Dose: psychoses, initially 80–120 mg daily in divided doses adjusted according to the response; max. 300 mg daily

Severe anxiety, initially 10 mg 3–4 times daily preferably after meals

Integrin® (Sterling Research)

Capsules, oxypertine 10 mg. Price 20 caps = **D**

Tablets, scored, oxypertine 40 mg. Price 20 tabs = **F**

PERICYAZINE

Indications: tranquillisation in behavioural disturbances, schizophrenia and related psychoses, short-term adjunctive treatment of severe anxiety

Cautions; Contra-indications; Side-effects: see under Chlorpromazine Hydrochloride, but more sedating. Extrapyramidal symptoms occur only with high doses

Dose: psychoses, initially 15–30 mg (reduced in elderly patients to 10 mg) daily divided into 2 doses, taking the larger dose at bedtime, adjusted according to the response; CHILD, initially 500 micrograms per year of age, adjusted according to the response; max. in children over 15 years 30 mg daily

Neulactil® (M&B)

Tablets, yellow, scored, pericyazine 2.5 mg. Price 20 tabs = **B**

Tablets, yellow, scored, pericyazine 10 mg. Price 20 tabs = **C**

Tablets, yellow, scored, pericyazine 25 mg. Price 20 tabs = **E**

Syrup (= elixir), green, pericyazine 2.5 mg/5 ml. Diluent syrup, life of diluted elixir 14 days. Price 100 ml = **C**

Syrup forte (= strong elixir), brown, pericyazine 10 mg/5 ml. Diluent as above. Price 100 ml = **D**

PERPHENAZINE

Indications: schizophrenia and related psychoses, tranquillisation and emergency control in behavioural disturbances, short-term adjunctive treatment of severe anxiety, terminal disease, intractable hiccup

Cautions; Contra-indications; Side-effects: see under Chlorpromazine Hydrochloride, but it is less sedating; extrapyramidal symptoms, especially dystonia, are more frequent, particularly at high dosage, tardive dyskinesia also occurs. Avoid in children

Dose: *by mouth,* psychoses and severe anxiety, initially 4 mg 3 times daily adjusted according to the response; max. 24 mg daily

By intramuscular injection (for relief of acute symptoms), 5–10 mg, followed if necessary by 5 mg every 6 hours; max. 15 mg daily

Fentazin® (A&H)

Tablets, s/c, perphenazine 2 mg. Price 20 tabs = **C**

Tablets, s/c, perphenazine 4 mg. Price 20 tabs = **C**

Tablets, s/c, perphenazine 8 mg. Price 20 tabs = **C**

Liquid concentrate (= elixir concentrate), perphenazine 2 mg/ml. Diluent syrup (without preservative), life of diluted concentrate 14 days. Price 100 ml = **C** (Hosp. only)

Injection, perphenazine 5 mg/ml. Price 1-ml amp = **A**

PIMOZIDE

Indications: schizophrenia and related psychoses, where thought disorders and inertia are prominent but not mania or psychomotor hyperactivity

Cautions; Side-effects: see under Chlorpromazine Hydrochloride, but less sedating and extrapyramidal symptoms are less frequent except with higher doses. May aggravate endogenous depression, parkinsonism, and epilepsy

Dose: initially 4–10 mg daily, adjusted according to the response; usual dose 2–20 mg daily, max. 20 mg daily

Orap® (Janssen)

Tablets, scored, pimozide 2 mg. Price 20 tabs = **E**

Tablets, green, scored, pimozide 4 mg. Price 20 tabs = **F**
Tablets, scored, pimozide 10 mg. Price 20 tabs = **I**

PROCHLORPERAZINE

Indications: schizophrenia and related psychoses, short-term adjunctive treatment of severe anxiety
Cautions; Contra-indications; Side-effects: see under Chlorpromazine Hydrochloride, but it is less sedating although extrapyramidal symptoms, particularly dystonic reactions, are more frequent; tardive dyskinesia also occurs. Avoid in children (but see section 4.6 for use as anti-emetic)
Dose: *by mouth,* prochlorperazine maleate or mesylate, psychoses, 12.5 mg twice daily for 7 days adjusted according to the response; max. 75–100 mg daily
Severe anxiety, 15–40 mg daily
By deep intramuscular injection, psychoses, prochlorperazine mesylate 12.5–25 mg 2–3 times daily
By rectum in suppositories, psychoses, the equivalent of prochlorperazine maleate 25 mg 2–3 times daily

Preparations
Section 4.6

PROMAZINE HYDROCHLORIDE

Indications: tranquillisation in disturbed behaviour particularly in the elderly, short-term adjunctive treatment of severe anxiety and terminal disease
Cautions; Contra-indications; Side-effects: see under Chlorpromazine Hydrochloride. With intravenous injection, thrombophlebitis
Dose: *by mouth,* initially 25–100 mg 3–4 times daily, adjusted according to response
By intramuscular or intravenous injection, 50 mg (reduced to 25 mg in elderly and debilitated patients) 6–8 hourly. Intravenous injections should be no stronger than 25 mg/ml

Sparine® (Wyeth)
Tablets, yellow, s/c, promazine hydrochloride 25 mg. Price 20 tabs = **A**
Tablets, orange, s/c, promazine hydrochloride 50 mg. Price 20 tabs = **B**
Tablets, red, s/c, promazine hydrochloride 100 mg. Price 20 tabs = **C**
Suspension (= mixture), yellow, promazine hydrochloride 50 mg (as embonate)/5 ml. Diluent syrup, life of diluted mixture 14 days. Price 150 ml = **C**
Injection, promazine hydrochloride 50 mg/ml. Price 1-ml amp = **A**; 2-ml amp = **B**

THIOPROPAZATE HYDROCHLORIDE

Indications: schizophrenia and related psychoses, tranquillisation in behavioural disturbances, short-term adjunctive treatment of severe anxiety
Cautions; Contra-indications; Side-effects: see under Chlorpromazine Hydrochloride, but less sedating
Dose: psychoses, initially 10 mg 3 times daily, adjusted according to the response; max. 100 mg daily
Severe anxiety, initially 5 mg 3 times daily, adjusted according to the response

Dartalan® (Searle)
Tablets, thiopropazate hydrochloride 5 mg. Price 20 tabs = **B**
Tablets, thiopropazate hydrochloride 10 mg. Price 20 tabs = **C**

THIORIDAZINE

Indications: schizophrenia and related psychoses, tranquillisation and emergency control in behavioural disturbances, agitation in elderly patients, short-term adjunctive treatment of severe anxiety
Cautions; Contra-indications; Side-effects: see under Chlorpromazine Hydrochloride, but less sedating and extrapyramidal symptoms and hypothermia rarely occur; more likely to induce hypotension. Caution in depression. Pigmentary retinopathy (with reduced visual acuity, brownish colouring of vision, and impaired night vision) occurs rarely with high doses
Dose: psychoses, 150–600 mg daily in divided doses, adjusted according to the response; max. 600 mg daily for up to 4 weeks. Usual maintenance dose 100–200 mg daily
Severe anxiety, 30–100 mg daily in divided doses; CHILD under 5 years 1 mg/kg, 6–12 years $\frac{1}{4}$–$\frac{1}{2}$ adult dose
Note: 100 mg thioridazine ≡ 110 mg thioridazine hydrochloride

Melleril® (Sandoz)
Tablets, s/c, thioridazine hydrochloride 10 mg. Price 20 tabs = **A**
Tablets, s/c, thioridazine hydrochloride 25 mg. Price 20 tabs = **B**
Tablets, s/c, thioridazine hydrochloride 50 mg. Price 20 tabs = **C**
Tablets, s/c, thioridazine hydrochloride 100 mg. Price 20 tabs = **C**
Suspension 25 mg/5 ml (= mixture), thioridazine 25 mg/5 ml. Price 100 ml = **B**
Suspension 100 mg/5 ml (= strong mixture), thioridazine 100 mg/5 ml. Price 100 ml = **E**. These suspensions should not be diluted but the two preparations may be mixed with each other to provide intermediate doses
Syrup (= elixir), orange, thioridazine 25 mg/5 ml. Diluent syrup (without preservative), life of diluted elixir 14 days. Price 100 ml = **B**
Concentrate for syrup (= elixir concentrate), orange, thioridazine 750 mg/5 ml for dilution with syrup (without preservative) or sorbitol

solution, life of diluted concentrate 6 months (Hosp. only)

TRIFLUOPERAZINE

Indications: schizophrenia and related psychoses, tranquillisation in behavioural disturbances, short-term adjunctive treatment of severe anxiety

Cautions; Contra-indications; Side-effects: see under Chlorpromazine Hydrochloride but less sedating, and hypotension, hypothermia, and anticholinergic side-effects occur less frequently. Extrapyramidal symptoms, particularly dystonic reactions and akathisia, are more frequent (particularly when the daily dose exceeds 6 mg). Caution in children

Dose: by mouth, psychoses, initially 5 mg twice daily, *or* 10 mg daily in slow-release form, adjusted according to the response; CHILD under 12 years, initially 5 mg daily in divided doses, adjusted according to the response

Severe anxiety, 2–4 mg daily in divided doses *or* 2–4 mg daily in slow-release form; CHILD 3–5 years up to 1 mg, 6–12 years up to 4 mg daily in divided doses

By deep intramuscular injection (for acute symptoms), 1–3 mg daily in divided doses to a max. of 6 mg daily; CHILD 50 micrograms/kg daily in divided doses

Stelazine® (SK&F)

Tablets, blue, s/c, trifluoperazine 1 and 5 mg (as hydrochloride). Price 20 tabs (both) = **B**

Spansules® (= capsules s/r), clear/yellow, enclosing dark blue, light blue, and white pellets, trifluoperazine 2 mg (as hydrochloride). Price 20 caps = **C**

Spansules® (= capsules s/r), clear/yellow, enclosing dark blue, light blue, and white pellets, trifluoperazine 10 mg (as hydrochloride). Price 20 caps = **C**

Spansules® (= capsules s/r), clear/yellow, enclosing dark blue, light blue, and white pellets, trifluoperazine 15 mg (as hydrochloride). Price 20 caps = **D**

Syrup (= elixir), yellow, trifluoperazine 1 mg (as hydrochloride)/5 ml. Diluent syrup, life of diluted elixir 14 days. Price 100 ml = **B**

Liquid concentrate, yellow, trifluoperazine 10 mg (as hydrochloride)/ml for dilution before use. Diluent syrup or water for preparations, life of diluted elixir 12 weeks or 1 week respectively. (Hosp. only)

Injection, trifluoperazine 1 mg (as hydrochloride)/ml. Price 1-ml amp = **B**

4.2.2 Antipsychotic depot injections

When transferring patients from one depot injection to another the following approximate equivalents may be used:

Clopenthixol decanoate	200 mg
Flupenthixol decanoate	40 mg
Fluphenazine decanoate	25 mg
Fluphenazine enanthate	25 mg

For notes on depot preparations of antipsychotic drugs see section 4.2.1.

CLOPENTHIXOL DECANOATE

Indications: maintenance in schizophrenia and related psychoses, particularly with aggression and agitation

Cautions; Side-effects: see under Chlorpromazine Hydrochloride (section 4.2.1) but it is less sedating. Treatment requires careful monitoring for optimum effect; extrapyramidal symptoms occur frequently. When transferring from oral to depot therapy, dosage by mouth should be gradually phased out. Caution in arteriosclerosis, and in renal and hepatic impairment. Pain at injection site may occur. Doses greater than 400 mg should be distributed between 2 injection sites

Contra-indications: children, coma caused by CNS depressants, senile confusional states, parkinsonism, intolerance to oral antipsychotics

Dose: by deep intramuscular injection into the gluteal muscle, test dose 100 mg, then after 7–28 days 100–200 mg or more, followed by 200–400 mg repeated at intervals of 2–4 weeks, adjusted according to the response

▼ **Clopixol®** (Lundbeck)

Injection (oily), clopenthixol decanoate 200 mg/ml. Price 1-ml amp = **E**

FLUPENTHIXOL DECANOATE

Indications: maintenance in schizophrenia and related psychoses

Cautions; Contra-indications; Side-effects: see under Clopenthixol Decanoate but it may have a mood elevating effect. Treatment requires careful monitoring, particularly when adjusting dosages; extrapyramidal symptoms occur frequently. They usually appear 1–3 days after administration and continue for about 5 days but may be delayed. With high doses, periodic blood counts are advisable. An alternative antipsychotic drug may be necessary if symptoms such as aggression or agitation appear. Avoid use in confusional states and in children

Dose: by deep intramuscular injection into the gluteal muscle, test dose 20 mg, then after 5–10 days 20–40 mg repeated at intervals of 2–4 weeks, adjusted according to the response

Depixol® (Lundbeck)

Injection (oily), flupenthixol decanoate 20 mg/ml. Price 1-ml amp or syringe = **D**; 2-ml amp or syringe = **E**

Depixol Conc® (Lundbeck)

Injection (oily), flupenthixol decanoate 100 mg/ml. Price 1-ml amp = **G**

FLUPHENAZINE DECANOATE

Indications: maintenance in schizophrenia and related psychoses

Cautions; Contra-indications; Side-effects: see under Clopenthixol Decanoate, but may be used in children. Extrapyramidal symptoms occur; patients require careful monitoring, particularly when adjusting dosage. Extrapyramidal symptoms usually appear a few hours after the dose has been administered and continue for about 2 days but may be delayed

Dose: *by deep intramuscular injection* into the gluteal muscle, test dose 12.5 mg (6.25 mg in children and elderly patients), then after 4–7 days 25 mg repeated at intervals of 14–40 days, adjusted according to the response

Modecate® (Squibb)
Injection (oily), fluphenazine decanoate 25 mg/ml. Price 0.5-ml amp = **D**; 1-ml amp or syringe = **E**; 2-ml amp or syringe = **F**; 10-ml vial = **J**

Modecate Concentrate® (Squibb)
Injection (oily), fluphenazine decanoate 100 mg/ml. Price 0.5-ml amp = **F**; 1-ml amp = **H**

FLUPHENAZINE ENANTHATE

Indications; Cautions; Contra-indications; Side-effects: see under Fluphenazine Decanoate but it has less prolonged effect and higher incidence of extrapyramidal symptoms

Dose: *by intramuscular injection* into the gluteal muscle, test dose 12.5 mg (6.25 mg in children and elderly patients), then after 4–7 days 25 mg repeated at intervals of 10–28 days, adjusted according to the response

Moditen Enanthate® (Squibb)
Injection (oily), fluphenazine enanthate 25 mg/ml. Price 1-ml amp = **E**; 10-ml vial = **J**

FLUSPIRILENE

Indications: maintenance in schizophrenia and related psychoses

Cautions; Contra-indications; Side-effects: see under Chlorpromazine Hydrochloride (section 4.2.1.), but less sedating. Extrapyramidal symptoms are less frequent than for the oily preparations (see above). They usually appear 12 hours after the dose and continue for about 2 days but may be delayed. Contra-indicated in children. Common side-effects are restlessness, and sweating. With prolonged use, tissue damage may occur

Dose: *by deep intramuscular injection,* 2 mg, increased by 2 mg at weekly intervals, adjusted according to the response; max. 20 mg weekly

Redeptin® (SK&F)
Injection (aqueous suspension), fluspirilene 2 mg/ml. Price 1-ml amp = **C**; 3-ml amp = **D**; 6-ml vial = **E**

4.2.3. Lithium salts

Lithium salts are used for their mood-regulating action in the treatment of manic illness and in the prevention of manic and depressive illnesses. Lithium treatment quietens the overactive euphoric patient. The decision to give prophylactic treatment usually requires specialist advice, and must be based on careful consideration of the likelihood of recurrence in the individual patient, and the benefit weighed against the risks.

Lithium salts have a narrow therapeutic/toxic ratio and should therefore not be prescribed unless facilities for monitoring plasma concentrations are available. Patients should be carefully selected. Doses are adjusted to achieve plasma concentrations of 0.6 to 1.2 mmol/litre (lower end of the range for maintenance therapy and elderly patients) on samples taken 12 hours after the preceding dose. Overdosage, usually with plasma concentrations over 1.5 mmol/litre, may be fatal and toxic effects include tremor, ataxia, dysarthria, nystagmus, renal impairment, and fits. If these potentially hazardous signs occur, treatment should be stopped, plasma-lithium concentrations redetermined, and steps taken to reverse lithium toxicity.

Lithium toxicity is made worse by sodium depletion. Concurrent use of diuretics that inhibit the uptake of sodium by the distal tubule (for example thiazides) should be avoided. In mild cases withdrawal of lithium and administration of generous amounts of sodium and fluid will reverse the toxicity. Plasma concentrations in excess of 2.5 mmol/litre are usually associated with serious toxicity requiring emergency treatment as indicated under Emergency Treatment of Poisoning, section 13. When toxic concentrations are reached there may be a delay of 1 or 2 days before maximum toxicity occurs.

In long-term use, therapeutic concentrations of lithium have been thought to cause histological and functional changes in the kidney. The significance of such changes is not clear but is of sufficient concern to discourage long-term use of lithium unless it is definitely indicated. Conventional and sustained-release tablets are available but it should be noted that **different preparations vary widely in bioavailability.**

Treatment should be discontinued only if relief from affective illness is absent or insignificant.

In the initial stages supplementary treatment with antipsychotic drugs (section 4.2.1) may be required because it may take a few days for lithium to exert its effect.

High doses of haloperidol, fluphenazine, or flupenthixol may be hazardous when used with lithium; irreversible toxic encephalopathy has been reported.

LITHIUM CARBONATE

Indications: prophylaxis in manic-depressive illness, treatment of mania

Cautions: plasma concentrations must be measured regularly (every 10 weeks on stabilised regimens), and thyroid function monitored; maintain adequate sodium and fluid intake. Avoid in impaired renal function, cardiac disease, and conditions with sodium imbalance (dose adjustment may be necessary in diarrhoea, vomiting, and heavy sweating). Caution in pregnancy (foetal intoxication), breast-feeding, elderly patients (reduce dose), diuretic treatment. Drug interactions: see Appendix 1

Side-effects: gastro-intestinal disturbances, fine tremor, polyuria and polydipsia (may disappear with continued treatment); also weight gain and oedema (may respond to dose reduction). Signs of lithium intoxication are blurred vision, increasing gastro-intestinal disturbances (anorexia, vomiting, diarrhoea), increasing CNS disturbances (mild drowsiness and sluggishness increasing to giddiness with ataxia, coarse tremor, lack of co-ordination, dysarthria) require withdrawal of treatment. With severe overdosage (plasma concentrations above 2 mmol/litre) hyperreflexia and hyperextension of limbs, fits, toxic psychoses, syncope, oliguria, circulatory failure, coma, and occasionally, death. Goitre, hypothyroidism, hypokalaemia, ECG changes, and kidney changes may also occur

Dose: 0.25–2 g daily, adjusted by daily tests on samples taken 12 hours after the preceding dose, to achieve a plasma concentration of 0.6–1.2 mmol/litre. Not suitable for children

Camcolit 250® (Norgine)
Tablets, f/c, lithium carbonate 250 mg (6.8 mmol Li^+). Price 20 tabs = **B**

Camcolit 400® (Norgine)
Tablets, f/c, scored, lithium carbonate 400 mg (10.8 mmol Li^+). Price 20 tabs = **B**

Liskonum® (SK&F)
Tablets, s/r, f/c, scored, lithium carbonate 450 mg (12.2 mmol Li^+). Price 20 tabs = **C**

Phasal® (Pharmax)
Tablets, s/r, lithium carbonate 300 mg (8.1 mmol Li^+). Price 20 tabs = **B**

Priadel® (Delandale)
Tablets, s/r, scored, lithium carbonate 400 mg (10.8 mmol Li^+). Price 20 tabs = **B**

4.3 Antidepressant drugs

The two main pharmacological types of antidepressant drugs are the tricyclic antidepressants and related compounds, for example amitriptyline and imipramine (section 4.3.1), and the monoamine-oxidase inhibitors (MAOIs), for example phenelzine and tranylcypromine (section 4.3.2).

Tricyclic and related antidepressants are the drugs of choice in the treatment of depressive illness, unless it is so severe that electroconvulsive therapy is immediately indicated. They are preferred to MAOIs because they are more effective antidepressants and do not show the dangerous interactions with some foods and drugs that are characteristic of the MAOIs.

The increasing trend towards prescribing more than one antidepressant of the tricyclic type is **not** recommended. It may constitute a hazard and there is no evidence that side-effects are minimised.

Mixtures of antidepressants with tranquillisers are included in section 4.3.3; their use is **not** recommended.

Other drugs used to treat depression (flupenthixol, tofenacin, and tryptophan) are included in section 4.3.4.

Lithium (section 4.2.3) has a mood-regulating action and is used specifically in the treatment of manic depressive illnesses.

Central nervous system stimulants (section 4.4) should **not** be used to treat depression. They may temporarily improve mood but may induce dependence and confusional states, or even a schizophrenia-like psychosis.This applies particularly with the amphetamines.

It should be noted that although anxiety is often present in depressive illness and may be the presenting symptom, the use of antipsychotics or anxiolytics may mask the true diagnosis. They should therefore be used with caution though they are useful aids in the management of agitated depression.

4.3.1 Tricyclic and related antidepressant drugs

The term 'tricyclic' is misleading as there are now 1-, 2-, and 4-ring structured drugs with broadly similar properties.

These drugs are most effective for treating moderate to severe depressive illness associated with psychomotor and physiological changes such as loss of appetite and eating and sleeping disturbances; improvement in sleep is usually the first benefit of therapy. There may be an interval of 2 or 3 weeks before the antidepressant action takes place so that electroconvulsive treatment may be required in severe depression when delay is hazardous or intolerable.

POSOLOGY. It is important to achieve plasma concentrations which are sufficiently high for effective treatment but not high enough to cause toxic effects. Optimum dosage varies between individuals, and patients taking similar daily doses may have markedly different plasma concentrations. These factors may account for some of the failures in therapy. Monitoring of plasma concentrations may be helpful if facilities are available. About 10 to 20% of patients fail to respond to these drugs.

MANAGEMENT. The patient's condition must be checked frequently, especially in the early weeks of treatment, to detect any suicidal tendencies. Limited quantities of antidepressant drugs should be prescribed at any one time as they are dangerous in overdosage. Some of the newer antidepressants, for example mianserin, nomifensine, and trazodone seem less dangerous in overdose than the older tricyclic compounds.

Treatment should be continued for 2 to 3 weeks before suppression of symptoms can be expected and thereafter should be maintained at the optimum level for at least another month before any attempt is made at dose reduction. Treatment should not be withdrawn prematurely, otherwise symptoms are likely to recur. The natural history of depressive illness suggests that remission usually occurs after 3 months to a year or more and some patients appear to benefit from maintenance therapy with about half the therapeutic dosage for several months to prevent relapse. It is often appropriate during the early stages of treatment to add a hypnotic (section 4.1.1) to correct the sleeping pattern and an anxiolytic (section 4.1.2) to allay anxiety or agitation.

SELECTION. Antidepressant drugs can be roughly divided into those with additional sedative properties, for example **amitriptyline**, and those with less, for example **imipramine**. Agitated and anxious patients, particularly women, tend to respond best to the sedative compounds. Retarded patients will often obtain most benefit from less sedating compounds.

Amitriptyline may be given in divided doses or the entire daily dose may be given at night to promote sleep and avoid daytime drowsiness. **Imipramine** can also be given once daily but as it has much less sedative action there is less advantage.

Imipramine or the more sedating amitriptyline are well established and relatively safe and effective, but have more marked anticholinergic or cardiac side-effects than some of the newer compounds (**doxepin, mianserin, nomifensine,** and **trazodone**); this may be important in individual patients.

Clomipramine has been used with some success in depressed patients who show marked obsessional or phobic features.

Antidepressants with **sedative** properties include amitriptyline (Tryptizol®, Lentizol® etc.), dothiepin (Prothiaden®), doxepin (Sinequan®), mianserin (Bolvidon®, Norval®), trazodone (Molipaxin®), and trimipramine (Surmontil®).

Less sedative antidepressants include butriptyline (Evadyne®), clomipramine (Anafranil®), desipramine (Pertofran®), imipramine (Tofranil® etc.), maprotiline (Ludiomil®), nomifensine (Merital®), nortriptyline (Allegron®, Aventyl®), and viloxazine (Vivalan®). Protriptyline has a **stimulant** action.

SIDE-EFFECTS. Cardiac arrhythmias and heart block occasionally follow the use of tricyclic antidepressants, particularly amitriptyline, and may be a factor in the sudden death of patients with cardiac disease. Other side-effects are troublesome rather than serious and may include drowsiness, dry mouth, blurred vision, constipation, urinary retention, and sweating, attributed to anticholinergic activity. The patient should be encouraged to persist with treatment as some tolerance to these side-effects seems to develop. They are further reduced if, when initiating therapy, low doses (for example 10 to 25 mg of amitriptyline 3 times daily) are given and then gradually increased but it is important to achieve full therapeutic doses as adequate plasma concentrations must be attained.

This gradual introduction of treatment is particularly important in the elderly, who, because of the hypotensive effects of these drugs, are prone to attacks of dizziness or even syncope. The tricyclic antidepressants should be prescribed with caution in epilepsy as they lower the convulsive threshold.

HYPERTENSIVE PATIENTS. Antidepressants may interfere with antihypertensive therapy. They diminish the action of bethanidine, clonidine, debrisoquine, and guanethidine. Beta-adrenoceptor blocking drugs may be used in conjunction with antidepressants as this combination does not interact. Alternatively, **mianserin** may be used with most antihypertensive agents (except for clonidine) as it does not interfere with re-uptake of amines into the neurone.

LACK OF RESPONSE. In patients who do not respond to antidepressants, the diagnosis, dosage, compliance, and possible continuation of psychosocial or physical aggravating causes should all be carefully reviewed; other drug treatment may be successful. The patient may respond to low-dose **flupenthixol** (Fluanxol®, section 4.3.4) or MAOIs (section 4.3.2). **Tryptophan** (section 4.3.4) appears to benefit some patients when given alone or as adjunctive therapy.

NOCTURNAL ENURESIS IN CHILDREN. Certain tricyclic antidepressants (**amitriptyline, imipramine,** and less often **nortriptyline**) are used to treat nocturnal enuresis in children. Their use should be reserved for when alternative methods have failed. Although they are effective, relapse occurs commonly after withdrawal of the drug. Also, behavioural disturbances may occur and cases of poisoning have been reported. It is recommended that they should be avoided in children under 6 years of age, and that treatment should not exceed 3 months unless a full physical examination (including an electrocardiogram) is given.

AMITRIPTYLINE HYDROCHLORIDE

Indications: depressive illness, particularly with anxiety, nocturnal enuresis in children

Cautions: initially, sedation may affect the ability to drive or operate machinery; effects of alcohol may be increased; caution in diabetes, cardiac disease (particularly with arrhythmias see contra-indications below), epilepsy, pregnancy, hepatic impairment, thyroid disease, psychoses (may aggravate mania), glaucoma, urinary retention. Avoid abrupt cessation of therapy. Also caution in anaesthesia (increased risk of cardiac arrhythmias). See notes above for nocturnal enuresis. Drug interactions: see Appendix 1

Contra-indications: recent myocardial infarction, heart block, mania

Side-effects: dry mouth, sedation, blurred vision, constipation, difficulty with micturition (due to anticholinergic action). Other common side-effects are cardiovascular (postural hypotension, tachycardia, syncope, particularly with high doses), sweating, tremor, rashes, behavioural disturbances (particularly with children), interference with sexual function. Less commonly, convulsions, agranulocytosis, leucopenia, eosinophilia, purpura, thrombocytopenia, and jaundice

Dose: *by mouth,* initially 30-75 mg (elderly patients 25–50 mg) daily in divided doses *or* as a single dose at bedtime increased gradually as necessary to a max. of 225 mg; usual maintenance dose 50–100 mg daily

Sustained-release preparations 50–150 mg at bedtime (50 mg s/r daily ≈ 25 mg amitriptyline 3 times daily)

Nocturnal enuresis, CHILD 6–10 years 10–20 mg, 11–16 years 25–50 mg half an hour before bedtime

By intramuscular or intravenous injection, 20–30 mg 4 times daily

Amitriptyline Tablets, f/c or s/c, amitriptyline hydrochloride 10 mg, price 20 tabs = **A**; 25 mg, price 20 tabs = **A**; 50 mg, price 20 tabs = **B**

Domical® (Berk)

Tablets, blue, f/c, amitriptyline hydrochloride 10 mg. Price 20 tabs = **A**

Tablets, orange, f/c, amitriptyline hydrochloride 25 mg. Price 20 tabs = **A**

Tablets, brown, f/c, amitriptyline hydrochloride 50 mg. Price 20 tabs = **C**

Elavil® (DDSA)

Tablets, blue, f/c, amitriptyline hydrochloride 10 mg. Price 20 tabs = **A**

Tablets, yellow, f/c, amitriptyline hydrochloride 25 mg. Price 20 tabs = **A**

Lentizol® (Warner)

Capsules, s/r, pink, enclosing white pellets, amitriptyline hydrochloride 25 mg. Price 20 caps = **C**

Capsules, s/r, pink/red, enclosing white pellets, amitriptyline hydrochloride 50 mg. Price 20 caps = **D**

Saroten® (Warner)

Tablets, red, s/c, amitriptyline hydrochloride 10 mg. Price 20 tabs = **A**

Tablets, red, s/c, amitriptyline hydrochloride 25 mg. Price 20 tabs = **B**

Tryptizol® (Morson)

Capsules, s/r, orange, amitriptyline hydrochloride 75 mg. Price 20 caps = **D**

Tablets, blue, f/c, amitriptyline hydrochloride 10 mg. Price 20 tabs = **A**

Tablets, yellow, f/c, amitriptyline hydrochloride 25 mg. Price 20 tabs = **B**

Tablets, brown, f/c, amitriptyline hydrochloride 50 mg. Price 20 tabs = **C**

Mixture, pink, amitriptyline 10 mg (as embonate)/5 ml. Diluent syrup, life of diluted mixture 14 days. Price 100 ml = **C**

Injection, amitriptyline hydrochloride 10 mg/ml. Price 10-ml vial = **B**

IMIPRAMINE HYDROCHLORIDE

Indications: depressive illness, nocturnal enuresis in children

Cautions; Contra-indications; Side-effects: see under Amitriptyline Hydrochloride, but less sedating; side-effects occur more frequently

Dose: *by mouth,* initially 75 mg daily in divided doses or as a single dose at bedtime increased gradually as necessary to a max. of 225 mg; usual maintenance dose 75–100 mg daily; elderly patients 10–25 mg 1–3 times daily

Nocturnal enuresis, CHILD 6–10 years 25–35 mg, over 11 years 50–75 mg half an hour before bedtime

By intramuscular injection, 25 mg up to 6 times daily or more as necessary

Imipramine Tablets, s/c, imipramine hydrochloride 10 and 25 mg. Price 20 tabs (both) = **A**

Berkomine® (Berk)

Tablets, brown, s/c, imipramine hydrochloride 10 mg. Price 20 tabs = **A**

Praminil® (DDSA)

Tablets, brownish-pink, s/c, imipramine hydrochloride 10 mg. Price 20 tabs = **A**

Tablets, brown, s/c, imipramine hydrochloride 25 mg. Price 20 tabs = **A**

Tofranil® (Geigy)

Tablets, brown, s/c, imipramine hydrochloride 10 mg. Price 20 tabs = **B**

Tablets, brown, s/c, imipramine hydrochloride 25 mg. Price 20 tabs = **C**

Syrup (= mixture), imipramine hydrochloride 25 mg/5 ml. Diluent purified water, freshly boiled and cooled, for dilutions above 15 mg/5 ml; equal parts of syrup and tragacanth mucilage (freshly prepared) for dilutions below 15 mg/5 ml, life of diluted mixture 14 days. Price 150 ml = **E**

Injection, imipramine hydrochloride 12.5 mg/ml. Price 2-ml amp = **A**

BUTRIPTYLINE

Indications: depressive illness, particularly with anxiety

Cautions; Contra-indications; Side-effects: see under Amitriptyline Hydrochloride, but side-effects are fewer and milder. Sedative effect between amitriptyline and imipramine

Dose: 25 mg 3 times daily, increased gradually as necessary to a max. of 150 mg; usual maintenance dose 25 mg 3 times daily

Evadyne® (Ayerst)
Tablets, orange, f/c, butriptyline 25 mg (as hydrochloride). Price 20 tabs = **C**
Tablets, pink, f/c, butriptyline 50 mg (as hydrochloride). Price 20 tabs = **D**

CLOMIPRAMINE HYDROCHLORIDE

Indications: depressive illness, adjunctive treatment of phobic and obsessional states
Cautions; Contra-indications; Side-effects: see under Amitriptyline Hydrochloride. Sedative action intermediate between amitriptyline and imipramine. Tremor and anticholinergic effects are common. Postural hypotension may occur on intravenous infusion
Dose: *by mouth,* initially 10–50 mg (elderly patients 10 mg) daily in divided doses *or* as a single dose at bedtime, increased gradually as necessary to 75 mg or more in severe depression and 150 mg daily in phobic and obsessional states; usual maintenance dose 50–100 mg daily
By intramuscular injection, up to 25 mg 6 times daily or more as necessary
By intravenous infusion, initially to assess tolerance, 25–50 mg over 45–120 minutes, adjusted as required

Anafranil® (Geigy)
Capsules, yellow/caramel, clomipramine hydrochloride 10 mg. Price 20 caps = **C**
Capsules, orange/caramel, clomipramine hydrochloride 25 mg. Price 20 caps = **D**
Capsules, blue/caramel, clomipramine hydrochloride 50 mg. Price 20 caps = **E**
Syrup (= elixir), orange, clomipramine hydrochloride 25 mg/5 ml. Diluent purified water, freshly boiled and cooled, for dilutions above 15 mg/5 ml; equal parts of syrup and tragacanth mucilage (freshly prepared) for dilutions below 15 mg/5 ml, life of diluted elixir few days only. Price 150 ml = **G**
Injection, clomipramine hydrochloride 12.5 mg/ml. Price 2-ml amp = **B**

DESIPRAMINE HYDROCHLORIDE

Indications: depressive illness
Cautions; Contra-indications; Side-effects: see under Amitriptyline Hydrochloride, but less sedating. Most common side-effects are anticholinergic effects, insomnia, and tremor
Dose: 25 mg 3 times daily, taken not later than 4 p.m., increased as necessary to a max. of 50 mg 3–4 times daily. Usual maintenance dose 100–150 mg daily in divided doses

Pertofran® (Geigy)
Tablets, pink, s/c, desipramine hydrochloride 25 mg. Price 20 tabs = **C**

DOTHIEPIN HYDROCHLORIDE

Indications: depressive illness, particularly with anxiety
Cautions; Contra-indications; Side-effects: see under Amitriptyline Hydrochloride. Most common side-effects are sedation, postural hypotension, tremor, and blurred vision
Dose: initially 75 mg daily in divided doses *or* as a single dose at bedtime, increased gradually as necessary to 150 mg daily

Prothiaden® (Boots)
Capsules, red/brown, dothiepin hydrochloride 25 mg. Price 20 caps = **B**
Tablets, red, s/c, dothiepin hydrochloride 75 mg. Price 28 tabs = **D**

DOXEPIN

Indications: depressive illness, particularly with anxiety
Cautions; Contra-indications; Side-effects: see under Amitriptyline Hydrochloride, but cardiac effects may occur less frequently
Dose: initially 30–75 mg daily in divided doses *or* as a single dose at bedtime, increased gradually to a max. of 300 mg daily in divided doses

Sinequan® (Pfizer)
Capsules, orange, doxepin 10 mg (as hydrochloride). Price 20 caps = **C**
Capsules, orange/blue, doxepin 25 mg (as hydrochloride). Price 20 caps = **C**
Capsules, blue, doxepin 50 mg (as hydrochloride). Price 20 caps = **D**
Capsules, yellow/blue, doxepin 75 mg (as hydrochloride). Price 20 caps = **E**

IPRINDOLE

Indications: depressive illness
Cautions; Contra-indications; Side-effects: see under Amitriptyline Hydrochloride, but less sedating, and fewer and milder side-effects, particularly anticholinergic and cardiovascular effects. Rarely, jaundice occurs, usually in the first 14 days of treatment
Dose: initially 15–30 mg 3 times daily, increased gradually as necessary to a max. of 60 mg 3 times daily; usual maintenance dose 30 mg 3 times daily

Prondol® (Wyeth)
Tablets, yellow, iprindole 15 mg (as hydrochloride). Price 20 tabs = **B**
Tablets, yellow, iprindole 30 mg (as hydrochloride). Price 20 tabs = **C**

MAPROTILINE HYDROCHLORIDE

Indications: depressive illness, particularly with anxiety
Cautions; Contra-indications; Side-effects: see under Amitriptyline Hydrochloride, but less sedating. Rashes commonly occur and there is an increased risk of convulsions at higher dosage
Dose: initially 25–75 mg daily in divided doses *or* as a single dose at bedtime, increased gradually as necessary to a max. of 150 mg daily

Ludiomil® (Ciba)
Tablets, peach, f/c, maprotiline hydrochloride 10 mg. Price 20 tabs = **C**
Tablets, orange, f/c, maprotiline hydrochloride 25 mg. Price 20 tabs = **C**
Tablets, dark orange, f/c, maprotiline hydrochloride 50 mg. Price 20 tabs = **E**
Tablets, orange-red, f/c, maprotiline hydrochloride 75 mg. Price 28 tabs = **F**

MIANSERIN HYDROCHLORIDE

Indications: depressive illness, particularly with anxiety
Cautions; Contra-indications; Side-effects: see under Amitriptyline Hydrochloride, but fewer and milder side-effects, particularly anticholinergic and cardiovascular effects, and many of the drug interactions of the tricyclic antidepressants are absent
Dose: initially 30–40 mg daily in divided doses *or* as a single dose at bedtime, increased gradually as necessary; usual dose range 30–90 mg, max. 200 mg daily in divided doses

Bolvidon® (Organon)
Tablets, yellow, f/c, mianserin hydrochloride 10 mg. Price 20 tabs = **D**
Tablets, f/c, mianserin hydrochloride 20 mg. Price 20 tabs = **E**
Tablets, f/c, mianserin hydrochloride 30 mg. Price 20 tabs = **F**
Norval® (Bencard)
Tablets, orange, f/c, mianserin hydrochloride 10 mg. Price 20 tabs = **D**
Tablets, orange, f/c, mianserin hydrochloride 20 mg. Price 20 tabs = **E**
Tablets, orange, f/c, mianserin hydrochloride 30 mg. Price 20 tabs = **F**

NOMIFENSINE HYDROGEN MALEATE

Indications: depressive illness
Cautions; Contra-indications; Side-effects: see under Amitriptyline Hydrochloride, but less sedating, and fewer and milder side-effects, particularly anticholinergic and cardiovascular effects; avoid in renal impairment
Dose: initially 25–50 mg 2–3 times daily, increased gradually as necessary to a max. of 200 mg daily in divided doses

▼ Merital® (Hoechst)
Capsules, orange, nomifensine hydrogen maleate 25 mg. Price 20 caps = **E**
Capsules, orange/caramel, nomifensine hydrogen maleate 50 mg. Price 20 caps = **F**

NORTRIPTYLINE

Indications: depressive illness, nocturnal enuresis in children
Cautions; Contra-indications; Side-effects: see under Amitriptyline Hydrochloride but less sedating. Anticholinergic effects occur more frequently
Dose: initially 10 mg 2–4 times daily, increased gradually as necessary to a max. of 100 mg daily in divided doses; usual maintenance dose 30–75 mg daily
Nocturnal enuresis, CHILD, 10–75 mg (1–2 mg/kg) daily in divided doses

Allegron® (Dista)
Tablets, yellow, nortriptyline 10 mg (as hydrochloride). Price 20 tabs = **B**
Tablets, orange, scored, nortriptyline 25 mg (as hydrochloride). Price 20 tabs = **C**
Aventyl® (Lilly)
Pulvules® (= capsules), yellow/white, nortriptyline 10 mg (as hydrochloride). Price 20 caps = **B**
Pulvules® (= capsules), yellow/white, nortriptyline 25 mg (as hydrochloride). Price 20 caps = **C**
Liquid (= elixir), nortriptyline 10 mg (as hydrochloride)/5 ml. Diluent syrup, life of diluted elixir 14 days. Price 120 ml = **C**

PROTRIPTYLINE HYDROCHLORIDE

Indications: depressive illness, particularly with apathy and withdrawal
Cautions; Contra-indications; Side-effects: see under Amitriptyline Hydrochloride but less sedating. Cardiovascular side-effects are more common. May aggravate anxiety and tension and cause insomnia. Also rashes associated with photosensitisation may occur (avoid direct exposure to sunlight). Caution in the elderly, particularly when daily dose exceeds 20 mg
Dose: initially 5–10 mg 3–4 times daily taken not later than 4 p.m., increased gradually as necessary in severe depression to 60 mg daily

Concordin® (MSD)
Tablets, pink, f/c, protriptyline hydrochloride 5 mg. Price 20 tabs = **B**
Tablets, f/c, protriptyline hydrochloride 10 mg. Price 20 tabs = **B**

TRAZODONE HYDROCHLORIDE

Indications: depressive illness, particularly with anxiety
Cautions; Contra-indications; Side-effects: see under Amitriptyline Hydrochloride but fewer and milder side-effects, particularly anticholinergic and cardiovascular effects
Dose: initially 100–150 mg daily in divided doses preferably after meals *or* as a single dose at bedtime; usual maintenance dose 200–300 mg daily; max. 600 mg daily

▼ Molipaxin® (Roussel)
Capsules, violet/green, trazodone hydrochloride 50 mg. Price 20 caps = **E**
Capsules, violet/fawn, trazodone hydrochloride 100 mg. Price 20 caps = **F**

TRIMIPRAMINE

Indications: depressive illness, particularly with anxiety and insomnia

Cautions; Contra-indications; Side-effects: see under Amitriptyline Hydrochloride but more sedating. Anticholinergic and cardiovascular side-effects commonly occur and occasionally paraesthesia. Caution in hepatic impairment

Dose: initially 50–75 mg daily in divided doses *or* as a single dose 2 hours before bedtime, increased as necessary to a max. of 300 mg daily; usual maintenance dose 75–150 mg daily

Surmontil® (M&B)

Capsules, green/white, trimipramine 50 mg (as maleate). Price 20 caps = **D**

Tablets, trimipramine 10 mg (as maleate). Price 20 tabs = **B**

Tablets, trimipramine 25 mg (as maleate). Price 20 tabs = **C**

VILOXAZINE HYDROCHLORIDE

Indications: depressive illness

Cautions; Contra-indications; Side-effects: see under Amitriptyline Hydrochloride, but less sedating and anticholinergic and cardiovascular side-effects are fewer and milder; nausea and headache may occur

Dose: initially 50–100 mg 2–3 times daily after meals not later than 6 p.m. or 100 mg daily in elderly patients, increased gradually as necessary; max. 400 mg daily

Vivalan® (ICI)

Tablets, yellow, f/c, viloxazine 50 mg (as hydrochloride). Price 20 tabs = **D**

4.3.2 Monoamine-oxidase inhibitors (MAOIs)

Monoamine-oxidase inhibitors are used much less frequently than tricyclic and related antidepressants because of the dangers of dietary and drug interactions and the fact that it is easier to prescribe MAOIs when tricyclic antidepressants have been unsuccessful than vice versa. **Tranylcypromine** (Parnate®) is the most **hazardous** of the MAOIs because of its stimulant action. The drugs of choice are **phenelzine** or **isocarboxazid** which are less stimulant and therefore safer.

Phobic patients and depressed patients with atypical, hypochondriacal, or hysterical features are said to respond best to MAOIs. However, MAOIs should be tried in any patients who are refractory to treatment with other antidepressants as there is occasionally a dramatic response. Response to treatment may be delayed for 3 weeks or more and may take an additional 1 or 2 weeks to become maximal.

MAOIs act by inhibiting monoamine oxidase, thereby causing an accumulation of amine neurotransmitters. The metabolism of some amine drugs such as sympathomimetics and tricyclic and related antidepressants is also inhibited and their pressor action may therefore be potentiated. The pressor effect of the tyramine present in some foods may also be dangerously potentiated.

Sympathomimetics are present in many proprietary cough mixtures and decongestant nasal drops. See Appendix 1, and Treatment Card. These interactions may cause a dangerous rise in blood pressure. An early warning symptom may be a throbbing headache. The danger of interaction persists for about 10–14 days after treatment with MAOIs is discontinued. Treatment cards which list the necessary precautions are given to patients at pharmacies etc.

Tricyclic and related antidepressants should **not** be given to patients for 14 days after treatment with MAOIs has been discontinued. Some psychiatrists use selected tricyclics in conjunction with MAOIs but this is hazardous, indeed potentially lethal, except in experienced hands and there is no evidence that the combination is more effective than when either constituent is used alone. The combination of tranylcypromine with clomipramine is particularly **dangerous**.

TREATMENT CARD

Carry this card with you at all times. Show it to any doctor who may treat you other than the doctor who prescribed this medicine, and to your dentist if you require dental treatment.

INSTRUCTIONS TO PATIENTS

Please read carefully

While taking this medicine and for 10 days after your treatment finishes you must observe the following simple instructions:–

1 Do not eat CHEESE, PICKLED HERRING OR BROAD BEAN PODS.

2 Do not eat or drink BOVRIL, OXO, MARMITE or ANY SIMILAR MEAT OR YEAST EXTRACT.

3 Do not take any other MEDICINES (including tablets, capsules, nose drops, inhalations or suppositories) whether purchased by you or previously prescribed by your doctor, without first consulting your doctor or your pharmacist.

NB *Treatment for coughs and colds, pain relievers and tonics are medicines.*

4 Drink ALCOHOL only in moderation and avoid CHIANTI WINE completely.

Report any severe symptoms to your doctor and follow any other advice given by him.

M.A.O.I. Prepared by The Pharmaceutical Society and the British Medical Association on behalf of the Health Departments of the United Kingdom.

PHENELZINE

Indications: depressive illness

Cautions: may affect mental concentration and ability to drive or operate machinery. Avoid abrupt discontinuation of treatment, certain drugs and foods (see Treatment Card above). Drug interactions: see Appendix 1

Contra-indications: hepatic, renal, cardiovascular, or cerebrovascular disease, epilepsy, children, elderly and debilitated patients
Side-effects: dizziness, postural hypotension, less commonly agitation, headache, tremor, constipation, dry mouth, blurred vision, difficulty in micturition, liver damage, rashes, psychotic episodes in susceptible patients; severe hypertensive reactions to certain drugs and foods
Dose: 15 mg 3 times daily, increased if necessary to 4 times daily after 2 weeks

Nardil® (Warner)
Tablets, orange, s/c, phenelzine 15 mg (as sulphate). Price 20 tabs = **C**

IPRONIAZID

Indications: depressive illness
Cautions; Contra-indications: see under Phenelzine
Side-effects: see under Phenelzine, but more toxic; rarely vasculitis and peripheral neuritis
Dose: 100–150 mg daily as a single dose, reducing to a maintenance dose of 25–50 mg daily

Marsilid® (Roche)
Tablets, orange, scored, iproniazid 25 mg (as phosphate). Price 20 tabs = **B**
Tablets, yellow, scored, iproniazid 50 mg (as phosphate). Price 20 tabs = **C**

ISOCARBOXAZID

Indications: depressive illness
Cautions; Contra-indications: see under Phenelzine
Side-effects: see under Phenelzine; rarely anaemia, hepatitis, peripheral oedema, and rashes
Dose: initially up to 30 mg daily in single or divided doses; usual maintenance dose 10–20 mg daily

Marplan® (Roche)
Tablets, pink, scored, isocarboxazid 10 mg. Price 20 tabs = **B**

TRANYLCYPROMINE

Indications: depressive illness
Cautions; Contra-indications: see under Phenelzine
Side-effects: insomnia, dizziness, muscular weakness, dry mouth, hypotension; hypertensive crises with throbbing headache requiring discontinuation of treatment occur more frequently than with other MAOIs; liver damage occurs less frequently than with phenelzine
Dose: initially 10 mg twice daily not later than 4 p.m., increasing if necessary to 10 mg 3 times daily after 1 week; usual maintenance dose 10 mg daily

Parnate® (SK&F)
Tablets, red, s/c, tranylcypromine 10 mg (as sulphate). Price 20 tabs = **C**

4.3.3 Compound antidepressant preparations

Antipsychotic drugs such as the phenothiazine derivatives or anxiolytics can be usefully given with antidepressants but the use of preparations listed below is **not** recommended because the dosage of the individual components should be adjusted separately to be appropriate for the individual patient. Whereas antidepressants are given continuously over several months, the phenothiazines and anxiolytics are usually prescribed intermittently in the lowest effective dosage.

Limbitrol 5® (Roche)
Capsules, pink/green, amitriptyline 12.5 mg (as hydrochloride), chlordiazepoxide 5 mg. Price 20 caps = **C**
Limbitrol 10® (Roche)
Capsules, pink/green, amitriptyline 25 mg (as hydrochloride), chlordiazepoxide 10 mg. Price 20 caps = **C**
Motipress® (Squibb)
Tablets, yellow, s/c, fluphenazine hydrochloride 1.5 mg, nortriptyline 30 mg (as hydrochloride). Price 28 tabs = **E**
Motival® (Squibb)
Tablets, pink, s/c, fluphenazine hydrochloride 500 micrograms, nortriptyline 10 mg (as hydrochloride). Price 20 tabs = **C**
Parstelin® (SK&F)
Tablets, green, s/c, tranylcypromine 10 mg (as sulphate), trifluoperazine 1 mg (as hydrochloride). Price 20 tabs = **C**
Triptafen-DA® (A&H)
Tablets, pink, s/c, amitriptyline hydrochloride 25 mg, perphenazine 2 mg. Price 20 tabs = **C**
Triptafen-Minor® (A&H)
Tablets, pink, s/c, amitriptyline hydrochloride 10 mg, perphenazine 2 mg. Price 20 tabs = **B**
Triptafen-Forte® (A&H)
Tablets, red, s/c, amitriptyline hydrochloride 25 mg, perphenazine 4 mg. Price 20 tabs = **C**

4.3.4 Other antidepressant drugs

Flupenthixol (Fluanxol®) has antidepressant properties, and low doses (1.5 to 3 mg daily) are given by mouth for this purpose. Its advantage over the tricyclic and related antidepressants is that, with the low doses employed, side-effects are fewer and overdosage less toxic.

Tryptophan appears to benefit some patients when given alone or as adjunctive therapy. Its antidepressant effect may take up to 4 weeks to develop. **Tofenacin** is of doubtful value.

FLUPENTHIXOL

Indications: depressive illness. For use in psychoses, see section 4.2.1
Cautions: cardiovascular disease (including cardiac disorders and cerebral arteriosclerosis), senile confusional states, parkinsonism, renal and hepatic disease; avoid in excitable and overactive patients
Side-effects: restlessness, insomnia, rarely extrapyramidal symptoms
Dose: 1 mg twice daily not later than 4 p.m., increased gradually as necessary to a max. of 3 mg daily

Fluanxol® (Lundbeck)
Tablets, red, s/c, flupenthixol 500 micrograms (as dihydrochloride). Price 20 tabs = **D**

TOFENACIN HYDROCHLORIDE

Indications: depressive illness
Cautions: drug interactions: see Appendix 1
Contra-indications: glaucoma, urinary retention, suicidal tendencies
Side-effects: dry mouth, blurred vision, tremor
Dose: up to 240 mg daily in divided doses

Elamol® (Brocades)
Capsules, grey/orange, tofenacin hydrochloride 80 mg. Price 20 caps = **B**

TRYPTOPHAN

Indications: adjunctive treatment of depressive illness, alone or in conjunction with other antidepressants
Cautions: active bladder disease, disorders of tryptophan metabolism. May initially affect ability to drive or operate machinery. Reduce dose when used in conjunction with MAOIs and discontinue if blurred vision or headache occur during tryptophan/MAOI therapy
Side-effects: nausea, anorexia, drowsiness
Dose: 1–2 g 3 times daily, preferably after meals

Optimax® (Merck)
Tablets, tryptophan 500 mg, pyridoxine hydrochloride 5 mg, ascorbic acid 10 mg. Price 20 tabs = **D**
Optimax WV® (Merck)
Tablets, tryptophan 500 mg. Price 20 tabs = **D**
Pacitron® (Berk)
Tablets, orange, f/c, tryptophan 500 mg. Price 20 tabs = **D**

4.4 Central nervous stimulants

4.4.1 Weak central nervous stimulants
4.4.2 Amphetamines and cocaine
See section 3.5 for respiratory stimulants.

4.4.1 Weak central nervous stimulants

Caffeine is a weak, widely used, stimulant present in tea and coffee. It is included in many analgesic preparations (see section 4.7.1.3) but does not contribute to their analgesic or anti-inflammatory effect. Over-indulgence may lead to a state of arousal and anxiety.

Pemoline may be useful in the management of hyperactive children. Other weak central nervous stimulants are **fencamfamin, meclofenoxate**, and **prolintane** (which is included in some vitamin preparations). Their value is doubtful but they have been advocated for the management of senility and relief of fatigue. They should not be used to treat depression.

PEMOLINE

Indications: debility and fatigue, hyperkinesia in children
Cautions: cardiovascular disease, insomnia. Drug interactions: see Appendix 1
Contra-indications: glaucoma, extrapyramidal disorders, hyperexcitable states (thyrotoxicosis)
Side-effects: insomnia, tachycardia, agitation
Dose: 20 mg in the morning and midday, gradually increased to a max. of 120 mg daily; CHILD over 6 years (also elderly patients), 10–20 mg morning and midday. Doses are best taken after meals

Ronyl® (Rona)
Tablets, pemoline 20 mg. Price 20 tabs = **B**
Volital® (LAB)
Tablets, pemoline 20 mg. Price 25 tabs = **B**

FENCAMFAMIN HYDROCHLORIDE

Indications: debility, fatigue
Cautions; Contra-indications; Side-effects: see under Pemoline

Reactivan® (Merck)
Tablets, yellow, s/c, fencamfamin hydrochloride 10 mg, ascorbic acid 100 mg, cyanocobalamin 10 micrograms, pyridoxine phosphate 20 mg, thiamine phosphate 10 mg. Price 20 tabs = **C**
Dose: 2 tablets in the morning and 1 at midday if necessary

MECLOFENOXATE HYDROCHLORIDE

Indications: mental deterioration associated with ageing, recovery after stroke
Cautions; Contra-indications; Side-effects: see under Pemoline
Dose: 300 mg 3–5 times daily, preferably one hour before meals and not later than 4 p.m.

Lucidril® (R&C)
Tablets, cream, f/c, meclofenoxate hydrochloride 300 mg. Price 20 tabs = **D**

4.4.2 Amphetamines and cocaine

The **amphetamines** (amphetamine, dexamphetamine, methylamphetamine, and methylphenidate) have a limited field of usefulness and their use should be **discouraged** as they may cause dependence and psychotic states. Combinations of amphetamines and barbiturates are more euphoriant than amphetamines alone and therefore more dangerous.

Patients with narcolepsy may derive benefit from treatment with amphetamines. They have also been advocated for the management of hyperactive children; beneficial effects have been described. However, they must be used very selectively as they retard growth and the effect of long-term therapy has not been evaluated.

Amphetamines have **no place** in the management of **depression** or **obesity**.

Cocaine is a drug of addiction which causes central nervous stimulation. Its clinical use is mainly as a topical local anaesthetic (section 15.2). Occasionally, it has been included in the traditional 'Brompton Cocktail' mixtures which are used for the relief of pain in terminal care. Its use for this indication is **decreasing**, but elixirs of diamorphine and morphine with cocaine are described in section 4.7.2.

DEXAMPHETAMINE SULPHATE

Indications: narcolepsy, hyperkinesia in children
Cautions: anorexia, insomnia, impaired renal function, unstable personality. Drug interactions: see Appendix 1
Contra-indications: cardiovascular disease, hyperexcitable states (thyrotoxicosis), glaucoma, extrapyramidal disorders
Side-effects: dependence and tolerance occur readily, also agitation, restlessness, insomnia, headache, dizziness, tremor, personality change, anorexia, cardiac arrhythmias, dry mouth, diarrhoea, or constipation. In children, anorexia, weight loss, growth inhibition, and tearfulness. Large doses cause disorientation and aggression, leading to paranoid psychosis, convulsions, and coma
Dose: narcolepsy, 5–60 mg daily in divided doses. Hyperkinesia, CHILD over 3 years, initially 2.5 mg in the morning gradually increased according to the response to a max. of 40 mg daily in 2 doses

CD Dexedrine® (SK&F)
Tablets, yellow, scored, dexamphetamine sulphate 5 mg. Price 20 tabs = **A**

METHYLPHENIDATE HYDROCHLORIDE

Indications: narcolepsy, hyperkinesia in children
Cautions; Contra-indications; Side-effects: see under Dexamphetamine Sulphate, but causes less elation and excitement. In children doses over 20 mg may cause weight loss and growth inhibition. Drug interactions: see Appendix 1
Dose: by mouth, usually 20–30 mg daily divided into 2 doses, given morning and midday; CHILD, 300–500 micrograms/kg daily *or* in children over 5 years initially 5 mg 2–3 times daily adjusted according to the response
By subcutaneous, intramuscular, or intravenous injection, 10–20 mg; CHILD, 5–10 mg, repeated if necessary

CD Ritalin® (Ciba)
Tablets, scored, methylphenidate hydrochloride 10 mg. Price 20 tabs = **A**
Injection, powder for reconstitution, methylphenidate hydrochloride. Price 20-mg amp = **A** (Hosp. only)

4.5 Appetite suppressants

4.5.1 Bulk-forming drugs
4.5.2 Centrally-acting appetite suppressants

The development of obesity appears to be multifactorial. Aggravating factors may be depression or other psychosocial problems or drug treatment.

The main treatment of the obese patient is an appropriate diet, carefully explained to the patient, with support and encouragement from the doctor. Attendance at groups (for example 'weight-watchers') helps some individuals. Drugs can play only a limited role and should never be used as the sole element of treatment as their effects tend to be disappointing.

Centrally-acting appetite suppressants (section 4.5.2) carry the risk of dependence and other adverse effects. They should **not** be given to patients with a past history of drug abuse or psychiatric illness. Also they are **not recommended** for periods of treatment beyond 3 to 6 months because of the risks of dependence and lack of efficacy in extended use.

4.5.1 Bulk-forming drugs

The most commonly used bulk-forming drug is **methylcellulose.** It is claimed to reduce intake by producing feelings of satiety but there is little evidence to support this claim.

METHYLCELLULOSE

Indications: obesity
Cautions: maintain adequate fluid intake
Side-effects: flatulence, abdominal distension, intestinal obstruction

Celevac® (WBP)
Tablets, pink, methylcellulose '450' 500 mg. Price 20 tabs = **A**
Dose: 3 tablets chewed or crushed with a tumblerful of liquid half an hour before meals or when hungry

Cellucon® (Medo)
Tablets, buff, methylcellulose '2500' 500 mg. Price 20 tabs = **A**
Dose: 1–4 tablets, chewed or crushed with a tumblerful of liquid half an hour before meals or when hungry

Nilstim® (De Witt)
Tablets, green, cellulose (microcrystalline) 220 mg, methylcellulose '2500' 400 mg. Price 20 tabs = **B**
Dose: 2 tablets, chewed or crushed, with a tumblerful of liquid 15 minutes before the 2 main meals or when hungry

STERCULIA

Indications; Cautions; Side-effects: see under Methylcellulose

Prefil® (Norgine)
Granules, brown, coated, sterculia 55%, guar gum 5%. Price 500 g = **F**
Dose: two 5-ml spoonfuls followed by a tumblerful of liquid ½–1 hour before meals, reduced in patients accustomed to a low-residue diet

4.5.2 Centrally-acting appetite suppressants

The use of amphetamine-like drugs, including **phenmetrazine,** in the treatment of obesity is **not** justified as any possible benefits are outweighed by the risks involved.

The centrally-acting appetite suppressants below may be used as adjunctive treatment in some patients with moderate to severe obesity. Patients should be given close support and supervision and treatment should be limited to short periods. These drugs should be avoided in children because of the possibility of growth suppression, and should not be used for cosmetic purposes in mild obesity.

Diethylpropion (Apisate®, Tenuate Dospan®), **mazindol** (Teronac®), and **phentermine** are used as appetite suppressants. They have anorectic properties comparable with amphetamine but their stimulant action and risk of dependence is considerably less. Drug abuse, particularly with diethylpropion, is, however, an increasing problem. They are preferred for their stimulant action in lethargic, rather depressed patients.

Fenfluramine (Ponderax®) differs from most other appetite suppressants in not being stimulant; indeed it has some sedative properties. Dependence is rare but abrupt withdrawal may induce depression.

Thyroid hormones have no place in the treatment of obesity except in hypothyroid patients.

DIETHYLPROPION HYDROCHLORIDE

Indications: short-term adjunct in moderate to severe obesity

Cautions: cardiovascular disease, diabetes, unstable personality. Drug interactions: see Appendix 1

Contra-indications: glaucoma, hyperexcitable states (thyrotoxicosis)

Side-effects: agitation, insomnia, tachycardia, gastro-intestinal disturbances, dizziness, tremor, restlessness, dry mouth, headache, chills; tolerance and amphetamine-type dependence may occur. Also psychotic episodes in predisposed patients

Apisate® (Wyeth)

Tablets, s/r, yellow, diethylpropion hydrochloride 75 mg, thiamine hydrochloride 5 mg, pyridoxine hydrochloride 2 mg, riboflavine 4 mg, nicotinamide 30 mg. Price 20 tabs = **B**

Dose: 1 tablet, morning and/or mid-afternoon

Tenuate Dospan® (Merrell)

Tablets, s/r, scored, diethylpropion hydrochloride 75 mg. Price 20 tabs = **C**

Dose: one tablet mid-morning

FENFLURAMINE HYDROCHLORIDE

Indications: short-term adjunct in moderate to severe obesity

Cautions: depression; may affect mental concentration and ability to drive or operate machinery and increase the effects of alcohol. Drug interactions: see Appendix 1

Side-effects: sedation, headache, dizziness, and gastro-intestinal disturbances. Less commonly, dry mouth, sleep disturbances, tachycardia, fluid retention, urinary frequency, chills, alopecia, and haemolytic anaemia. Dosage should be discontinued gradually as rebound depression can occur rarely when therapy is discontinued abruptly. Tolerance may also occur

Dose: initially 20 mg morning and evening, increasing to a max. of 120 mg daily in divided doses

Ponderax® (Servier)

Tablets, pale blue, s/c, fenfluramine hydrochloride 20 mg. Price 20 tabs = **C**

Tablets, s/c, fenfluramine hydrochloride 40 mg. Price 20 tabs = **D**

Pacaps® (= capsules s/r), clear/blue, enclosing white pellets, fenfluramine hydrochloride 60 mg. Price 20 caps = **E**

Dose: 1–2 capsules daily, preferably before breakfast

MAZINDOL

Indications: short-term adjunct in moderate to severe obesity

Cautions; Contra-indications; Side-effects: see under Diethylpropion Hydrochloride. Avoid in peptic ulceration

Dose: 2 mg after breakfast

Teronac® (Wander)

Tablets, scored, mazindol 2 mg. Price 20 tabs = **E**

PHENTERMINE

Indications: short-term adjunct in moderate to severe obesity

Cautions; Contra-indications; Side-effects: see under Diethylpropion Hydrochloride

Dose: as resin complex, at breakfast time, 15–30 mg

Duromine® (Carnegie)

Capsules, s/r, green/grey, phentermine 15 mg (as resin complex). Price 30 caps = **E**

Capsules, s/r, maroon/grey, phentermine 30 mg (as resin complex). Price 30 caps = **E**

Ionamin® (Lipha)

Capsules, s/r, grey/yellow, phentermine 15 mg (as resin complex). Price 20 caps = **C**

Capsules, s/r, yellow, phentermine 30 mg (as resin complex). Price 20 caps = **D**

COMPOUND PREPARATIONS

CD Durophet® (Riker)

Capsules, s/r, amphetamine 3.75 mg, dexamphetamine 3.75 mg (both resin complexes). Price 30 caps = **D**

Capsules, s/r, white/grey, amphetamine 6.25 mg, dexamphetamine 6.25 mg (both resin complexes). Price 30 caps = **D**

Capsules, s/r, grey, amphetamine 10 mg, dexamphetamine 10 mg (both resin complexes). Price 30 caps = **D**

4.6 Drugs used in nausea and vertigo

Drug treatment of nausea and vertigo is discussed under the following headings: Vestibular disorders; Nausea of pregnancy; Symptomatic relief of nausea from underlying disease.

Anti-emetics should be prescribed only when the cause of vomiting is known, particularly in children, otherwise the symptomatic relief that they produce may delay identification and treatment of the underlying disease. When the cause can be treated (as in diabetic ketoacidosis and digitalis intoxication), anti-emetics are generally unnecessary. If drug treatment is indicated the choice of drugs depends on the aetiology of vomiting.

VESTIBULAR DISORDERS

Anti-emetics may be required in motion sickness, Ménière's disease, positional vertigo, labyrinthitis, and operative manipulation of the otovestibular apparatus. **Hyoscine** and the **antihistamines** are the drugs of choice. If possible they should be administered prophylactially at least 30 minutes before the emetic stimulus. Patients should be **warned** that these compounds may cause drowsiness, impair driving performance, and enhance the effects of alcohol and central nervous depressants.

MOTION SICKNESS. The most effective drug for the prevention of motion sickness is **hyoscine**. Adverse effects (drowsiness, blurred vision, dry mouth, urinary retention) are more frequent than with the **antihistamines** but are not generally prominent at the doses employed.

Antihistamines such as **cinnarizine, cyclizine, dimenhydrinate, mepyramine,** and **promethazine** are slightly less effective but generally better tolerated. There is no evidence that one antihistamine is superior to another but their duration of action and incidence of adverse effects (drowsiness and anticholinergic effects) differ. If a sedative effect is desired promethazine and dimenhydrinate are useful, but generally a less sedating antihistamine like cyclizine or cinnarizine is preferred. To prevent motion sickness the first dose is usually taken half an hour (2 hours for cinnarizine) before the start of the journey. Metoclopramide and the phenothiazine derivatives (except promethazine) are ineffective in motion sickness.

OTHER LABYRINTHINE DISORDERS. Vertigo and nausea associated with Ménière's disease and middle-ear surgery disorders may be difficult to treat. **Hyoscine, antihistamines,** and **phenothiazine derivatives** (such as chlorpromazine, prochlorperazine, and thiethylperazine) are effective in the prophylaxis and treatment of such conditions. **Betahistine** and **cinnarizine** have been promoted as specific treatment for Ménière's disease but are no more effective than the other drugs. In the acute attack **chlorpromazine, cyclizine, prochlorperazine,** or **thiethylperazine** may be given rectally or by intramuscular injection.

Treatment of vertigo in its chronic forms is seldom fully effective but antihistamines (such as dimenhydrinate) or phenothiazine derivatives (such as prochlorperazine) may help.

NAUSEA OF PREGNANCY

Nausea and vomiting in the first trimester of pregnancy does **not** generally require drug therapy. Although they respond to antihistamines, phenothiazine derivatives, metoclopramide, and doxylamine, none of these drugs should be used unless vomiting is a major problem. If vomiting is troublesome, an antihistamine or a phenothiazine derivative (promethazine or thiethylperazine) may be useful.

Pyridoxine has been used for the treatment of nausea and vomiting in pregnancy but its value has not been established.

SYMPTOMATIC RELIEF OF NAUSEA FROM UNDERLYING DISEASE

A **phenothiazine derivative,** in low doses, is the drug of choice for the prophylaxis and treatment of nausea and vomiting associated with uraemia, diffuse neoplastic disease, radiation sickness, acute viral gastro-enteritis, and the emesis caused by drugs such as oestrogens, narcotics, general anaesthetics, and cytotoxic drugs. Rectal or parenteral administration is required if the vomiting has already started. **Chlorpromazine** is usually suitable and although a sedative effect is common, adverse extrapyramidal effects are not generally prominent at the doses required for full anti-emetic action.

Prochlorperazine, perphenazine, trifluoperazine, and **thiethylperazine** are less sedating than chlorpromazine but severe dystonic reactions sometimes occur, especially in children.

Metoclopramide is an effective anti-emetic with a spectrum of activity closely resembling that of the phenothiazine derivatives but it may be less potent. It has a peripheral action in addition to its central effect and therefore may be superior to the phenothiazine derivatives in the emesis associated with gastroduodenal, hepatic, and biliary disease. Acute dystonic reactions may occur, particularly with children, but they are less frequent than with phenothiazine derivatives.

Although antihistamines are active in most of these conditions, they are not usually drugs of choice.

ATROPINE SULPHATE

Indications: nausea, vomiting
Cautions; Contra-indications: see under Hyoscine Hydrobromide
Side-effects: dry mouth, confusion, tachycardia

Dose: by mouth or by subcutaneous or intramuscular injection, 0.25–2 mg daily in single or divided doses; CHILD up to 1 year 250 micrograms, 1–5 years 250–500 micrograms, 6–12 years 0.5–1 mg

Atropine Sulphate Tablets, atropine sulphate 600 micrograms. Price 20 tabs = **A**
Atropine Sulphate Injection: see section 2.3.2

BETAHISTINE HYDROCHLORIDE

Indications: vertigo and hearing disturbances in labyrinthine disorders
Cautions: asthma, peptic ulcer, rhinitis, urticaria
Contra-indications: phaeochromocytoma
Side-effects: nausea, headache, rashes
Dose: 8–16 mg 3 times daily, preferably after meals, increased as necessary to a max. of 48 mg daily

Serc® (Duphar)
Tablets, scored, betahistine hydrochloride 8 mg. Price 20 tabs = **D**

BUCLIZINE HYDROCHLORIDE

Indications: nausea, vertigo, labyrinthine disorders
Cautions; Side-effects: see under Cyclizine. Avoid in children

Equivert® (Pfizer)
Tablets, yellow, buclizine hydrochloride 25 mg, nicotinic acid 25 mg. Price 20 tabs = **D**
Dose: 1 tablet 3 times daily before meals

CHLORPROMAZINE HYDROCHLORIDE

Indications: severe nausea and vomiting (see notes above)
Cautions; Contra-indications; Side-effects: see section 4.2.1. Side-effects occur infrequently with anti-emetic doses
Dose: by mouth, 25–50 mg 3 times daily
By subcutaneous or intramuscular injection, 12.5–50 mg 3 times daily
By rectum in suppositories, chlorpromazine 100 mg up to 3 times daily

Preparations
Section 4.2.1

CINNARIZINE

Indications: nausea, vertigo, labyrinthine disorders, motion sickness
Cautions; Side-effects: see under Cyclizine. Rarely hypersensitivity
Dose: 15–30 mg 3 times daily; CHILD half the adult dose

Stugeron® (Janssen)
Tablets, scored, cinnarizine 15 mg. Price 20 tabs = **C**

Stugeron Forte: see section 2.6.3

CYCLIZINE

Indications: nausea, vomiting, vertigo, motion sickness, labyrinthine disorders
Cautions: patient's ability to drive or operate machinery may be impaired; alcohol increases CNS depression; liver disease. Drug interactions: see Appendix 1
Side-effects: drowsiness, headache, dry mouth, gastro-intestinal disturbances, blurred vision
Dose: by mouth, cyclizine hydrochloride 50 mg 3 times daily; CHILD 3 times daily, 1–5 years 12.5 mg, 6–12 years 25 mg
By intramuscular injection, cyclizine lactate 50 mg 3 times daily; CHILD 6–12 years 25 mg

Valoid® (Calmic)
Tablets, scored, cyclizine hydrochloride 50 mg. Price 20 tabs = **C**
Injection, cyclizine lactate 50 mg/ml. Price 1-ml amp = **B**

DIMENHYDRINATE

Indications: nausea, vomiting, vertigo, motion sickness, labyrinthine disorders
Cautions; Side-effects: see under Cyclizine but more sedating
Dose: by mouth or by intramuscular or slow intravenous injection, 50–100 mg 3–6 times daily; max. in 24 hours 400 mg; CHILD, 2–3 times daily, 1–5 years 12.5–25 mg, 6–12 years 25–50 mg
By rectum in suppositories, 100 mg up to 4 times daily; CHILD 2–3 times daily, up to 1 year 25 mg, 1–5 years 25–50 mg, 6–12 years 100 mg

Dramamine® (Searle)
Tablets, yellow, scored, dimenhydrinate 50 mg. Price 20 tabs = **B**
Injection, dimenhydrinate 50 mg/ml in solvent. Price 1-ml amp = **B**
Gravol® (Pharmax)
Tablets, orange, scored, dimenhydrinate 50 mg. Price 20 tabs = **B**
Suppositories, dimenhydrinate 100 mg. Price 10 suppos = **D**
Paediatric suppositories, dimenhydrinate 50 mg. Price 10 suppos = **D**

DIPHENHYDRAMINE HYDROCHLORIDE

Indications: nausea, vertigo, labyrinthine disorders
Cautions; Side-effects: see under Cyclizine
Dose: 25–50 mg 3–4 times daily; CHILD 1–5 years 12.5–25 mg, 6–12 years 25–50 mg

Preparations
See section 3.4.1

DOXYLAMINE SUCCINATE

Indications: nausea
Cautions; Side-effects: see under Cyclizine

Debendox® (Merrell)
Tablets, s/r, doxylamine succinate 10 mg, dicyclomine hydrochloride 10 mg, pyridoxine hydrochloride 10 mg. Price 20 tabs = **C**
Dose: severe nausea in pregnancy, 2 tablets at bedtime, then if necessary 1 on rising and 1 mid-afternoon

HYOSCINE HYDROBROMIDE

Indications: nausea, vomiting, vertigo, labyrinthine disorders, motion sickness
Cautions: elderly patients, urinary retention, cardiovascular disease, paralytic ileus, pyloric stenosis
Contra-indications: glaucoma
Side-effects: drowsiness, dry mouth, dizziness, blurred vision, difficulty with micturition
Dose: by mouth or by subcutaneous injection, 300–600 micrograms 4 times daily; CHILD 3–5 years 75–100 micrograms, 6–12 years 100–300 micrograms

Hyoscine Tablets, hyoscine hydrobromide 300 and 600 micrograms. Price 20 tabs (both) = **A**
Hyoscine Injection, hyoscine hydrobromide 400 and 600 micrograms/ml. Price 1-ml amp (both) = **B**

MECLOZINE HYDROCHLORIDE

Indications: nausea
Cautions; Side-effects: see under Cyclizine

Ancoloxin® (DF)
Tablets, meclozine hydrochloride 25 mg, pyridoxine hydrochloride 50 mg. Price 20 tabs = **C**
Dose: severe nausea and vomiting of pregnancy, 2 tablets at bedtime and if necessary 1 in the morning

MEPYRAMINE MALEATE

Indications: nausea, vomiting, vertigo, labyrinthine disorders, motion sickness
Cautions; Side-effects: see under Cyclizine
Dose: by mouth, 100 mg 3 times daily, increased if necessary to 1 g daily; CHILD 3 times daily, up to 5 years 12.5–25 mg, 6–12 years 25–75 mg
By deep intramuscular or slow intravenous injection, 25–50 mg, repeated when necessary

Preparations
See section 3.4.1

METOCLOPRAMIDE HYDROCHLORIDE

Indications: nausea and vomiting, particularly in gastro-intestinal disorders
Cautions; Side-effects: see section 1.2
Dose: by mouth, or by intramuscular or intravenous injection, up to 10 mg (5 mg in young adults up to 20 years) 3 times daily; CHILD (see cautions) up to 1 year 1 mg twice daily, 1–2 years 1 mg 2–3 times daily, 3–5 years 2 mg 2–3 times daily, 6–14 years 2·5–5 mg 3 times daily

Preparations
See section 1.2

PERPHENAZINE

Indications: severe nausea, vomiting (see notes above)
Cautions; Contra-indications; Side-effects: see section 4.2.1. Side-effects infrequent with anti-emetic doses
Dose: by mouth, 4 mg 3 times daily, increased if necessary to a max. of 24 mg in 24 hours
By intramuscular injection, 5–10 mg initially, then 5 mg every 6 hours, max. 15 mg in 24 hours

Preparations
Section 4.2

PROCHLORPERAZINE

Indications: severe nausea, vomiting, vertigo, labyrinthine disorders (see notes above)
Cautions; Contra-indications: see under Chlorpromazine Hydrochloride (section 4.2.1). Avoid in children weighing less than 10 kg
Side-effects: dry mouth, drowsiness, which may affect the ability to drive or operate machinery or increase the CNS depressant effect of alcohol. Side-effects are rare with anti-emetic doses, but with high doses extrapyramidal symptoms may occur, particularly in children, elderly, and debilitated patients
Dose: by mouth, prochlorperazine maleate or mesylate 5–25 mg repeated as required; max. 30 mg in 24 hours; CHILD daily in divided doses, 1–5 years 5 mg, 6–12 years 10–15 mg
By deep intramuscular injection, 12.5 mg when required
By rectum, in suppositories, 25 mg; CHILD daily in divided doses, 1–2 years up to 7.5 mg, 3–5 years up to 10 mg, 6–12 years up to 15 mg

Stemetil® (M&B)
Tablets, prochlorperazine maleate 5 mg. Price 20 tabs = **B**
Tablets, scored, prochlorperazine maleate 25 mg. Price 20 tabs = **D**
Syrup (= elixir), green, prochlorperazine mesylate 5 mg/5 ml. Diluent syrup, life of diluted elixir 14 days. Price 125 ml = **C**
Injection, prochlorperazine mesylate 12.5 mg/ml. Price 1-ml amp = **A**; 2-ml amp = **B**
Suppositories, prochlorperazine maleate 5 and 25 mg (as prochlorperazine). Price 5 suppos (both) = **D**

Vertigon® (SK&F)
Spansules® (= capsules s/r), clear/purple, enclosing yellowish-green and white pellets, prochlorperazine 10 and 15 mg (as maleate). Price 20 caps (both) = **C**
Dose: initially 10–15 mg once or twice daily. Maintenance 10–15 mg daily

PROMETHAZINE HYDROCHLORIDE

Indications: nausea, vomiting, vertigo, labyrinthine disorders, motion sickness
Cautions; Side-effects: see under Cyclizine but more sedating; intramuscular injection may be painful
Dose: *by mouth,* 25–50 mg daily in single or divided doses; CHILD, daily, up to 1 year 5–10 mg, 1–5 years 10–15 mg, 6–12 years 15–25 mg
By deep intramuscular injection, half oral dose

Preparations
See section 3.4.1

PROMETHAZINE THEOCLATE

Indications: nausea, vertigo, labyrinthine disorders, motion sickness (acts longer than the hydrochloride)
Cautions; Side-effects: see under Cyclizine but more sedating
Dose: 25–75 mg daily; CHILD 5–10 years 12.5–37.5 mg daily
For severe nausea and vomiting in pregnancy, 25 mg at bedtime, increased if necessary to a max. of 100 mg daily

Avomine® (M&B)
Tablets, scored, promethazine theoclate 25 mg. Price 10 tabs = **B**

THIETHYLPERAZINE

Indications: severe nausea, vomiting, vertigo, labyrinthine disorders (see notes above)
Cautions; Contra-indications: see under Chlorpromazine Hydrochloride (section 4.2.1)
Side-effects: dry mouth, postural hypotension, drowsiness (which may affect the ability to drive or operate machinery and increase CNS effects of alcohol). Extrapyramidal effects are rare but females under 30 years are particularly susceptible
Dose: *by mouth,* thiethylperazine maleate 10 mg 2–3 times daily
By intramuscular injection, thiethylperazine 6.5 mg when necessary
By rectum, in suppositories, thiethylperazine 6.5 mg night and morning

Torecan® (Sandoz)
Tablets, s/c, thiethylperazine *maleate* 10 mg. Price 20 tabs = **C**
Injection, thiethylperazine 6.5 mg (as *malate*)/ml. Price 1-ml amp = **A**
Suppositories, thiethylperazine 6.5 mg (as *maleate*). Price 6 suppos = **C**

THIOPROPAZATE HYDROCHLORIDE

Indications: severe nausea and vomiting (see notes above)
Cautions; Contra-indications; Side-effects: see section 4.2.1. Side-effects occur infrequently with anti-emetic doses
Dose: 5–10 mg 3 times daily

Preparations
Section 4.2.1

TRIFLUOPERAZINE

Indications: severe nausea and vomiting (see notes above)
Cautions; Contra-indications; Side-effects: see section 4.2.1. Side-effects occur infrequently with anti-emetic doses
Dose: *by mouth,* 2–4 mg daily in divided doses *or* as a single dose of a sustained-release preparation; CHILD 3–5 years up to 1 mg daily, 6–12 years up to 4 mg daily
By deep intramuscular injection, 1–3 mg daily in divided doses; CHILD 50 micrograms/kg daily in divided doses

Preparations
Section 4.2.1

4.7 Analgesics

4.7.1 Analgesics used for mild to moderate pain

The non-narcotic drugs (aspirin and paracetamol) are particularly suited to the relief of pain in musculoskeletal conditions, whereas the narcotic analgesics are more suited for the relief of severe pain of visceral origin.

Analgesic requirements may be profoundly affected by the attitude of both the patient and the prescriber to the pain; in many cases where analgesics might normally have been given a placebo has provided substantial relief.

4.7.1.1 NON-NARCOTIC ANALGESICS

Aspirin and paracetamol are the main drugs in this group.

Aspirin is the analgesic of choice for headache and transient musculoskeletal pain. It also has anti-inflammatory properties which may sometimes be useful. Aspirin tablets or dispersible aspirin tablets are adequate for most purposes as they act rapidly and are inexpensive.

Gastric irritation may be a problem; it is minimised by taking the dose after meals. Numerous formulations are available which improve gastric tolerance, for example the buffered aspirin preparations such as aloxiprin, micro-encapsulated aspirin (Levius®) and enteric-coated aspirin (Nu-Seals®). Some of these preparations have a slow onset of action and are therefore unsuitable for single-dose analgesic use though their prolonged action may be useful for the relief of night pain.

Aspirin is **not** recommended for use in infants under one year because of the danger of metabolic acidosis and fatal poisoning which may occur after repeated dosage, but single doses may be used for minor infections in young children.

Aspirin Mixture BPC 1963 is an unstable mixture that should **not** be prescribed. The appropriate quantity of aspirin in the form of dispersible tablets should be ordered to be taken in water.

Paracetamol is similar in efficacy to aspirin, but it is less irritant to the stomach. Paediatric paracetamol elixir is preferable to aspirin in infants. Overdosage with paracetamol is particularly dangerous as it may cause hepatic damage which is sometimes not apparent for 4 to 6 days.

Benorylate is an aspirin–paracetamol ester which releases paracetamol slowly and so hepatotoxicity in overdosage may be reduced.

Anti-inflammatory analgesics (section 10.1.1.2) are particularly useful for the treatment of patients with chronic disease accompanied by pain and inflammation. Some of them are also used in the short-term treatment of mild to moderate pain including transient musculoskeletal pain. They may be particularly suitable for the relief of pain in dysmenorrhoea because of their ability to inhibit prostaglandin synthetase.

ASPIRIN

Indications: mild to moderate pain, pyrexia (see notes above); see also section 10.1.1.1

Cautions: asthma, impaired renal or hepatic function, dehydration, pregnancy. Drug interactions: see Appendix 1

Contra-indications: gastro-intestinal ulceration (see notes above), haemophilia, concurrent anticoagulant therapy

Side-effects: generally mild and infrequent but high incidence of gastro-intestinal irritation with slight asymptomatic blood loss, increased bleeding time, bronchospasm and skin reactions in hypersensitive patients. Prolonged administration, see section 10.1.1.1

Dose: 300–900 mg every 4–6 hours when necessary; max. 4 g daily; CHILD 1–2 years 75–150 mg every 6 hours, 3–5 years 225–300 mg every 8 hours, 6–12 years 300–400 mg every 6 hours. Not suitable for children under 1 year

Aspirin Tablets, aspirin 300 mg. Price 20 tabs = **A**

Aspirin Tablets, Dispersible, aspirin 300 mg. Price 20 tabs = **A**

Aspirin Tablets, Paediatric Dispersible, aspirin 75 mg. Price 20 tabs = **A**

Aspergum® (Plough)

Tablets, chewing gum, s/c, aspirin 227 mg. Price 20 tabs = **B**

Dose: 1–2 tablets chewed every 4–6 hours when necessary; max. 8 tablets daily; CHILD 6–9 years up to 3 tablets daily, 10–14 years up to 5 tablets daily

Breoprin® (Sterling Research)

Tablets, s/r, scored, aspirin 648 mg (for intestinal release). Price 20 tabs = **C**

Caprin® (Sinclair)

Tablets, s/r, pink, aspirin 324 mg (for intestinal release). Price 20 tabs = **B**

Claradin® (Nicholas)

Tablets, effervescent, scored, aspirin 300 mg. Price 20 tabs = **B**

Laboprin® (LAB)

Tablets, mottled white/brown, aspirin 300 mg with lysine 245 mg. Price 24 tabs = **B**

Levius® (Farmitalia Carlo Erba)

Tablets, s/r, aspirin 500 mg. Price 30 tabs = **B**

Nu-Seals Aspirin® (Lilly)

Tablets, red, e/c, aspirin 300 mg. Price 20 tabs = **B**

Tablets, red, e/c, aspirin 600 mg. Price 20 tabs = **B**

Palaprin Forte® (Nicholas)

Tablets, orange, scored, aloxiprin 600 mg ≡ aspirin 500 mg. To be taken dispersed in water, chewed, sucked, or swallowed whole. Price 20 tabs = **B**

Paynocil® (Beecham)

Tablets, scored, aspirin 600 mg, glycine 300 mg. To be dissolved on the tongue. Price 18 tabs = **B**

Solprin® (R&C)

Tablets, dispersible, aspirin 300 mg. Price 20 tabs = **A**

PARACETAMOL

Indications: mild to moderate pain, pyrexia

Cautions: renal or hepatic impairment, alcoholism. Drug interactions: see Appendix 1

Side-effects: liver damage in prolonged use or overdosage

Dose: 0.5–1 g every 4–6 hours to a max. of 4 g daily; CHILD up to 1 year 60–120 mg, 1–5 years 120–250 mg, 6–12 years 250–500 mg; these doses may be repeated every 4–6 hours when necessary

Paracetamol Tablets, paracetamol 500 mg. Price 20 tabs = **A**

Paracetamol Elixir, Paediatric, red, paracetamol 120 mg/5 ml. Do not dilute. Price 100 ml = **B**

Calpol® (Calmic)
Suspension (= mixture), pink, paracetamol 120 mg/5 ml. Diluent syrup, life of diluted elixir 14 days. Price 100 ml = **C**

Panadol® (Winthrop)
Caplets® (= tablets), paracetamol 500 mg. Price 20 tabs = **B**
Tablets, paracetamol 500 mg. Price 20 tabs = **A**
Soluble (= effervescent tablets), paracetamol 500 mg. Price 12 tabs = **B**
Elixir, yellow, paracetamol 120 mg/5 ml. Diluent syrup, life of diluted elixir 14 days. Price 60 ml = **B**

Panasorb® (Winthrop)
Tablets, paracetamol 500 mg in sorbitol basis. Price 20 tabs = **C**

Salzone® (Wallace Mfg)
Syrup (= elixir), paracetamol 120 mg/5 ml. Diluent syrup, life of diluted elixir 14 days. Price 75 ml = **C**

AZAPROPAZONE

Indications: mild to moderate pain; see also section 10.1.1.2
Cautions; Side-effects: see section 10.1.1.2
Dose: 300–600 mg 2–4 times daily, preferably after meals

Preparations
See section 10.1.1.2

BENORYLATE

Aspirin-paracetamol ester
Indications: mild to moderate pain; pyrexia; see also section 10.1.1.1
Cautions; Contra-indications; Side-effects: see under Aspirin and under Paracetamol
Dose: 1–1.5 g every 6–8 hours, preferably after meals; CHILD, see section 10.1.1.1

Benoral® (Winthrop)
Tablets, benorylate 750 mg. Price 20 tabs = **C**
Sachets, benorylate 2 g. Price 10 sachets = **D**
Suspension (= mixture), benorylate 2 g/5 ml. Diluent syrup, life of diluted mixture 14 days. Price 150 ml = **F**

DIFLUNISAL

Indications: mild to moderate pain; see also section 10.1.1.2
Cautions; Contra-indications; Side-effects: see under Aspirin; also section 10.1.1.2. Drug interactions: see Appendix 1
Dose: 250–500 mg twice daily

▼ Dolobid® (Morson)
Tablets, peach, f/c, diflunisal 250 mg. Price 20 tabs = **D**
Tablets, orange, f/c, diflunisal 500 mg. Price 20 tabs = **F**

FENOPROFEN

Indications: mild to moderate pain, pyrexia; see also section 10.1.1.2
Cautions; Contra-indications; Side-effects: see under Aspirin; also section 10.1.1.2
Dose: 200–400 mg 3–4 times daily, preferably after meals; max. 3 g daily

Progesic® (Lilly)
Tablets, yellow, fenoprofen 200 mg (as calcium salt). Price 20 tabs = **C**

Fenopron: see section 10.1.1.2

FLUFENAMIC ACID

Indications: mild to moderate pain; pyrexia; see also section 10.1.1.2
Cautions; Contra-indications; Side-effects: see under Mefenamic Acid (below)
Dose: 200 mg 3 times daily after meals

Meralen® (Merrell)
Capsules, blue, flufenamic acid 100 mg. Price 20 caps = **D**

IBUPROFEN

Indications: mild to moderate pain; see also section 10.1.1.2
Cautions; Side-effects: see section 10.1.1.2
Dose: 200–400 mg 3 times daily preferably after meals, max. 2.4 g daily; CHILD, section 10.1.1.2

Preparations
See section 10.1.1.2

MEFENAMIC ACID

Indications: mild to moderate pain, pyrexia in children; see also section 10.1.1.2
Cautions: allergic disease, particularly asthma, blood tests needed during long-term therapy. Drug interactions: see Appendix 1
Contra-indications: peptic ulceration, inflammatory bowel disease, impaired renal and hepatic function, pregnancy
Side-effects: drowsiness, dizziness, gastro-intestinal disturbances; rarely rashes, thrombocytopenia, haemolytic anaemia. See also section 10.1.1.2
Dose: 500 mg 3 times daily after meals; CHILD over 6 months 6.5 mg/kg 3–4 times daily for not longer than 7 days, except in juvenile chronic arthritis

Ponstan® (P-D)
Capsules, ivory/blue, mefenamic acid 250 mg. Price 20 caps = **C**
Tablets forte, yellow, f/c, mefenamic acid 500 mg. Price 20 tabs = **D**
Paediatric suspension (= mixture), mefenamic acid 50 mg/5 ml. Diluent syrup, life of diluted mixture 14 days. Price 125 ml = **D**

NAPROXEN SODIUM

Indications: mild to moderate pain; see also Naproxen, section 10.1.1.2
Cautions; Side-effects: see under Naproxen, section 10.1.1.2

Dose: 550 mg initially, then 275 mg 6–8 hourly when necessary, after meals
Note: 275 mg naproxen sodium ≡ 250 mg naproxen but the sodium salt has a more rapid action

▼ **Synflex®** (Syntex)
Capsules, orange, naproxen sodium 275 mg. Price 20 caps = **E**

SALSALATE

Indications: mild to moderate pain, pyrexia; see also section 10.1.1.1
Cautions; Contra-indications; Side-effects: see under Aspirin (above)
Dose: 500 mg every 6–8 hours when necessary

Disalcid® (Riker)
Capsules, orange/grey, salsalate 500 mg. Price 20 caps = **D**

SODIUM SALICYLATE

Indications: mild to moderate pain, pyrexia
Cautions; Contra-indications; Side-effects: see under Aspirin (above), but gastric irritation and hearing disturbances occur more frequently
Dose: 0.5–1 g every 4 hours, when required, after meals

Sodium Salicylate Mixture, sodium salicylate 250 mg/5 ml (see Formulary). Price 100 ml = **A**
Sodium Salicylate Mixture, Strong, sodium salicylate 500 mg/5 ml (see Formulary). Price 100 ml = **A**
Entrosalyl® (Cox-Continental)
Tablets, gluten-coated, sodium salicylate 500 mg. Price 20 tabs = **B**

ZOMEPIRAC

Indications: moderate pain; see also section 10.1.1.2
Cautions; Side-effects: see section 10.1.1.2
Dose: 100 mg every 4–6 hours. Max. 600 mg daily

▼ **Zomax®** (Ortho)
Tablets, yellow, scored, zomepirac 100 mg (as sodium salt dihydrate). Price 20 tabs = **E**

4.7.1.2 NARCOTIC ANALGESICS USED IN MILD TO MODERATE PAIN

The risk of addiction, though possible, occurs rarely with drugs of this group. However they should be prescribed with caution in patients with a history of drug abuse; there is an increasing problem of drug abuse with dextropropoxyphene/paracetamol compound preparations (Distalgesic® etc.). Narcotic analgesics used in severe pain are listed in section 4.7.2 and have an appreciable risk of addiction.

The narcotic analgesics listed below and in section 4.7.2 share many of the same side-effects (listed in section 4.7.2).

The temptation to prescribe these drugs freely should be **avoided;** the non-narcotic analgesics, though freely available to the public, are adequate for most purposes.

Codeine is used for the relief of mild to moderate pain but is too constipating for long-term use.

Dihydrocodeine (DF 118®) is a more potent analgesic than codeine. It is suitable for use in ambulant patients with moderate pain but may cause dizziness and constipation. It may be given by mouth or by injection.

Pentazocine (Fortral®) is more potent than dihydrocodeine or codeine. Disadvantages are that hallucinations and thought disturbances may sometimes occur. It should be avoided after myocardial infarction as it may increase pulmonary and aortic blood pressure as well as cardiac work. Several formulations are available but it is usually given orally for mild pain and parenterally for severe pain.

Dextropropoxyphene given alone is a very mild analgesic and is somewhat less potent than codeine. Combinations of dextropropoxyphene and paracetamol (Distalgesic® etc.) or aspirin have a more potent effect. However the chief disadvantage of combinations with paracetamol is that overdosage is complicated by respiratory depression due to dextropropoxyphene and hepatoxicity due to paracetamol.

CODEINE PHOSPHATE

Indications: mild to moderate pain
Cautions: liver disease; avoid in pregnancy and in children under 1 year. Drug interactions: see Appendix 1
Side-effects: tolerance and dependence, particularly on injection, sedation, dizziness, nausea, constipation; may enhance the effects of alcohol
Dose: by mouth, 10–60 mg every 4 hours when necessary, to a max. of 200 mg daily; CHILD, 3 mg/kg daily in divided doses
By injection, up to 30 mg when necessary

Codeine Phosphate Tablets, codeine phosphate 15 mg, price 20 tabs = **B**; 30 mg, price 20 tabs = **C**; 60 mg, price 20 tabs = **D**
Codeine Phosphate Syrup, codeine phosphate 25 mg/5 ml. Price 100 ml = **C**
CD **Codeine Phosphate Injection,** (USP), codeine phosphate 60 mg/ml. Price 1-ml amp = **C**
For compound proprietary preparations containing codeine phosphate see section 4.7.1.3

DEXTROPROPOXYPHENE

Indications: mild to moderate pain
Cautions: see under Codeine Phosphate; caution in renal impairment
Side-effects: see under Codeine Phosphate; with daily doses above 720 mg toxic psychoses and convulsions may occur
Dose: 60 mg every 6–8 hours when necessary

Note: 60 mg dextropropoxyphene ≡ 65 mg dextropropoxyphene hydrochloride ≡ 100 mg dextropropoxyphene napsylate

Depronal SA® (Warner)
Capsules, s/r, clear/orange, dextropropoxyphene hydrochloride 150 mg. Price 20 caps = **C**
Dose: 1 capsule every 8–12 hours; max. 2 daily

Doloxene® (Lilly)
Pulvules® (= capsules), orange, the equivalent of dextropropoxyphene hydrochloride 65 mg (as napsylate). Price 20 caps = **C**

DIHYDROCODEINE TARTRATE

Indications: moderate to severe pain

Cautions; Side-effects: see under Codeine Phosphate. Caution in respiratory disease; reduce dose in elderly and debilitated patients, hypothyroidism, impaired renal function. Side-effects more frequent with doses above 30 mg

Dose: *by mouth, subcutaneous, or intramuscular injection,* 30–60 mg every 4–6 hours when necessary; CHILD over 4 years, 0.5–1 mg/kg. Oral doses should preferably be taken after food

DF 118® (DF)
Tablets, dihydrocodeine tartrate 30 mg. Price 20 tabs = **C**
Elixir, brown, dihydrocodeine tartrate 10 mg/5 ml. Diluent syrup (without preservative), life of diluted elixir 14 days. Price 150 ml = **D**
CD *Injection,* dihydrocodeine tartrate 50 mg/ml. Price 1-ml amp = **B**

PENTAZOCINE

Indications: moderate to severe pain

Cautions; Side-effects: see under Codeine Phosphate. Occasionally hallucinations occur. Avoid in patients dependent on narcotics and in arterial or pulmonary hypertension and cardiac failure. Drug interactions: see Appendix 1

Dose: *by mouth,* pentazocine hydrochloride 25–100 mg every 3–4 hours; CHILD 6–12 years 25 mg

By subcutaneous or intramuscular injection, pentazocine 30–60 mg every 3–4 hours

By intravenous injection, pentazocine 30 mg every 3–4 hours

By rectum in suppositories, pentazocine 50 mg up to 4 times daily

CHILD over 1 year, *by subcutaneous, intramuscular, or intravenous injection,* pentazocine 0.5–1 mg/kg every 3–4 hours

Fortral® (Winthrop)
Capsules, grey/yellow, pentazocine hydrochloride 50 mg. Price 20 caps = **E**
Tablets, yellow, f/c, pentazocine hydrochloride 25 mg. Price 20 tabs = **D**
Injection, pentazocine 30 mg (as lactate)/ml. Price 1-ml amp = **B**; 2-ml amp = **C**
Suppositories, pentazocine 50 mg (as lactate). Price 20 suppos = **F**

4.7.1.3 COMPOUND ANALGESIC PREPARATIONS

Compound analgesic preparations of, for example, aspirin, paracetamol, and codeine are **not** recommended. Single-ingredient preparations (sections 4.7.1.1 and 4.7.1.2) should be prescribed in preference because compound preparations rarely have any advantage; they may increase the cost of treatment unnecessarily and complicate the treatment of overdosage.

It is even more desirable to **avoid** mixtures of analgesics with laxatives, corticosteroids, or hypnotics; the individual components should be prescribed separately so that the dose of each can be adjusted as appropriate. Some analgesic preparations are combinations of analgesics with barbiturates, sedatives, or amphetamines. Their use is likewise undesirable.

Compound analgesic preparations containing muscle relaxants are discussed in section 10.2.2.

Caffeine is a weak stimulant that is often included, in small doses, in analgesic preparations. It does not contribute to the analgesic or anti-inflammatory effect of the preparation and may possibly aggravate the gastric irritation caused by aspirin.

Phenacetin is no longer used because of the dangers of renal damage.

Aspirin and Codeine Tablets, aspirin 400 mg, codeine phosphate 8 mg. Price 20 tabs = **A**
Dose: 1–2 tablets every 4–6 hours when necessary

Aspirin and Codeine Tablets, Dispersible, as for Aspirin and Codeine Tablets (above) but in an effervescent basis. Price 20 tabs = **B**

Aspirin, Paracetamol, and Codeine Tablets, aspirin 250 mg, paracetamol 250 mg, codeine phosphate 6.8 mg. Price 20 tabs = **B**
Dose: 1–2 tablets every 4–6 hours when necessary

Codeine and Paracetamol Tablets, codeine phosphate 8 mg, paracetamol 500 mg (sorbitol basis). Price 20 tabs = **B**
Dose: 1–2 tablets every 4–6 hours when necessary; max. 8 tablets daily

Dihydrocodeine and Paracetamol Tablets, dihydrocodeine tartrate 10 mg, paracetamol 500 mg. Price 20 tabs = **B**
Dose: 1–2 tablets every 4–6 hours when necessary; max. 8 tablets daily

Antoin® (Cox-Continental)
Dispersible tablets, aspirin 400 mg, codeine phosphate 5 mg, caffeine citrate 15 mg. Price 20 tabs = **B**

Cafadol® (Typharm)
Tablets, yellow, scored, paracetamol 500 mg, caffeine 30 mg. Price 20 tabs = **B**

Carisoma Co® (Pharmax)
Tablets, orange, carisoprodol 175 mg, paracetamol 350 mg. Price 20 tabs = **B**

Codis® (R&C)
Dispersible tablets, aspirin 500 mg, codeine phosphate 8 mg. Price 20 tabs = **B**

Cosalgesic® (Cox-Continental)
Tablets, dextropropoxyphene hydrochloride 32.5 mg, paracetamol 325 mg. Price 20 tabs = **A**

Delimon® (Consolidated)
Tablets, morazone hydrochloride 150 mg, paracetamol 50 mg, salicylamide 200 mg. Price 20 tabs = **C**

Dextrogesic® (Unimed)
Tablets, dextropropoxyphene hydrochloride 32.5 mg, paracetamol 325 mg. Price 20 tabs = **B**

Distalgesic® (Dista)
Tablets, dextropropoxyphene hydrochloride 32.5 mg, paracetamol 325 mg. Price 20 tabs = **B**

Distalgesic Soluble® (Dista)
Dispersible tablets, dextropropoxyphene napsylate 50 mg, paracetamol 325 mg. Price 20 tabs = **C**

Dolasan® (Lilly)
Tablets, orange, dextropropoxyphene napsylate 100 mg, aspirin 325 mg. Price 20 tabs = **C**

Doloxene Compound® (Lilly)
Capsules, grey/red, dextropropoxyphene napsylate 100 mg, aspirin 375 mg, caffeine 30 mg. Price 20 caps = **C**

Equagesic® (Wyeth)
Tablets, pink/white/yellow, ethoheptazine citrate 75 mg, meprobamate 150 mg, aspirin 250 mg. Price 20 tabs = **B**

Femerital® (MCP)
Tablets, scored, ambucetamide 100 mg, paracetamol 250 mg. Price 20 tabs = **C**

Fortagesic® (Winthrop)
Tablets, pentazocine 15 mg (as hydrochloride), paracetamol 500 mg. Price 20 tabs = **C**

Hypon® (Calmic)
Tablets, yellow, aspirin 325 mg, caffeine 10 mg, codeine phosphate 5 mg. Price 20 tabs = **B**

Lobak® (Winthrop)
Tablets, scored, chlormezanone 100 mg, paracetamol 450 mg. Price 20 tabs = **D**

Medised® (Martindale)
Suspension (= mixture), paracetamol 120 mg, promethazine hydrochloride 2.5 mg/5 ml. Price 100 ml = **C**

Medocodene® (Medo)
Tablets, yellow, scored, paracetamol 500 mg, codeine phosphate 8 mg. Price 20 tabs = **B**

Myolgin® (Cox-Continental)
Dispersible tablets, scored, paracetamol 200 mg, aspirin 200 mg, codeine phosphate 5 mg, caffeine citrate 15 mg. Price 20 tabs = **B**

Napsalgesic® (Dista)
Tablets, f/c, yellow, dextropropoxyphene napsylate 50 mg, aspirin 500 mg. Price 20 tabs = **B**

Neurodyne® (Rorer)
Capsules, paracetamol 500 mg, codeine phosphate 8 mg. Price 20 caps = **C**

Norgesic® (Riker)
Tablets, scored, orphenadrine citrate 35 mg, paracetamol 450 mg. Price 20 tabs = **C**

Onadox-118® (DF)
Dispersible tablets, aspirin 300 mg, dihydrocodeine tartrate 10 mg. Price 20 tabs = **B**

Paedo-Sed® (Pharmax)
Syrup (= elixir), pale straw, dichloralphenazone 200 mg, paracetamol 100 mg/5 ml. Diluent syrup, life of diluted elixir 14 days. Price 100 ml = **C**

Panadeine Co® (Winthrop)
Tablets, scored, codeine phosphate 8 mg, paracetamol 500 mg. Price 20 tabs = **B**

Paracodol® (Fisons)
Effervescent tablets, paracetamol 500 mg, codeine phosphate 8 mg. Price 20 tabs = **B**

Paradeine® (Scotia)
Tablets, paracetamol 500 mg, codeine phosphate 10 mg, phenolphthalein 2.5 mg. Price 20 tabs = **C**

Parahypon® (Calmic)
Tablets, pink, scored, paracetamol 500 mg, codeine phosphate 5 mg, caffeine 10 mg. Price 20 tabs = **C**

Parake® (Galen)
Tablets, paracetamol 500 mg, codeine phosphate 8 mg. Price 20 tabs = **B**

Paralgin® (Norton)
Tablets, scored, paracetamol 450 mg, caffeine 20 mg, codeine phosphate 6 mg. Price 20 tabs = **B**

Paramol-118® (DF)
Tablets, scored, paracetamol 500 mg, dihydrocodeine tartrate 10 mg. Price 20 tabs = **B**

Para-seltzer® (Wander)
Effervescent tablets, paracetamol 500 mg, caffeine 20 mg. Price 20 tabs = **C**

Parazolidin® (Geigy)
Tablets, scored, phenylbutazone 50 mg, paracetamol 500 mg. Price 20 tabs = **B**

Pardale® (Martindale)
Tablets, scored, paracetamol 400 mg, codeine phosphate 9 mg, caffeine hydrate 10 mg. Price 20 tabs = **C**

Paxidal® (Wallace Mfg)
Tablets, paracetamol 325 mg, meprobamate 135 mg, caffeine 65 mg. Price 12 tabs = **B**

Pharmidone® (Farmitalia Carlo Erba)
Tablets, scored, yellow, codeine phosphate 10 mg, diphenhydramine hydrochloride 5 mg, paracetamol 400 mg, caffeine 50 mg. Price 12 tabs = **B**

Propain® (Luitpold-Werk)
Tablets, yellow, scored, codeine phosphate 10 mg, diphenhydramine hydrochloride 5 mg, paracetamol 400 mg, caffeine 50 mg. Price 20 tabs = **C**

Robaxisal Forte® (Robins)
Tablets, pink/white, scored, methocarbamol 400 mg, aspirin 325 mg. Price 20 tabs = **B**

Safapryn® (Pfizer)
Tablets, pink, s/c, paracetamol 250 mg, aspirin e/c 300 mg. Price 20 tabs = **B**

Safapryn-Co® (Pfizer)
Tablets, green, s/c, paracetamol 250 mg, codeine phosphate 8 mg, aspirin e/c 300 mg. Price 20 tabs = **B**

Solpadeine® (Winthrop)
Effervescent tablets, paracetamol 500 mg, codeine phosphate 8 mg, caffeine 30 mg. Price 20 tabs = **C**

Syndol® (Merrell)
Tablets, yellow, scored, paracetamol 450 mg, codeine phosphate 10 mg, doxylamine succinate 5 mg, caffeine 30 mg. Price 20 tabs = **D**

Tandalgesic® (Geigy)
Tablets, scored, oxyphenbutazone 50 mg, paracetamol 500 mg. Price 20 tabs = **C**

Trancoprin® (Sterling Research)
Tablets, scored, aspirin 300 mg, chlormezanone 100 mg. Price 20 tabs = **C**

Unigesic® (Unimed)
Capsules, grey/yellow, paracetamol 500 mg, caffeine 30 mg. Price 20 caps = **D**

Veganin® (Warner)
Tablets, aspirin 250 mg, paracetamol 250 mg, codeine phosphate 6.8 mg. Price 20 tabs = **B**

Zactipar® (Wyeth)
Tablets, yellow, ethoheptazine citrate 75 mg, paracetamol 400 mg. Price 20 tabs = **C**

Zactirin® (Wyeth)
Tablets, ethoheptazine citrate 75 mg, aspirin 325 mg. Price 20 tabs = **B**

4.7.2 Narcotic and other analgesics used for severe pain

These analgesics are used to relieve moderate to severe pain, but with repeated administration they cause tolerance and dependence. This is no deterrent in the control of pain in terminal disease and the recommended practice is to adjust both the dose and frequency of administration so that the patient never suffers pain; both dose and frequency may need to be gradually increased as tolerance develops, to maintain adequate analgesia.

The narcotic analgesics used for severe pain and those used in mild to moderate pain (section 4.7.1.2) share many side-effects though qualitative and quantitative differences exist. They all cause constipation (by reduction of intestinal motility), respiratory depression, cough suppression, urinary retention, nausea, and tolerance, and are liable to cause dependence. Drug interactions: see Appendix 1. Combining two or more narcotic analgesics is unnecessary; a higher dose of one will be as effective.

In general all narcotic analgesics should be used with caution, if at all, in patients taking monoamine-oxidase inhibitors, those with a history of drug abuse, and those with hypotension, asthma, decreased respiratory reserve, hepatic impairment, raised intracranial pressure, or head injury, and during pregnancy and lactation.

Morphine remains the most valuable narcotic analgesic for severe pain although it frequently causes nausea and vomiting, and it is the standard against which other narcotic analgesics are compared.

The initial dose depends largely on the patient's previous treatment. To replace a weak narcotic analgesic 5–10 mg of morphine should be prescribed, for an intermediate narcotic 10 mg, and for a strong narcotic 20 mg or more. If the first dose of morphine is no more effective than the previous medicine it should be increased by 50%.

Morphine often confers a state of euphoria and mental detachment which may enhance the sense of well-being. Concurrent administration of chlorpromazine or other phenothiazine derivatives (section 4.6) reduces the tendency to nausea and vomiting. Preparations containing morphine with an anti-emetic such as cyclizine (Cyclimorph®) are available. Mixed opium alkaloids such as **papaveretum** (Omnopon®) do not appear to have any advantage over morphine. Morphine is often formulated as an elixir for oral use (see below).

Diamorphine (heroin) is a powerful narcotic analgesic. It is more likely to produce euphoria and addiction than morphine but causes relatively less nausea, constipation, and hypotension. It is often formulated as an elixir for oral use (see below) but has little advantage over morphine as such preparations are chemically unstable, the diamorphine being gradually deacetylated to morphine. The greater solubility of diamorphine hydrochloride allows effective doses to be injected in smaller volumes and this is important in the emaciated patient.

Phenazocine (Narphen®) may also be effective in severe pain. It is particularly useful in biliary colic as it has less tendency to increase biliary pressure than other narcotic analgesics but its respiratory depressant properties are very marked.

Pethidine produces a prompt but short-lasting analgesia and even in high doses it is a less potent analgesic than morphine. It is unsuitable for the relief of pain in terminal disease. It remains the drug of choice for the relief of pain when intracranial damage is known or suspected and for analgesia in labour. In the neonate it is associated with less respiratory depression than other narcotic analgesics but this is probably because its pharmacological actions are, in general, weaker. See also section 15.1.4.1 for its use in surgical anaesthesia.

Dextromoramide (Palfium®), **dipipanone, levorphanol** (Dromoran®), and **methadone** (Physeptone®) are less sedating than morphine and are satisfactory drugs for the oral treatment of chronic pain in terminal disease.

Oxycodone pectinate has a prolonged action; a single dose (by rectum in suppositories) may be sufficient to provide relief throughout the night. A suppository containing 30 mg of oxycodone (as pectinate) is as effective as 20 mg of morphine by mouth and acts for about 8 hours.

The use of **fentanyl** (Sublimaze®) and **phenoperidine** (Operidine®) to produce surgical analgesia and postoperative analgesia is discussed in section 15.1.4. **Piritramide** (Dipidolor®) is used in postoperative analgesia.

Pentazocine and **dihydrocodeine** injections (section 4.7.1.2) are also used in severe pain.

Dextromoramide, morphine, and oxycodone pectinate are all available as **suppositories.**

NEWER ANALGESICS. **Buprenorphine** (Temgesic®) is a new analgesic for sublingual or parenteral use. It has not been fully evaluated. It has a much longer duration of action than morphine and is thought to have a low dependence potential. Its main disadvantage is that unlike most narcotic analgesics its effects cannot be reversed by naloxone. **Butorphanol** (Stadol®) has similar properties.

Nefopam (Acupan®) is a new analgesic unrelated to the narcotic analgesics, with an unknown mode of action. Nefopam has not been fully evaluated but may have a place for the relief of persistent pain unresponsive to non-narcotic analgesics, before pethidine is tried. It should be avoided in patients taking paracetamol because of the possible risk of hepatotoxicity.

MORPHINE SALTS

Indications: severe pain, left ventricular failure, pulmonary oedema

Cautions; Contra-indications; Side-effects: see notes (above). Drug interactions: see Appendix 1

Dose: *by mouth or by subcutaneous, intramuscular or intravenous injection,* morphine hydrochloride, sulphate, or tartrate 10–20 mg; CHILD up to 1 month 150 micrograms/kg, 1–12 months 200 micrograms/kg, 1–5 years 2.5–5 mg, 6–12

years 5–10 mg; these doses may be repeated every 4 hours, or more in terminal pain. See also notes above
Left ventricular failure and pulmonary oedema, *by intravenous injection,* morphine sulphate 5–10 mg as a single dose
By rectum, in suppositories, morphine hydrochloride or sulphate, 15–30 mg every 4 hours

CD **Morphine Sulphate Injection,** morphine sulphate 10, 15, and 20 mg/ml, price 1-ml amp (all) = **A**; 30 mg/ml, price 1- and 2-ml amp (both) = **B**

CD **Morphine Suppositories,** morphine hydrochloride or sulphate 15 mg, price 12 suppos = **E**; 30 mg, price 12 suppos = **G**. The strength of the suppositories and the morphine salt contained in them must be specified by the prescriber

CD **Opium Tincture,** morphine 1% (10 mg/ml). Price 10 ml = **A**
Dose: 1–2 ml; CHILD 1–5 years 0.25–0.5 ml, 6–12 years 0.5–1 ml

CD **Cyclimorph-10**® (Calmic)
Injection, morphine tartrate 10 mg, cyclizine tartrate 50 mg/ml. Price 1-ml amp = **B**
Dose: as for morphine salts (above)

CD **Cyclimorph-15**® (Calmic)
Injection, morphine tartrate 15 mg, cyclizine tartrate 50 mg/ml. Price 1-ml amp = **B**
Dose: as for morphine salts (above)

CD **Duromorph**® (LAB)
Injection, s/r, morphine 64 mg/ml. Price 1-ml amp = **C**
Dose: by subcutaneous or intramuscular injection, in terminal pain, 1–1.5 ml every 9 hours

CD **MST-1 Continus**® (Napp)
Tablets, s/r, brown, f/c, morphine sulphate 10 mg. Price 20 tabs = **E**
Dose: 1–2 tablets twice daily

CD **Nepenthe**® (Evans)
Oral solution (= elixir), brown, anhydrous morphine 8.4 mg/ml (500 micrograms from opium tincture, 7.9 mg from morphine). Diluent syrup, life of diluted elixir 4 weeks. Price 100 ml = **E**
Dose: 1–2 ml, repeated every 4 hours when necessary; CHILD 1–5 years 0.25–0.5 ml, 6–12 years 0.5–1 ml, as a single dose
Injection, anhydrous morphine 8.4 mg/ml (500 micrograms from papaveretum, 7.9 mg from morphine hydrochloride). Price 0.6-ml amp = **B**
Dose: 1–2 ml, repeated every 4 hours when necessary; CHILD 1–5 years 0.25–0.5 ml, 6–12 years 0.5–1 ml as a single dose

BUPRENORPHINE

Indications: moderate to severe pain
Cautions; Contra-indications; Side-effects: see notes (above), but side-effects are less marked than for morphine and the risk of dependence is lower. Commonest side-effects are drowsiness, respiratory depression, nausea, dizziness, and sweating. Effects only partially reversed by naloxone
Dose: *by sublingual administration,* 400 micrograms every 6-8 hours
By intramuscular or slow intravenous injection, 300–600 micrograms every 6–8 hours

▼ **Temgesic**® (R&C)
Tablets (sublingual), buprenorphine 200 micrograms (as hydrochloride). Price 20 tabs = **E**
Injection, buprenorphine 300 micrograms (as hydrochloride)/ml. Price 1- and 2-ml amp (both) = **C**

BUTORPHANOL TARTRATE

Indications: moderate to severe pain
Cautions; Contra-indications; Side-effects: see under Buprenorphine. Avoid in acute myocardial infarction
Dose: *by intramuscular injection,* 1–4 mg every 3–4 hours
By intravenous injection, 0.5–2 mg every 3–4 hours

▼ **Stadol**® (Mead Johnson)
Injection, butorphanol tartrate 2 mg/ml. Price 1-ml vial = **B**; 2-ml vial = **C**

DEXTROMORAMIDE

Indications: moderate to severe pain, particularly chronic pain in terminal disease
Cautions; Contra-indications; Side-effects: see notes (above) but less sedating than morphine and development of tolerance and dependence is slower. Avoid in obstetric analgesia (increased risk of neonatal depression)
Dose: *by mouth,* 5 mg increasing to 20 mg, every 6 hours
By subcutaneous or intramuscular injection, 5 mg increasing to 15 mg, every 6 hours
By rectum in suppositories, 10 mg every 6 hours

CD **Palfium**® (MCP)
Tablets, scored, dextromoramide 5 mg (as tartrate). Price 20 tabs = **D**
Tablets, peach, scored, dextromoramide 10 mg (as tartrate). Price 20 tabs = **E**
Injection, dextromoramide 5 mg (as tartrate)/ml. Price 1-ml amp = **A**
Injection, dextromoramide 10 mg (as tartrate)/ml. Price 1-ml amp = **B**
Suppositories, dextromoramide 10 mg (as tartrate). Price 10 suppos = **E**

DIAMORPHINE HYDROCHLORIDE

Indications: severe pain
Cautions; Contra-indications; Side-effects: see notes (above) but more potent than morphine, causes greater respiratory depression, and is more liable to induce dependence. Drug interactions: see Appendix 1
Dose: *by mouth, or by subcutaneous, intramuscular or intravenous injection,* 5–10 mg every 4 hours

CD **Diamorphine Tablets,** diamorphine hydrochloride 10 mg (for oral administration). Price 20 tabs = **C**

CD **Diamorphine Injection,** powder for reconstitution, diamorphine hydrochloride 5, 10, and 30 mg (incompatible with sodium chloride). Price per amp (all) = **B**

DIPIPANONE HYDROCHLORIDE

Indications: moderate to severe pain, particularly chronic pain in terminal disease

Cautions; Contra-indications; Side-effects: see notes (above) but less sedating than morphine

CD **Diconal**® (Calmic)

Tablets, pink, scored, dipipanone hydrochloride 10 mg, cyclizine hydrochloride 30 mg. Price 20 tabs = **C**

Dose: 1 tablet gradually increased to 3 tablets every 6 hours

LEVORPHANOL TARTRATE

Indications: severe pain

Cautions; Contra-indications; Side-effects: see notes (above), but causes less sedation than morphine and effects are longer-lasting

Dose: *by mouth,* 1.5–4.5 mg 1–2 times daily

By subcutaneous or intramuscular injection, 2–4 mg, repeated when necessary

By slow intravenous injection, 1–2 mg, repeated when necessary

CD **Dromoran**® (Roche)

Tablets, levorphanol tartrate 1.5 mg. Price 20 tabs = **C**

Injection, levorphanol tartrate 2 mg/ml. Price 1-ml amp = **A**

METHADONE HYDROCHLORIDE

Indications: severe pain

Cautions; Contra-indications; Side-effects: see notes (above), but less sedating than morphine. Injections may cause local pain and tissue damage

Dose: *by mouth or by subcutaneous or intramuscular injection,* 5–10 mg every 4 hours

CD **Physeptone**® (Wellcome)

Tablets, scored, methadone hydrochloride 5 mg. Price 20 tabs = **B**

Injection, methadone hydrochloride 10 mg/ml. Price 1-ml amp = **B**

NEFOPAM HYDROCHLORIDE

Indications: moderate pain

Cautions: hepatic disease, glaucoma, urinary retention

Contra-indications: convulsive disorders, myocardial infarction

Side-effects: nausea, nervousness, insomnia, dry mouth; less frequently blurred vision, drowsiness, sweating, tachycardia, headache; on intravenous injection, syncope

Dose: *by mouth,* 30 mg, gradually increased to 90 mg, up to 3 times daily

By intramuscular or slow intravenous injection, 20 mg every 6 hours

Note: 20 mg by injection ≈ 60 mg by mouth

▼ **Acupan**® (Carnegie)

Tablets, f/c, nefopam hydrochloride 30 mg. Price 20 tabs = **E**

Injection, nefopam hydrochloride 20 mg/ml. Price 1-ml amp = **C**

OXYCODONE

Indications: prolonged relief of severe pain

Cautions; Contra-indications; Side-effects: see notes (above)

Dose: *by rectum* in suppositories, 30 mg (as pectinate), effective for about 8 hours

CD **Proladone**® (Boots)

Suppositories, oxycodone 30 mg (as pectinate) (supplied only to special order)

PAPAVERETUM

Indications: moderate to severe pain

Cautions; Contra-indications; Side-effects: see notes (above)

Dose: *by mouth or by subcutaneous, intramuscular, or intravenous injection,* 10–20 mg; CHILD up to 1 month 150 micrograms/kg, 1–12 months 200 micrograms/kg, 1–5 years 2.5–5 mg, 6–12 years 5–10 mg; these doses may be given every 4 hours

Note: Papaveretum contains anhydrous morphine 50% as hydrochloride with the hydrochlorides of other opium alkaloids. 10 mg papaveretum is equivalent in morphine content to 6.25 mg of morphine sulphate.

CD **Papaveretum Injection,** papaveretum 10 mg/ml, price 1-ml amp = **B**; 20 mg/ml, price 1-ml amp = **A**

CD **Omnopon**® (Roche)

Tablets, buff, papaveretum 10 mg. Price 20 tabs = **B**

Injection, papaveretum 20 mg/ml. Price 1-ml amp = **A**

PETHIDINE HYDROCHLORIDE

Indications: moderate to severe pain, obstetric analgesia

Cautions; Contra-indications; Side-effects: see notes (above). Drug interactions: see Appendix 1

Dose: *by mouth,* 50–100 mg every 4 hours

By subcutaneous or intramuscular injection, 25–100 mg; CHILD, *by intramuscular injection,* up to 1 year 1–2 mg/kg, 1–5 years 12.5–25 mg, 6–12 years 25–50 mg

By slow intravenous injection, 25–50 mg

Obstetric analgesia, *by intramuscular injection,* 100 mg, repeated 1–3 hours later if necessary; max. 400 mg in 24 hours

CD Pethidine Tablets, pethidine hydrochloride 25 and 50 mg. Price 20 tabs (both) = **B**

CD Pethidine Injection, pethidine hydrochloride 50 mg/ml. Price 1- and 2-ml amp (both) = **A**

CD Pamergan P100® (M&B)

Injection, pethidine hydrochloride 50 mg, promethazine hydrochloride 25 mg/ml. Price 2-ml amp = **B**

Dose: by intramuscular injection, for obstetric analgesia, 1–2 ml every 4 hours if necessary; severe pain 1–2 ml up to 4 times daily

CD Pethilorfan® (Roche)

Injection, pethidine hydrochloride 50 mg, levallorphan tartrate 625 micrograms/ml. Price 1- and 2-ml amp (both) = **A**

Dose: by intramuscular injection, for obstetric analgesia, 2–4 ml every 3–4 hours if necessary; severe pain, as for pethidine hydrochloride (above)

PHENAZOCINE HYDROBROMIDE

Indications: severe pain

Cautions; Contra-indications; Side-effects: see notes (above), but less sedating than morphine and dependence is slower to develop

Dose: 5 mg every 4 hours when necessary; single doses may be increased to 20 mg

CD Narphen® (S&N Pharm.)

Tablets, scored, phenazocine hydrobromide 5 mg. Price 20 tabs = **D**

PIRITRAMIDE

Indications: postoperative pain

Cautions; Contra-indications; Side-effects: see notes (above), but may be more sedating than morphine

Dose: *by intramuscular injection,* 20 mg repeated every 6 hours to a max. of 4 doses

CD Dipidolor® (Janssen)

Injection, piritramide 10 mg/ml. Price 2-ml amp = **C**

ANALGESIC ELIXIRS OF DIAMORPHINE AND MORPHINE

Both **morphine** and **diamorphine** are suitable for oral use in the relief of pain in terminal care. Many patients are adequately treated with morphine hydrochloride (or diamorphine hydrochloride). Routine administration of **cocaine** with the opiates is no longer recommended.

Prochlorperazine (Stemetil®) may be used for its anti-emetic and tranquillising action; **chlorpromazine** is an alternative but is more depressant. Such mixtures are usually preferable to the traditional 'Brompton Cocktail' elixirs (see below) which contain diamorphine or morphine with cocaine in a sweetened alcoholic basis. Many patients dislike the alcohol; the inclusion of chlorpromazine in such elixirs opposes the stimulant action of cocaine.

Simple Elixirs

Simple elixirs of **morphine** or **diamorphine** should be prescribed by writing the formula in full, for example:

Morphine hydrochloride	5 mg
Chloroform water to	5 ml

The total quantity to be supplied should be added in both words and figures, together with the other details required for controlled drug prescriptions (see Controlled Drugs and Drug Dependence). It is usual to adjust the strength so that the dose volume is 5 or 10 ml. These simple elixirs are now generally preferred to the traditional compound elixirs given below.

Traditional Compound Elixirs in a sweetened alcoholic basis

CD Diamorphine and Cocaine Elixir, diamorphine hydrochloride 5 mg, cocaine hydrochloride 5 mg/5 ml (see Formulary). Price 100 ml = **C**

CD Diamorphine, Cocaine, and Chlorpromazine Elixir, as above with chlorpromazine hydrochloride 6.25 mg/5 ml (see Formulary). Price 100 ml = **C**

* **Morphine and Cocaine Elixir,** morphine hydrochloride 5 mg, cocaine hydrochloride 5 mg/5 ml (see Formulary). Price 100 ml = **C**

* **Morphine, Cocaine, and Chlorpromazine Elixir,** as above with chlorpromazine hydrochloride 6.25 mg/5 ml (see Formulary). Price 100 ml = **C**

*CD if morphine content is increased

When these preparations are ordered without qualification the proportion of diamorphine hydrochloride or of morphine hydrochloride is as stated above, but it may be varied when specified by the prescriber. For details see Formulary.

4.7.3 Other drugs used for the relief of pain

In certain painful conditions, drugs that have no marked general analgesic effect may be of value.

TRIGEMINAL NEURALGIA. **Carbamazepine** (Tegretol®) reduces the frequency and severity of attacks if given continuously. It has no effect on other forms of headache. A dose of 100 mg once or twice a day should be given initially and the dose slowly increased until the best response is obtained. Occasionally extreme dizziness is encountered which is a further reason for starting treatment with a small dose and increasing it slowly. Drug interactions: see Appendix 1. See section 4.8.1 for preparations.

Some cases of trigeminal neuralgia also respond to **phenytoin** which may also be of value for the pain of *diabetic neuropathy*.

4.7.4 Antimigraine drugs

These drugs are discussed under treatment of the acute migraine attack (section 4.7.4.1) and prophylaxis of migraine (section 4.7.4.2).

4.7.4.1 TREATMENT OF THE ACUTE MIGRAINE ATTACK

Most migraine headaches respond to analgesics

such as **aspirin** or **paracetamol** (section 4.7.1.1) but as peristalsis is often reduced during migraine attacks the medication may not be sufficiently well absorbed to be effective; dispersible or effervescent preparations should therefore preferably be used.

Ergotamine is used in patients who do not respond to analgesics. It relieves migraine headache by constricting cranial arteries but visual and other symptoms are not affected and vomiting may be made worse. This can be relieved by the addition of an anti-emetic (see below).

The value of ergotamine is limited by difficulties in absorption and the frequency of its side-effects, particularly nausea, vomiting, abdominal pain, and muscular cramps. In some patients repeated administration may cause habituation to ergotamine and attempts to withdraw the drug provoke severe withdrawal headaches which may resemble the original migraine. Ergotamine treatment should **not** be repeated at intervals of less than 4 days and it should **never** be prescribed prophylactically.

There are various ergotamine preparations designed to improve absorption and best results are obtained when the dose is given early in an attack. An aerosol form (Medihaler-Ergotamine®) is acceptable to some patients. Sublingual ergotamine (Lingraine®) probably has no advantage over oral treatment. **Isometheptene** (present in Midrid®) is as effective as ergotamine and has fewer side-effects.

Dihydroergotamine (Dihydergot®) is much less effective than ergotamine but is less likely to produce side-effects.

Anti-emetics, such as **metoclopramide** (section 4.6) by mouth or, if vomiting is likely, by intramuscular injection, or the phenothiazine and antihistamine anti-emetics, relieve the nausea associated with migraine attacks and metoclopramide has the added advantage of promoting gastric emptying and normal peristalsis. A single dose should be given at the onset of symptoms. Oral analgesic preparations containing metoclopramide are available but there is little evidence that the presence of the anti-emetic promotes absorption once gastric stasis is established because both compounds will remain in the stomach; the same applies with preparations containing buclizine. If metoclopramide is to be used it should be given separately, by intramuscular injection if necessary.

Diazepam and similar anxiolytics may be useful adjuvant medication to counteract muscle spasm and anxiety often present in a migraine attack.

ERGOTAMINE TARTRATE

Indications: migraine attack, vascular headache
Cautions: renal, hepatic, and cardiovascular disease, hyperthyroidism, sepsis; unsuitable for prophylaxis. Drug interactions: see Appendix 1
Contra-indications: pregnancy, breast feeding
Side-effects: headache, nausea, and vomiting; repeated dosage may cause ergotism with gangrene and mental derangement
Dose: *by mouth,* 1–2 mg at onset of attack, repeated every 30 minutes if necessary; **max.** 6–8 mg per attack and 12 mg per week
By rectum in suppositories, 2 mg, repeated after 1 hour if necessary; **max.** 6–8 mg per attack and 12 mg per week
By aerosol inhalation (oral), 360 micrograms, repeated after 5 minutes if necessary; **max.** 6 inhalations daily and 15 weekly

Cafergot® (Wander)
Tablets, pink, s/c, ergotamine tartrate 1 mg, caffeine 100 mg. Price 20 tabs = **D**
Suppositories, ergotamine tartrate 2 mg, caffeine 100 mg, butalbital 100 mg, belladonna alkaloids 250 micrograms. Price 6 suppos = **D**

Effergot® (Wander)
Tablets, effervescent, scored, ergotamine tartrate 2 mg, caffeine 50 mg. Price 20 tabs = **E**

Lingraine® (Winthrop)
Tablets (for sublingual use), green, ergotamine tartrate 2 mg. Price 12 tabs = **F**

Medihaler-Ergotamine® (Riker)
Aerosol inhalation (oral), ergotamine tartrate 360 micrograms/metered inhalation. Price 75-dose unit = **F**

Migril® (Wellcome)
Tablets, scored, ergotamine tartrate 2 mg, cyclizine hydrochloride 50 mg, caffeine hydrate 100 mg. Price 20 tabs = **F**

DIHYDROERGOTAMINE MESYLATE

Indications: migraine attack, vascular headache
Cautions; Contra-indications; Side-effects: see under Ergotamine Tartrate, but less effective and side-effects are milder. Avoid injection in coronary disease and uncontrolled hypertension
Dose: *by mouth,* mild attacks, 2–3 mg repeated every 30 minutes if necessary to a max. of 10 mg daily
By subcutaneous or intramuscular injection, 1–2 mg repreated after 30 minutes if necessary

Dihydergot® (Sandoz)
Tablets, scored, dihydroergotamine mesylate 1 mg. Price 20 tabs = **D**
Oral solution, dihydroergotamine mesylate 2 mg/ml. 20 drops ≈ 1 ml. Do not dilute. Price 15-ml dropper bottle = **E**
Injection, dihydroergotamine mesylate 1 mg/ml. Price 1-ml amp = **B**

ISOMETHEPTENE MUCATE

Indications: migraine attack, vascular headache
Cautions: hepatic, renal, and cardiovascular disease
Contra-indications: glaucoma
Side-effects: dizziness, circulatory disturbances

Midrid® (Carnrick)

Capsules, red, isometheptene mucate 65 mg, dichloralphenazone 100 mg, paracetamol 325 mg. Price 20 caps = **E**

Dose: 1–2 capsules every 4 hours when necessary; max. 8 daily

ANALGESICS

Aspirin Preparations

Section 4.7.1.1

Paracetamol Preparations

Section 4.7.1.1

ANALGESICS WITH ANTI-EMETICS

Migraleve® (International Labs)

Tablets, all f/c, *pink tablets*, buclizine hydrochloride 6.25 mg, paracetamol 500 mg, codeine phosphate 8 mg, dioctyl sodium sulphosuccinate 10 mg; *yellow tablets*, paracetamol 500 mg, codeine phosphate 8 mg, dioctyl sodium sulphosuccinate 20 mg. Price 12 tabs (pink or yellow) = **C**; 16 pink + 8 yellow = **D**

Dose: 2 pink tablets at onset of attack, or at night during periods of impending attack then 2 yellow tablets every 3–4 hours if necessary; max. in 24 hours 2 pink and 6 yellow

Migravess® (Dome)

Tablets, effervescent, scored, metoclopramide hydrochloride 5 mg, aspirin 325 mg. Price 20 tabs = **E**

Dose: 2 tablets dissolved in water at onset of attack then every 4 hours when necessary; max. 6 tablets in 24 hours; CHILD 10–15 years, half the adult dose

Paramax® (Beecham)

Tablets, scored, paracetamol 500 mg, metoclopramide hydrochloride 5 mg. Price 20 tabs = **D**

Sachets, the contents of 1 sachet = 1 tablet; to be dissolved in ¼ tumblerful of liquid before administration. Price 30 sachets = **F**

Dose: 1–2 tablets at onset of attack then every 4 hours when necessary to a max. of 6 tablets in 24 hours; CHILD max. in 24 hours 12–14 years 3 tablets, 15–20 years 5 tablets

4.7.4.2 PROPHYLAXIS OF MIGRAINE

Prophylaxis is rarely indicated in patients who have one attack per month or less. A small dose of a benzodiazepine anxiolytic (section 4.1.2) is the first line of treatment in patients in whom nervous tension is playing a part. Depression is sometimes a provocative factor and should be treated with a tricyclic antidepressant. Combined oral contraceptives may precipitate migraine or worsen the pre-existing disease.

Clonidine (Dixarit®) is helpful in about 70% of patients but may aggravate depression and cause insomnia. It appears to diminish the responsiveness of the cranial vessels to either dilatation or constriction.

Pizotifen (Sanomigran®) is an antiserotonergic drug which is structurally related to the tricyclic antidepressants. Its efficacy is similar to that of clonidine but it causes anticholinergic side-effects and weight gain.

Methysergide (Deseril®) is also an antiserotonergic drug, but chronic use can cause retroperitoneal fibrosis and fibrosis of the heart valves and pleura, and for this reason its use is seldom justified. It should not be used for longer than 6 months without a break of 1 month to reassess the patient, who should be advised to report immediately any loin pain, urinary symptoms, or dypsnoea.

Some (but not all) beta-adrenoceptor blocking drugs are effective in about 60% of patients. These are propranolol, acebutolol, and atenolol. **Propranolol** is the most commonly used.

Experimental work suggests that beta-adrenoceptor blocking drugs may act paradoxically by causing dilatation of constricted cerebral vessels but may also prevent dilatation of the extracranial vessels which occurs in migraine. The value of these drugs is limited by their contra-indications (see section 2.4) and by interaction with ergotamine (see Appendix 1).

Dihydroergotamine (Dihydergot®) has been prescribed prophylactically but its value is uncertain.

CLONIDINE HYDROCHLORIDE

Indications: prevention of recurrent migraine, menopausal flushing

Cautions: depressive illness, concurrent antihypertensive therapy. Drug interactions: see Appendix 1

Side-effects: depression, dry mouth, sedation, dizziness, headache, circulatory disturbances, rarely nausea

Dose: 50 micrograms twice daily, increased after 2 weeks to 75 micrograms twice daily if necessary

Dixarit® (WBP)

Tablets, blue, s/c, clonidine hydrochloride 25 micrograms. Price 20 tabs = **D**

DIHYDROERGOTAMINE MESYLATE

Indications: prevention of recurrent migraine (see notes above)

Cautions; Contra-indications; Side-effects: section 4.7.4.1

Dose: by mouth, 1–2 mg 3 times daily

Preparations

Section 4.7.4.1

METHYSERGIDE

Indications: prevention of severe recurrent migraine and migrainous neuralgia

Cautions: peptic ulceration; avoid abrupt withdrawal of treatment; withdraw treatment for reassessment after 6 months

Contra-indications: renal, hepatic, pulmonary, and cardiovascular disease, collagen disorders, pregnancy

Side-effects: nausea, drowsiness, and dizziness occur frequently in initial treatment; psychic reactions, oedema, arterial spasm, paraesthesias of extremities, postural hypotension, and tachycardia also occur. Retroperitoneal and other abnormal fibrotic reactions may occur on prolonged administration, requiring immediate withdrawal of treatment

Dose: 1 mg at bedtime, gradually increased to 1–2 mg 2–3 times daily

Deseril® (Wander)

Tablets, yellow, s/c, methysergide 1 mg (as hydrogen maleate). Price 20 tabs = **E**

PIZOTIFEN

Indications: prevention of recurrent migraine, vascular headache

Cautions: may affect the ability to drive or operate machinery and increase effects of alcohol

Contra-indications: urinary retention; closed-angle glaucoma

Side-effects: anticholinergic effects, drowsiness, weight gain; occasionally nausea, dizziness, muscle pain

Dose: initially 1.5 mg daily as a single dose at night or in divided doses, increased if necessary to 3 mg daily (6 mg daily in resistant patients) in divided doses

Sanomigran® (Wander)

Tablets, s/c, pizotifen 500 micrograms (as hydrogen malate). Price 20 tabs = **D**

Tablets, ivory, s/c, pizotifen 1.5 mg (as hydrogen malate). Price 28 tabs = **G**

PROCHLORPERAZINE

Indications: prevention of severe recurrent migraine

Cautions; Contra-indications; Side-effects: see section 4.6

Dose: 5 mg 3–4 times daily

Preparations

Section 4.6

PROPRANOLOL HYDROCHLORIDE

Indications: prevention of severe recurrent migraine

Cautions; Contra-indications; Side-effects: see section 2.4

Dose: by mouth, 40–80 mg 2–3 times daily; CHILD 20 mg 2–3 times daily

Preparations

Section 2.4

4.7.5 Drugs for urinary-tract pain

Phenazopyridine (Pyridium®) may allay pain and irritability in the urinary tract in cystitis, prostatitis, and urethritis.

Emepronium (Cetiprin®) and less frequently **flavoxate** (Urispas®) are used to alleviate dysuria and urinary frequency by reducing bladder muscle tone. They are often used in the elderly but should be used with caution as anticholinergic effects occur, particularly with emepronium.

Potassium citrate mixture, by its alkalinising action, can relieve discomfort caused by mild urinary-tract infection.

See also Table 1, section 5.1 for antibacterial drugs used in urinary-tract infections. Parasympathomimetic drugs, such as neostigmine, used in postoperative urinary retention are described in section 1.6.2.

EMEPRONIUM BROMIDE

Indications: urinary frequency and incontinence, dysuria

Cautions: glaucoma

Contra-indications: achalasia, obstructive intestinal lesions, oesophagitis

Side-effects: oesophageal ulceration. Also mild peripheral anticholinergic side-effects, see under Atropine Sulphate, section 1.2

Dose: frequency and severe incontinence, 200 mg 3 times daily; nocturnal frequency, 200–400 mg before bedtime with 100 ml of fluid

Cetiprin® (KabiVitrum)

Tablets, emepronium bromide 100 mg. Price 20 tabs = **D**

Tablets, emepronium bromide 200 mg. Price 20 tabs = **E**

FLAVOXATE HYDROCHLORIDE

Indications; Cautions; Contra-indications; Side-effects: see under Emepronium Bromide

Dose: 200 mg 3 times daily

Urispas® (Syntex)

Tablets, s/c, flavoxate hydrochloride 100 mg. Price 20 tabs = **C**

PHENAZOPYRIDINE HYDROCHLORIDE

Indications: urinary tract pain

Contra-indications: renal and hepatic impairment

Side-effects: gastro-intestinal disturbances, headache, vertigo; in high dosage methaemoglobinaemia; rarely haemolytic anaemia. Colours the urine red

Dose: 200 mg 3 times daily before meals; CHILD over 8 years 100 mg

Pyridium® (Warner)

Tablets, brown, s/c, phenazopyridine hydrochloride 100 mg. Price 20 tabs = **B**

POTASSIUM CITRATE

Indications: relief of discomfort in mild infections of the urinary tract by rendering the urine alkaline

Side-effects: hyperkalaemia on prolonged high dosage

Potassium Citrate Mixture, potassium citrate 1.5 g/5 ml (see Formulary). Price 100 ml = **A**

Dose: 10–20 ml with water

4.8 Antiepileptics

In this section drugs are discussed under the following subsections:

4.8.1 Control of epilepsy
4.8.2 Drugs used in status epilepticus

4.8.1 Control of epilepsy

The object of treatment is to suppress fits by maintaining an effective concentration of the drug in the plasma and hence brain tissue at all times. Dose and frequency are determined by the plasma half-life. Painstaking adjustment of doses is necessary, starting with low doses and increasing gradually until fits are controlled or there are overdose effects.

Frequency of administration should be kept as low as possible to encourage better patient compliance. Most antiepileptics, when used in average dosage, may be given twice daily. Phenobarbitone, which has a long half-life, may often be given as a daily dose at bedtime. However, with large doses, antiepileptics may need to be administered 3 or 4 times daily to avoid adverse effects associated with high peak plasma concentrations. Young children metabolise antiepileptics more rapidly than adults and therefore require more frequent dosing as well as higher doses per kilogram body-weight.

Therapy with several drugs concurrently should be avoided. Patients are best controlled with one antiepileptic. Combinations of drugs have been used on the grounds that their therapeutic effects were additive while their individual toxicity was reduced but there is no evidence for this. A second drug should only be added to the regimen if fits continue despite high plasma concentrations or toxic effects. The use of more than two antiepileptics is rarely justified for one type of fit.

Another disadvantage of multiple therapy is that drug interactions occur between the various antiepileptics. By inducing liver microsomal enzymes, phenobarbitone, phenytoin, and primidone increase each other's metabolism and can reduce plasma concentrations of carbamazepine. Also, primidone is partially metabolised to phenobarbitone. Compound preparations should be avoided because the dose of each antiepileptic should be adjusted separately.

Adequate control for most types of fits is usually provided by the correct use of phenytoin, carbamazepine, phenobarbitone, primidone, sodium valproate, ethosuximide, or clonazepam.

Once a regimen is established it should be maintained until there is freedom from fits for at least two years. Treatment should not be withdrawn abruptly as this may precipitate convulsions. Change-over from one antiepileptic to another should be made cautiously over several weeks.

DRIVING. Patients suffering from epilepsy may drive a motor vehicle (but not a heavy goods or public service vehicle) provided that they have had a fit-free period of three years or that fits have occurred only during sleep. Patients affected by drowsiness should not drive or operate machinery.

PREGNANCY. Although several antiepileptics are teratogenic in *animals,* the increased risk of congenital malformations is in practice slight. Abrupt withdrawal of antiepileptics also carries risk of increased seizure frequency or status epilepticus.

Drug treatment of epilepsy is discussed under the headings tonic-clonic (grand mal) seizures; partial (focal) seizures; absence seizures (petit mal); myoclonic-atonic seizures (myoclonic jerks) (all in section 4.8.1) and status epilepticus (section 4.8.2).

Neonatal fits, infantile spasms (West's syndrome), and febrile convulsions are outside the scope of this book.

TONIC-CLONIC (GRAND MAL) AND PARTIAL (FOCAL) SEIZURES

The same range of drugs is used to treat both tonic-clonic seizures and partial fits. Phenytoin and carbamazepine are the drugs of choice as they usually give adequate control and the use of the more sedating compounds such as phenobarbitone or primidone is usually unnecessary. Carbamazepine is preferred to phenytoin in patients with partial seizures, particularly complex partial (temporal lobe or psychomotor) seizures because it is more effective and less likely to cause confusion in these patients.

Phenytoin (Epanutin®) is as effective as carbamazepine in tonic-clonic seizures but is ineffective in absence seizures. Disadvantages are that it has a narrow therapeutic index and readily produces nystagmus, slurred speech, and ataxia in overdose. Monitoring of plasma concentrations greatly assists dosage adjustment. A few missed doses or a small change in drug absorption will result in a marked change in plasma concentration.

Phenytoin may cause coarse facies, acne, hirsutes, and gingival hyperplasia and for these reasons may be particularly undesirable in adolescent patients. Carbamazepine is often used as an alternative for this reason.

Carbamazepine (Tegretol®) is the drug of choice in controlling partial seizures. It is effective in controlling tonic-clonic fits regardless of whether they are primary (idiopathic) or secondary to a focal discharge. Minor fits of focal origin, including complex partial seizures, also respond. It is less sedating than phenobarbitone, but side-effects such as diplopia and dizziness may be dose-limiting. Monitoring plasma carbamazepine concentrations is helpful in determining the optimum dosage.

Phenobarbitone is an effective drug but it is sedative in adults and may cause behavioural disturbances and hyperkinesia in children. Rebound fits may be a problem on withdrawal. Monitoring plasma concentrations is less useful than with other drugs because tolerance occurs. **Methylphenobarbitone** is largely converted to phenobarbitone in the liver and has no advantages. **Primidone** (Mysoline®) is partially converted to phenobarbitone, but the unchanged drug and a second metabolite (both with short half-lives) may also be active. A small starting dose is essential.

Sodium valproate (Epilim®) is active in controlling tonic-clonic fits, particularly if they are primary (idiopathic), but its efficacy compared with the longer-established drugs has still to be evaluated. It has little effect on partial seizures. Routine monitoring is unjustified at present because the activity of the drug may not be accurately reflected by its plasma concentration.

Ethotoin (Peganone®) is less toxic but also less effective than phenytoin.

Sulthiame (Ospolot®) is a weak antiepileptic but readily causes drug interactions by inhibition of metabolism, particularly with phenytoin. Hyperventilation is common.

Clonazepam (Rivotril®) and other **benzodiazepines** are, in general, too sedating for chronic use in doses which control tonic-clonic or partial fits. They are the drugs of choice for major status epilepticus (section 4.8.2 below).

ABSENCE SEIZURES (PETIT MAL)

Ethosuximide (Emeside®, Zarontin®) and **sodium valproate** are the drugs of choice in children who have simple absence seizures. In complex absences with co-existing tonic-clonic fits, against which ethosuximide is not active, additional treatment with another suitable drug (see above) may be necessary. Monitoring plasma ethosuximide concentrations is helpful in determining the optimum dosage.

Sodium valproate (Epilim®) is effective in simple absence seizures and since, unlike ethosuximide, it will also treat tonic-clonic fits, it may be preferred for absences associated with tonic-clonic fits.

Troxidone (Tridione®) and **paramethadione** (Paradione®) are **less effective** and more toxic than ethosuximide or sodium valproate. They are rarely used.

MYOCLONIC-ATONIC SEIZURES (MYOCLONIC JERKS)

There are a variety of syndromes occurring in childhood in which myoclonic jerks and atonic seizures occur. They have responded poorly to the traditional drugs.

Sodium valproate (Epilim®) and **clonazepam** (Rivotril®) are the drugs of first choice. Sodium valproate should be tried before clonazepam, which is more sedating.

BECLAMIDE

Indications: behavioural disorders, tonic-clonic and partial seizures

Cautions: previous antiepileptic medication should be maintained for 4 weeks

Side-effects: dizziness, nervousness, rashes, and renal and gastro-intestinal disturbances are uncommon

Dose: 0.5–1 g 3–4 times daily; CHILD up to 5 years 0.75–1 g daily in divided doses, 6–12 years 1.5 g daily in divided doses

Nydrane® (Rona)

Tablets, scored, beclamide 500 mg. Price 20 tabs = **C**

CARBAMAZEPINE

Indications: tonic-clonic and partial seizures

Contra-indications: previous sensitivity to carbamazepine, atrioventricular conduction abnormalities; patients on monamine-oxidase inhibitors or within 2 weeks of MAOI therapy

Side-effects: dizziness, drowsiness, visual, and gastro-intestinal disturbances; a generalised erythematous rash may occur in about 3% of patients; leucopenia and other blood disorders have occurred rarely

Dose: initially, 100–200 mg 1–2 times daily, increased slowly to a usual dose of 0.8–1.2 g daily in divided doses, according to the patient's needs; in some cases 1.6 g daily may be needed; CHILD daily in divided doses, up to one year 100–200 mg, 1–5 years 200–400 mg, 5–10 years 400–600 mg, 10–15 years 0.6–1 g

Note: plasma concentration for optimum response 5–12 micrograms/ml

Tegretol® (Geigy)

Tablets, carbamazepine 100 mg. Price 20 tabs = **B**

Tablets, scored, carbamazepine 200 mg. Price 20 tabs = **C**

Tablets, scored, carbamazepine 400 mg. Price 20 tabs = **E**

Syrup (= mixture), carbamazepine 100 mg/5 ml. Diluent tragacanth mucilage for 1 + 1 dilution, life of diluted mixture 14 days. Price 100 ml = **D**

CLONAZEPAM

Indications: all forms of epilepsy and seizures. For status epilepticus see section 4.8.2

Cautions: may affect the ability to drive or operate machinery and increase the effects of alcohol; withdraw treatment slowly to prevent status epilepticus

Side-effects: drowsiness, fatigue, dizziness, muscle hypotonia, hypersalivation in infants, paradoxical aggression, irritability and mental changes

Dose: 1 mg, initially at night for 4 nights, increased over 2–4 weeks to a daily maintenance dose of 4–8 mg; CHILD up to 1 year 250 micrograms increased as above to 0.5–1 mg, 1–5 years 250 micrograms increased to 1–3 mg, 6–12 years 500 micrograms increased to 3–6 mg. Daily maintenance doses should be given in 3–4 divided doses

Rivotril® (Roche)
Tablets, orange, scored, clonazepam 500 micrograms. Price 20 tabs = **B**
Tablets, scored, clonazepam 2 mg. Price 20 tabs = **C**

ETHOSUXIMIDE

Indications: absence seizures
Side-effects: gastro-intestinal disturbances, drowsiness, dizziness, ataxia, headache, depression, and mild euphoria. Psychotic states, rashes, liver changes, and haematological disorders such as leucopenia and agranulocytosis occur rarely
Dose: initially, 500 mg daily, increased according to patient's needs by 250 mg at intervals of 4–7 days to a max. of 2 g daily; CHILD up to 6 years 250 mg daily, over 6 years 500 mg, increased gradually to a max. of 1 g daily
Note: plasma concentration for optimum response 50–100 micrograms/ml

Ethosuximide Capsules, ethosuximide 250 mg. Price 20 caps = **C**
Ethosuximide Elixir, ethosuximide 250 mg/5 ml. Diluent water for preparations for Emeside, syrup for Zarontin, life of diluted elixir 14 days. Price 100 ml = **D**
Emeside® (LAB)
Capsules, yellow, ethosuximide 250 mg. Price 20 caps = **C**
Syrup (= elixir), blackcurrant or orange, ethosuximide 250 mg/5 ml. Diluent syrup, life of diluted elixir 14 days. Price 100 ml = **C**
Zarontin® (P-D)
Capsules, orange, ethosuximide 250 mg. Price 20 caps = **D**
Syrup (= elixir), red, ethosuximide 250 mg/5 ml. Diluent syrup, life of diluted elixir 14 days. Price 100 ml = **D**

ETHOTOIN

Indications: tonic-clonic and partial seizures
Cautions; Side-effects: see under Phenytoin Sodium. Change-over from other drugs should be made cautiously over several weeks
Dose: initially, 1 g daily in divided doses after food, increased by 500 mg at intervals of several days to 2–3 g daily in 4–6 divided doses after food; CHILD initially 500 mg daily in divided doses increased gradually to 1 g daily, according to the patient's needs

Peganone® (Abbott)
Tablets, scored, ethotoin 500 mg. Price 20 tabs = **D**

METHYLPHENOBARBITONE

Indications: tonic-clonic and partial seizures
Cautions; Contra-indications; Side-effects: see under Phenobarbitone
Dose: 100–600 mg daily, according to the patient's needs

Prominal® (Winthrop)
Tablets, methylphenobarbitone 30 mg. Price 20 tabs = **B**
Tablets, methylphenobarbitone 60 mg. Price 20 tabs = **B**
Tablets, methylphenobarbitone 200 mg. Price 20 tabs = **C**

PARAMETHADIONE

Indications: absence seizures
Cautions; Contra-indications; Side-effects: see under Troxidone, but side-effects are less common
Dose: adults and children over 6 years, initially, 900 mg daily in divided doses increased according to the patient's needs by 300 mg per day every 1–2 weeks to a max. of 1.8 g daily; CHILD 2–6 years, initially 600 mg daily in divided doses increased by 300 mg per day every 1–2 weeks to a max. of 1.2 g daily

Paradione® (Abbott)
Capsules, red, paramethadione 300 mg. Price 20 caps = **B**

PHENOBARBITONE

Indications: tonic-clonic and partial seizures
Cautions: elderly, impaired renal or hepatic function, severe respiratory depression, breast feeding; avoid sudden withdrawal, or use with other CNS sedatives, particularly alcohol; prolonged dosage may produce dependence. Drug interactions: see Appendix 1
Contra-indications: acute intermittent porphyria
Side-effects: drowsiness, lethargy, ataxia and allergic skin reactions; paradoxical excitement, restlessness and confusion in the elderly and hyperkinesia in children
Dose: *by mouth*, daily, as a single dose at night *or* in divided doses, 90–375 mg, to a max. of 600 mg daily; CHILD up to 2 years 25–45 mg, 2–5 years 45–90 mg, 6–12 years 90–375 mg
By subcutaneous, intramuscular, or intravenous injection, 50–200 mg as a single dose
By intramuscular or intravenous injection, CHILD up to 1 year 30–60 mg, 1–5 years 90 mg, 6–12 years 120 mg, *or* 3–5 mg/kg intramuscularly
Note: for therapeutic purposes phenobarbitone and phenobarbitone sodium may be considered equivalent in effect

Phenobarbitone Tablets, phenobarbitone 15, 30, 60, and 100 mg. Price 20 tabs (all) = **A**
Phenobarbitone Sodium Tablets, phenobarbitone sodium 30 and 60 mg. Price 20 tabs (both) = **A**
Phenobarbitone Elixir, yellow, phenobarbitone 30 mg/10 ml (see Formulary). Price 100 ml = **B**
Phenobarbitone Injection, phenobarbitone sodium 200 mg/ml in propylene glycol 90% and water for injections 10%. Price 1-ml amp = **B**
Luminal® (Winthrop)
Tablets, phenobarbitone 15 mg. Price 20 tabs = **A**

Tablets, phenobarbitone 30 mg. Price 20 tabs = **A**
Tablets, phenobarbitone 60 mg. Price 20 tabs = **A**

Phenobarbitone Spansules® (SK&F)
Spansules® (=capsules s/r), clear/blue enclosing blue and white pellets, phenobarbitone 60 mg and 100 mg. Price 20 caps (both) = **B**

Parabal® (Sinclair)
Tablets, lilac, phenobarbitone 10 mg (as phenobarbitone sodium dihydroxyaluminiumaminoacetate) and claimed to be therapeutically equivalent to phenobarbitone 60 mg. Price 20 tabs = **D**

PHENYTOIN

Indications: tonic-clonic and partial seizures
Cautions; Side-effects: see under Phenytoin Sodium (below)
Dose: 250 mg daily increased to 400 mg daily according to patient's response; CHILD, twice daily, up to 1 year 25 mg, 1–5 years 25–50 mg increasing to 75 mg, 6–12 years 50–100 mg increasing to 150 mg
See also under Phenytoin Sodium (below)
Note: phenytoin 100 mg ≡ phenytoin sodium 108 mg; this difference may be significant when the dosage is critical

Epanutin® (P-D)
Suspension (=mixture), red, phenytoin 30 mg/5 ml. Diluent syrup, life of diluted mixture 14 days. Price 100 ml = **B**
Infatabs® (= tablets, chewable), yellow, scored, phenytoin 50 mg. Price 20 tabs = **C**

PHENYTOIN SODIUM

Indications: tonic-clonic and partial seizures
Cautions: breast feeding, change-over from other drugs should be made cautiously; avoid sudden withdrawal. Drug interactions: see Appendix 1
Side-effects: solutions are alkaline and may be irritant; nausea, vomiting, mental confusion, dizziness, headache, tremor, insomnia occur commonly. Ataxia, slurred speech, nystagmus and blurred vision are signs of overdosage. Skin eruptions, sometimes severe, coarse facies, acne and hirsutism, fever and hepatitis; lupus erythematosus, erythema multiforme; lymphadenopathy; gingival hypertrophy and tenderness; haematological effects, including megaloblastic anaemia due to folate deficiency, leucopenia, thrombocytopenia, agranulocytosis, and aplastic anaemia are rare. Serum calcium may be lowered
Dose: *by mouth,* daily as a single dose or 2 divided doses, 150–300 mg increased gradually to 600 mg according to the patient's needs; CHILD up to 5 years 50 mg increased gradually to 150 mg, 6–12 years 100 mg increased to 300 mg. Alternatively, 5–8 mg/kg daily in 1 or 2 doses
By intravenous injection—section 4.8.2
Note: plasma concentration for optimum response 10–20 micrograms/ml

Phenytoin Tablets, s/c, phenytoin sodium 50 and 100 mg. Price 20 tabs (both) = **A**

Epanutin® (P-D)
Capsules, white/purple, phenytoin sodium 25 mg. Price 20 caps = **B**
Capsules, white/pink, phenytoin sodium 50 mg. Price 20 caps = **B**
Capsules, white/orange, phenytoin sodium 100 mg. Price 20 caps = **B**

PRIMIDONE

Indications: tonic-clonic and partial seizures
Cautions: renal impairment, breast feeding. Drug interactions: see Appendix 1
Side-effects: drowsiness, ataxia, nausea, visual disturbances, and rashes, particularly at first, but usually reversible on continued administration. Megaloblastic anaemia may be treated with folic acid
Dose: initially, 125 mg at bedtime, increased by 125 mg every 3 days to 500 mg daily in divided doses then increased by 250 mg every 3 days to a max. of 1.5 g daily in divided doses; CHILD daily in divided doses, initially, 125 mg increasing, for a child up to 2 years, to 250–500 mg, 2–5 years 500–750 mg, 6–12 years 0.75–1 g, according to the patient's needs

Mysoline® (ICI)
Tablets, scored, primidone 250 mg. Price 20 tabs = **B**
Oral suspension (=mixture), primidone 250 mg/5 ml. Diluent propyl hydroxybenzoate 0.015%, methyl hydroxybenzoate 0.15%, sodium carboxymethylcellulose '50' 1%, sucrose 20%, in freshly boiled and cooled purified water. Price 100 ml = **B**

SODIUM VALPROATE

Indications: tonic-clonic, absence and myoclonic-atonic seizures
Cautions: monitor liver function before and at 2-month intervals during first 6 months of therapy; monitor platelet function before major surgery; may give false positive urine tests for ketones in diabetes. Drug interactions: see Appendix 1
Side-effects: gastric irritation, nausea (use e/c tablets); transient hair loss, oedema, thrombocytopenia; impaired hepatic function leading rarely to fatal hepatic failure
Dose: initially, 200 mg 3 times daily, increasing by 200 mg per day at 3-day intervals to a max. of 2.6 g daily in divided doses, according to the patient's needs; CHILD up to 20 kg (about 4 years) initially 20 mg/kg daily in divided doses increased gradually to a max. of 50 mg/kg daily, over 20 kg initially 400 mg daily in divided doses increased gradually to 30 mg/kg daily, according to the patient's needs

Epilim® (Labaz)
Tablets, scored, sodium valproate 200 mg. Price 20 tabs = **D**

Tablets, e/c, lilac, sodium valproate 200 mg. Price 20 tabs = **D**
Tablets, e/c, lilac, sodium valproate 500 mg. Price 20 tabs = **F**
Syrup (= elixir), red, sodium valproate 200 mg/5 ml. Diluent syrup (without preservative), life of diluted elixir 14 days. Price 100 ml = **E**

SULTHIAME

Indications: myoclonic seizures, partial seizures, hyperkinesia, and possibly tonic-clonic seizures
Cautions: history of renal disease; change-over from other drugs should be made cautiously over several weeks. Drug interactions: see Appendix 1
Side-effects: paraesthesias of face and extremities, gastric disturbances, headache, vertigo, ataxia, hyperventilation, anorexia, and loss of weight
Dose: initially 100 mg twice daily increased to 200 mg 3 times daily according to the patient's needs; CHILD, daily in divided doses, 3–5 mg/kg increasing to 10–15 mg/kg

Ospolot® (Bayer)
Tablets, f/c, sulthiame 50 mg. Price 20 tabs = **B**
Tablets, f/c, scored, sulthiame 200 mg. Price 20 tabs = **C**
Suspension (= mixture), yellow, sulthiame 50 mg/5 ml. Diluent tragacanth mucilage, life of diluted mixture 14 days; *or* sodium carboxymethylcellulose 1% with methyl hydroxybenzoate 0.07%. Price 100 ml = **C**

TROXIDONE

Indications: absence seizures
Cautions: should be withdrawn at once if any skin disorder, neutropenia (less than 2500 per mm^3), albuminuria or jaundice appears—strict medical supervision is required; avoid use of other toxic drugs. Blood counts and urine should be examined monthly
Contra-indications: severe hepatic or renal impairment, anaemia, blood dyscrasias, diseases of the retina or optic nerve, drug hypersensitivity
Side-effects: occasionally nausea, hiccups, vertigo, headache, sedation, photophobia, hemeralopia; rarely, rashes, neutropenia, aplastic anaemia, nephrotic syndrome, hepatitis
Dose: daily in divided doses, initially, 900 mg increased at intervals of 1–2 weeks by 300 mg per day until toxicity develops, control is achieved, or a max. of 1.8 g is reached; CHILD up to 2 years, initially 300 mg, increased as above to a max. of 600 mg, 2–6 years 600 mg increased as above to a max. of 1.2 g, over 6 years as for adults

Tridione® (Abbott)
Capsules, troxidone 300 mg. Price 20 caps = **B**

COMPOUND PREPARATIONS

Compound preparations in fixed proportions should be **avoided** because the dose of each antiepileptic should be adjusted separately according to the patient's response.

Epanutin with Phenobarbitone® (P-D) *capsules,* yellow/white, phenytoin sodium, phenobarbitone. Price 20 caps = **B**
Garoin® (M&B) *tablets,* scored, phenytoin sodium, phenobarbitone sodium. Price 20 tabs = **B**

4.8.2 Drugs used in status epilepticus

Major status epilepticus should be treated first with intravenous **diazepam** or **clonazepam** (Rivotril®) but they should be used with caution because of the risk of respiratory depression; there may be a high incidence of venous thrombophlebitis. Intramuscular injection is unsatisfactory as the drugs are too slowly absorbed. When diazepam is given intravenously the risk of thrombophlebitis is claimed to be minimised by using an emulsion (Diazemuls®) but this has not been substantiated. If status epilepticus continues or returns, an intravenous infusion of **chlormethiazole** (Heminevrin®) should be used.

Paraldehyde also remains a valuable drug. It may be given diluted with sodium chloride 0.9% by intravenous injection or may be given by intramuscular or rectal administration.

Phenobarbitone sodium (section 4.8.1) is less satisfactory for urgent treatment because it enters the brain too slowly, but slow intravenous injections of **phenytoin sodium** may be tried in patients who are not taking it by mouth.

Intravenous infusion of **lignocaine** may also be tried if the above drugs fail.

DIAZEPAM

Indications: status epilepticus, convulsions due to poisoning
Cautions; Side-effects: see under anxiolytics (section 4.1.2). When given intravenously facilities for reversing respiratory depression with mechanical ventilation should be at hand
Dose: *by slow intravenous injection,* as a 0.5% solution, 150–250 micrograms/kg at a rate of 0.5 ml (2.5 mg) per 30 seconds, repeated if necessary after 30–60 minutes; may be followed by *slow intravenous infusion* to a max. of 3 mg/kg over 24 hours

Diazemuls® (KabiVitrum)
Injection (emulsion), diazepam 5 mg/ml. May be mixed with dextrose intravenous infusion 5% to a concentration of 400 micrograms/ml and used within 6 hours. May also be mixed with Intralipid 10% or 20% (use within 24 hours). May be given through the drip-tubing during infusion with sodium chloride 0.9%, dextrose 5%, and dextrose 10% intravenous infusions. Price 2-ml amp = **B**

Valium® (Roche)
Injection, diazepam 5 mg/ml in solvent. This injection should not be diluted except that up to 8 ml (40 mg) may be added to 500 ml of dextrose intravenous infusion 5% or sodium chloride intravenous infusion 0.9% for slow intravenous infusion. Such dilutions must be used within 6 hours. Price 2- and 4-ml amp (both) = **B**

CLONAZEPAM

Indications: status epilepticus
Cautions; Side-effects: see section 4.8.1. Hypotension and apnoea may occur and resuscitation facilities must be available
Dose: *by slow intravenous injection or infusion,* 1 mg over 30 seconds; CHILD all ages 500 micrograms

Rivotril® (Roche)
Injection, clonazepam 1 mg/ml in solvent, for dilution with 1 ml water for injections immediately before injection. Up to 3 mg may be mixed with 250 ml of dextrose intravenous infusion 5% or sodium chloride intravenous infusion 0.9% and used within 12 hours. Price 1-ml amp (with diluent) = **B**

CHLORMETHIAZOLE EDISYLATE

Indications: status epilepticus
Cautions: obstructive pulmonary disease; sedative effects may be enhanced by other central depressants, phenothiazines or butyrophenones; during continuous infusion deep sleep may quickly lapse into unconsciousness and patients must be constantly observed
Side-effects: tingling in the nose, sneezing, conjunctival irritation, headache, slight hypotension, respiratory depression, local thrombophlebitis at site of continuous infusion
Dose: *by intravenous infusion,* as a 0.8% solution, 40–100 ml (320–800 mg) at a rate of 60–150 drops per minute

Heminevrin® (Astra)
Intravenous infusion 0.8%, chlormethiazole edisylate 8 mg/ml. Price 500-ml bottle = **F**

LIGNOCAINE HYDROCHLORIDE

Indications: status epilepticus
Cautions; Contra-indications; Side-effects: see section 2.3.3. Fits may be caused by overdosage
Dose: *by slow intravenous infusion,* 200–300 mg/hour as a 0.2% solution
By intravenous bolus injection, 30 mg, repeated according to the patient's needs

Preparations
See section 2.3.3

PARALDEHYDE

Indications: status epilepticus
Cautions: bronchopulmonary disease, hepatic impairment
Side-effects: rashes; injections are painful
Dose: *by intramuscular injection,* as a single dose, 5–10 ml; not more than 5 ml at any one site; CHILD up to 3 months 0.5 ml, 3–6 months 1 ml, 6–12 months 1.5 ml, 1–2 years 2 ml, 3–5 years 3–4 ml, 6–12 years 5–6 ml
By slow intravenous injection, diluted with several times its volume of sodium chloride intravenous infusion 0.9%, up to 4–5 ml
By rectum, 4–5 ml, administered as a 10% enema in isotonic sodium chloride solution; CHILD as for intramuscular dose
Note: do not use paraldehyde if it has a brownish colour or an odour of acetic acid

Paraldehyde Injection, sterile paraldehyde. Avoid contact with rubber and plastics. Price 5-ml amp = **B**; 10-ml amp = **C**

PHENYTOIN SODIUM

Indications: status epilepticus; prophylaxis of seizures in neurosurgery
Cautions; Side-effects: see under Phenytoin Sodium, section 4.8.1
Contra-indications: should not be given intravenously in patients with bradycardia or heart block
Dose: *by slow intravenous injection,* up to 250 mg at a rate not exceeding 50 mg per minute, repeated if nesessary, after 30 minutes; CHILD up to 5 mg/kg
By intramuscular injection, as for intravenous injection but absorption is not reliable

Epanutin® (P-D)
Ready Mixed Parenteral (= injection), phenytoin sodium 50 mg/ml with propylene glycol 40% and alcohol 10% in water for injections. Price 5-ml amp = **E**

4.9 Drugs used in parkinsonism and related disorders

4.9.1 Dopaminergic drugs used in parkinsonism
4.9.2 Anticholinergic drugs used in parkinsonism
4.9.3 Drugs used in choreas, tics, and related disorders

In idiopathic Parkinson's disease, progressive degeneration of pigment-containing cells of the substantia nigra leads to deficiency of the inhibitory neurotransmitter dopamine. This, in turn, results in a neurohumoral imbalance in the basal ganglia, causing the characteristic signs and symptoms of the illness to appear. The pathogenesis of this process is still obscure and current therapy aims simply to correct the imbalance. Although this approach fails to prevent the progression of the disease, it greatly improves the quality and expectancy of life of most patients.

Levodopa, used in conjunction with dopa-decarboxylase inhibitors (section 4.9.1), is the treatment of choice for patients disabled by idiopathic Parkinson's disease. It is less effective in patients with post-encephalitic parkinsonism and should be avoided in neuroleptic-induced parkinsonism.

Parkinsonism caused by generalised degenerative brain disease does not respond to levodopa.

Anticholinergic drugs (section 4.9.2) are the other main class of drugs used in Parkinson's disease. They are less effective than dopamine in idiopathic Parkinson's disease although they often usefully supplement its action. Patients with mild symptoms may be treated with anticholinergic drugs before they are eventually transferred to levodopa therapy as symptoms progress. Anticholinergic drugs are particularly valuable in treating drug-induced parkinsonism or in patients with post-encephalitic parkinsonism.

Other antiparkinsonian drugs include amantadine and bromocriptine (section 4.9.1).

The patient should be advised at the outset of the limitations of treatment and possible side-effects. About 10 to 20% of patients are unresponsive to treatment.

4.9.1 Dopaminergic drugs used in parkinsonism

Levodopa is the treatment of choice for disabled patients. It is least valuable in elderly patients and in those with long-standing disease who rarely tolerate a dose large enough to overcome their deficit. It is also less valuable in patients with post-encephalitic disease who are particularly susceptible to the side-effects.

Levodopa, the amino-acid precursor of dopamine, acts mainly by replenishing depleted striatal dopamine. It improves bradykinesia and rigidity more rapidly than tremor. It is generally administered in conjunction with an extra-cerebral dopa-decarboxylase inhibitor (**carbidopa**, as in Sinemet® or **benserazide**, as in Madopar®) which prevents the peripheral degradation of levodopa to dopamine so enabling more of the drug to enter the brain.

The presence of the inhibitor enables the effective dose of levodopa to be greatly reduced, and peripheral side-effects such as nausea and vomiting and cardiovascular effects to be minimised. In addition, there is less delay in onset of therapeutic effect and a smoother clinical response is obtained. A disadvantage is that there is an increased incidence of abnormal involuntary movements. When Sinemet® is used in low dosage the dose of carbidopa may be insufficient to achieve full inhibition of extracellular dopa decarboxylase; Sinemet Plus® (containing 25 mg of carbidopa for each 100 mg of levodopa) should then be used so that the daily dose of carbidopa is at least 75 mg. This will ensure maximum effectiveness of the levodopa with a minimum of adverse effects.

Treatment with levodopa should be initiated with low doses and gradually increased, by small increments, at intervals of 2 to 3 days. (It is rarely necessary to exceed a daily dose of 1 gram when levodopa is used in conjunction with a dopa-decarboxylase inhibitor.) When titrated in this way the final dose is usually a compromise between increased mobility and dose-limiting side-effects. Nausea and vomiting are rarely dose-limiting if levodopa is given in this way but doses should be taken after meals. The most frequent dose-limiting side-effects are involuntary movements and psychiatric complications.

Treatment with levodopa should not be discontinued abruptly. As the patient ages, the maintenance dose may need to be reduced. When substituting the combined levodopa-decarboxylase inhibitor preparations for levodopa alone, treatment should be discontinued for 12 hours (24 hours for slow-release preparations) before starting therapy with the combined preparation.

During the first 6 to 18 months of levodopa therapy there is a slow improvement in the response of the patient which is maintained for 1½ to 2 years; thereafter a slow decline occurs. Particularly troublesome is the 'on-off' effect the incidence of which increases as the treatment progresses. This is characterised by fluctuations in performance with normal performance during the 'on' period and weakness and akinesia lasting for 2 to 4 hours during the 'off' period.

Monoamine-oxidase inhibitors must be withdrawn at least 14 days before treatment. Close observation is especially necessary in patients with a past history of psychiatric illness, dementia, open-angle glaucoma, or skin melanoma. Antipsychotic drugs should not be administered concurrently.

Bromocriptine (Parlodel®) acts by direct stimulation of surviving dopamine receptors. Although effective, it has no advantages over levodopa. Its use should be restricted to the treatment of previously untreated disabled patients and those who despite careful titration cannot tolerate levodopa. When used with levodopa, abnormal involuntary movements and confusional states are common.

Amantadine (Symmetrel®) has modest antiparkinsonian effects. It improves mild bradykinetic disabilities as well as tremor and rigidity. Unfortunately only a small proportion of patients derive benefit from this drug and tolerance to its effects occurs. However it has the advantage of being relatively free from side-effects.

LEVODOPA

Indications: parkinsonism (but not drug-induced extrapyramidal symptoms), see notes above

Cautions: pulmonary disease, peptic ulceration, renal, hepatic, or cardiovascular disease, diabetes, open-angle glaucoma, skin melanoma, psychiatric illness. In prolonged therapy, psychiatric, hepatic, haematological, renal, and cardiovascular surveillance is advisable. Avoid in pregnant and nursing mothers. Discontinue treatment 8 hours before surgery (increased risk of cardiac arrhythmias). Warn patients who benefit from therapy to resume normal activities gradually. Drug interactions: see Appendix 1

Contra-indications: closed-angle glaucoma

Side-effects: anorexia, nausea, insomnia, agitation, postural hypotension, dizziness, tachycardia, cardiac arrhythmias, abdominal pain, polyuria, incontinence, difficulty with micturition, discoloration of urine and other body fluids, rarely hypersensitivity; abnormal involuntary movements and psychiatric symptoms may be dose-limiting

Dose: initially 125–500 mg daily in divided doses after meals, increased according to response (see notes above)

Levodopa Capsules, levodopa 250 mg, price 20 caps = **C**; 500 mg, price 20 caps = **D**

Levodopa Tablets, levodopa 500 mg. Price 20 tabs = **C**

Berkdopa® (Berk)

Capsules, levodopa 250 mg. Price 20 caps = **C**

Capsules, levodopa 500 mg. Price 20 caps = **D**

Tablets, scored, levodopa 500 mg. Price 20 tabs = **C**

Brocadopa® (Brocades)

Capsules, levodopa 125 mg. Price 20 caps = **B**

Capsules, levodopa 250 mg. Price 20 caps = **C**

Capsules, levodopa 500 mg. Price 20 caps = **D**

Tablets, scored, levodopa 500 mg. Price 20 tabs = **D**

Temtabs® (= tablets s/r), scored, levodopa 500 mg. Price 20 tabs = **D**

Larodopa® (Roche)

Tablets, scored, levodopa 500 mg. Price 20 tabs = **D**

Madopar® (Roche)

Capsules (Madopar 62.5), blue/grey, levodopa 50 mg, benserazide 12.5 mg (as hydrochloride). Price 20 caps = **C**

Capsules (Madopar 125), blue/pink, levodopa 100 mg, benserazide 25 mg (as hydrochloride). Price 20 caps = **D**

Dose: initially 1 capsule twice daily, adjusted according to the response; usual maintenance dose 4–8 capsules daily in divided doses. Similar quantities of levodopa and benserazide may be given as Madopar 62.5 or Madopar 250

Capsules (Madopar 250), blue/caramel, levodopa 200 mg, benserazide 50 mg (as hydrochloride). Price 20 caps = **E**

Sinemet® (MSD)

Tablets (Sinemet 110), blue, scored, levodopa 100 mg, carbidopa 10 mg (as monohydrate). Price 20 tabs = **D**

Tablets (Sinemet 275), blue, scored, levodopa 250 mg, carbidopa 25 mg (as monohydrate). Price 20 tabs = **E**

Dose: initial dose, see Sinemet Plus, below; maintenance 3–6 tablets daily in divided doses. Similar quantities of levodopa and carbidopa may be given as Sinemet 110

Sinemet Plus® (MSD)

Tablets, yellow, scored, levodopa 100 mg, carbidopa 25 mg (as monohydrate). Price 20 tabs = **E**

Dose: initially 1 tablet 3 times daily, adjusted according to response to 8 daily in divided doses; larger doses by gradual substitution of Sinemet for Sinemet Plus

AMANTADINE HYDROCHLORIDE

Indications: parkinsonism (but not drug-induced extrapyramidal symptoms)

Cautions: cardiovascular, hepatic, or renal disease, recurrent eczema and psychosis, elderly patients. Avoid abrupt discontinuation of treatment. Drug interactions: see Appendix 1

Contra-indications: epilepsy, peptic ulceration, breast-feeding

Side-effects: nervousness, inability to concentrate, insomnia, dizziness, gastro-intestinal disturbances, skin discoloration, dry mouth, oedema; rarely leucopenia

Dose: 100 mg daily increased if necessary to 100 mg twice daily (not later than early evening), usually in conjunction with other treatment

Symmetrel® (Geigy)

Capsules, brownish-red, amantadine hydrochloride 100 mg. Price 20 caps = **F**

Syrup (= elixir), amantadine hydrochloride 50 mg/5 ml. Diluent syrup, life of diluted elixir 4 weeks. Price 150 ml = **F**

BROMOCRIPTINE

Indications: parkinsonism (but not drug-induced extrapyramidal symptoms)

Cautions; Side-effects: see section 6.7.1

Dose: initially 1.25 mg at night with food, gradually increased to 40-100 mg daily

Parlodel® (Sandoz)

Tablets, scored, bromocriptine 2.5 mg (as mesylate). Price 20 tabs = **G**

Capsules, bromocriptine 10 mg (as mesylate). Price 20 caps = **J**

4.9.2 Anticholinergic drugs used in parkinsonism

These drugs exert their antiparkinsonian effect by correcting the relative cholinergic excess which is thought to occur in parkinsonism as a result of dopamine deficiency. They produce at most only a 20% reduction in disability from tremor and rigidity, and do not significantly help bradykinesia. Anticholinergic drugs exert a synergistic effect when used with levodopa and are useful in reducing sialorrhoea. They are particularly valuable in treating patients with post-encephalitic parkinsonism who are also taking antipsychotic drugs.

The anticholinergic drugs also reduce drug-induced symptoms of parkinsonism as for example with antipsychotic drugs (section 4.2.1). There is no justification for giving anticholinergic drugs simultaneously with antipsychotics unless parkinsonian adverse effects occur. Tardive dyskinesia is not improved by the anticholinergic drugs and may be made worse.

No important differences exist between the many synthetic drugs available. The most commonly used are **orphenadrine** (Disipal®) and **benzhexol** (Artane®). They may have a mood-elevating effect which is useful in the management of phenothiazine-induced parkinsonism.

Benztropine (Cogentin®) and **procyclidine** (Kemadrin®) are also used. Benztropine is similar to benzhexol but is excreted more slowly; changes in dose therefore need to be carried out very gradually. Both benztropine and procyclidine may be given parenterally and are effective treatments for antipsychotic-induced acute dystonic reactions.

BENZHEXOL HYDROCHLORIDE

Indications: parkinsonism, particularly with apathy and depression; drug-induced extrapyramidal symptoms.
Cautions: urinary retention, glaucoma, cardiovascular disease, hepatic or renal impairment; avoid abrupt discontinuation of treatment. Drug interactions: see Appendix 1
Contra-indications: tardive dyskinesia
Side-effects: dry mouth, gastro-intestinal disturbances, dizziness, blurred vision; less commonly tachycardia, hypersensitivity, nervousness, and with high doses in susceptible patients, mental confusion, excitement, and psychiatric disturbances which may necessitate discontinuation of treatment
Dose: 1–2 mg daily, gradually increased; usual maintenance dose 5–15 mg daily in divided doses

Benzhexol Tablets, benzhexol hydrochloride 2 mg, price 20 tabs = **B**; 5 mg, price 20 tabs = **C**
Artane® (Lederle)
Tablets, scored, benzhexol hydrochloride 2 mg. Price 20 tabs = **B**
Tablets, scored, benzhexol hydrochloride 5 mg. Price 20 tabs = **C**
Sustets® (= capsules s/r), turquoise, benzhexol hydrochloride 5 mg. Price 20 caps = **C**
Dose: 1–3 capsules daily in divided doses or as a single dose in the morning

ORPHENADRINE HYDROCHLORIDE

Indications: parkinsonism, particularly with apathy and depression; drug-induced extrapyramidal symptoms
Cautions; Contra-indications; Side-effects: see under Benzhexol Hydrochloride, but more euphoric; may cause insomnia; less effective in controlling tremor
Dose: *by mouth,* daily in divided doses, 150 mg gradually increased; max. 400 mg daily
By intramuscular injection, 20–40 mg when necessary; max. 120 mg daily

Disipal® (Brocades)
Tablets, yellow, s/c, orphenadrine hydrochloride 50 mg. Price 20 tabs = **B**
Injection, orphenadrine hydrochloride 20 mg/ml. Price 2-ml amp = **B**

BENZTROPINE MESYLATE

Indications: parkinsonism, drug-induced extrapyramidal symptoms
Cautions; Contra-indications; Side-effects: see under Benzhexol Hydrochloride, but causes sedation rather than stimulation; persons affected should not drive or operate machinery; avoid alcohol (CNS depression); avoid in children under 3 years
Dose: *by mouth,* 500 micrograms daily, gradually increased; usual maintenance dose 1–4 mg daily in divided doses
By intramuscular or intravenous injection, 1–2 mg, repeated if symptoms reappear

Cogentin® (MSD)
Tablets, scored, benztropine mesylate 2 mg. Price 20 tabs = **B**
Injection, benztropine mesylate 1 mg/ml. Price 2-ml amp = **B**

BIPERIDEN

Indications: parkinsonism, drug-induced extrapyramidal symptoms
Cautions; Contra-indications; Side-effects: see under Benzhexol Hydrochloride
Dose: *by mouth,* biperiden hydrochloride 1 mg twice daily, gradually increased if necessary; usual maintenance dose 2–6 mg daily in divided doses
By intramuscular or slow intravenous injection, biperiden lactate 5–20 mg daily in divided doses

Akineton® (Abbott)
Tablets, scored, biperiden hydrochloride 2 mg. Price 20 tabs = **B**
Injection, biperiden lactate 5 mg/ml. Price 1-ml amp = **B**

METHIXENE HYDROCHLORIDE

Indications: parkinsonism, drug-induced extrapyramidal symptoms, more effective in controlling tremor than rigidity
Cautions; Contra-indications; Side-effects: see under Benzhexol Hydrochloride
Dose: 2.5 mg 3 times daily gradually increased; usual maintenance dose 15–60 mg daily in divided doses

Tremonil® (Wander)
Tablets, scored, methixene hydrochloride 5 mg. Price 20 tabs = **C**

PROCYCLIDINE HYDROCHLORIDE

Indications: parkinsonism, drug-induced extrapyramidal symptoms
Cautions; Contra-indications; Side-effects: see under Benzhexol Hydrochloride; may cause drowsiness
Dose: by mouth, 2.5 mg 3 times daily, gradually increased; max. 60 mg daily
By intramuscular or intravenous injection, 5–10 mg, repeated if necessary after 20 minutes; max. 20 mg daily

Kemadrin® (Wellcome)
Tablets, scored, procyclidine hydrochloride 5 mg. Price 20 tabs = **C**
Injection, procyclidine hydrochloride 5 mg/ml. Price 2-ml amp = **C**

4.9.3 Drugs used in choreas, tics, and related disorders

Tetrabenazine (Nitoman®) is mainly used to control movement disorders in Huntington's chorea and related disorders. It may act by depleting nerve endings of dopamine. It was formerly used as an antipsychotic drug.

Haloperidol may be useful in improving motor tics, stuttering, hiccup, and symptoms of Gilles de la Tourette syndrome and related choreas. Other antipsychotic drugs such as **chlorpromazine** and **perphenazine** are used to relieve intractable hiccup (section 4.2.1).

Propranolol or another beta-adrenoceptor blocking drug (see section 2.4) may be useful in treating essential tremor or tremors associated with anxiety or thyrotoxicosis.

HALOPERIDOL

Indications: motor tics, stuttering, adjunctive treatment in choreas and Gilles de la Tourette syndrome
Cautions; Contra-indications; Side-effects: see section 4.2.1
Dose: 0.5–1.5 mg 3 times daily adjusted according to the response; 10 mg daily or more may occasionally be necessary

Preparations
Section 4.2.1

TETRABENAZINE

Indications: movement disorders due to Huntington's chorea, senile chorea, and related neurological conditions
Side-effects: drowsiness, rarely depression, extrapyramidal dysfunction
Dose: initially 25 mg 3 times daily, gradually increased; maximum 200 mg daily

Nitoman® (Roche)
Tablets, yellow, scored, tetrabenazine 25 mg. Price 20 tabs = **C**

5: Drugs used in the treatment of INFECTIONS

In this chapter, drug treatment is discussed under the following headings:

5.1 Antibacterial drugs

CHOICE OF A SUITABLE DRUG. Before selecting an antibiotic for the treatment of an infection the clinician must first consider two factors—the patient and the known or likely causative organism. Factors related to the patient which must be considered include history of allergy to antibiotics, renal and hepatic function, resistance to infection (i.e. whether a compromised host), ability to tolerate oral drugs, severity of illness, race, age and, if female, whether pregnant or taking an oral contraceptive.

The known or likely organism and its antibiotic sensitivity, considered in association with the above factors, should guide the prescriber towards one or more antibiotics, the final choice depending on the microbiological, pharmacological, and toxicological properties of the various possible drugs for any particular infection.

An example of a rational approach to the selection of an antibiotic is the treatment of a urinary-tract infection in a patient complaining of nausea in early pregnancy. The causative organism is reported as being resistant to ampicillin but sensitive to nitrofurantoin (which can cause nausea), gentamicin (which can only be given by injection and is best avoided in pregnancy), tetracycline and co-trimoxazole (which are both contra-indicated in pregnancy), and cephalexin. The safest antibiotics in pregnancy are the penicillins and cephalosporins and, therefore, cephalexin would be indicated for this patient.

The principles involved in the selection of an antibiotic must allow for a number of variables including changing renal function, increasing bacterial resistance, and new information on side-effects of drugs. Duration of therapy, dosage, and route of administration of the drug depend on the type of infection and its severity.

BEFORE STARTING THERAPY. The following precepts should be considered before starting antibiotic therapy:

Viral infections should not be treated with antibiotics.

The **'blind'** prescribing of an antibiotic for a patient ill with unexplained pyrexia usually leads to further difficulty in establishing the diagnosis.

An up-to-date knowledge of **prevalent organisms** and their current sensitivity is of great help in choosing an antibiotic before bacteriological confirmation is available.

The **dose** of an antibiotic will vary according to a number of factors including age, weight, renal function and severity of infection. The prescribing of the so-called 'standard' dose in serious infections may result in failure of treatment or even death of the patient.

The **route** of administration of an antibiotic will often depend on the severity of the infection. Life-threatening infections require intravenous therapy.

Duration of therapy depends on the nature of the infection and the response to treatment. Courses should not be unduly prolonged as they are wasteful and may lead to side-effects. However, in certain infections such as endocarditis or tuberculosis it is necessary to continue treatment for relatively long periods.

Suggested antibacterial therapy for various infections is shown in Table 1. Sites of infection are arranged in the same order as the chapters of this book.

The possible infections for which antibacterial prophylaxis is useful are listed in Table 2.

Where *ampicillin* is suggested in the tables *amoxycillin* may be used, and where *flucloxacillin* is suggested *cloxacillin* may be used.

Table 1. Summary of antibacterial therapy

Infection	Suggested antibacterial	Comment
1: Gastro-intestinal system		
Gastro-enteritis	Antibiotic not indicated	Frequently nonbacterial aetiology

Table 1. Summary of antibacterial therapy (*continued*)

Infection	Suggested antibacterial	Comment
Bacillary dysentery	Antibiotic usually not indicated	Co-trimoxazole in severe illness
Invasive salmonellosis	Co-trimoxazole *or* ampicillin	
Typhoid fever	Chloramphenicol *or* co-trimoxazole	
Biliary tract infection	Gentamicin *or* a cephalosporin	
Peritonitis	Gentamicin + metronidazole (*or* clindamycin)	
2: Cardiovascular system		
Endocarditis caused by:		
Strep. viridans	Benzylpenicillin (+ gentamicin)	Treat for at least 4 weeks
Strep. faecalis	Benzylpenicillin (*or* ampicillin) + gentamicin	Treat for at least 4 weeks
Staph. aureus	Flucloxacillin + fusidic acid (*or* clindamycin)	Treat for at least 4 weeks
3: Respiratory system		
Exacerbations of chronic bronchitis	Tetracycline *or* ampicillin *or* ampicillin derivative *or* co-trimoxazole	Note that 20% of pneumococci are tetracycline-resistant
Pneumonia:		
Previously healthy chest	Penicillin *or* ampicillin *or* ampicillin derivative	Add flucloxacillin if *Staphylococcus* suspected e.g. in influenza or measles
Previously unhealthy chest	Flucloxacillin + ampicillin (*or* co-trimoxazole)	
4: Central nervous system		
Meningitis caused by:		
Meningococcus	Benzylpenicillin	Intrathecal therapy not usually necessary
Pneumococcus	Benzylpenicillin	
Haemophilus influenzae	Chloramphenicol	
Urinary tract		
Acute pyelonephritis and prostatitis	Co-trimoxazole *or* gentamicin	Do not give co-trimoxazole in pregnancy. Treat prostatitis with co-trimoxazole for 4 weeks
'Lower' UTI	1 Sulphonamide *or* 2 Ampicillin *or* 3 Co-trimoxazole	Select in order
Recurrent UTI	Ampicillin *or* Co-trimoxazole *or* Cephalexin	
Genital system		
Syphilis	Procaine penicillin (*or* tetracycline *or* erythromycin if penicillin-allergic)	Treat for 10–21 days
Gonorrhoea	Procaine penicillin with probenecid *or* ampicillin with probenecid (*or* co-trimoxazole, spectinomycin, *or* cefuroxime if penicillin-allergic)	Single-dose treatment
Non-gonococcal urethritis	Tetracycline	Treat for 10–21 days

Table 1. Summary of antibacterial therapy (*continued*)

Infection	Suggested antibacterial	Comment
10: Musculoskeletal system		
Osteomyelitis and septic arthritis	Clindamycin *or* flucloxacillin *or* fusidic acid. If *H. influenzae* give ampicillin *or* co-trimoxazole	Under 5 years of age may be *H. influenzae*. Treat acute disease for at least 6 weeks and chronic infection for at least 12 weeks
11: Eye		
Purulent conjunctivitis	Chloramphenicol eye-drops	
12: Ear, nose, and oropharynx		
Tonsillitis	Benzylpenicillin Penicillin V	Initial therapy with i/m benzylpenicillin in severe infection, then change to oral penicillin V. Most infections are caused by viruses
Otitis media	Benzylpenicillin Penicillin V	Initial therapy with i/m benzylpenicillin if possible, then change to oral penicillin V
	Ampicillin if under 5 years (*or* erythromycin if penicillin-allergic)	Under 5 years of age may be *H. influenzae*
Sinusitis	Erythromycin *or* co-trimoxazole	
13: Skin		
Impetigo	Topical chlortetracycline *or* oral flucloxacillin if systemic toxicity	
Erysipelas	Benzylpenicillin Penicillin V	Initial therapy with i/m benzylpenicillin if possible, then change to oral penicillin V
Cellulitis and wound infection	Flucloxacillin (*or* clindamycin if penicillin-allergic)	
Acne	Tetracycline	

Table 2. Summary of antibacterial prophylaxis

Infection	Antibacterial and adult dose
Prevention of recurrence of rheumatic fever	Penicillin V 500 mg daily *or* benzathine penicillin (Penidural LA) 900 mg every 4 weeks
Prevention of secondary case of meningococcal meningitis	Rifampicin 600 mg twice daily for 2 days; *or* minocycline 100 mg twice daily for 5 days; *or* sulphadimidine 2 g/day for 5 days (if strain known to be sensitive)
Prevention of secondary case of diphtheria in non-immune patient	Erythromycin 500 mg 4 times a day for 5 days
Prevention of endocarditis in patients with heart-valve lesion	*Dental procedures*—in-patients, i/m benzylpenicillin 1.2 g 30 minutes before procedure, *or* if already taking a penicillin *or* if penicillin-allergic i/v vancomycin 1 g 30 minutes before procedure;

Table 2. Summary of antibacterial prophylaxis (*continued*)

Infection	Antibacterial and adult dose
Prevention of endocarditis in patients with heart-valve lesion (*continued*)	out-patients, oral amoxycillin 3 g 1 hour before procedure, *or* if already taking a penicillin *or* if penicillin-allergic oral erythromycin 1 g (as stearate) 45 minutes before procedure, then 500 mg every 6 hours for 24 hours; patients with prosthetic heart valves, i/m benzylpenicillin 1.2 g + i/v gentamicin 1.5 mg/kg 30 minutes before procedure, *or* if already taking a penicillin *or* if penicillin-allergic i/v vancomycin 1 g + gentamicin 30 minutes before procedure. *Genito-urinary and colonic procedures*—i/v gentamicin 1.5 mg/kg (reduce dose in renal impairment) + i/v ampicillin 1 g 30 minutes before procedure and repeated twice at 8-hourly intervals, *or* if penicillin-allergic i/v erythromycin 500 mg (as lactobionate); metronidazole may also be added
Prevention of gas-gangrene in high lower-limb amputations or following major trauma	Benzylpenicillin 300–600 mg every 6 hours for 5 days; *or* procaine penicillin 2.4 g every 12 hours for 5 days; *or* if penicillin-allergic give erythromycin 500 mg every 6 hours
Prevention of tuberculosis in susceptible close contacts	Isoniazid alone for 12 months *or* isoniazid + ethambutol for 6–9 months

5.1.1 Penicillins

The penicillins are bactericidal and act by interfering with bacterial cell wall synthesis. They diffuse well into body tissues and fluids, but penetration into the cerebrospinal fluid is poor except when the meninges are inflamed. They are excreted in the urine in therapeutic concentrations. Probenecid blocks the renal tubular excretion of the penicillins, producing higher and more prolonged blood concentrations.

The most important side-effect of the penicillins is hypersensitivity, which causes rashes and, occasionally, anaphylaxis, which can be fatal. Patients who are allergic to one penicillin will be allergic to all as the hypersensitivity is related to the basic penicillin structure. A rare but serious toxic effect of the penicillins is encephalopathy due to cerebral irritation. This may result from excessively high doses but can also develop with normal doses given to patients with renal failure. Encephalopathy may follow intrathecal injection of the penicillins and this route of administration is best **avoided**, unless absolutely necessary, as chemical irritation of the brain can produce convulsions and sometimes death.

A second problem relating to high doses of penicillin, or normal doses given to patients with renal failure, is the accumulation of electrolyte since the injectable penicillins contain either sodium or potassium.

UNITS. International units are no longer used for penicillins and all doses are stated in milligrams.

5.1.1.1 PENICILLINASE-SENSITIVE PENICILLINS

Benzylpenicillin (Penicillin G, Crystapen®), the first of the penicillins, remains an important and useful antibiotic; it is inactivated by bacterial penicillinases (beta-lactamases). It is the drug of choice for streptococcal, pneumococcal, gonococcal, and meningococcal infections and also for actinomycosis, anthrax, diphtheria, gas-gangrene, syphilis, tetanus, and yaws. Pneumococci and gonococci have recently been isolated which have decreased sensitivity to penicillin. Benzylpenicillin is destroyed by gastric acid and absorption from the gut is low; therefore it is best given by injection.

Procaine penicillin (Depocillin®) is a sparingly soluble salt of benzylpenicillin. It is used in intramuscular depot preparations which provide therapeutic tissue concentrations for up to 24 hours. It is commonly used for the treatment of syphilis and gonorrhoea.

Benethamine penicillin and **benzathine penicillin** are benzylpenicillin salts with a very low solubility which give a prolonged action after intramuscular injection, though producing low serum concentrations, and so can be used for prophylaxis, combined with soluble and procaine benzylpenicillin.

Phenoxymethylpenicillin (Penicillin V) has a similar antibacterial spectrum to benzylpenicillin, but is less active. It is gastric acid-stable, so is suitable for oral administration. It should not be used for serious infections because absorption can be unpredictable and blood concentrations variable. It is indicated principally for respiratory-tract infections in children, for streptococcal tonsillitis, and for continuing treatment after one or more injections of benzylpenicillin when clinical response has begun. Phenoxymethylpenicillin is used for prophylaxis against streptococcal infections following rheumatic fever.

Penamecillin and **phenethicillin** have similar antibacterial activity, but they are no more effective than phenoxymethylpenicillin.

BENZYLPENICILLIN

(Penicillin G)

Indications: tonsillitis, otitis media, erysipelas, streptococcal endocarditis, meningococcal and pneumococcal meningitis, prophylaxis in limb amputation

Cautions: history of allergy

Contra-indications: penicillin hypersensitivity

Side-effects: sensitivity reactions including urticaria, fever, joint pains; angioneurotic oedema; anaphylactic shock in hypersensitive patients; convulsions after high doses by intravenous or intrathecal injection or in renal failure; diarrhoea after administration by mouth

Dose: *by intramuscular injection,* 300–600 mg 2–4 times daily; CHILD up to 12 years, 10–20 mg/kg daily; NEONATE, 30 mg/kg daily

By intravenous infusion, up to 24 g daily

By intrathecal injection, 6–12 mg daily

Crystapen® (Glaxo)

Injection, powder for reconstitution, benzylpenicillin sodium (unbuffered). Price 300- and 600-mg vial (both) = **A**

Injection, powder for reconstitution, benzylpenicillin sodium (buffered). Price 3-g vial = **B**; 6-g vial = **C**

Crystapen G® (Glaxo)

Tablets, yellow, f/c, benzylpenicillin potassium 250 mg. Price 20 tabs = **B**

Syrup (= elixir), orange, benzylpenicillin potassium 125 mg/5 ml when reconstituted with water for preparations. Diluent syrup, life of diluted elixir 7 days. Price 100 ml = **C**

Syrup (= elixir), orange, benzylpenicillin potassium 250 mg/5 ml when reconstituted with water for preparations. Diluent as above. Price 100 ml = **C**

BENETHAMINE PENICILLIN

Indications: penicillin-sensitive infections; prophylaxis

Cautions; Contra-indications; Side-effects: see under Benzylpenicillin

Triplopen® (Glaxo)

Injection, powder for reconstitution, benethamine penicillin 475 mg, procaine penicillin 250 mg, benzylpenicillin sodium 300 mg. Price per vial = **B**

Dose: by deep intramuscular injection, 1 vial every 2–3 days

BENZATHINE PENICILLIN

Indications: penicillin-sensitive infections; rheumatic fever prophylaxis

Cautions; Contra-indications; Side-effects: see under Benzylpenicillin

Dose: *by mouth,* 458 mg every 6–8 hours

By intramuscular injection, treatment of infections 229–916 mg every 5–7 days; rheumatic fever prophylaxis 916 mg every 3 weeks

Penidural (Oral)® (Wyeth)

Suspension (= mixture), pink, benzathine penicillin 229 mg/5 ml. Price 100 ml = **D**

Paediatric drops, pink, benzathine penicillin 115 mg/ml. Measure with pipette. Price 10 ml = **D**

Penidural-AP® (Wyeth)

Injection, powder for reconstitution, benzathine penicillin 458 mg, procaine penicillin 300 mg, benzylpenicillin potassium 190 mg. Price per vial = **C**

Dose: by deep intramuscular injection, 1 vial every 2–3 days

Penidural-LA® (Wyeth)

Injection (long-acting), benzathine penicillin 229 mg/ml. Price 10-ml vial = **E**

PENAMECILLIN

Indications: penicillin-sensitive infections

Cautions; Contra-indications; Side-effects: see under Benzylpenicillin

Dose: 350 mg every 8 hours

Havapen® (Wyeth)

Tablets, penamecillin 350 mg. Price 20 tabs = **D**

PHENETHICILLIN

Indications: penicillin-sensitive infections

Cautions; Contra-indications; Side-effects: see under Benzylpenicillin

Dose: 250 mg every 6 hours, at least 30 minutes before food

Broxil® (Beecham)

Capsules, black/ivory, phenethicillin 250 mg (as potassium salt). Price 20 caps = **D**

Tablets, yellow, scored, phenethicillin 250 mg (as potassium salt). Price 20 tabs = **D**

Syrup (= elixir), phenethicillin 125 mg (as potassium salt)/5 ml when reconstituted with water for preparations. Diluent syrup, life of diluted elixir 7 days. Price 100 ml = **D**

PHENOXYMETHYLPENICILLIN

(Penicillin V)

Indications: tonsillitis, otitis media, erysipelas, rheumatic fever prophylaxis, endocarditis prophylaxis

Cautions; Contra-indications; Side-effects: see under Benzylpenicillin. Drug interactions: see Appendix 1

Dose: 250–500 mg every 6 hours, at least 30 minutes before food; CHILD, $\frac{1}{4}$–$\frac{1}{2}$ adult dose

Phenoxymethylpenicillin Potassium Capsules, phenoxymethylpenicillin 250 mg (as potassium salt). Price 20 caps = **B**

Phenoxymethylpenicillin Potassium Tablets, phenoxymethylpenicillin 125 mg (as potassium salt), price 20 tabs = **A**; 250 mg, price 20 tabs = **B**

Phenoxymethylpenicillin Elixir, phenoxymethylpenicillin 62.5 mg (as potassium salt)/5 ml when reconstituted with water for preparations. Diluent syrup, life of diluted elixir 7 days. Price 100 ml = **B**

Phenoxymethylpenicillin 125 mg (as potassium salt)/5 ml when reconstituted with water for preparations. Diluent as above. Price 100 ml = **B**

Phenoxymethylpenicillin 250 mg (as potassium salt)/5 ml when reconstituted with water for preparations. Diluent as above. Price 100 ml = **C**

Phenoxymethylpenicillin Mixture, phenoxymethylpenicillin 125 mg (as calcium or potassium salt)/5 ml. Diluent fractionated coconut oil, life of diluted mixture 14 days. Price 100 ml = **C**

Apsin VK® (APS)

Tablets, scored, phenoxymethylpenicillin 250 mg (as potassium salt). Price 20 tabs = **B**

Syrup (= elixir), phenoxymethylpenicillin 125 mg (as potassium salt)/5 ml when reconstituted with water for preparations. Diluent syrup, life of diluted elixir 7 days. Price 100 ml = **B**

Syrup (= elixir), phenoxymethylpenicillin 250 mg (as potassium salt)/5 ml when reconstituted with water for preparations. Diluent as above. Price 100 ml = **C**

Crystapen V® (Glaxo)

Tablets, orange, f/c, phenoxymethylpenicillin 250 mg (as potassium salt). Price 20 tabs = **B**

Suspension (= mixture), phenoxymethylpenicillin 125 mg (as calcium salt)/5 ml. Diluent fractionated coconut oil, life of diluted mixture 14 days. Price 100 ml = **C**

Syrup (= elixir), red, phenoxymethylpenicillin 125 mg (as potassium salt)/5 ml when reconstituted with water for preparations. Diluent syrup, life of diluted elixir 7 days. Price 100 ml = **C**

Syrup (= elixir), red, phenoxymethylpenicillin 250 mg (as potassium salt)/5 ml when reconstituted with water for preparations. Diluent as above. Price 100 ml = **C**

Distaquaine V-K® (Dista)

Tablets, scored, phenoxymethylpenicillin 125 mg (as potassium salt). Price 20 tabs = **A**

Tablets, scored, phenoxymethylpenicillin 250 mg (as potassium salt). Price 20 tabs = **B**

Elixir, orange, phenoxymethylpenicillin 62.5 mg (as potassium salt)/5 ml when reconstituted with water for preparations. Diluent syrup, life of diluted elixir 7 days. Price 100 ml = **B**

Syrup (= elixir), orange, phenoxymethylpenicillin 125 mg (as potassium salt)/5 ml when reconstituted with water for preparations. Diluent as above. Price 100 ml = **B**

Syrup (= elixir), orange, phenoxymethylpenicillin 250 mg (as potassium salt)/5 ml when reconstituted with water for preparations. Diluent as above. Price 100 ml = **C**

Econocil VK® (DDSA)

Capsules, pink, phenoxymethylpenicillin 250 mg (as potassium salt). Price 20 caps = **A**

Tablets, phenoxymethylpenicillin 125 mg (as potassium salt). Price 20 tabs = **A**

Tablets, phenoxymethylpenicillin 250 mg (as potassium salt). Price 20 tabs = **A**

Icipen® (ICI)

Tablets, scored, phenoxymethylpenicillin 300 mg (as potassium salt). Price 20 tabs = **B**

Stabillin V-K® (Boots)

Tablets, phenoxymethylpenicillin 250 mg (as potassium salt). Price 20 tabs = **B**

Elixir, phenoxymethylpenicillin 62.5 mg (as potassium salt)/5 ml when reconstituted with water for preparations. Diluent syrup, life of diluted elixir 7 days. Price 100 ml = **B**

Elixir, phenoxymethylpenicillin 125 mg (as potassium salt)/5 ml when reconstituted with water for preparations. Diluent as above. Price 100 ml = **B**

Elixir, phenoxymethylpenicillin 250 mg (as potassium salt)/5 ml when reconstituted with water for preparations. Diluent as above. Price 100 ml = **C**

V-Cil-K® (Lilly)

Capsules, pink, phenoxymethylpenicillin 250 mg (as potassium salt). Price 20 caps = **B**

Tablets, phenoxymethylpenicillin 125 mg (as potassium salt). Price 20 tabs = **A**

Tablets, phenoxymethylpenicillin 250 mg (as potassium salt). Price 20 tabs = **B**

Pedipacs®, granules, phenoxymethylpenicillin 125 mg (as potassium salt)/single-dose sachet. Price 12 sachets = **B**

Paediatric syrup (= elixir), phenoxymethylpenicillin 62.5 mg (as potassium salt)/5 ml when reconstituted with water for preparations. Diluent syrup, life of diluted elixir 7 days. Price 100 ml = **B**

Paediatric syrup (= elixir), phenoxymethylpenicillin 125 mg (as potassium salt)/5 ml when reconstituted with water for preparations. Diluent as above. Price 100 ml = **B**

Syrup (= elixir), phenoxymethylpenicillin 250 mg (as potassium salt)/5 ml when reconstituted with water for preparations. Diluent as above. Price 100 ml = **C**

PROCAINE PENICILLIN

Indications: prevention of endocarditis during dental procedures, gas-gangrene following amputation; syphilis, gonorrhoea

Cautions; Contra-indications; Side-effects: see under Benzylpenicillin

Dose: *by intramuscular injection,* 300 mg 1–2 times daily

Gonorrhoea, men, 2.4 g; women, 4.8 g as a single dose

Syphilis, 1.2 g daily for 10 days

See also section 5.1, Table 1

Bicillin® (Brocades)

Injection, powder for reconstitution, procaine penicillin 3 g, benzylpenicillin sodium 600 mg. Price per vial = **B**

Dose: when reconstituted with 7.5 ml water for injections, 1 ml 1–2 times daily

Depocillin® (Brocades)

Injection, powder for reconstitution, procaine penicillin. Price 3-g vial = **B**

Aqueous injection, procaine penicillin 300 mg/ml. Price 10-ml vial = **B**

5.1.1.2 PENICILLINASE-RESISTANT PENICILLINS

Most staphylococci are now resistant to benzylpenicillin because they produce penicillinases. **Cloxacillin** (Orbenin®) and **flucloxacillin** (Floxapen®), however, are not inactivated by these enzymes and are thus effective in infections caused by penicillin-resistant *Staphylococcus aureus,* which is the sole indication for their use. They are acid-stable and can, therefore, be given by mouth as well as by injection. The antibacterial activity of both is identical, as are blood concentrations following injection.

Flucloxacillin is approximately twice as well absorbed from the gut as cloxacillin and is, therefore, to be preferred for oral therapy.

Methicillin (Celbenin®) is also effective against penicillin-resistant *Staph. aureus,* but can only be given by injection because it is not acid-stable.

CLOXACILLIN

Indications: infections due to penicillinase-producing staphylococci

Cautions; Contra-indications; Side-effects: see under Benzylpenicillin (section 5.1.1.1)

Dose: *by mouth,* 500 mg every 6 hours, at least 30 minutes before food

By intramuscular injection, 500 mg every 4–6 hours

By intravenous injection, 0.5–1 g every 4–6 hours

CHILD, any route, ¼-½ adult dose

Orbenin® (Beecham)

Capsules, orange/black, cloxacillin 250 mg (as sodium salt). Price 20 caps = **F**

Capsules, orange/black, cloxacillin 500 mg (as sodium salt). Price 20 caps = **G**

Syrup (= elixir), cloxacillin 125 mg (as sodium salt)/5 ml when reconstituted with water for preparations. Diluent syrup, life of diluted elixir 7 days. Price 100 ml = **E**

Injection, powder for reconstitution, cloxacillin (as sodium salt). Price 250-mg vial = **C**; 500-mg vial = **D**; 1-g vial = **F**

FLUCLOXACILLIN

Indications: infections due to penicillinase-producing staphylococci

Cautions; Contra-indications; Side-effects: see under Benzylpenicillin (section 5.1.1.1)

Dose: *by mouth,* 250 mg every 6 hours, at least 30 minutes before food

By intramuscular injection, 250 mg every 6 hours

By slow intravenous injection, 250–500 mg every 6 hours

CHILD, any route, ¼–½ adult dose

Floxapen® (Beecham)

Capsules, black/caramel, flucloxacillin 250 mg (as sodium salt). Price 20 caps = **F**

Capsules, black/caramel, flucloxacillin 500 mg (as sodium salt). Price 20 caps = **H**

Syrup (= elixir), flucloxacillin 125 mg (as sodium salt)/5 ml when reconstituted with water for preparations. Diluent syrup, life of diluted elixir 7 days. Price 100 ml = **F**

Injection, powder for reconstitution, flucloxacillin (as sodium salt). Price 250-mg vial = **C**; 500-mg vial = **D**

METHICILLIN SODIUM

Indications: infections due to penicillinase-producing staphylococci

Cautions; Contra-indications; Side-effects: see under Benzylpenicillin (section 5.1.1.1)

Dose: *by intramuscular or slow intravenous injection,* 1 g every 4–6 hours

Celbenin® (Beecham)

Injection, powder for reconstitution, methicillin sodium. Price 1-g vial = **D**

5.1.1.3 BROAD-SPECTRUM PENICILLINS

Ampicillin (Penbritin®) is active against certain Gram-positive and Gram-negative organisms but is inactivated by penicillinases including those produced by *Staph. aureus* and by common Gram-negative bacilli such as *Escherichia coli.* Almost all staphylococci, one-third of *E. coli* strains and up to one-tenth of *H. influenzae* strains are now resistant.

It can be given by mouth before food, and by injection, and is well excreted in the bile and urine. It is principally indicated for the treatment of exacerbations of chronic bronchitis and middle ear infections, both of which are usually due to *Streptococcus pneumoniae* and *Haemophilus influenzae,* and for urinary-tract infections.

Less than half the dose of ampicillin is absorbed after oral administration, and absorption is further decreased by the presence of food in the gut. Higher blood concentrations are obtained with the ampicillin derivatives **bacampicillin** (Ambaxin®), **ciclacillin** (Calthor®), **pivampicillin** (Pondocillin®), and **talampicillin** (Talpen®); their absorption is little affected by the presence of food, and the incidence of diarrhoea is less than with ampicillin.

Maculo-papular rashes commonly occur with the ampicillins but are not usually related to true penicillin allergy. They are almost invariable in patients with glandular fever or chronic lymphatic leukaemia who are given these antibiotics.

Amoxycillin (Amoxil®) is a derivative of ampicillin which differs by only one hydroxyl group and has a similar antibacterial spectrum. It is, however, twice as well absorbed when given by mouth, producing higher blood and tissue concentrations.

Augmentin® consists of amoxycillin with the beta-lactamase inhibitor **clavulanic acid**, which itself has no antibacterial activity but which, by inactivating penicillinases, increases the activity of the product against penicillinase-producing bacteria that are normally resistant to amoxycillin.

Mezlocillin (Baypen®) is a derivative of ampicillin which is active against certain ampicillin-resistant bacteria. However, like ampicillin, it is inactivated by beta-lactamases.

AMOXYCILLIN

Indications: urinary-tract infections, otitis media, chronic bronchitis, gonorrhoea

Cautions; Contra-indications; Side-effects: see under Benzylpenicillin (section 5.1.1.1); also erythematous rashes in glandular fever and chronic lymphatic leukaemia

Dose: *by mouth,* 250 mg every 8 hours, doubled in severe infections; CHILD up to 10 years, 125 mg every 8 hours

By intramuscular injection, 500 mg every 8 hours; CHILD, 50–100 mg/kg daily in divided doses

By intravenous injection or infusion (in severe infections), 1 g every 6 hours; CHILD, 50–100 mg/kg daily in divided doses

Amoxil® (Bencard)

Capsules, maroon/gold, amoxycillin 250 mg (as trihydrate). Price 20 caps = **F**

Capsules, maroon/gold, amoxycillin 500 mg (as trihydrate). Price 20 caps = **G**

Dispersible tablets, amoxycillin 500 mg (as trihydrate). Price 20 tabs = **H**

Syrup (= mixture), amoxycillin 125 mg (as trihydrate)/5 ml when reconstituted with water for preparations. Diluent syrup, life of diluted mixture 14 days. Price 100 ml = **D**

Syrup forte (= strong mixture), amoxycillin 250 mg (as trihydrate)/5 ml when reconstituted with water for preparations. Diluent as above. Price 100 ml = **F**

Paediatric suspension, amoxycillin 125 mg (as trihydrate)/1.25 ml when reconstituted with water for preparations. Measure with pipette. Price 20 ml = **E**

▼ *Sachets,* powder, amoxycillin (as trihydrate). Price per 3-g sachet = **D**

Dose: urinary-tract infections, 3 g in water, repeated after 12 hours

▼ *Injection,* powder for reconstitution, amoxycillin (as sodium salt). Price 250-mg vial = **B**; 500-mg vial = **C**; 1-g vial = **D**

▼ **Augmentin®** (Beecham)

Tablets, f/c, amoxycillin 250 mg (as trihydrate), clavulanic acid 125 mg (as potassium salt). Price 20 tabs = **G**

Dispersible tablets, amoxycillin 250 mg (as trihydrate), clavulanic acid 125 mg (as potassium salt). Price 20 tabs = **G**

Dose: 1 tablet every 8 hours, increased to 2 tablets in severe infections

---

AMPICILLIN

Indications: see under Amoxycillin

Cautions; Contra-indications; Side-effects: see under Benzylpenicillin (section 5.1.1.1); also erythematous rashes in glandular fever and chronic lymphatic leukaemia

Dose: *by mouth,* 0.25–1 g every 6 hours, at least 30 minutes before food

By intramuscular or intravenous injection, 500 mg every 4–6 hours; higher doses in meningitis

CHILD, any route, ½ adult dose

Ampicillin Capsules, ampicillin 250 mg, price 20 caps = **C**; 500 mg, price 20 caps = **D**

Ampicillin Mixture, ampicillin 125 mg/5 ml when reconstituted with water for preparations. Diluent syrup, life of diluted mixture 7 days. Price 100 ml = **C**

Ampicillin Mixture, Strong, ampicillin 250 mg/5 ml when reconstituted with water for preparations. Diluent as above. Price 100 ml = **D**

Amfipen® (Brocades)

Capsules, red/grey, ampicillin 250 mg. Price 20 caps = **C**

Capsules, red/grey, ampicillin 500 mg. Price 20 caps = **D**

Syrup (= mixture), pink, ampicillin 125 mg/5 ml when reconstituted with water for preparations. Diluent syrup, life of diluted mixture 7 days. Price 100 ml = **C**

Syrup forte (= strong mixture), pink, ampicillin 250 mg/5 ml when reconstituted with water for preparations. Diluent as above. Price 100 ml = **D**

Britcin® (DDSA)

Capsules, red/grey, ampicillin 250 mg (as trihydrate). Price 20 caps = **C**

Capsules, red/grey, ampicillin 500 mg (as trihydrate). Price 20 caps = **D**

Penbritin® (Beecham)

Capsules, black/red, ampicillin 250 mg (as trihydrate). Price 20 caps = **D**

Capsules, black/red, ampicillin 500 mg (as trihydrate). Price 20 caps = **E**

Paediatric tablets, scored, ampicillin 125 mg (as trihydrate). Price 20 tabs = **C**

Syrup (= mixture), ampicillin 125 mg (as trihydrate)/5 ml when reconstituted with water for preparations. Diluent syrup, life of diluted mixture 7 days. Price 100 ml = **D**

Syrup forte (= strong mixture), ampicillin 250 mg (as trihydrate)/5 ml when reconstituted with water for preparations. Diluent as above. Price 100 ml = **E**

Paediatric suspension, pink, ampicillin 125 mg (as trihydrate)/1.25 ml. Measure with pipette. Price 25 ml = **E**

Injection, powder for reconstitution, ampicillin (as sodium salt). Price 250-mg vial = **B**; 500-mg vial = **C**

Pentrexyl® (Bristol)

Capsules, red/grey, ampicillin 250 mg (as trihydrate). Price 20 caps = **C**

Capsules, red/grey, ampicillin 500 mg (as trihydrate). Price 20 caps = **D**

Vidopen® (Berk)

Capsules, pink/red, ampicillin 250 mg (as trihydrate). Price 20 caps = **C**

Capsules, pink/red, ampicillin 500 mg (as trihydrate). Price 20 caps = **D**

Syrup (= mixture), pink, ampicillin 125 mg (as trihydrate)/5 ml when reconstituted with water for preparations. Diluent syrup, life of diluted mixture 7 days. Price 100 ml = **C**

Syrup forte (= strong mixture), pink, ampicillin 250 mg (as trihydrate)/5 ml when reconstituted with water for preparations. Diluent as above. Price 100 ml = **D**

Preparations containing ampicillin and a penicillinase-resistant penicillin

Ampiclox® (Beecham)

Injection, ampicillin 250 mg (as sodium salt), cloxacillin 250 mg (as sodium salt). Price per vial = **D**

Dose: by intramuscular or intravenous injection, 1–2 vials every 4–6 hours; CHILD up to 2 years ¼ adult dose, 2–10 years ½ adult dose

Ampiclox Neonatal® (Beecham)

Suspension, ampicillin 60 mg (as trihydrate), cloxacillin 30 mg (as sodium salt)/0.6 ml when reconstituted with water for preparations. Price 10 ml = **D**

Dose: 0.6 ml every 4 hours. Measure with pipette

Injection, powder for reconstitution, ampicillin 50 mg (as sodium salt), cloxacillin 25 mg (as sodium salt). Price per vial = **B**

Dose: by intramuscular or intravenous injection, 1 vial every 8 hours

Magnapen® (Beecham)

Capsules, black/turquoise, ampicillin 250 mg (as trihydrate), flucloxacillin 250 mg (as sodium salt). Price 20 caps = **F**

Dose: 1 capsule every 6 hours

Syrup (= mixture), ampicillin 125 mg (as trihydrate), flucloxacillin 125 mg (as sodium salt)/5 ml when reconstituted with water for preparations. Diluent syrup, life of diluted mixture 7 days. Price 100 ml = **F**

Dose: 10 ml every 6 hours; CHILD up to 2 years ¼ adult dose, 2–10 years ½ adult dose

Injection 500 mg, powder for reconstitution, ampicillin 250 mg (as sodium salt), flucloxacillin 250 mg (as sodium salt). Price per vial = **C**

Dose: by intramuscular or intravenous injection, 1 vial every 6 hours; CHILD up to 2 years ¼ adult dose, 2–10 years ½ adult dose; doses may be doubled in severe infections

Injection 1 g, powder for reconstitution, ampicillin 500 mg (as sodium salt), flucloxacillin 500 mg (as sodium salt). Price per vial = **E**

BACAMPICILLIN HYDROCHLORIDE

Indications: urinary-tract infections, chronic bronchitis, invasive salmonellosis

Cautions; Contra-indications; Side-effects: see under Benzylpenicillin (section 5.1.1.1); also erythematous rashes in glandular fever and chronic lymphatic leukaemia

Dose: 400 mg 2–3 times daily, doubled in severe infections

▼Ambaxin® (Upjohn)

Tablets, scored, bacampicillin hydrochloride 400 mg. Price 20 tabs = **F**

CICLACILLIN

Indications: bronchitis, urinary-tract infections, soft-tissue infections

Cautions; Contra-indications; Side-effects: see under Benzylpenicillin (section 5.1.1.1); also erythematous rashes in glandular fever and chronic lymphatic leukaemia

Dose: 250–500 mg every 6 hours; longer interval between doses in renal impairment

▼Calthor® (Ayerst)

Tablets, scored, ciclacillin 250 mg. Price 20 tabs = **E**

Tablets, scored, ciclacillin 500 mg. Price 20 tabs = **G**

Suspension (= mixture), ciclacillin 125 mg/5 ml when reconstituted with water for preparations. Price 120 ml = **E**

Suspension (= mixture), orange, ciclacillin 250 mg/5 ml when reconstituted with water for preparations. Price 120 ml = **F**

MEZLOCILLIN

Indications: infections due to *E. coli, Pseudomonas,* and *Proteus* spp.

Cautions; Contra-indications; Side-effects: see under Benzylpenicillin (section 5.1.1.1); increase interval between doses in renal impairment
Dose: *by intravenous injection,* 2 g every 6–8 hours
By intravenous infusion, in serious infections, 5 g every 6–8 hours
By intramuscular injection, 0.5–2 g

▼ **Baypen®** (Bayer)
Injection, powder for reconstitution, mezlocillin (as sodium salt). Price 500-mg vial = **D**; 1-g vial = **E**; 2-g vial = **F**; 5-g infusion vial = **I**

PIVAMPICILLIN

Indications: urinary-tract infections, chronic bronchitis, gonorrhoea
Cautions; Contra-indications; Side-effects: see under Benzylpenicillin (section 5.1.1.1); also erythematous rashes in chronic lymphatic leukaemia; liver- and kidney-function tests required in long-term use
Dose: 500 mg every 12 hours, doubled in severe infections

▼ **Pondocillin®** (Burgess)
Tablets, f/c, pivampicillin 500 mg. Price 20 tabs = **F**
Suspension (= mixture), pivampicillin 162 mg /5 ml when reconstituted with water for preparations. Price 50 ml = **D**; 100 ml = **E**

TALAMPICILLIN HYDROCHLORIDE

Indications: urinary-tract infections, chronic bronchitis, invasive salmonellosis
Cautions; Contra-indications; Side-effects: see under Benzylpenicillin (section 5.1.1.1); caution in severe renal or hepatic impairment; also erythematous rashes in glandular fever and chronic lymphatic leukaemia
Dose: 250–500 mg every 8 hours

Talpen® (Beecham)
Tablets, red, f/c, talampicillin hydrochloride 250 mg. Price 20 tabs = **E**
Syrup (= mixture), talampicillin hydrochloride 125 mg (as napsylate)/5 ml when reconstituted with water for preparations. Diluent syrup, life of diluted mixture 7 days. Price 100 ml = **E**
Syrup forte (= strong mixture), talampicillin hydrochloride 250 mg (as napsylate)/5 ml when reconstituted with water for preparations. Diluent as above. Price 100 ml = **F**

5.1.1.4 ANTIPSEUDOMONAL PENICILLINS

Carbenicillin (Pyopen®) is active against *Pseudomonas aeruginosa* and also against certain other Gram-negative organisms including *Proteus* species. It is not absorbed when given by mouth. Its phenyl ester, **carfecillin** (Uticillin®) is absorbed, carbenicillin being released into the blood in only low concentration although urinary concentrations are adequate.

The only specific indication for carbenicillin is in the treatment of *Pseudomonas* infections but because this organism is only moderately sensitive, large doses are necessary for systemic infections and must be given by intravenous injection or infusion. Carfecillin can only be used for *Pseudomonas* and *Proteus* infections of the lower urinary tract.

Side-effects of intravenous carbenicillin include hypokalaemia and alteration in platelet function.

Ticarcillin (Ticar®) is more active than carbenicillin against *Ps. aeruginosa.*

Both carbenicillin and ticarcillin can be given with gentamicin, as the combination is synergistic.

Azlocillin (Securopen®), a derivative of ampicillin, has slightly greater activity than ticarcillin against *Ps. aeruginosa.*

AZLOCILLIN

Indications: infections due to *Pseudomonas aeruginosa*
Cautions; Contra-indications; Side-effects: see under Benzylpenicillin (section 5.1.1.1); also longer dose interval in renal impairment
Dose: *by intravenous injection,* 2 g every 8 hours
By intravenous infusion, in serious infections, 5 g every 8 hours

▼ **Securopen®** (Bayer)
Injection, powder for reconstitution, azlocillin (as sodium salt). Price 500-mg vial = **E**; 1-g vial = **F**; 2-g vial = **H**; 5-g infusion vial = **J**

CARBENICILLIN

Indications: infections due to *Pseudomonas aeruginosa* and *Proteus* spp.
Cautions; Contra-indications; Side-effects: see under Benzylpenicillin (section 5.1.1.1)
Dose: *by slow intravenous injection or rapid infusion,* severe systemic infections, 5 g every 4–6 hours; CHILD 250–400 mg/kg daily in divided doses
By intramuscular injection, urinary-tract infections, 2 g every 6 hours; CHILD 50–100 mg/kg daily in divided doses

Pyopen® (Beecham)
Injection, powder for reconstitution, carbenicillin (as sodium salt). Price 1-g vial = **D**; 5-g vial = **H**
Infusion set, powder for reconstitution, carbenicillin 5 g (as sodium salt) in infusion bottle, with transfer needle and diluent. Price (complete unit) = **H**

CARFECILLIN SODIUM

Indications: urinary-tract infections due to *Pseudomonas* and *Proteus* spp.
Cautions; Contra-indications; Side-effects: see under Benzylpenicillin (section 5.1.1.1)
Dose: 0.5–1 g 3 times daily

Uticillin® (Beecham)
Tablets, carfecillin sodium 500 mg. Price 20 tabs = **G**

TICARCILLIN

Indications: infections due to *Pseudomonas* and *Proteus* spp.
Cautions; Contra-indications; Side-effects: see under Benzylpenicillin (section 5.1.1.1)
Dose: by intramuscular or slow intravenous injection, or rapid intravenous infusion, 15–20 g daily in divided doses

▼Ticar® (Beecham)
Injection, powder for reconstitution, ticarcillin (as sodium salt). Price 1-g vial = **E**; 3-g vial = **G**; 5-g vial = **I**
Infusion, powder for reconstitution, ticarcillin 5 g (as sodium salt) in infusion bottle, with transfer needle and diluent. Price complete unit = **J**

5.1.1.5 OTHER PENICILLINS

Mecillinam (Selexidin®) and **pivmecillinam** (Selexid®) have a similar antibacterial spectrum to ampicillin, but are more active against enteric bacteria, notably salmonellae. Pivmecillinam is given by mouth and subsequently hydrolysed to mecillinam, which is the active agent and must itself be given by injection.

MECILLINAM

Indications: severe infections due to Gram-negative enteric bacteria
Cautions; Contra-indications; Side-effects: see under Benzylpenicillin (section 5.1.1.1); also liver- and kidney-function tests required in long-term use
Dose: by intramuscular or slow intravenous injection, 5–15 mg/kg every 6–8 hours

▼Selexidin® (Leo)
Injection, powder for reconstitution, mecillinam. Price 200-mg vial = **C**; 400-mg vial = **D**

PIVMECILLINAM HYDROCHLORIDE

Indications: urinary-tract infections due to enterobacteria, salmonellosis
Cautions; Contra-indications; Side-effects: see under Benzylpenicillin (section 5.1.1.1); also liver- and kidney-function tests required in long-term use
Dose: salmonellosis, 1.2–2.4 g daily
Urinary-tract infections, 200–400 mg every 6–8 hours

▼Selexid® (Leo)
Tablets, f/c, pivmecillinam hydrochloride 200 mg. Price 20 tabs = **F**
Suspension, granules, pivmecillinam hydrochloride 100 mg/single-dose sachet. Price 20 sachets = **F**

5.1.2 Cephalosporins and cephamycins

The cephalosporins are broad-spectrum antibiotics, but in spite of the number of cephalosporins currently available there are few absolute indications for their use. All have a similar antibacterial spectrum although individual agents have differing activity against certain organisms. The pharmacology of the cephalosporins is similar to that of the penicillins, excretion being principally renal and blocked by probenecid. Cephalexin, cephradine, and cefaclor are the only available cephalosporins that are active when given by mouth.

The principal side-effect of the cephalosporins is hypersensitivity and about 10% of penicillin-sensitive patients will also be allergic to the cephalosporins. **Cephaloridine** can cause renal tubular necrosis especially if given in large doses (over 6 g per day) and this nephrotoxicity is potentiated by potent tubular diuretics such as frusemide and ethacrynic acid.

The first cephalosporins were **cephaloridine** (Ceporin®) and **cephalothin** (Keflin®). Cephalothin is less active and less stable than cephaloridine necessitating relatively high doses given by intravenous injection. These two have been replaced by the newer cephalosporins, **cephradine** (Velosef®), **cephazolin** (Kefzol®), **cefuroxime** (Zinacef®), and **cephamandole** (Kefadol®).

Cefuroxime and cephamandole are 'second generation' cephalosporins and are less susceptible than the other cephalosporins to inactivation by penicillinases. They are, therefore, active against certain bacteria which are resistant to the other drugs. Apart from this, and the greater activity of cefuroxime against *H.influenzae* and *Neisseria gonorrhoeae,* there is little to choose between these four antibiotics and it is suggested that the prescriber should become familiar with one and use it when a cephalosporin is indicated.

Cefotaxime (Claforan®) is a 'third generation' cephalosporin. It is similar to cefuroxime and cephamandole but is more active against certain Gram-negative bacilli and also has some activity against *Ps. aeruginosa*. It is less active than cefuroxime and cephamandole against *Staph. aureus*.

Cefoxitin (Mefoxin®) is the first of the **cephamycins**, a new group of antibiotics closely related to the cephalosporins and with the same basic structure and side-effects. It is active against *Bacteroides fragilis* and because of this it has been recommended for the treatment of abdominal sepsis such as peritonitis.

CEFACLOR

Indications: infections due to sensitive Gram-positive and Gram-negative bacteria, but see notes above
Cautions: penicillin sensitivity

Contra-indications: cephalosporin hypersensitivity
Side-effects: allergic reactions including urticaria and rashes; hypersensitivity reactions including anaphylaxis; nausea, vomiting, diarrhoea
Dose: 250 mg every 8 hours; max. 2 g daily; CHILD, 20–40 mg/kg daily in divided doses; max. 1 g daily

▼ Distaclor® (Dista)
Capsules, violet/white, cefaclor 250 mg. Price 20 caps = **G**
Suspension (= mixture), pink, cefaclor 125 mg/5 ml when reconstituted with water for preparations. Diluent water for preparations or syrup, life of diluted mixture 14 days. Price 100 ml = **F**
Suspension (= mixture), pink, cefaclor 250 mg/5 ml when reconstituted with water for preparations. Diluent as above. Price 100 ml = **G**

CEFOTAXIME

Indications: see under Cefaclor; see also notes above
Cautions; Contra-indications; Side-effects: see under Cefaclor; also reduce doses in severe renal impairment, false-positive results for glucose in urine with reducing substances. Drug interactions: see Appendix 1
Dose: *by intramuscular or intravenous injection,* 1 g every 12 hours; in severe infections up to 12 g in 3–4 divided doses. NEONATE, 50 mg/kg daily in 2–4 divided doses; in severe infections 150–200 mg/kg daily. CHILD, 100–150 mg/kg daily in 2–4 divided doses; in severe infections, up to 200 mg/kg daily. In severe renal impairment, doses to be halved
By intravenous infusion, 1–2 g over 20–60 minutes

▼ Claforan® (Roussel)
Injection, powder for reconstitution, cefotaxime (as sodium salt). Price 500-mg vial = **E**; 1-g vial = **F**; 2-g vial = **H**

CEFOXITIN

Indications: see under Cefaclor; more active against Gram-negative bacteria
Cautions; Contra-indications; Side-effects: see under Cefaclor; also reduced doses in renal impairment, false-positive results for glucose in urine with reducing substances
Dose: *by intramuscular injection or slow intravenous injection or infusion,* 1–2 g every 8 hours; CHILD over 2 years, 80–160 mg/kg daily in divided doses

▼ Mefoxin® (MSD)
Injection, powder for reconstitution, cefoxitin (as sodium salt). Price 1-g vial = **F**; 2-g vial = **H**

CEFUROXIME

Indications: see under Cefaclor; more active against *H. influenzae* and *N. gonorrhoeae*
Cautions; Contra-indications; Side-effects: see under Cefaclor; also positive Coombs' test may develop; reduce dose in renal impairment
Dose: *by intramuscular or intravenous injection,* 750 mg every 8 hours
By intravenous injection or infusion, in severe infections, 1.5 g every 6–8 hours
CHILD, 30–100 mg/kg daily in divided doses

▼ Zinacef® (Glaxo)
Injection, powder for reconstitution, cefuroxime (as sodium salt). Price 250-mg vial = **C**; 750-mg vial = **E**; 1.5-g vial = **G**

CEPHALEXIN

Indications: see under Cefaclor; not for severe infections
Cautions; Contra-indications; Side-effects: see under Cefaclor; also reduced doses in renal impairment, false-positive results for glucose in urine with reducing substances
Dose: 250–500 mg every 6 hours; CHILD, 25–50 mg/kg daily in divided doses

Cephalexin Capsules, cephalexin 250 mg, price 20 caps = **E**; 500 mg, price 20 caps = **G**
Cephalexin Tablets, cephalexin 250 mg, price 20 tabs = **E**; 500 mg, price 20 tabs = **G**
Cephalexin Mixture, cephalexin 125 mg/5 ml when reconstituted with water for preparations. Diluent, see below under Ceporex or Keflex. Price 100 ml = **D**
Cephalexin 250 mg/5 ml when reconstituted with water for preparations. Diluent as above. Price 100 ml = **E**
Ceporex® (Glaxo)
Capsules, caramel/grey, cephalexin 250 mg. Price 20 caps = **E**
Capsules, caramel/grey, cephalexin 500 mg. Price 20 caps = **G**
Tablets, pink, f/c, cephalexin 250 mg. Price 20 tabs = **E**
Tablets, pink, f/c, cephalexin 500 mg. Price 20 tabs = **G**
Paediatric drops, orange, cephalexin 125 mg/1.25 ml when reconstituted with water for preparations. Measure with dropper. Price 10 ml = **D**
Suspension, yellow, cephalexin 125 mg/5 ml. Do not dilute. Price 100 ml = **D**
Suspension, yellow, cephalexin 250 mg/5ml. Do not dilute. Price 100 ml = **E**
Syrup (= mixture), orange, cephalexin 125 mg/5 ml when reconstituted with water for preparations. Diluent water for preparations, life of diluted mixture 7 days. Price 100 ml = **D**
Syrup (= mixture), orange, cephalexin 250 mg/5 ml when reconstituted with water for preparations. Diluent as above. Price 100 ml = **E**
Syrup (= mixture), orange, cephalexin 500 mg/5 ml when reconstituted with water for preparations. Diluent as above. Price 100 ml = **G**
Keflex® (Lilly)
Capsules, green/white, cephalexin 250 mg. Price 20 caps = **F**

Capsules, green, cephalexin 500 mg. Price 20 caps = **G**
Tablets, peach, cephalexin 250 mg. Price 20 tabs = **F**
Tablets, peach, cephalexin 500 mg. Price 20 tabs = **G**
Suspension (= mixture), pink, cephalexin 125 mg/5 ml after reconstitution with water for preparations. Diluent syrup, life of diluted mixture 10 days. Price 100 ml = **D**
Suspension (= mixture), orange, cephalexin 250 mg/5 ml after reconstitution with water for preparations. Diluent as above. Price 100 ml = **F**

CEPHALORIDINE

Indications: see under Cefaclor
Cautions; Contra-indications; Side-effects: see under Cefaclor; also acute renal failure and positive Coombs' test may develop. Drug interactions: see Appendix 1
Dose: *by intramuscular or intravenous injection,* 0.5–1 g every 8–12 hours; max. 6 g daily; CHILD, 20–40 mg/kg daily in divided doses, max. 4 g daily

Ceporin® (Glaxo)
Injection, powder for reconstitution, cephaloridine. Price 250-mg vial = **B**; 500-mg vial = **C**; 1-g vial = **D**

CEPHALOTHIN

Indications: see under Cefaclor
Cautions; Contra-indications; Side-effects: see under Cefaclor; also reduced doses in renal impairment, intramuscular injections painful. Drug interactions: see Appendix 1
Dose: *by intravenous injection or infusion,* 1 g every 4 hours; max. 12 g daily; CHILD, 12.5–25 mg/kg every 6 hours

Keflin® (Lilly)
Injection, powder for reconstitution, cephalothin (as sodium salt). Price 1-g vial = **D**; 4-g vial = **G**

CEPHAMANDOLE

Indications: see under Cefaclor
Cautions; Contra-indications; Side-effects: see under Cefaclor; also reduce doses in renal impairment, false-positive results for glucose in urine with reducing substances
Dose: *by intramuscular injection or intravenous injection or infusion,* 0.5–2 g every 4–8 hours; CHILD, 50–100 mg/kg daily in divided doses

▼ Kefadol® (Lilly)
Injection, powder for reconstitution, cephamandole (as nafate) with sodium carbonate. Price 500-mg vial = **D**; 1-g vial = **E**; 2-g vial = **G** (Hosp. only)

CEPHAZOLIN

Indications: see under Cefaclor
Cautions; Contra-indications; Side-effects: see under Cefaclor; also reduce doses in renal impairment, false-positive results for glucose in urine with reducing substances
Dose: *by intramuscular injection or intravenous injection or infusion,* 0.5–1 g every 6–12 hours; CHILD, 125–250 mg every 8 hours

Kefzol® (Lilly)
Injection, powder for reconstitution, cephazolin (as sodium salt). Price 500-mg vial = **D**; 1-g vial = **E**

CEPHRADINE

Indications: see under Cefaclor
Cautions; Contra-indications; Side-effects: see under Cefaclor; also reduce doses in renal impairment, false-positive results for glucose in urine with reducing substances
Dose: *by mouth,* 250–500 mg every 6 hours; CHILD, 25–50 mg/kg daily in divided doses
By intramuscular injection or intravenous injection or infusion, 0.5–1 g every 6 hours; CHILD, 50–100 mg/kg daily in 4 divided doses

Velosef® (Squibb)
Capsules, orange/blue, cephradine 250 mg. Price 20 caps = **F**
Capsules, blue, cephradine 500 mg. Price 20 caps = **G**
Syrup (= elixir), orange, cephradine 125 mg/5 ml when reconstituted with water for preparations. Diluent syrup, life of diluted elixir 7 days. Price 100 ml = **E**
Syrup (= elixir), red, cephradine 250 mg/5 ml when reconstituted with water for preparations. Diluent as above. Price 100 ml = **F**
Injection, powder for reconstitution, cephradine. Price 500-mg vial = **C**; 1-g vial = **D**

5.1.3 Tetracyclines

The tetracyclines are broad-spectrum antibiotics whose usefulness has decreased as a result of increasing bacterial resistance. They remain, however, the treatment of choice for infections caused by chlamydia (causing trachoma, psittacosis, and lymphogranuloma venereum), rickettsia (including Q-fever), mycoplasma (respiratory and genital tract infections), and brucella. They are also used for the treatment of exacerbations of chronic bronchitis because of their activity against *H.influenzae.*

Microbiologically, there is little to choose between the various tetracyclines, the only exception being **minocycline** (Minocin®) which has a broader spectrum, is active against *Neisseria meningitidis* and is used for meningococcal prophylaxis.

The tetracyclines are deposited in growing bone and teeth (being bound to calcium) causing staining and occasionally dental hypoplasia, and should **not** be given to children under 12 years or to pregnant women. With the exception of **doxycycline** (Vibramycin®) and **minocycline** the tetracyclines may exacerbate renal failure and should **not** be given to patients with kidney disease. Absorption of tetracyclines is decreased by milk (except minocycline), antacids, and calcium, iron, and magnesium salts.

Super-infection with *Candida, Proteus,* or *Pseudomonas* may occur; overgrowth with staphylococci, causing fulminating enterocolitis, is an uncommon complication.

TETRACYCLINE

Indications: exacerbations of chronic bronchitis; infections due to brucella, chlamydia, mycoplasma, and rickettsia; severe acne vulgaris

Cautions: rarely causes photosensitivity. Drug interactions: see Appendix 1

Contra-indications: renal failure, pregnancy, children under 12 years of age

Side-effects: nausea, vomiting, diarrhoea; super-infection with resistant organisms; rarely allergic reactions

Dose: *by mouth,* 250–500 mg every 6 hours

By intramuscular injection, 100–200 mg every 6–8 hours

By intravenous infusion, 500 mg every 12 hours

Tetracycline Capsules, tetracycline hydrochloride 250 mg. Price 20 caps = **B**

Tetracycline Tablets, f/c or s/c, tetracycline hydrochloride 250 mg. Price 20 tabs = **B**

Tetracycline Mixture, tetracycline hydrochloride 125 mg (as tetracycline)/5 ml. Diluent syrup, life of diluted mixture 14 days. Price 100 ml = **D**

Achromycin® (Lederle)

Capsules, orange, tetracycline hydrochloride 250 mg. Price 20 caps = **C**

Tablets, orange, f/c, tetracycline hydrochloride 250 mg. Price 20 tabs = **C**

Powder, tetracycline hydrochloride. Price 25-g bottle = **H**

Syrup (= mixture), red, tetracycline hydrochloride 125 mg (as tetracycline)/5 ml. Diluent syrup, life of diluted mixture 14 days. Price 100 ml = **D**

Intramuscular injection, powder for reconstitution, tetracycline hydrochloride 100 mg, procaine hydrochloride 40 mg. Price per vial = **C**

Intravenous injection, powder for reconstitution, tetracycline hydrochloride. Price 250- and 500-mg vial (both) = **D**

Achromycin V® (Lederle)

Capsules, pink, tetracycline hydrochloride 250 mg (as tetracycline) with buffer. Price 20 caps = **E**

Syrup (= mixture), red, tetracycline hydrochloride 125 mg (as tetracycline)/ 5 ml with buffer. Do not dilute. Price 100 ml = **D**

Deteclo® (Lederle)

Tablets, blue, f/c, tetracycline hydrochloride 115.4 mg, chlortetracycline hydrochloride 115.4 mg, demeclocycline hydrochloride 69.2 mg. Price 20 tabs = **D**

Syrup (= mixture), red, tetracycline hydrochloride 28.85 mg (as tetracycline), chlortetracycline hydrochloride 28.85 mg (as chlortetracycline), and demeclocycline hydrochloride 17.3 mg (as demeclocycline)/5 ml when reconstituted with water for preparations. Do not dilute. Price 100 ml = **D**

Dose: 1 tablet or 20 ml mixture every 12 hours

Economycin® (DDSA)

Capsules, orange, tetracycline hydrochloride 250 mg. Price 20 caps = **B**

Tablets, orange, f/c, tetracycline hydrochloride 250 mg. Price 20 tabs = **A**

Sustamycin® (MCP)

Capsules, s/r, blue, tetracycline hydrochloride 250 mg. Price 20 caps = **E**

Dose: 2 capsules initially, then 1 every 12 hours

Tetrabid® (Organon)

Capsules, s/r, purple/yellow, tetracycline hydrochloride 250 mg. Price 20 caps = **E**

Dose: 2 capsules initially, then 1 every 12 hours

Tetrachel® (Berk)

Capsules, orange, tetracycline hydrochloride 250 mg. Price 20 caps = **B**

Tablets, orange, f/c, tetracycline hydrochloride 250 mg. Price 20 tabs = **B**

Syrup (= mixture), red, tetracycline hydrochloride 125 mg (as tetracycline)/5 ml. Diluent syrup, life of diluted mixture 14 days. Price 100 ml = **B**

Tetracyn® (Pfizer)

Capsules, yellow/black, tetracycline 250 mg (as hydrochloride). Price 20 caps = **C**

Tablets, orange, s/c, tetracycline 250 mg (as hydrochloride). Price 20 tabs = **C**

Intramuscular injection, powder for reconstitution, tetracycline 100 mg (as hydrochloride), procaine hydrochloride 40 mg. Price per vial = **C**

Tetrex® (Bristol)

Capsules, yellow/orange, tetracycline 250 mg (as phosphate complex). Price 20 caps = **E**

CHLORTETRACYCLINE HYDROCHLORIDE

Indications: see under Tetracycline

Cautions; Contra-indications; Side-effects: see under Tetracycline

Dose: 250–500 mg every 6 hours

Aureomycin® (Lederle)

Capsules, yellow, chlortetracycline hydrochloride 250 mg. Price 20 caps = **F**

Powder, chlortetracycline hydrochloride. Price 25-g bottle = **H**

CLOMOCYCLINE SODIUM

Indications: see under Tetracycline

Cautions; Contra-indications; Side-effects: see under Tetracycline

Dose: 170–340 mg every 6–8 hours

Megaclor® (Pharmax)
Capsules, red, clomocycline sodium 170 mg. Price 20 caps = **E**

DEMECLOCYCLINE HYDROCHLORIDE

Indications: see under Tetracycline
Cautions; Contra-indications; Side-effects: see under Tetracycline, but photosensitivity is more common
Dose: 150 mg every 6 hours *or* 300 mg every 12 hours

Ledermycin® (Lederle)
Capsules, red, demeclocycline hydrochloride 150 mg. Price 20 caps = **F**
Tablets, red, f/c, demeclocycline hydrochloride 300 mg. Price 20 tabs = **H**
Drops, yellow, demeclocycline hydrochloride 60 mg (as demeclocycline)/ml. Price 10 ml = **E**
Syrup (= mixture), red, demeclocycline hydrochloride 75 mg (as demeclocycline)/5 ml. Do not dilute. Price 100 ml = **E**

DOXYCYCLINE

Indications: see under Tetracycline
Cautions; Contra-indications; Side-effects: see under Tetracycline, except renal failure
Dose: 200 mg on 1st day, then 100 mg daily

Vibramycin® (Pfizer)
Capsules, green, doxycycline 100 mg (as hydrochloride). Price 20 caps = **I**
Syrup (= mixture), red, doxycycline 50 mg (as calcium chelate)/5 ml. Diluent syrup, life of diluted mixture 14 days. Price 30 ml = **D**

LYMECYCLINE

Indications: see under Tetracycline
Cautions; Contra-indications; Side-effects: see under Tetracycline
Dose: 408 mg every 12 hours

Tetralysal® (Farmitalia Carlo Erba)
Capsules, lymecycline 204 mg. Price 20 caps = **D**

METHACYCLINE HYDROCHLORIDE

Indications: see under Tetracycline
Cautions; Contra-indications; Side-effects: see under Tetracycline
Dose: 150 mg every 6 hours *or* 300 mg every 12 hours

Rondomycin® (Pfizer)
Capsules, red/white, methacycline hydrochloride 150 mg. Price 20 caps = **E**

MINOCYCLINE

Indications: see under Tetracycline; also meningococcal carrier state
Cautions; Contra-indications; Side-effects: see under Tetracycline; also dizziness and vertigo
Dose: 200 mg initially, then 100 mg every 12 hours

Acne, initially 100–200 mg daily, then 50 mg twice daily

Minocin® (Lederle)
Tablets, beige, f/c, minocycline 50 mg (as hydrochloride). Price 20 tabs = **F**
Tablets, orange, f/c, minocycline 100 mg (as hydrochloride). Price 20 tabs = **H**

OXYTETRACYCLINE

Indications: see under Tetracycline
Cautions; Contra-indications; Side-effects: see under Tetracycline
Dose: *by mouth,* 250–500 mg every 6 hours
By intramuscular injection, 100 mg every 8–12 hours

Oxytetracycline Capsules, oxytetracycline hydrochloride 250 mg. Price 20 caps = **B**
Oxytetracycline Tablets, f/c or s/c, oxytetracycline dihydrate 250 mg. Price 20 tabs = **B**
Oxytetracycline Mixture, oxytetracycline 125 mg (as calcium salt)/5 ml. Diluent syrup, life of diluted mixture 14 days. Price 100 ml = **C**
Abbocin® (Abbott)
Tablets, yellow, s/c, oxytetracycline dihydrate 250 mg. Price 20 tabs = **B**
Berkmycen® (Berk)
Capsules, red/yellow, oxytetracycline hydrochloride 250 mg. Price 20 caps = **B**
Tablets, yellow, f/c, oxytetracycline dihydrate 250 mg. Price 20 tabs = **B**
Chemocycline® (Consolidated)
Tablets, yellow, s/c, oxytetracycline dihydrate 250 mg. Price 20 tabs = **B**
Syrup (= mixture), oxytetracycline 125 mg (as calcium salt)/5 ml. Diluent syrup, life of diluted mixture 14 days. Price 100 ml = **C**
Galenomycin® (Galen)
Tablets, brown, s/c, oxytetracycline dihydrate 250 mg. Price 20 tabs = **B**
Imperacin® (ICI)
Tablets, yellow, f/c, oxytetracycline dihydrate 250 mg. Price 20 tabs = **B**
Oxymycin® (DDSA)
Tablets, oxytetracycline dihydrate 250 mg. Price 20 tabs = **A**
Terramycin® (Pfizer)
Capsules, yellow, oxytetracycline 250 mg (as hydrochloride). Price 20 caps = **C**
Tablets, yellow, s/c, oxytetracycline 100 mg (as dihydrate). Price 20 tabs = **B**
Tablets, yellow, s/c, oxytetracycline 250 mg (as dihydrate). Price 20 tabs = **C**
Syrup (= mixture), oxytetracycline 125 mg (as calcium salt)/5 ml. Diluent syrup, life of diluted mixture 14 days. Price 100 ml = **C**
Intramuscular injection, powder for reconstitution, oxytetracycline 100 mg (as hydrochloride), procaine hydrochloride 40 mg. Price per vial = **C**
Unimycin® (Unigreg)
Capsules, yellow/red, oxytetracycline hydrochloride 250 mg. Price 20 caps = **C**

COMPOUND PREPARATIONS

Bisolvomycin® (Boehringer Ingelheim)
Capsules, turquoise/grey, oxytetracycline hydrochloride 250 mg, bromhexine hydrochloride 8 mg. Price 20 caps = **D**

Chymocyclar® (Armour)
Capsules, pink, tetracycline hydrochloride 250 mg, pancreatic concentrate 50 000 Armour units. Price 20 caps = **D**

Mysteclin® (Squibb)
Capsules, pink/brown, tetracycline hydrochloride 250 mg, nystatin 250 000 units. Price 20 caps = **D**
Tablets, orange, s/c, tetracycline hydrochloride 250 mg, nystatin 250 000 units. Price 20 tabs = **D**
Syrup, orange, tetracycline 125 mg, amphotericin 25 mg/5 ml. Price 100 ml = **D**

Terra-Bron® (Pfizer)
Syrup, oxytetracycline 250 mg (as calcium salt), ephedrine hydrochloride 7.5 mg, ipecacuanha liquid extract 0.03 ml/5 ml. Price 100 ml = **D**

Terramycin SF® (Pfizer)
Capsules, red, oxytetracycline 250 mg (as hydrochloride), ascorbic acid 75 mg, nicotinamide 25 mg, riboflavine 2.5 mg, thiamine mononitrate 2.5 mg. Price 20 caps = **D**

Tetracyn SF® (Pfizer)
Capsules, maroon, tetracycline 250 mg (as hydrochloride), ascorbic acid 75 mg, nicotinamide 25 mg, riboflavine 2.5 mg, thiamine mononitrate 2.5 mg. Price 20 caps = **C**

5.1.4 Aminoglycosides

This group includes amikacin, gentamicin, kanamycin, neomycin, netilmicin, streptomycin, and tobramycin. All are bactericidal and active against Gram-positive and Gram-negative organisms. Streptomycin and kanamycin are also active against *Mycobacterium tuberculosis* while amikacin, gentamicin, and tobramycin have activity against *Strep. faecalis* and *Ps. aeruginosa*, and tobramycin has activity against *Ps. aeruginosa*.

The aminoglycosides are not absorbed from the gut unless there is inflammatory bowel disease or liver failure and must, therefore, be given by injection to treat systemic infections. Excretion is principally via the kidney and if there is renal impairment accumulation occurs in the blood with increased risk of side-effects which are dose-related.

The important side-effects are ototoxicity, and to a lesser degree nephrotoxicity, and occur most commonly in the elderly and in patients with renal failure. Where possible, the aminoglycosides should be avoided in pregnancy as they cross the placenta and can cause foetal eighth nerve damage. Care must therefore be taken with the dose of this group of antibiotics and, if possible, serum concentrations should be monitored to prevent toxicity and, at the same time, ensure efficacy.

Serum concentrations are measured by microbiological methods, blood being taken approximately one hour after an intramuscular injection and also just before the next dose. One-hour concentrations of **gentamicin** should not exceed 10 micrograms/ml while the pre-dose (trough) concentrations should be less than 2 micrograms/ml.

Simultaneous administration of the aminoglycosides with the potentially ototoxic diuretics, frusemide, ethacrynic acid, and related compounds should be avoided. If it is necessary to administer an aminoglycoside and one of these diuretics to a patient the doses should be separated by as long a period as practicable.

Gentamicin (Cidomycin®, Genticin®) is the most important of the aminoglycosides and is widely used for the treatment of serious infections. It has a broad spectrum but is inactive against anaerobes and has poor activity against haemolytic streptococci and pneumococci. When used for the 'blind' therapy of undiagnosed serious infections it is frequently given in conjunction with a penicillin, such as carbenicillin, and/or metronidazole.

The daily dose is up to 5 mg/kg. Higher doses are occasionally indicated for serious infections, especially in the neonate or compromised host. When high doses are being given or if there is renal failure, serum concentrations **must** be measured. If renal function is normal gentamicin is given in divided doses every 8 hours.

If there is impairment of renal function the time between doses must be increased and if uraemia is severe the individual dose should also be reduced. Nomograms are available for the calculation of the dose, which depends on the patient's age, weight, and renal function.

Kanamycin (Kannasyn®, Kantrex®) has been replaced by gentamicin as the drug of first choice for serious infections caused by Gram-negative bacilli.

Amikacin (Amikin®) is a derivative of kanamycin and has one important advantage over gentamicin in that it is stable to 8 of the 9 classified aminoglycoside-inactivating enzymes whereas gentamicin is inactivated by 5. It is principally indicated for the treatment of serious infections caused by Gram-negative bacilli which are resistant to gentamicin, and is given by intramuscular or intravenous injection.

Tobramycin (Nebcin®) is similar to gentamicin. It is slightly more active against *Ps. aeruginosa* but shows less activity against certain other Gram-ve bacteria. Recent studies indicate that it is less nephrotoxic than gentamicin.

Netilmicin (Netillin®) also has similar activity to gentamicin, but is claimed to cause less ototoxicity and nephrotoxicity than other aminoglycosides.

Neomycin is too toxic for parenteral administration and can only be used for infections of the skin or mucous membranes or to reduce the bacterial population of the colon prior to bowel surgery or in hepatic failure. Topical application may lead to hypersensitivity, and oral administration to malabsorption. Small amounts of neomycin may be absorbed from the gut in patients with hepatic failure and, as these patients may also be uraemic, cumulation may occur with resultant ototoxicity. Similarly, ototoxicity may result from topical application to large areas, for example burns. **Framycetin** is almost identical with neomycin in its actions and uses.

Streptomycin is today almost entirely reserved for the treatment of tuberculosis (section 5.1.9) as other sensitive organisms, principally Gram-negative bacilli, can rapidly become resistant.

GENTAMICIN

Indications: septicaemia and neonatal sepsis; meningitis and other CNS infections; biliary tract infection, acute pyelonephritis or prostatitis, endocarditis caused by *Strep. viridans* or *faecalis* (with a penicillin)

Cautions: increase dose interval in renal impairment. Drug interactions: see Appendix 1

Contra-indications: pregnancy

Side-effects: vestibular damage, reversible nephrotoxicity

Dose: by intramuscular injection, 2–5 mg/kg daily, in divided doses every 8 hours. In renal impairment the interval between successive doses should be increased to 12 hours when the creatinine clearance is 30–70 ml/minute, 24 hours for 10–30 ml/minute, 48 hours for 5–10 ml/minute, and 3–4 days after dialysis for less than 5 ml/minute

CHILD, up to 2 weeks, 3 mg/kg every 12 hours; 2 weeks–12 years, 2 mg/kg every 8 hours

By intrathecal injection, 1 mg daily, with 2–4 mg/kg daily *by intramuscular injection* in divided doses every 8 hours

Gentamicin Injection, gentamicin 40 mg (as sulphate)/ml, price 2-ml amp or vial = **D**; 60 mg (as sulphate)/ml, price 2-ml amp = **E**

Gentamicin Injection, Paediatric, gentamicin 5 mg (as sulphate)/ml, price 2-ml amp = **B**; 10 mg (as sulphate)/ml, price 2-ml vial = **C**

Gentamicin Injection, powder for reconstitution, gentamicin (as sulphate). Price 1-g vial = **J**

Cidomycin® (Roussel)

Injection, gentamicin 40 mg (as sulphate)/ml. Price 2-ml amp or vial = **D**; 2-ml syringe = **E**

Injection, gentamicin 80 mg (as sulphate)/ml. Price 1.5-ml syringe = **F**

Paediatric injection, gentamicin 10 mg (as sulphate)/ml. Price 2-ml vial = **C**

Intrathecal injection, gentamicin 5 mg (as sulphate)/ml. Price 1-ml amp = **C**

Powder (for preparing injections), gentamicin (as sulphate). Price 1-g bottle = **J**

Garamycin® (Kirby-Warrick)

Injection, gentamicin 40 mg (as sulphate)/ml. Price 2-ml amp or vial = **D** (Hosp. only)

Paediatric injection, gentamicin 10 mg (as sulphate)/ml. Price 2-ml vial = **C** (Hosp. only)

Genticin® (Nicholas)

Injection, gentamicin 40 mg (as sulphate)/ml. Price 2-ml amp or vial = **D**

Paediatric injection, gentamicin 10 mg (as sulphate)/ml. Price 2-ml vial = **C**

Intrathecal injection, gentamicin 1 mg (as sulphate)/ml. Price 2-ml amp = **C**

Powder (for preparing injections), gentamicin (as sulphate). Price 1-g vial = **J**

AMIKACIN

Indications: serious Gram-negative infections resistant to gentamicin

Cautions; Contra-indications; Side-effects: see under Gentamicin

Dose: by intramuscular or intravenous injection, 15 mg/kg daily in 2 divided doses

Amikin® (Mead Johnson)

Injection, amikacin 250 mg (as sulphate)/ml. Price 2-ml vial = **I**

Paediatric injection, amikacin 50 mg (as sulphate)/ml. Price 2-ml amp = **E**

FRAMYCETIN SULPHATE

Indications: see under Neomycin Sulphate

Cautions; Contra-indications; Side-effects: see under Gentamicin

Dose: by mouth, 2–4 g daily

Soframycin® (Roussel)

Tablets, scored, framycetin sulphate 250 mg. Price 20 tabs = **F**

Powder (for preparing intrathecal or subconjunctival injections and topical solutions), framycetin sulphate. Price 500-mg vial = **E**

KANAMYCIN

Indications: serious Gram-negative infections resistant to gentamicin

Cautions; Contra-indications; Side-effects: see under Gentamicin

Dose: by mouth, 250–500 mg every 6 hours

By intramuscular injection, 250 mg every 6 hours *or* 500 mg every 12 hours

By slow intravenous infusion, 15–30 mg/kg daily in divided doses every 8–12 hours

Kannasyn® (Winthrop)

Solution (=injection), kanamycin 250 mg (as sulphate)/ml. Price 4-ml vial = **I**

Powder (for preparing injections), kanamycin (as acid sulphate). Price 1-g vial = **I**

Kantrex® (Bristol)

Capsules, yellow, kanamycin 250 mg (as sulphate). Price 20 caps = **G**

Injection, kanamycin 333 mg (as sulphate)/ml. Price 3-ml vial (1 g) = **F**

NEOMYCIN SULPHATE

Indications: bowel sterilisation prior to surgery

Cautions; Contra-indications; Side-effects: see under Gentamicin

Dose: by mouth, 1 g every 4 hours

Neomycin Elixir, neomycin sulphate 100 mg/5 ml. Price 100 ml = **C**

Mycifradin® (Upjohn)
Powder (for preparing injections and topical solutions), neomycin sulphate. Price 500-mg vial = **D**
Nivemycin® (Boots)
Tablets, neomycin sulphate 500 mg. Price 20 tabs = **E**
Elixir, neomycin sulphate 100 mg/5 ml. Price 100 ml = **C**

NETILMICIN

Indications: serious Gram-negative infections resistant to gentamicin
Cautions; Contra-indications; Side-effects: see under Gentamicin
Dose: *by intramuscular or intravenous injection or infusion,* 4–6 mg/kg daily, in divided doses every 8 or 12 hours; in severe infections, up to 7.5 mg/kg daily in divided doses every 8 hours (usually for 48 hours)
INFANT age up to 1 week, 3 mg/kg every 12 hours; age over 1 week, 2.5–3 mg/kg every 12 hours; CHILD 2–2.5 mg/kg every 8 hours

▼ **Netillin®** (Kirby-Warrick)
Injection, netilmicin 10 mg (as sulphate)/ml. Price 1.5-ml amp = **D**
Injection, netilmicin 50 mg (as sulphate)/ml. Price 1-ml amp = **E**
Injection, netilmicin 100 mg (as sulphate)/ml. Price 1-ml amp = **E**; 1.5-ml amp or vial = **F**; 2-ml amp or vial = **G**

TOBRAMYCIN

Indications: infections caused by *Ps. aeruginosa* (see notes above)
Cautions; Contra-indications; Side-effects: see under Gentamicin
Dose: *by intramuscular injection or intravenous injection or infusion,* 3–5 mg/kg daily in divided doses every 8 hours; INFANT age up to 1 week 2 mg/kg twice daily; age over 1 week 2–2.5 mg/kg every 8 hours

Nebcin® (Lilly)
Injection, tobramycin 10 mg (as sulphate)/ml. Price 2-ml vial = **C**
Injection, tobramycin 40 mg (as sulphate)/ml. Price 1-ml vial = **C**; 2-ml vial = **D**

5.1.5 Macrolides

Erythromycin has a similar, although not identical, antibacterial spectrum to that of penicillin and is thus an alternative in penicillin-allergic patients. Indications include respiratory infections in children, legionnaire's disease and campylobacter enteritis. It has activity against gut anaerobes and has been used with neomycin for prophylaxis prior to bowel surgery.

Erythromycin is a relatively insoluble antibiotic and the volume required for intramuscular injection is large (10 ml for 500 mg)—this route of administration is, therefore, best avoided, the drug being given by mouth or intravenous injection.

Erythromycin estolate, if given for more than 14 days, may cause cholestatic jaundice. This may rarely occur with other erythromycin preparations.

ERYTHROMYCIN

Indications: alternative to penicillin in hypersensitive patients; sinusitis, diphtheria and whooping cough prophylaxis; legionnaire's disease
Cautions: hepatic impairment
Contra-indications: estolate contra-indicated in liver disease
Side-effects: nausea, vomiting, diarrhoea after large doses
Dose: *by mouth,* 250–500 mg every 6 hours; CHILD, 125–250 mg every 6 hours
By intramuscular injection, 100 mg every 4–8 hours
By slow intravenous injection or infusion, 300 mg every 6 hours *or* 600 mg every 8 hours; CHILD, 30–50 mg/kg daily in divided doses every 6 hours

Erythromycin Tablets, e/c, s/c or f/c, erythromycin 250 mg. Price 20 tabs = **C**
Erycen® (Berk)
Tablets, orange, e/c, f/c, erythromycin 250 mg. Price 20 tabs = **C**
Erythrocin® (Abbott)
Tablets, f/c, erythromycin 250 mg (as stearate). Price 20 tabs = **E**
Tablets, f/c, erythromycin 500 mg (as stearate). Price 20 tabs = **F**
Suspension (=mixture), erythromycin 100 mg (as stearate)/5 ml. Diluent syrup (without preservative), life of diluted mixture 14 days. Price 100 ml = **D**
Intramuscular injection, erythromycin 50 mg (as ethylsuccinate)/ml. Price 2-ml amp = **C**
Intravenous injection, powder for reconstitution, erythromycin (as lactobionate). Price 300-mg vial = **D**; 1-g vial = **G**
Erythromid® (Abbott)
Tablets, orange, e/c, f/c, erythromycin 250 mg. Price 20 tabs = **D**
Erythroped® (Abbott)
Suspension PI (=paediatric mixture), erythromycin 125 mg (as ethylsuccinate)/5 ml when reconstituted with water for preparations. Diluent syrup, life of diluted mixture 5 days. Price 100 ml = **D**
Suspension (=mixture), erythromycin 250 mg (as ethylsuccinate)/5 ml when reconstituted with water for preparations. Diluent as above. Price 100 ml = **E**
Suspension Forte (=strong mixture), erythromycin 500 mg (as ethylsuccinate)/5 ml when reconstituted with water for preparations. Diluent as above. Price 100 ml = **F**
Ilosone® (Dista)
Capsules, ivory/red, erythromycin 250 mg (as estolate). Price 20 caps = **E**

Tablets, pink, erythromycin 500 mg (as estolate). Price 20 tabs = **F**
Suspension (=mixture), orange, erythromycin 125 mg (as estolate)/5 ml. Diluent syrup, life of diluted mixture 14 days. Price 100 ml = **D**
Suspension forte (=strong mixture), orange, erythromycin 250 mg (as estolate)/5 ml. Diluent as above. Price 100 ml = **F**

Ilotycin® (Lilly)
Tablets, red, e/c, erythromycin 250 mg. Price 20 tabs = **D**

Retcin® (DDSA)
Tablets, red, e/c, erythromycin 250 mg. Price 20 tabs = **C**

5.1.6 Clindamycin and lincomycin

These antibiotics have a very limited use because of their serious side-effects.

Clindamycin (Dalacin C®), which is more active and better absorbed from the gut, has generally replaced **lincomycin** (Lincocin®).

They are active against Gram-positive cocci, including penicillin-resistant staphylococci and also against many anaerobes, especially *Bacteroides fragilis*. They are well concentrated in bone and excreted in bile and urine.

Clindamycin is recommended for staphylococcal bone and joint infections, and intra-abdominal sepsis.

The most serious toxic effect of clindamycin and lincomycin is pseudomembranous colitis which may be fatal and is commonest in middle-aged and elderly females, especially following operation. This complication may occur with most antibiotics but is more frequently seen with clindamycin and is due to a toxin produced by *Clostridium difficile,* an anaerobic organism resistant to many antibiotics including clindamycin. It is sensitive to vancomycin administered by mouth (section 5.1.7).

CLINDAMYCIN

Indications: staphylococcal bone and joint infections, peritonitis
Cautions: discontinue immediately if diarrhoea or colitis develops; impaired hepatic or renal function. Drug interactions: see Appendix 1
Contra-indications: diarrhoeal states
Side-effects: diarrhoea (discontinue treatment), nausea, vomiting, pseudomembranous colitis
Dose: *by mouth,* 150–300 mg every 6 hours; CHILD, 75–150 mg every 6 hours
By intramuscular injection or slow intravenous infusion, 0.6–2.7 g daily in 2–4 divided doses; CHILD, 15–40 mg/kg daily in 3–4 divided doses

Dalacin C® (Upjohn)
Capsules, lavender, clindamycin 75 mg (as hydrochloride). Price 20 caps = **E**
Capsules, lavender/maroon, clindamycin 150 mg (as hydrochloride). Price 20 caps = **G**
Paediatric suspension (=mixture), pink, clindamycin 75 mg (as palmitate hydrochloride)/5 ml when reconstituted with purified water, freshly boiled and cooled. Diluent purified water, freshly boiled and cooled, life of diluted mixture 14 days. Price 100 ml = **F**
Injection, clindamycin 150 mg (as phosphate)/ml. Price 2-ml amp = **E**; 4-ml amp = **F**

LINCOMYCIN

Indications: see under Clindamycin, also notes above
Cautions; Contra-indications; Side-effects: see under Clindamycin
Dose: *by mouth,* 500 mg every 6–8 hours
By intramuscular injection, 600 mg every 12–24 hours
By slow intravenous infusion, 600 mg every 8–12 hours

Lincomycin Injection, lincomycin 300 mg (as hydrochloride)/ml. Price 2-ml amp = **B**

Lincocin® (Upjohn)
Capsules, blue, lincomycin 500 mg (as hydrochloride). Price 20 caps = **H**
Syrup (=elixir), red, lincomycin 250 mg (as hydrochloride)/5 ml. Diluent syrup, life of diluted elixir 14 days. Price 100 ml = **F**
Injection, lincomycin 300 mg (as hydrochloride)/ml. Price 2-ml amp = **D**

Mycivin® (Boots)
Injection, lincomycin 300 mg (as hydrochloride)/ml. Price 2-ml amp = **B**

5.1.7 Other antibiotics

Antibiotics discussed in this section include chloramphenicol, colistin, fusidic acid, novobiocin, polymyxin B, spectinomycin, and vancomycin.

Chloramphenicol is a potent, potentially toxic, broad-spectrum antibiotic which should be reserved for the treatment of life-threatening infections particularly those caused by *Haemophilus influenzae* or *Klebsiella pneumoniae* and also for typhoid fever.

Eye-drops of chloramphenicol (see section 11.3.1) are useful for the treatment of bacterial conjunctivitis.

CHLORAMPHENICOL

Indications: see notes above
Cautions: avoid repeated courses and prolonged treatment; reduce doses in hepatic or renal impairment; periodic blood counts required; interferes with development of immunity; caution in neonates (may cause 'grey syndrome'). Drug interactions: see Appendix 1
Side-effects: leucopenia, thrombocytopenia, irreversible aplastic anaemia, peripheral neuritis, optic neuritis, erythema multiforme, nausea, vomiting, diarrhoea
Dose: *by mouth,* 500 mg every 6 hours
By intravenous or intramuscular injection, 1 g every 6–8 hours; CHILD, pyogenic meningitis, 50–100 mg/kg daily in divided doses every 6

hours; INFANTS under 1 month 25 mg/kg daily in divided doses every 6 hours

Chloromycetin® (P-D)
Capsules, white/grey, chloramphenicol 250 mg. Price 20 caps = **D**
Suspension (=mixture), chloramphenicol 125 mg (as palmitate)/5 ml. Diluent syrup, life of diluted mixture 14 days. Price 100 ml = **D**
Injection, powder for reconstitution, chloramphenicol (as sodium succinate). Price 300 mg vial = **C**; 1.2-g vial = **D**
Powder, chloramphenicol. Price 5-g vial = **D**

Kemicetine® (Farmitalia Carlo Erba)
Injection, powder for reconstitution, chloramphenicol (as sodium succinate). Price 1-g vial = **C**
Powder, chloramphenicol. Price 1-g vial = **D**

Colistin is a polymyxin antibiotic active against Gram-negative organisms including *Ps. aeruginosa* but there are very few, if any, indications for its use in the treatment of systemic infection.

It is **not** absorbed when given by mouth but is sometimes prescribed in infantile gastro-enteritis and used topically for skin infection and also as ear drops.

COLISTIN

Indications: see notes above
Cautions: reduce dose in renal impairment. Drug interactions: see Appendix 1
Side-effects: perioral paraesthesia, vertigo, muscle weakness, apnoea
Dose: *by mouth,* 1.5–3 million units every 8 hours
By intravenous or intramuscular injection, 2 million units every 8 hours

Colomycin® (Pharmax)
Tablets, scored, colistin sulphate 1.5 million units. Price 20 tabs = **J**
Syrup (=elixir), pink, colistin sulphate 250 000 units/5 ml when reconstituted with water for preparations. Diluent syrup, life of diluted elixir 14 days. Price 80 ml = **E**
Injection, powder for reconstitution, colistin sulphomethate sodium. Price 500 000-unit vial = **C**; 1 million-unit vial = **D**

Fusidic acid and its salts are narrow-spectrum antibiotics. The only indication for their use is in infections caused by penicillin-resistant staphylococci, especially osteomyelitis, as they are well concentrated in bone.

SODIUM FUSIDATE

Indications: see notes above
Cautions: liver-function tests required
Side-effects: nausea, vomiting, rashes, jaundice, reversible change in liver function
Dose: *by mouth,* 500 mg every 8 hours
By slow intravenous infusion, 500 mg over 6 hours, 3 times daily

Fucidin® (Leo)
Capsules, yellow, sodium fusidate 250 mg. Price 20 caps = **I**
Tablets, e/c, sodium fusidate 250 mg. Price 20 tabs = **I**
Suspension (=mixture), orange, fusidic acid 250 mg (≡sodium fusidate 175 mg)/5 ml. Do not dilute. Price 25 ml = **E**
Intravenous infusion, powder for reconstitution, diethanolamine fusidate 580 mg (≡sodium fusidate 500 mg), with buffer. Price per vial (with diluent) = **D**

Novobiocin has limited use owing to the frequent incidence of adverse effects and the development of bacterial resistance.

NOVOBIOCIN

Indications: see notes above
Cautions: periodic blood counts required
Contra-indications: infants under 6 months
Side-effects: nausea, vomiting, diarrhoea, rashes, erythema multiforme, leucopenia, eosinophilia, thrombocytopenia, haemolytic anaemia

Albamycin T® (Upjohn)
Capsules, blue/grey, novobiocin 125 mg (as sodium salt), tetracycline 125 mg (as hydrochloride). Price 20 caps = **E**
Paediatric suspension, granules for reconstitution, novobiocin 62.5 mg (as calcium salt), tetracycline 62.5 mg/5 ml. Price 100 ml = **D**

Polymyxin B sulphate is effective against Gram-negative organisms, particularly *Ps. aeruginosa.*

POLYMYXIN B SULPHATE

Indications: see notes above
Cautions: impaired renal function, may cause muscular weakness and respiratory depression. Drug interactions: see Appendix 1
Side-effects: dizziness, ataxia, circumoral and peripheral paraesthesia; haematuria, proteinuria, and tubular necrosis
Dose: *by slow intravenous infusion,* 15 000–25 000 units/kg daily in divided doses

Aerosporin® (Calmic)
Injection, powder for reconstitution, polymyxin B sulphate. Price 500 000-unit vial = **G**

Polybactrin® (Calmic)
Soluble GU, powder for reconstitution, polymyxin B sulphate 75 000 units, neomycin sulphate 20 000 units, bacitracin 1000 units. For bladder irrigation. Price per vial = **E**
Aerosol spray, polymyxin B sulphate 150 000 units, neomycin sulphate 495 000 units, bacitracin zinc 37 500 units. Price per pack = **I**

Spectinomycin is active against Gram-negative organisms, including *N. gonorrhoeae.* Its only indication is the treatment of gonorrhoea caused by penicillin-resistant organisms or in a penicillin-allergic patient.

SPECTINOMYCIN

Indications: see notes above
Side-effects: nausea, vomiting, headache, dizziness, urticaria, fever
Dose: by intramuscular injection, 2 g in men and 4 g in women

Trobicin® (Upjohn)
Injection, powder for reconstitution, spectinomycin (as hydrochloride). Price 2-g vial (with diluent) = **F**

Vancomycin is a bactericidal antibiotic. It is the drug of choice for antibiotic-associated pseudomembranous colitis, for which it is given by mouth, and also has a limited use by the intravenous route in the prophylaxis and treatment of endocarditis caused by Gram-positive cocci.

VANCOMYCIN

Indications: see notes above
Cautions: extravasation at injection site may cause necrosis and thrombophlebitis, blood counts and liver- and kidney-function tests required
Contra-indications: parenteral administration in renal insufficiency, deafness
Side-effects: after parenteral administration nausea, chills, fever, urticaria, rashes, eosinophilia, tinnitus (discontinue use), renal impairment
Dose: by mouth, 500 mg every 6 hours
By intravenous infusion, 500 mg over 20–30 minutes every 6 hours

Vancocin® (Lilly)
Powder (for oral use), vancomycin (as hydrochloride). Price 10-g bottle = **J**
Injection, powder for reconstitution, vancomycin (as hydrochloride). Price 500-mg vial = **I**

5.1.8 Co-trimoxazole and sulphonamides

The importance of the sulphonamides as chemotherapeutic agents has decreased as a result of increasing bacterial resistance and their replacement by antibiotics which are generally more active and less toxic.

The principal indication for sulphonamides used alone is urinary-tract infections caused by sensitive organisms and for this purpose **sulphamethizole** is effective.

The addition of the folic acid antagonist trimethoprim to sulphamethoxazole (co-trimoxazole), to sulphamoxole (co-trifamole), or to sulphadiazine (co-trimazine) increases the activity of the sulphonamides against Gram-negative bacteria except *Pseudomonas.*

Indications for **co-trimoxazole** (Bactrim®, Septrin® etc.) include urinary-tract infections, prostatitis, exacerbations of chronic bronchitis, invasive salmonella infections, brucellosis, and *Pneumocystis carinii* infections; **co-trifamole** (Co-Fram®) has similar antibacterial activity. **Co-trimazine** (Coptin®) is only indicated for urinary-tract infections.

Trimethoprim is described in section 5.1.11.3.

Side-effects of the sulphonamides include rashes, which are common, the Stevens-Johnson syndrome (erythema multiforme), renal failure (especially with the less soluble preparations), and blood dyscrasias, notably marrow depression and agranulocytosis.

Side-effects of co-trimoxazole, co-trifamole, and co-trimazine are similar to those of the sulphonamides but a particular watch should be kept for haematological effects and special care should be taken in patients who may be folate deficient such as the elderly and chronic sick. The effect on the foetus is unknown and the drugs should not be used in pregnancy.

The **longer-acting sulphonamides** (sulfametopyrazine, sulphadimethoxine, and sulphamethoxypyridazine) which are usually highly bound to plasma proteins, have the advantage of less frequent administration, but toxic effects due to accumulation are more likely to occur.

The **poorly-absorbed sulphonamides** (calcium sulphaloxate, phthalylsulphathiazole, and sulphaguanidine) have been widely used for the treatment of intestinal infections and pre-operative bowel preparation but can no longer be recommended for these indications (for use in acute and chronic diarrhoeas see sections 1.4.3 and 1.5).

For *topical preparations* of sulphonamides used in the treatment of burns see section 13.10.1.1.

CO-TRIMOXAZOLE

A mixture of sulphamethoxazole 5 parts, trimethoprim 1 part
Indications: invasive salmonellosis, typhoid fever, bone and joint infections due to *H. influenzae,* urinary-tract infections, sinusitis, exacerbations of chronic bronchitis, gonorrhoea in penicillin-allergic patients
Cautions: blood counts in prolonged treatment, maintain adequate fluid intake, renal impairment. Drug interactions: see Appendix 1
Contra-indications: pregnancy, infants under 6 weeks, renal or hepatic failure, jaundice, blood disorders
Side-effects: nausea, vomiting, rashes, erythema multiforme, epidermal necrolysis, eosinophilia, agranulocytosis, granulocytopenia, purpura, leucopenia; megaloblastic anaemia due to trimethoprim
Dose: by mouth, 960 mg every 12 hours, increased to 1.44 g in severe infections; 480 mg every 12 hours if treated for more than 14 days; CHILD, every 12 hours, 6 weeks to 5 months, 120 mg; 6 months to 5 years, 240 mg; 6–12 years, 480 mg
By intramuscular injection or intravenous infusion, 960 mg every 12 hours
Note: 480 mg of co-trimoxazole consists of sulphamethoxazole 400 mg and trimethoprim 80 mg

Co-trimoxazole Tablets, co-trimoxazole 480 mg. Price 20 tabs = **D**

Co-trimoxazole Tablets, Dispersible, co-trimoxazole 480 mg. Price 20 tabs = **D**

Co-trimoxazole Tablets, Double-strength, co-trimoxazole 960 mg. Price 20 tabs = **E**

Co-trimoxazole Tablets, Paediatric, co-trimoxazole 120 mg. Price 20 tabs = **B**

Co-trimoxazole Mixture, co-trimoxazole 480 mg/5 ml. Diluent syrup, life of diluted mixture 14 days. Price 100 ml = **E**

Co-trimoxazole Mixture, Paediatric, co-trimoxazole 240 mg/5 ml. Diluent as above. Price 100 ml = **D**

Co-trimoxazole Intramuscular Injection, co-trimoxazole 320 mg/ml in solvent. Price 3-ml amp = **D**

Co-trimoxazole Solution, Strong Sterile, co-trimoxazole 96 mg/ml. **Co-trimoxazole Injection** is prepared by diluting this solution with 25 to 35 times its volume of dextrose intravenous infusion or sodium chloride intravenous infusion before use. Price 5-ml amp = **C**

Bactrim® (Roche)
Drapsules®(=tablets), orange, f/c, co-trimoxazole 480 mg. Price 20 tabs = **D**
Tablets (dispersible), yellow, scored, co-trimoxazole 480 mg. Price 20 tabs = **D**
Double-strength tablets, scored, co-trimoxazole 960 mg. Price 20 tabs = **E**
Paediatric tablets, co-trimoxazole 120 mg. Price 20 tabs = **B**
Adult suspension (=mixture), yellow, co-trimoxazole 480 mg/5 ml. Diluent syrup, life of diluted mixture 14 days. Price 100 ml = **E**
Paediatric syrup (=paediatric mixture), pink, co-trimoxazole 240 mg/5 ml. Diluent as above. Price 100 ml = **D**
Intramuscular injection, co-trimoxazole 320 mg/ml. Price 3-ml amp = **D**
Intravenous infusion, co-trimoxazole 96 mg/ml. To be diluted before use. Price 5-ml amp = **C** (Hosp. only)

Cotrimox® (Unimed)
Tablets, co-trimoxazole 480 mg. Price 20 tabs = **E**

Fectrim® (DDSA)
Tablets (dispersible), co-trimoxazole 480 mg. Price 20 tabs = **D**
Forte tablets (dispersible), co-trimoxazole 960 mg. Price 20 tabs = **E**
Paediatric tablets, co-trimoxazole 120 mg. Price 20 tabs = **B**

Septrin® (Wellcome)
Tablets, scored, co-trimoxazole 480 mg. Price 20 tabs = **E**
Dispersible tablets, orange, scored, co-trimoxazole 480 mg. Price 20 tabs = **E**
Forte tablets, scored, co-trimoxazole 960 mg. Price 20 tabs = **E**
Paediatric tablets, scored, co-trimoxazole 120 mg. Price 20 tabs = **C**
Adult suspension (=mixture), co-trimoxazole 480 mg/5 ml. Diluent syrup, life of diluted mixture 14 days. Price 100 ml = **E**
Paediatric suspension (=paediatric mixture), pink, co-trimoxazole 240 mg/5 ml. Diluent as above. Price 100 ml = **D**
Intramuscular injection, co-trimoxazole 320 mg/ml. Price 3-ml amp = **D**
Intravenous infusion, co-trimoxazole 96 mg/ml. To be diluted before use. Price 5-ml amp = **C**

CALCIUM SULPHALOXATE

Indications: see notes on poorly-absorbed sulphonamides
Cautions; Contra-indications; Side-effects: see under Co-trimoxazole; side-effects less common because of limited absorption
Dose: 1 g every 8 hours

Enteromide® (Consolidated)
Tablets, calcium sulphaloxate 500 mg. Price 20 tabs = **C**

CO-TRIFAMOLE

A mixture of sulphamoxole 5 parts and trimethoprim 1 part
Indications; Cautions; Contra-indications; Side-effects: see under Co-trimoxazole
Dose: 960 mg initially, then 480 mg every 12 hours; CHILD, 6–12 years, 480–720 mg initially, then 240–480 mg
Note: 480 mg of co-trifamole consists of sulphamoxole 400 mg and trimethoprim 80 mg

▼ Co-Fram® (Abbott)
Tablets, scored, co-trifamole 480 mg. Price 20 tabs = **E**

CO-TRIMAZINE

A mixture of sulphadiazine approx. 5 parts, trimethoprim 1 part
Indications: urinary-tract infections
Cautions; Contra-indications; Side-effects: see under Co-trimoxazole
Dose: 500 mg every 12 hours; CHILD, 125–250 mg every 12 hours
Note: 500 mg of co-trimazine consists of sulphadiazine 410 mg and trimethoprim 90 mg.

Coptin® (Pfizer)
Tablets, scored, co-trimazine 500 mg. Price 20 tabs = **E**
Suspension (=mixture), co-trimazine 250 mg/5 ml. Diluent syrup, life of diluted mixture 14 days. Price 100 ml = **E**

PHTHALYLSULPHATHIAZOLE

Indications: see notes on poorly-absorbed sulphonamides
Cautions; Contra-indications; Side-effects: see under Co-trimoxazole; side-effects less common because of limited absorption
Dose: 2–12 g daily in divided doses

Thalazole® (M&B)
Tablets, scored, phthalylsulphathiazole 500 mg. Price 20 tabs = **A**

SULFAMETOPYRAZINE

Indications: urinary-tract infections, chronic bronchitis
Cautions; Contra-indications; Side-effects: see under Co-trimoxazole
Dose: 2 g once weekly; CHILD, 30 mg/kg once weekly

Kelfizine W® (Farmitalia Carlo Erba)
Tablets, sulfametopyrazine 2 g. Tablets to be taken in water. Price 1 tab = **C**
Suspension (=mixture), sulfametopyrazine 500 mg/5 ml. Diluent syrup, life of diluted mixture 14 days. Price 20 ml (adult dose) = **C**; 10 ml (paediatric dose) = **C**

SULPHADIAZINE

Indications: meningococcal meningitis (for use with trimethoprim, see under Co-trimazine)
Cautions; Contra-indications; Side-effects: see under Co-trimoxazole
Dose: *by intramuscular injection or intravenous infusion,* 1–1.5 g every 4 hours

Sulphadiazine (M&B)
Injection, sulphadiazine 250 mg (as sodium salt)/ml. Price 4-ml amp = **B**

Streptotriad® (M&B)
Tablets, pink, scored, sulphadiazine 100 mg, streptomycin 65 mg (as sulphate), sulphadimidine 100 mg, sulphathiazole 100 mg. Price 20 tabs = **C**

Sulphatriad® (M&B)
Tablets, scored, sulphadiazine 185 mg, sulphamerazine 130 mg, sulphathiazole 185 mg. Price 20 tabs = **B**
Suspension (= mixture), sulphadiazine 185 mg, sulphamerazine 130 mg, sulphathiazole 185 mg/5 ml. Diluent syrup (without preservative), life of diluted mixture 14 days. Price 125 ml = **C**

SULPHADIMETHOXINE

Indications: urinary-tract infections, bronchitis
Cautions; Contra-indications; Side-effects: see under Co-trimoxazole
Dose: 1–2 g initially, then 0.5–1 g daily

Madribon® (Roche)
Tablets, scored, sulphadimethoxine 500 mg. Price 20 tabs = **C**

SULPHADIMIDINE

Indications: urinary-tract infections
Cautions; Contra-indications; Side-effects: see under Co-trimoxazole
Dose: *by intravenous or intramuscular injection,* 2 g initially, then 0.5–1 g every 6–8 hours

Sulphamezathine® (ICI)
Injection, sulphadimidine sodium 333 mg/ml. Price 3-ml (l-g) amp = **B**

SULPHAFURAZOLE

Indications: urinary-tract infections
Cautions; Contra-indications; Side-effects: see under Co-trimoxazole
Dose: 2 g initially, then 1 g every 4–6 hours

Gantrisin® (Roche)
Tablets, sulphafurazole 500 mg. Price 20 tabs = **B**
Syrup (=mixture), sulphafurazole 500 mg (as acetyl derivative)/5 ml. Diluent syrup, life of diluted mixture 14 days. Price 100 ml = **C**

SULPHAGUANIDINE

Indications: see notes on poorly-absorbed sulphonamides
Cautions; Contra-indications; Side-effects: see under Co-trimoxazole; rashes frequent
Dose: 3 g every 6–8 hours for 3 days, then 3 g every 12 hours for 4 days

Sulphaguanidine Tablets, sulphaguanidine 500 mg. Price 20 tabs = **B**

SULPHAMETHIZOLE

Indications: urinary-tract infections
Cautions; Contra-indications; Side-effects: see under Co-trimoxazole
Dose: 200 mg 5 times daily; CHILD up to 5 years 50 mg; 6–12 years 100 mg

Sulphamethizole Tablets, sulphamethizole 100 mg. Price 20 tabs = **A**

Urolucosil® (Warner)
Tablets, scored, sulphamethizole 100 mg. Price 20 tabs = **A**
Suspension (=mixture), sulphamethizole 100 mg/5 ml. Diluent syrup, life of diluted mixture 28 days. Price 200 ml = **C**

SULPHAMETHOXYPYRIDAZINE

Indications: urinary-tract infections
Cautions; Contra-indications; Side-effects: see under Co-trimoxazole
Dose: 1–2 g initially, then 500 mg daily

Lederkyn® (Lederle)
Tablets, peach, sulphamethoxypyridazine 500 mg. Price 20 tabs = **E**

SULPHAPHENAZOLE

Indications: infections due to sensitive organisms
Cautions; Contra-indications; Side-effects: see under Co-trimoxazole
Dose: 1 g every 12 hours for 2 days, then 500 mg every 12 hours

Orisulf® (Ciba)
Tablets, scored, sulphaphenazole 500 mg. Price 20 tabs = **B**

SULPHAPYRIDINE

Indications: dermatitis herpetiformis unresponsive to dapsone

Cautions; Contra-indications; Side-effects: see under Co-trimoxazole
Dose: 3–4 g daily; maintenance, 0.5–1 g

M&B 693® (M&B)
Tablets, scored, sulphapyridine 500 mg. Price 20 tabs = **B**

SULPHATHIAZOLE

Indications: infections due to sensitive organisms
Cautions; Contra-indications; Side-effects: see under Co-trimoxazole; side-effects frequent
Dose: 2 g initially, then 1 g every 4–6 hours

Thiazamide® (M&B)
Tablets, scored, sulphathiazole 500 mg. Price 20 tabs = **B**

SULPHAUREA

Indications: urinary-tract infections
Cautions; Contra-indications; Side-effects: see under Co-trimoxazole

Uromide® (Consolidated)
Tablets, yellow, sulphaurea 500 mg, phenazopyridine hydrochloride 50 mg. Price 20 tabs = **C**

5.1.9 Antituberculous drugs

The treatment of tuberculosis has two phases—an *initial phase* using at least three drugs and a *continuation phase* with two drugs.

Treatment, at least in the initial stages, requires specialised knowledge. This applies particularly to infections caused by bacteria resistant to any of the first-line drugs, isoniazid, rifampicin, streptomycin, ethambutol, and pyrazinamide.

INITIAL PHASE. The concurrent use of at least three drugs during the initial phase is designed to reduce the population of viable bacteria as rapidly as possible and to minimise the risk of ineffective treatment in those patients infected by drug-resistant bacteria. Treatment of choice for the initial phase involves the daily use of isoniazid and rifampicin supplemented by ethambutol or streptomycin. These drugs should be continued for at least 8 weeks and preferably until the result of drug-sensitivity testing is known.

CONTINUATION PHASE. After the initial phase, treatment is continued with only two drugs, one of which, in the absence of contra-indications, should always be isoniazid. The second drug may be rifampicin, ethambutol, or streptomycin (which can be given twice weekly with a high dose of isoniazid to allow treatment to be fully supervised).

DURATION OF TREATMENT. Sufficient information is now available on the outcome of treatment with the initial phase described above, followed by a continuation phase comprising daily isoniazid and rifampicin, to confirm that a course of *9 months duration* gives satisfactory results in pulmonary tuberculosis regardless of the extent of the disease.

This regimen may also be used in the treatment of extrapulmonary tuberculosis but until more information is available on the frequency of relapse, a total treatment period of *12 months* should be employed. The major causes of treatment failure are incorrect prescribing by the physician and inadequate compliance by the patient.

Isoniazid (Rimifon®) is relatively free from side-effects in doses not exceeding 300 mg daily. Higher doses are used in twice-weekly dosage regimens and also for tuberculous meningitis. Side-effects with higher doses are mainly neurological, and their incidence is reduced by pyridoxine 20–50 mg daily.

Streptomycin, as with most drugs for the treatment of tuberculosis, is given once a day. Patients over the age of 40 years and small patients such as Asian females require lower doses; in these groups serum concentrations should be measured.

Rifampicin (Rifadin®, Rimactane®) is a highly effective bactericidal drug. It should be given in a single dose before breakfast. Young children require a higher dose relative to their weight.

On daily treatment regimens, signs of hepatic toxicity (raised serum transaminases) may occur but are usually transient; the drug should be used with care in alcoholics and patients with liver disease.

On intermittent treatment six toxicity syndromes have been recognised—influenzal, abdominal, and respiratory symptoms, shock, renal failure, and thrombocytopenic purpura—and can occur in 20–30% of patients.

Rifampicin induces hepatic enzymes which accelerate the metabolism of several drugs including oestrogens, corticosteroids, sulphonylureas, and anticoagulants. The effectiveness of oral contraceptives is reduced and, where appropriate, alternative family planning advice should be offered. The drug should be avoided in pregnancy as the effect on the foetus is unknown.

Ethambutol (Myambutol®) should be avoided in very young children and in the elderly. It may cause loss of visual acuity and colour vision. Ocular toxicity is more likely in patients with renal impairment given full doses. This is not always reversible on stopping the drug and routine pretreatment ophthalmic examination is only of limited value as early recognition of ocular toxicity depends on the patient's own observations.

Pyrazinamide (Zinamide®) is a bactericidal drug active against *Mycobacterium tuberculosis* but not *M. bovis*. It is particularly useful in tuberculous meningitis because of good meningeal penetration.

Second-line drugs available for infections caused by resistant organisms, or when first-line drugs cause unacceptable side-effects, include **capreomycin** (Capastat®), **cycloserine**, and **sodium aminosalicylate**.

CAPREOMYCIN

Indications: tuberculosis resistant to first-line drugs

Cautions: renal, hepatic, or auditory impairment; do not give with streptomycin or other ototoxic drugs

Side-effects: hypersensitivity reactions including urticaria and rashes, changes in liver function, renal damage, hearing loss with tinnitus and vertigo, pain and induration at injection site

Dose: *by intramuscular injection*, 1 g daily (not more than 20 mg/kg)

Capastat® (Dista)

Injection, powder for reconstitution, capreomycin sulphate 1 million units (capreomycin approx. 1 g). Price per vial = **D**

CYCLOSERINE

Indications: tuberculosis resistant to first-line drugs

Cautions: reduce dose in renal impairment

Contra-indications: epilepsy, depression, severe anxiety, psychotic states, alcoholism

Side-effects: mainly neurological, including headache, dizziness, vertigo, drowsiness, convulsions; allergic rashes

Dose: 250 mg every 12 hours, increased to 250 mg every 8 hours; max. 1 g daily

Cycloserine (Lilly)

Capsules, red/grey, cycloserine 125 mg. Price 20 caps = **F**

Capsules, red/grey, cycloserine 250 mg. Price 20 caps = **G**

ETHAMBUTOL HYDROCHLORIDE

Indications: tuberculosis, in combination with other drugs, usually rifampicin and/or isoniazid; prophylaxis—section 5.1, table 2

Cautions: reduce dose in renal impairment, warn patients to report visual changes—see notes above

Contra-indications: young children, elderly patients, optic neuritis

Side-effects: optic neuritis, red/green colour blindness, peripheral neuritis

Dose: 15 mg/kg daily; CHILD 25 mg/kg daily for 60 days, followed by 15 mg/kg daily

Paediatric prophylaxis 15 mg/kg daily (with isoniazid)

Myambutol® (Lederle)

Tablets, yellow, ethambutol hydrochloride 100 mg. Price 20 tabs = **D**

Tablets, grey, ethambutol hydrochloride 400 mg. Price 20 tabs = **F**

Mynah 200® (Lederle)

Tablets, ethambutol hydrochloride 200 mg, isoniazid 100 mg. Price 20 tabs = **E**

Mynah 250® (Lederle)

Tablets, yellow, ethambutol hydrochloride 250 mg, isoniazid 100 mg. Price 20 tabs = **F**

Mynah 300® (Lederle)

Tablets, orange, ethambutol hydrochloride 300 mg, isoniazid 100 mg. Price 20 tabs = **F**

Mynah 365® (Lederle)

Tablets, pink, ethambutol hydrochloride 365 mg, isoniazid 100 mg. Price 20 tabs = **G**

ISONIAZID

Indications: tuberculosis, in combination with other drugs; prophylaxis—section 5.1, table 2

Cautions: impaired liver and kidney function, epilepsy, alcoholism. Drug interactions: see Appendix 1

Contra-indications: drug-induced liver disease

Side-effects: nausea, vomiting, hypersensitivity reactions including rashes, peripheral neuritis with high doses (treat with pyridoxine 10–20 mg daily), convulsions, psychotic episodes, agranulocytosis

Dose: *by mouth or intramuscular injection,* pulmonary tuberculosis, up to 300 mg daily (adults 3 mg/kg, children 6 mg/kg); up to 1 g (14 mg/kg) twice weekly

Tuberculous meningitis, 10 mg/kg daily

Isoniazid Tablets, isoniazid 50 and 100 mg. Price 20 tabs (both) = **A**

Isoniazid Elixir, isoniazid 50 mg/5 ml (see Formulary). Price 100 ml = **A**

Rimifon® (Roche)

Injection, isoniazid 25 mg/ml. Price 2-ml amp = **A**

PYRAZINAMIDE

Indications: tuberculosis, especially tuberculous meningitis

Cautions: impaired renal function, diabetes, gout, liver-function tests required

Contra-indications: liver damage

Side-effects: hepatotoxicity including fever, anorexia, hepatomegaly, jaundice, fulminating liver failure; nausea, vomiting, arthralgia, sideroblastic anaemia, urticaria

Dose: 20–30 mg/kg daily; max. 3 g daily

Zinamide® (MSD)

Tablets, scored, pyrazinamide 500 mg. Price 20 tabs = **D**

RIFAMPICIN

Indications: tuberculosis, in combination with other drugs, usually isoniazid and ethambutol; leprosy (section 5.1.10)

Cautions: hepatic impairment, alcoholism. Drug interactions: see Appendix 1. Also see notes

Contra-indications: jaundice, pregnancy

Side-effects: gastro-intestinal symptoms including anorexia, nausea, vomiting, diarrhoea; influenzal syndrome including chills, fever, dizziness, bone pain; respiratory symptoms including shortness of breath, wheezing; collapse and shock; acute renal failure; thrombocytopenic purpura; hepatic reactions with alterations of

liver function, jaundice; urticaria and rashes; urine, saliva, and other body secretions coloured orange-red
Dose: 450–600 mg (about 10 mg/kg) daily preferably before breakfast; CHILD up to 20 mg/kg daily to a max. of 600 mg

Rifampicin Capsules, rifampicin 150 mg. Price 20 caps = **G**; 300 mg, price 20 caps = **I**
Rifampicin Mixture, rifampicin 100 mg/5ml. Price 100 ml = **F**
Rifampicin and Isoniazid 150 + 100 Tablets, rifampicin 150 mg, isoniazid 100 mg. Price 20 tabs = **G**
Rifampicin and Isoniazid 300 + 150 Tablets, rifampicin 300 mg, isoniazid 150 mg. Price 20 tabs = **I**
Rifadin® (Lepetit)
Capsules, blue/red, rifampicin 150 mg. Price 20 caps = **G**
Capsules, red, rifampicin 300 mg. Price 20 caps = **I**
Syrup (=mixture), red, rifampicin 100 mg/5 ml. Do not dilute. Price 120 ml = **F**
Rifinah 150® (Lepetit)
Tablets, pink, rifampicin 150 mg, isoniazid 100 mg. Price 20 tabs = **G**
Rifinah 300® (Lepetit)
Tablets, orange, rifampicin 300 mg, isoniazid 150 mg. Price 20 tabs = **I**
Rimactane® (Ciba)
Capsules, red, rifampicin 150 mg. Price 20 caps = **G**
Capsules, red/brown, rifampicin 300 mg. Price 20 caps = **I**
Syrup (=mixture), red, rifampicin 100 mg/5 ml. Do not dilute. Price 100 ml = **F**
Rimactazid 150® (Ciba)
Tablets, pink, s/c, rifampicin 150 mg, isoniazid 100 mg. Price 20 tabs = **G**
Rimactazid 300® (Ciba)
Tablets, orange, s/c, rifampicin 300 mg, isoniazid 150 mg. Price 20 tabs = **I**

SODIUM AMINOSALICYLATE

Indications: tuberculosis resistant to first-line drugs
Cautions; Contra-indications: see under Aspirin (section 10.1.1.1)
Side-effects: see under Aspirin, section 10.1.1.1; also jaundice, albuminuria, and haematuria
Dose: 8–15 g daily in divided doses

Inapasade® (S&N Pharm.)
Granules, pink, single-dose sachets, sodium aminosalicylate 6 g, isoniazid 150 mg. Price 20 sachets = **F**
Paediatric granules, pink, single-dose sachets, sodium aminosalicylate 2 g, isoniazid 50 mg. Price 20 sachets = **D**

STREPTOMYCIN

Indications: tuberculosis, especially in patients with impaired liver function
Cautions; Contra-indications; Side-effects: see under Aminoglycosides, section 5.1.4; also hypersensitivity reactions, paraesthesia of mouth
Dose: by intramuscular injection, 1 g daily; in patients over 40 years, 750 mg; in small patients, 500 mg

Streptomycin Sulphate (Evans)
Injection, powder for reconstitution, streptomycin (as sulphate). Price 1-g vial = **B**

5.1.10 Antileprotic drugs

Treatment of leprosy varies with the type of disease, and advice from a member of the Panel of Leprosy Opinion is essential. Details of the Panel can be found in *Memorandum on Leprosy,* DHSS, London, H. M. Stationery Office, 1977 [in Scotland, NHS Circular 1978(GEN)44].

Dapsone, a sulphone, is the most widely used drug for the treatment of leprosy. However, dapsone resistance has recently become an increasing problem, and if the patient has severe (multibacillary) infection dapsone should be given initially in combination with **rifampicin** (section 5.1.9) and **clofazimine** (Lamprene®). Rifampicin should be continued for at least 4 weeks, clofazimine for one year, and dapsone for life.

Patients with few organisms (paucibacillary) are treated with dapsone for from 3 to 10 years depending on precise classification of the disease and response to therapy.

Lepra reactions, fever, erythema nodosum, painful polyneuritis, and iritis may complicate treatment, especially with dapsone, and are treated with clofazimine (which has an anti-inflammatory action), or prednisolone. Neurological involvement commonly occurs in leprosy and therefore neuropathy resulting from treatment with dapsone may be overlooked.

DAPSONE

Indications: leprosy
Cautions: cardiac or pulmonary disease. Drug interactions: see Appendix 1
Side-effects: neuropathy, allergic dermatitis, anorexia, nausea, vomiting, headache, insomnia, tachycardia, anaemia, hepatitis, agranulocytosis, lepra reactions (discontinue if eye or nerve trunks affected)
Dose: 25–50 mg twice weekly, gradually increased to 400 mg twice weekly or 100 mg daily

Dapsone Tablets, dapsone 50 and 100 mg. Price 20 tabs (both) = **B**

CLOFAZIMINE

Indications: leprosy
Cautions: hepatic and renal impairment—function tests required
Side-effects: nausea, giddiness, headache, and diarrhoea with high doses, red coloration of

skin and urine, blue-black discoloration of lesions
Dose: previously untreated patients, 100 mg 3 times weekly; sulphone-resistant patients, 100 mg 6 times weekly
Lepra reactions, 200 mg daily

Lamprene® (Geigy)
Capsules, brown, clofazimine 100 mg. Price 20 caps = **D**

5.1.11 Other antimicrobial drugs

5.1.11.1 Metronidazole
5.1.11.2 Urinary antimicrobial drugs
5.1.11.3 Trimethoprim
5.1.11.4 Acrosoxacin

5.1.11.1 METRONIDAZOLE

Metronidazole (Flagyl®) is an antimicrobial drug with high activity against anaerobic bacteria and protozoa. Indications include surgical and gynaecological sepsis in which its activity against colonic anaerobes, especially *Bacteroides fragilis,* is important, trichomonal vaginitis (section 5.4.3), and *Entamoeba histolytica* and *Giardia lamblia* infections (section 5.4.2). Side-effects are uncommon but neuropathy can occur during prolonged therapy. Gastro-intestinal disturbances may be minimised by taking tablets with or after food, but the mixture (which contains benzoyl metronidazole) should be taken at least 1 hour before food.

METRONIDAZOLE

Indications: see notes above
Cautions: active CNS disease, disulfiram-like reaction with alcohol. Drug interactions: see Appendix 1
Side-effects: nausea, drowsiness, headache, rashes, leucopenia, darkening of urine, peripheral neuropathy in prolonged treatment, dizziness, ataxia, transient epileptiform seizures with high doses
Dose: anaerobic infections, *by mouth,* 400 mg every 8 hours; *by rectum,* 1 g every 8 hours for 3 days, then 1 g every 12 hours; *by intravenous infusion,* 500 mg every 8 hours for up to 7 days; CHILD, any route, 7.5 mg/kg every 8 hours
Trichomoniasis, *by mouth,* 200 mg every 8 hours for 7 days *or* 800 mg in the morning and 1.2 g at night for 2 days *or* 2 g as a single dose
Amoebiasis, *by mouth,* 2–2.4 g daily for 2–3 days *or* 800 mg every 8 hours for 5 days
Giardiasis, *by mouth,* 2 g daily for 3 days

Metronidazole Tablets, metronidazole 200 mg. Price 20 tabs = **D**
Flagyl® (M&B)
Tablets, scored, metronidazole 200 mg. Price 20 tabs = **E**
Tablets, yellow, scored, metronidazole 400 mg. Price 20 tabs = **F**
▼*Suppositories,* metronidazole 500 mg. Price 20 suppos = **I**
▼*Suppositories,* metronidazole 1 g. Price 20 suppos = **J**
Compak, tablets, scored, metronidazole 200 mg, with pessaries, yellow, nystatin 100000 units. Price 21 tablets and 14 pessaries (with applicator) = **F**
Intravenous infusion, metronidazole 5 mg/ml. Price 20-ml amp = **E**; 100-ml bottle = **G**
▼ **Flagyl S**® (M&B)
Suspension (= mixture), metronidazole 200 mg (as benzoyl metronidazole)/5 ml. Diluent syrup, life of diluted mixture 14 days. Price 100 ml = **F**
Vaginyl® (DDSA)
Tablets, scored, metronidazole 200 mg. Price 20 tabs = **D**

5.1.11.2 URINARY ANTIMICROBIAL DRUGS

Nitrofurantoin is active against many organisms causing urinary-tract infection and this is the only indication for its use. Blood concentrations are low and it should **not** be prescribed for acute pyelonephritis which may be associated with septicaemia.

Nalidixic acid (Negram®) has a narrower spectrum of activity than nitrofurantoin, and is effective against certain Gram-negative bacteria, but not against *Pseudomonas* spp. **Cinoxacin** (Cinobac®) has similar antibacterial activity to nalidixic acid.

Hexamine should **not** be used any longer as it is only bacteriostatic, requires acidification of urine, and frequently causes side-effects.

NITROFURANTOIN

Indications: urinary-tract infections
Cautions: drug interactions: see Appendix 1
Contra-indications: impaired renal function, infants less than 1 month old, glucose-6-phosphate dehydrogenase deficiency
Side-effects: nausea, vomiting, rashes, peripheral neuropathy, pulmonary infiltration, allergic liver damage
Dose: 100 mg every 6 hours with food

Nitrofurantoin Tablets, nitrofurantoin 50 mg, price 20 tabs = **C**; 100 mg, price 20 tabs = **D**
Berkfurin® (Berk)
Tablets, yellow, scored, nitrofurantoin 50 mg. Price 20 tabs = **C**
Tablets, yellow, scored, nitrofurantoin 100 mg. Price 20 tabs = **D**
Ceduran® (Tillotts) *tablets,* brown, scored, nitrofurantoin, deglycyrrhizinised extract of liquorice. Price 20 tabs = **D**
Furadantin® (Eaton)
Tablets, yellow, scored, nitrofurantoin 50 mg. Price 20 tabs = **D**
Tablets, yellow, scored, nitrofurantoin 100 mg. Price 20 tabs = **E**

Suspension (=mixture), yellow, nitrofurantoin 25 mg/5 ml. Do not dilute. Price 300 ml = **E**

Furan® (Chelsea)

Tablets, yellow, scored, nitrofurantoin 50 mg. Price 20 tabs = **A**

Tablets, yellow, scored, nitrofurantoin 100 mg. Price 20 tabs = **B**

Macrodantin® (Eaton)

Capsules, yellow/white, nitrofurantoin 50 mg. Price 20 caps = **D**

Capsules, yellow, nitrofurantoin 100 mg. Price 20 caps = **E**

Urantoin® (DDSA)

Tablets, yellow, scored, nitrofurantoin 50 mg. Price 20 tabs = **A**

Tablets, yellow, scored, nitrofurantoin 100 mg. Price 20 tabs = **B**

CINOXACIN

Indications: urinary-tract infections

Cautions: moderately impaired renal function

Contra-indications: severe renal impairment

Side-effects: gastro-intestinal symptoms including anorexia, nausea, vomiting, cramps, diarrhoea; hypersensitivity reactions including urticaria, rashes, peripheral and oral oedema; dizziness, headache, photophobia, tinnitus, perineal burning, changes in liver-function tests

Dose: 500 mg every 12 hours; prophylaxis, 500 mg at night

▼ **Cinobac**® (Lilly)

Capsules, green/orange, cinoxacin 500 mg. Price 20 caps = **H**

HEXAMINE

Indications: see notes above

Cautions: urine must be acidic

Contra-indications: impaired renal and hepatic function, dehydration, metabolic acidosis

Side-effects: gastro-intestinal disturbances, frequent and painful micturition, bladder irritation, haematuria, proteinuria, rashes

Dose: hexamine hippurate, 1 g every 12 hours; hexamine mandelate, 1 g every 6 hours

Hiprex® (Carnegie)

Tablets, hexamine hippurate 1 g. Price 20 tabs = **D**

Mandelamine® (Warner)

Tablets, brown, e/c, hexamine mandelate 250 mg. Price 20 tabs = **B.**

Tablets, brown, e/c, hexamine mandelate 500 mg. Price 20 tabs = **B**

NALIDIXIC ACID

Indications: urinary-tract infections

Cautions: impaired renal or hepatic function, avoid strong sunlight, interference with tests using copper salts (e.g. Benedict's test)

Contra-indications: pregnancy (1st trimester), infants under 3 months, epilepsy, CNS lesions

Side-effects: gastro-intestinal disturbances including nausea, vomiting, diarrhoea, haemorrhage; allergic reactions including urticaria, rashes, fever, arthralgia, eosinophilia; also myalgia, muscle weakness, phototoxicity, jaundice, visual disturbances, convulsions

Dose: 1 g every 6 hours for 7 days, reducing to 500 mg every 6 hours

Mictral® (Winthrop)

Granules, effervescent, nalidixic acid 660 mg, sodium citrate 3.75 g/sachet (Na^+ 41 mmol/sachet). Price 9 sachets = **E**

Dose: 1 sachet in water 3 times daily for 3 days.

Negram® (Sterling Research)

Tablets, beige, nalidixic acid 500 mg. Price 20 tabs = **E**

Suspension (=mixture), pink, nalidixic acid 300 mg/5 ml. Diluent syrup, life of diluted mixture 14 days. Price 100 ml = **G**

NITROFURAZONE

Indications: bladder infections

Cautions: sensitisation may develop

Dose: *as an irrigation or by instillation,* 1 in 6 solution

Furacin® (Eaton)

Solution, yellow, nitrofurazone 0.2%. Price 500 ml = **H**

NOXYTHIOLIN

Indications: bladder infections, irrigation of body cavities

Side-effects: burning sensation on application to bladder (relieved by addition of amethocaine)

Dose: *by irrigation,* 1–2.5% solution

Noxyflex® (Geistlich)

Solution, powder for reconstitution, noxythiolin 2.5 g, amethocaine hydrochloride 10 mg. Price per vial = **F**

Noxyflex S® (Geistlich)

Solution, powder for reconstitution, noxythiolin. Price 2.5-g vial = **F**

5.1.11.3 TRIMETHOPRIM

Trimethoprim is used alone in the treatment of respiratory-tract infections and acute and chronic urinary-tract infections. For use with sulphamethoxazole (as co-trimoxazole), sulphamoxole (as co-trifamole), or sulphadiazine (as co-trimazine) see section 5.1.8. For use in malaria see section 5.4.1.

TRIMETHOPRIM

Indications: urinary-tract infections, acute and chronic bronchitis

Cautions: moderately impaired renal function, predisposition to folate deficiency, blood counts required on long-term therapy

Contra-indications: severe renal failure, pregnancy, neonates

Side-effects: gastro-intestinal disturbances including nausea and vomiting, pruritus, rashes, depression of haemopoiesis

Dose: by mouth, acute infections, 200 mg every 12 hours *or* 300 mg once daily; chronic infections and prophylaxis, 100 mg at night; CHILD, twice daily, 2–5 months 25 mg, 6 months–5 years 50 mg, 6–12 years 100 mg
By slow intravenous injection, 150–250 mg every 12 hours

Trimethoprim Tablets, trimethoprim 100 mg. Price 20 tabs = **C**

Ipral® (Squibb)
Tablets, trimethoprim 100 mg. Price 20 tabs = **C**
Paediatric suspension (= mixture), sugar-free, trimethoprim 50 mg/5 ml. Diluents sorbitol solution, syrup, or water for preparations, life of diluted mixture 14 days. Price 100 ml = **D**

Monotrim® (Duphar)
Tablets, scored, trimethoprim 100 mg. Price 20 tabs = **C**
Tablets, trimethoprim 200 mg. Price 20 tabs = **E**
Suspension (= mixture), sugar-free, trimethoprim 50 mg/5ml. Diluents sorbitol solution, syrup, or water for preparations, life of diluted mixture 14 days. Price 100 ml = **D**

Syraprim® (Wellcome)
Tablets, scored, trimethoprim 100 mg. Price 28 tabs = **E**
Tablets, scored, trimethoprim 300 mg. Price 20 tabs = **G**
Injection, trimethoprim 20 mg (as lactate)/ml. Price 5-ml amp = **C**

Tiempe® (DDSA)
Tablets, trimethoprim 100 mg. Price 20 tabs = **C**

Trimopan® (Berk)
Tablets, scored, trimethoprim 100 mg. Price 20 tabs = **D**
Tablets, scored, trimethoprim 200 mg. Price 20 tabs = **E**

Unitrim® (Unimed)
Tablets, trimethoprim 100 mg. Price 20 tabs = **E**

5.1.11.4 ACROSOXACIN

Acrosoxacin (Eradacin®) is used in the treatment of gonorrhoea in patients allergic to penicillins or who have strains resistant to penicillins and other antibiotics.

ACROSOXACIN
(Rosoxacin)
Indications: gonorrhoea
Cautions: impaired renal or hepatic function; patient's ability to drive or operate machinery may be impaired
Side-effects: dizziness, drowsiness, headache, gastro-intestinal disturbances
Dose: 300 mg as a single dose on an empty stomach

▼**Eradacin®** (Sterling Research)
Capsules, red/yellow, acrosoxacin 150 mg. Price 2 caps = **E**

5.2 Antifungal drugs

It is important to remember that fungal infections are frequently associated with a defect in host resistance which should, if possible, be corrected otherwise drug therapy may fail. Similarly, treatment of dermatophyte infection may be unsuccessful until the animal source has been removed or controlled.

Amphotericin (Fungilin®) is not absorbed from the gut and is the only polyene antibiotic which can be given parenterally. It is the most important drug for the treatment of systemic fungal infections and is active against most fungi and yeasts. It is highly protein bound and penetrates poorly into body fluids and tissues. Amphotericin is a toxic drug and side-effects are common.

Flucytosine (Alcobon®) is a synthetic antifungal drug which is only active against yeasts and has been used for the treatment of systemic candidiasis, cryptococcosis, and torulopsosis. It is well absorbed from the gut and distributed widely in the body. Side-effects are uncommon but bone-marrow depression can occur and weekly blood counts are necessary during prolonged therapy. It can be given with amphotericin and synergy has been demonstrated. Resistance to flucytosine is not uncommon and can develop during therapy; sensitivity testing is, therefore, essential before treatment.

Griseofulvin is selectively concentrated in keratin and is the drug of choice for widespread or intractable dermatophyte infections—a topical imidazole or **Whitfield's ointment** is used for localised lesions. The drug is well absorbed from the gut but is inactive when applied topically. It is more effective in skin than in nail infections and treatment must be continued for several weeks or even months. Side-effects are uncommon.

The imidazole group of antifungal drugs includes **clotrimazole** (Canesten®), **miconazole,** and **econazole.** The imidazoles are active against a wide range of fungi and yeasts. The main indications for their use at present are vaginal candidiasis and dermatophyte infections. Miconazole is also available for oral and parenteral administration. **Ketoconazole** (Nizoral®), a recently introduced imidazole, is for oral administration only.

Nystatin (Nystan®) is a polyene antibiotic which is not absorbed when given by mouth and is too toxic for parenteral use. It is active against a number of yeasts and fungi but is principally used for *Candida albicans* infections of skin and mucous membranes.

For antifungal preparations used in genital infections see section 7.2.2 and in skin infections, see section 13.10.2.

AMPHOTERICIN
Indications: candidiasis, systemic fungal infections

Cautions: when given parenterally, renal-function tests required, frequent change of injection site, avoid other nephrotoxic drugs
Side-effects: when given parenterally, fever, anorexia, nausea, vomiting, hypokalaemia, nephrotoxicity (reduced by intravenous infusion of mannitol), tinnitus
Dose: by mouth, up to 200 mg every 6 hours
By intravenous infusion, 250 micrograms/kg daily, gradually increased if tolerated to 1 mg/kg daily; max. in severely ill patients 1.5 mg/kg daily or on alternate days

Fungilin® (Squibb)
Tablets, yellow, scored, amphotericin 100 mg. Price 20 tabs = **E**
Lozenges, yellow, amphotericin 10 mg. Price 20 lozenges = **C**
Dose: dissolve 1 lozenge in the mouth 4 times (increased if necessary to 8 times) daily
Suspension (=mixture), orange, amphotericin 100 mg/ml. Do not dilute. Measure with pipette. Price 12 ml = **D**
Fungizone® (Squibb)
Intravenous infusion, powder for reconstitution, amphotericin (as sodium deoxycholate complex). Price 50-mg vial = **E**

FLUCYTOSINE

Indications: systemic yeast infections
Cautions: renal and hepatic impairment, blood disorders, liver-function tests and blood counts required, blood concentrations monitored in renal impairment; pregnancy
Side-effects: nausea, vomiting, diarrhoea, rashes, thrombocytopenia, leucopenia
Dose: by mouth or intravenous infusion, 150–200 mg/kg daily in divided doses; reduce doses in renal impairment

Alcobon® (Roche)
Tablets, scored, flucytosine 500 mg. Price 20 tabs = **G** (Hosp. only)
Intravenous infusion, flucytosine 10 mg/ml. Price 250-ml infusion bottle and giving set = **I** (Hosp. only)

GRISEOFULVIN

Indications: severe dermatophyte infections
Cautions: drug interactions: see Appendix 1
Contra-indications: pregnancy, liver failure, porphyria
Side-effects: headache, nausea, vomiting, rashes, photosensitivity
Dose: 0.5–1 g daily, in divided doses or as a single dose; CHILD, 10 mg/kg daily in divided doses

Griseofulvin Tablets, griseofulvin 125 mg, price 20 tabs = **B**; 500 mg, price 20 tabs = **E**
Fulcin® (ICI)
Tablets, scored, griseofulvin 125 mg. Price 20 tabs = **B**
Tablets, f/c, griseofulvin 500 mg. Price 20 tabs = **E**
Suspension (=mixture), brown, griseofulvin 125 mg/5 ml. Diluent syrup, life of diluted mixture 14 days. Price 100 ml = **C**
Grisovin® (Glaxo)
Tablets, f/c, griseofulvin 125 mg. Price 20 tabs = **B**
Tablets, f/c, griseofulvin 500 mg. Price 20 tabs = **E**

KETOCONAZOLE

Indications: dermatophyte infections; systemic fungal infections, candidiasis unresponsive to topical treatment
Cautions: drug interactions: see Appendix 1
Contra-indications: pregnancy
Side-effects: rarely nausea, rashes, pruritus
Dose: 200 mg once daily with food, increased to max. of 400 mg once daily in severe infections: oral thrush—10 days; mycoses of skin and hair—1–2 months; systemic candidiasis—1–2 months; coccidioidomycosis and histoplasmosis—2–6 months; prophylaxis and maintenance treatment—6 months. CHILD, 3 mg/kg daily
Vaginal candidiasis, 200 mg with food every 12 hours for 5 days

▼ **Nizoral**® (Janssen)
Tablets, scored, ketoconazole 200 mg. Price 20 tabs = **I**

MICONAZOLE

Indications: systemic fungal infections, candidiasis, dermatophyte infections
Cautions: change infusion site to avoid phlebitis; pregnancy
Side-effects: nausea and vomiting, pruritus, rashes
Dose: by mouth, 250 mg every 6 hours
By intravenous infusion, initially, 600 mg every 8 hours

Daktarin® (Janssen)
Tablets, scored, miconazole 250 mg. Price 20 tabs = **J**
Oral gel, miconazole 25 mg/ml. Price 40 g = **E**
Intravenous solution, miconazole 10 mg/ml with Cremophor EL. Price 20-ml amp for preparing infusions = **D** (Hosp. only)

NATAMYCIN

Indications: candidiasis
Side-effects: nausea, vomiting, diarrhoea
Dose: by mouth, 10 drops of 1% suspension after meals; INFANTS, 4 drops
By inhalation, 2.5 mg every 8 hours

Pimafucin® (Brocades)
Oral suspension, natamycin 10 mg/ml. Price 5-ml dropper bottle = **C**
Suspension for inhalation, natamycin 25 mg/ml. Price 20 ml = **F**

C = 51-100p, **D** = 101-180p, **E** = 181-300p, **F** = 301-450p, **G** = 451-650p, **H** = 651-900p, **I** = 901-1200p, **J** = over 1200p.

NYSTATIN

Indications: candidiasis
Side-effects: nausea, vomiting, diarrhoea
Dose: *by mouth,* 500 000 units every 6 hours, doubled in severe infections

Nystatin Mixture, nystatin 100 000 units/ml. Do not dilute. Price 30 ml = **D**

Nystan® (Squibb)
Tablets, brown, s/c, nystatin 500 000 units. Price 20 tabs = **D**
Suspension (=mixture), yellow, nystatin 100 000 units/ml. Do not dilute. Measure with pipette. Price 30 ml with pipette = **D**

Nystatin-Dome® (Dome)
Oral suspension (= mixture), yellow, nystatin 100 000 units/ml. Price 30 ml = **E**

5.3 Antiviral drugs

The specific therapy of virus infections is generally unsatisfactory and treatment is, therefore, primarily symptomatic. Fortunately, the majority of infections resolve spontaneously.

Idoxuridine is active against herpes viruses; it is too toxic for systemic administration, a problem with many antiviral drugs, but has been used in the treatment of *Herpes simplex* lesions of the skin, eye, and external genitalia with variable results. Idoxuridine is also used for the topical treatment of shingles, in which it is claimed to reduce the duration of pain and lessen the incidence of post-herpetic neuralgia. However, to be effective, it must be applied early in the illness as soon as the first skin lesions appear. For use in herpetic skin diseases, see section 13.10.3; for use in herpetic conjunctivitis, see section 11.3.1; for use in oral lesions, see section 12.3.2.

Amantadine (Symmetrel®), given by mouth, has been used for the prophylaxis of influenza A infections and for the treatment of shingles.

Vidarabine (Vira-A®) is used in immunosuppressed patients for the treatment of serious infections caused by herpes viruses; these include varicella, zoster, and *Herpes simplex* infections. For use in herpetic conjunctivitis, see section 11.3.1.

AMANTADINE HYDROCHLORIDE

Indications: influenza A prophylaxis
Cautions; Contra-indications; Side-effects: see under section 4.9.1
Dose: 100 mg every 12 hours

Symmetrel® (Geigy)
Capsules, brown, amantadine hydrochloride 100 mg. Price 20 caps = **F**
Syrup (=elixir), amantadine hydrochloride 50 mg/5 ml. Diluent syrup, life of diluted elixir 28 days. Price 150 ml = **F**

VIDARABINE

Indications: chicken-pox and herpes zoster infections in immunosuppressed patients
Cautions: reduce dose in renal impairment; blood counts required
Side-effects: anorexia, nausea, vomiting, diarrhoea; tremor, ataxia, dizziness, confusion; decreased haematocrit, white cell count, and platelet count
Dose: *by slow intravenous infusion,* 10 mg/kg daily for at least 5 days

▼ **Vira-A**® (P-D)
Injection, vidarabine 200 mg/ml. To be diluted before use. Price 5-ml vial = **J**

5.4 Antiprotozoal drugs

Prophylaxis and treatment of protozoal infections frequently require expert management and advice is available from the Liverpool School of Tropical Medicine (051-708 9393), the London School of Hygiene and Tropical Medicine (01-636 8636), or the East Birmingham Hospital (021-772 4311).

Many of the drugs and proprietary preparations mentioned in the notes in section 5.4 are not generally available in the U.K. Details are given only for those which are available.

5.4.1 Antimalarials
5.4.2 Amoebicides
5.4.3 Trichomonacides
5.4.4 Antigiardial drugs
5.4.5 Leishmaniacides
5.4.6 Trypanocides
5.4.7 Drugs for toxoplasmosis

5.4.1 Antimalarials

TREATMENT OF BENIGN TERTIAN MALARIA. **Chloroquine** is the drug of choice for the treatment of benign tertian malaria, which is usually caused by *Plasmodium vivax* and less commonly by *P. ovale* and *P. malariae*. The dose by mouth is the equivalent of 600 mg of chloroquine followed after 6 hours by 300 mg, then 150 mg twice daily for a further 2 days. If the patient is vomiting or seriously ill, chloroquine sulphate can be given by intramuscular or slow intravenous injection in a dose equivalent to 200–300 mg of chloroquine. If after 6 hours the patient still cannot take tablets a second injection should be given. The drug should not be given intravenously to infants as it can have cardiovascular side-effects. Chloroquine causes cerebral and ocular changes if given in excessive dosage.

ERADICATION OF BENIGN TERTIAN MALARIA. **Primaquine** in a dose of 15 mg daily (7.5 mg for children) should be given for 14 days following the treatment of benign tertian malaria with chloroquine, to destroy parasites in the liver and prevent relapses. Before starting primaquine the blood should be tested for glucose-6-phosphate dehydrogenase (G-6-PD) activity as the drug can cause haemolysis in patients who are deficient in the enzyme.

TREATMENT OF MALIGNANT TERTIAN MALARIA. **Chloroquine** in the dosage schedule outlined above is also effective in malignant tertian malaria. However, strains of *P. falciparum* resistant to chloroquine are becoming increasingly common particularly in East Africa, in Asia east of Bangladesh, and in Central and South America. If the patient has come from one of these areas, or is seriously ill, **quinine** should be given by intravenous infusion over 4 hours in a dose of 5 to 10 mg/kg of base. The total dose should not normally exceed 500 mg and 4 doses should be given at intervals of from 12 to 24 hours depending on the size of the patient, severity of infection, and evidence of liver disease (when the intervals should be increased).

For patients who are not seriously ill quinine can be given by mouth in a dose of 600 mg every 8 hours for at least 4 doses. Quinine should not be given intravenously to infants but may be given by intramuscular injection in a dose not exceeding 5 mg/kg. Following a course of quinine the patient should be given Fansidar® (2 tablets) which is also an alternative to quinine for chloroquine-resistant falciparum malaria.

CHEMOPROPHYLAXIS. The chemoprophylaxis of malaria is becoming more complex as a result of drug resistance, and varies for different areas of the world. Advice may be obtained from the Bureau of Hygiene and Tropical Medicine in London (01-636 8636) on currently recommended drugs.

Prophylactic drugs should be taken from the day before travel into an endemic area until at least 4 weeks after leaving it. For the **Indian subcontinent** and the **Middle East**, give chloroquine 300 mg once weekly or proguanil 100–200 mg daily. For **South-east Asia** and **Central** and **South America**, give Maloprim® or Fansidar® 1 tablet once weekly. For **Africa**, give chloroquine 300 mg once weekly (except **Kenya** or **Tanzania**, where Fansidar® or Maloprim® should be used).

CHLOROQUINE

Indications: benign and malignant tertian malaria, amoebiasis.
Cautions: impaired renal or hepatic function, psoriasis, porphyria, ocular examinations in long-term treatment
Side-effects: headache, nausea, vomiting, diarrhoea, rashes; rarely psychotic episodes, convulsions; corneal and retinal changes with prolonged high dosage (may be irreversible)
Dose: see notes above
Note: Chloroquine base 100 mg≡chloroquine phosphate 160 mg≡chloroquine sulphate 137 mg

Avloclor® (ICI)
Tablets, scored, chloroquine phosphate 250 mg (≡chloroquine 155 mg). Price 20 tabs = **B**

Malarivon® (Wallace Mfg)
Syrup (=elixir), chloroquine phosphate 80 mg (≡chloroquine 50 mg)/5 ml. Price 75 ml = **C**

Nivaquine® (M&B)
Tablets, scored, chloroquine sulphate 200 mg (≡chloroquine 150 mg). Price 20 tabs = **B**
Syrup (=elixir), red, chloroquine sulphate 68 mg (≡chloroquine 50 mg)/5 ml. Diluent syrup, life of diluted elixir 14 days. Price 125 ml = **D**
Injection, chloroquine 40 mg (as sulphate)/ml. Price 5-ml amp = **B**

HYDROXYCHLOROQUINE SULPHATE

Indications: malaria
Cautions; Side-effects: see under Chloroquine
Dose: malaria, treatment, 800 mg initially, 400 mg after 6–8 hours, then 400 mg daily for 2 days
Prophylaxis, 400 mg 1–2 times weekly

Plaquenil® (Winthrop)
Tablets, orange, s/c, hydroxychloroquine sulphate 200 mg. Price 20 tabs = **F**

PRIMAQUINE

Indications: eradication of benign tertian malaria
Cautions: see notes above
Side-effects: anorexia, nausea, vomiting, jaundice; less commonly bone-marrow depression, methaemoglobinaemia, haemolytic anaemia
Dose: see notes above

Primaquine
Tablets, s/c, primaquine 7.5 mg (as phosphate). Price 20 tabs = **A**

PROGUANIL HYDROCHLORIDE

Indications: chemoprophylaxis of malaria
Side-effects: rarely vomiting, epigastric pain, haematuria, renal irritation
Dose: see notes above

Paludrine® (ICI)
Tablets, scored, proguanil hydrochloride 100 mg. Price 20 tabs = **A**

PYRIMETHAMINE

Indications: chemoprophylaxis of malaria
Cautions: hepatic or renal impairment, folate supplements in pregnancy, blood counts required with high doses
Side-effects: depression of haemopoiesis with prolonged treatment, rashes
Dose: see notes above

Daraprim® (Wellcome)
Tablets, scored, pyrimethamine 25 mg. Price 20 tabs = **C**

Fansidar® (Roche)
Tablets, scored, pyrimethamine 25 mg, sulfadoxine 500 mg. Price 20 tabs = **F**
Dose: see notes above

Maloprim® (Wellcome)
Tablets, scored, pyrimethamine 12.5 mg, dapsone 100 mg. Price 20 tabs = **C**
Dose: 1 tablet weekly

QUININE

Indications: malignant tertian malaria
Cautions: atrial fibrillation, conduction defects, heart block
Contra-indications: haemoglobinuria, optic neuritis
Side-effects: cinchonism, including tinnitus, headache, nausea, abdominal pain, rashes, visual disturbances, blindness; hypersensitivity reactions including angioneurotic oedema
Dose: see notes above
Note: Quinine 100 mg≡quinine bisulphate 145 mg≡quinine dihydrochloride 105 mg ≡quinine hydrochloride 105 mg≡quinine sulphate 103 mg

Quinine Bisulphate Tablets, s/c, or f/c, quinine bisulphate 300 mg. Price 20 tabs = **C**
Quinine Dihydrochloride Tablets, quinine dihydrochloride 300 mg. Price 20 tabs = **D**
Quinine Hydrochloride Tablets, quinine hydrochloride 300 mg. Price 20 tabs = **D**
Quinine Sulphate Tablets, s/c or f/c, quinine sulphate 125, 200, and 300 mg. Price 20 tabs (all) = **C**

TRIMETHOPRIM

Indications: prophylaxis of malaria resistant to pyrimethamine (for use with sulphamethoxazole, sulphamoxole, or sulphadiazine, see section 5.1.8; for use in urinary-tract infections, see section 5.1.11.3)
Cautions; Contra-indications; Side-effects: see section 5.1.11.3
Dose: up to 1.5 g daily for 7 days

Preparations
See section 5.1.11.3

5.4.2 Amoebicides

Metronidazole (section 5.1.11.1) is the drug of choice for acute invasive amoebic dysentery for it is very effective against vegetative amoebae in ulcers and also against amoebae which may have migrated to the liver. Much of it is absorbed and excreted in the urine, which becomes dark in colour. Side-effects include anorexia, giddiness, and lassitude. It is given either for 10 days, or for 5 days followed by a 10-day course of diloxanide furoate.

Metronidazole is relatively ineffective in chronic intestinal amoebiasis in which only cysts are present in the stool.

Diloxanide furoate (Furamide®) is the drug of choice in chronic infections in which only cysts and not vegetative forms of *E. histolytica* are present in the faeces. It is relatively free from toxic effects in therapeutic doses and the usual course is of 10 days, given alone for chronic infections or following 5 days of metronidazole in acute dysenteric infections.

Emetine hydrochloride and **emetine and bismuth iodide** have now been largely replaced by metronidazole and are rarely used for they are associated with more nausea and have a smaller margin of safety between the therapeutic and the cardiotoxic dose.

For the treatment of amoebic abscesses of the liver **metronidazole** is effective in doses of 800 mg 3 times daily for 10 days and the course may be repeated after 2 weeks if necessary.

If metronidazole is not available emetine may be used but its side-effects are more marked. Diloxanide is not effective against hepatic amoebiasis. **Chloroquine** (section 5.4.1) is concentrated in the liver and for adults a dosage of 600 mg (base) daily for 5 days followed by 300 mg (base) daily for 14 to 21 days is effective but is slower and less certain in its action than metronidazole. For abscesses containing more than 100 ml of pus (i.e. approximately 60 to 100 mm in diameter) aspiration carried out in conjunction with drug therapy will greatly reduce the period of disability.

DILOXANIDE FUROATE

Indications: chronic amoebiasis—see notes above
Side-effects: flatulence, vomiting, urticaria, pruritus
Dose: 500 mg every 8 hours for 10 days—see notes above

Furamide® (Boots)
Tablets, diloxanide furoate 500 mg

5.4.3 Trichomonacides

Metronidazole (section 5.1.11.1) is the treatment of choice for *Trichomonas vaginalis* infection. It is given by mouth after meals; 200 mg 3 times daily for 7 days, 800 mg in the morning and 1.2 g at night for 2 days, or a single 2-g dose have given satisfactory results.

If metronidazole is ineffective, **nimorazole** (Naxogin®) may be tried; usual doses are 250 mg every 12 hours for 6 days, 1 g every 12 hours for 3 doses, or a single 2-g dose, given with food.

Alcohol should be avoided during treatment with both metronidazole and nimorazole.

NIMORAZOLE

Indications: trichomoniasis
Contra-indications: active CNS disease, severe renal failure
Side-effects: nausea, vomiting, rashes, vertigo, drowsiness, ataxia (discontinue treatment), intolerance to alcohol
Dose: see notes above

Naxogin 500® (Farmitalia Carlo Erba)
Tablets, scored, nimorazole 500 mg. Price 4 tabs = **C**

5.4.4 Antigiardial drugs

Metronidazole (section 5.1.11.1) is the treatment of choice for *Giardia lamblia* infections, given by mouth in a dosage of 2 g daily for 3 days, or 400 mg every 8 hours for 7 days.

Alternative treatments are **chloroquine** base (section 5.4.1) 300 mg daily for 5 days or **mepacrine hydrochloride** 100 mg every 8 hours for 5–8 days or **furazolidone**.

FURAZOLIDONE

Indications: bacterial and protozoal gastroenteritis
Cautions: avoid alcohol during and for 4 days after treatment. MAOI—see section 4.3.2
Contra-indications: infants under 1 month
Side-effects: nausea, vomiting, headache, malaise, rashes, intolerance to alcohol, haemolytic anaemia in patients with glucose-6-phosphate dehydrogenase deficiency
Dose: 100 mg every 6 hours

Furoxone® (Eaton)
Tablets, brown, scored, furazolidone 100 mg. Price 20 tabs = **D**
Suspension, see section 1.4.3

5.4.5 Leishmaniacides

Cutaneous leishmaniasis frequently heals spontaneously without specific treatment. If the skin lesions are extensive or unsightly, treatment is indicated, as it is in visceral leishmaniasis (kala-azar).

Sodium stibogluconate (Pentostam®), an organic pentavalent antimony compound, is the treatment of choice. The dose is the equivalent of 600 mg of pentavalent antimony given daily by intramuscular or intravenous injection. Skin lesions are treated for 10 days and visceral disease for up to 4 weeks. An alternative drug is **pentamidine** which is toxic and should only be used on the advice of experts.

PENTAMIDINE ISETHIONATE

Indications: leishmaniasis, but see notes above

Pentamidine Isethionate (M&B)
Injection, powder for reconstitution, pentamidine isethionate. Price 200-mg amp = **D**

SODIUM STIBOGLUCONATE

Indications: leishmaniasis
Cautions: intravenous injections must be given slowly and stopped if coughing or substernal pain develops
Contra-indications: pneumonia, myocarditis, nephritis, hepatitis
Side-effects: anorexia, vomiting, coughing, substernal pain
Dose: see notes above

Pentostam® (Wellcome)
Injection, sodium stibogluconate equivalent to pentavalent antimony 100 mg/ml. Price 100-ml vial = **J**

5.4.6 Trypanocides

The prophylaxis and treatment of trypanosomiasis is difficult and differs according to the strain of organism. Expert advice should therefore be obtained.

5.4.7 Drugs for toxoplasmosis

Most infections caused by *Toxoplasma gondii* are self-limiting, and treatment is not necessary. Exceptions are patients with eye involvement, and those who are immunosuppressed. The treatment of choice is a combination of pyrimethamine and a sulphonamide, given for several weeks. Pyrimethamine is a folate antagonist, and adverse reactions to this combination are relatively common.

5.5 Anthelmintics

Prophylaxis and treatment of helminth infections frequently requires expert management and advice is available from the Liverpool School of Tropical Medicine (051-708 9393), the London School of Hygiene and Tropical Medicine (01-636 8636), or the East Birmingham Hospital (021-772 4311).

Many of the drugs and proprietary preparations mentioned in the notes in section 5.5 are not generally available in the U.K. Details are given only for those which are available.

5.5.1 Drugs for threadworms

(pinworms, *Enterobius vermicularis*)
Anthelmintics are relatively ineffective in threadworm infections, and their use should be combined with hygienic measures to break the cycle of auto-infection. All members of the family require treatment.

Adult threadworms do not live for longer than 6 weeks and for development of fresh worms, ova must be swallowed and exposed to the action of digestive juices in the upper intestinal tract. Direct multiplication of worms does not take place in the large bowel. Adult female worms lay ova on the peri-anal skin and cause pruritus by so doing; scratching the area then leads to ova being transmitted on fingers to the mouth, often via food eaten with unwashed hands. Washing the hands and fingers with the aid of a nail brush before each meal and after each visit to the toilet is essential. A bath taken immediately after rising will remove ova laid during the night and limit their dissemination.

Piperazine salts including the citrate and phosphate are used. Piperazine may be given in doses equivalent to the following quantities of ipierazine hydrate: up to 2 years 50–75 mg/kg, 2–4 years 750 mg, 5–12 years 1.5 g, adults and children over 12 years 2 g. These doses are given daily for 7 days.

Thiabendazole (Mintezol®) in 3 doses of 50 mg/kg at intervals of a week is also employed and **mebendazole** (Vermox®) has been used in a single dose of 100 mg for all ages.

MEBENDAZOLE

Indications: threadworm, roundworm, and hookworm infections
Contra-indications: pregnancy, children under 2 years
Side-effects: rarely abdominal pain, diarrhoea
Dose: see notes above

Vermox® (Janssen)
Tablets, pink, scored, chewable, mebendazole 100 mg. Price 6 tabs = **E**
Suspension (=mixture), mebendazole 100 mg/5 ml. Price 30 ml = **E**

PIPERAZINE

Indications: threadworm and roundworm infections
Cautions: impaired renal function, psychiatric states, neurological disease
Contra-indications: epilepsy, renal failure, liver disease
Side-effects: nausea, vomiting, diarrhoea, urticaria; rarely dizziness, paraesthesia, muscular incoordination
Dose: see notes above
Note: 100 mg piperazine hydrate≡125 mg piperazine citrate≡104 mg piperazine phosphate

Piperazine Citrate Elixir, green, piperazine citrate equivalent to piperazine hydrate 750 mg/5 ml. Diluent syrup, life of diluted elixir 14 days. Price 100 ml = **B**

Antepar® (Wellcome)
Tablets, yellow, scored, piperazine hydrate 500 mg (as phosphate). Price 28 tabs = **D**
Elixir, orange, piperazine hydrate 750 mg/5 ml (as hydrate and citrate). Diluent syrup, life of diluted elixir 14 days. Price 100 ml = **D**

Ascalix® (Wallace Mfg)
Syrup (=elixir), piperazine hydrate 750 mg (as citrate)/5 ml. Price 75 ml = **D**. Also 4g in 20-ml sachet, price each = **A**; 4 g in 30-ml bottle, price each = **B**

Pripsen® (R&C)
Oral powder, cream, piperazine phosphate 4 g (=4 g of hydrate) and sennosides 15.3 mg/sachet. Price per sachet = **B**

THIABENDAZOLE

Indications: threadworm, roundworm, hookworm, and strongyloid infections
Cautions: hepatic or renal impairment, if drowsiness occurs warn patients not to drive, discontinue if hypersensitivity reactions occur
Side-effects: anorexia, nausea, vomiting, dizziness, diarrhoea, headache, pruritus, drowsiness; hypersensitivity reactions including fever, chills, angioneurotic oedema, rashes, erythema multiforme; rarely tinnitus, collapse, parenchymal liver damage
Dose: see notes above

Mintezol® (MSD)
Tablets, pink, chewable, thiabendazole 500 mg. Price 6 tabs = **B**

5.5.2 Ascaricides

(common roundworm infections)

Piperazine salts (section 5.5.1) have been used for over a quarter of a century in the treatment of ascariasis and have proved to be highly effective in a single dose equivalent to 4 g of piperazine hydrate. There have been very occasional reports of confusional states, vertigo, and incoordination following their use but they remain among the safest anthelmintics known.

Bephenium (Alcopar®) is also effective; 2.5 g may be given as a single dose or divided into 2 doses separated by 2–3 days. In some patients it may produce nausea and vomiting. **Thiabendazole** (section 5.5.1) has a broad spectrum of anthelmintic activity which includes ascaris worms; it is usually given in doses of 25 mg/kg twice daily for 2–3 days and the course may need to be repeated after a week's interval. **Mebendazole** (section 5.5.1) is active against *Ascaris lumbricoides*; the usual dose is 100 mg twice daily for 3 days. **Pyrantel** is also an effective broad-spectrum anthelmintic and a single dose of 10 mg/kg is often sufficient to eradicate ascaris but the dose is usually repeated after 24–48 hours. It may occasionally produce mild nausea but experience shows it to be a very safe drug. **Tetramisole** is also effective against ascaris and is very well tolerated; mild nausea or vomiting has been reported in about 1% of treated patients.

BEPHENIUM

Indications: roundworm and hookworm infections
Side-effects: nausea, vomiting, diarrhoea, headache, vertigo
Dose: see notes above

Alcopar® (Wellcome)
Granules, yellow/green, bephenium 2.5 g (as hydroxynaphthoate)/sachet. Price per sachet = **B**

5.5.3 Taenicides

(tapeworms)

Niclosamide (Yomesan®) is the most widely used drug for tapeworm infections and side-effects are limited to occasional gastro-intestinal upset, light-headedness, and pruritus. Accurate identification of the worm is necessary before niclosamide is given for it causes partial digestion of the worm and may lead to release of ova in the patient's intestine. While this is of little or no consequence in infections with *Taenia saginata* or *Diphyllobothrium latum,* the release of *Taenia solium* ova in the intestine, particularly if associated with nausea and retrograde peristalsis, could lead to cysticercosis developing in the treated patient. Treatment with **mepacrine** or with **male fern extract** is preferable in patients with *T. solium* infections.

NICLOSAMIDE

Indications: tapeworm infections—see notes above
Side-effects: gastro-intestinal discomfort
Dose: 2 g on an empty stomach, followed by a purgative after 2 hours

Yomesan® (Bayer)
Tablets, yellow, chewable, niclosamide 500 mg. Price 4 tabs = **D**

5.5.4 Drugs for hookworms

(ancylostomiasis, necatoriasis)

Hookworms live in the upper small intestine and draw blood from the point of their attachment to their host. An iron-deficiency anaemia may thereby be produced and, if present, effective treatment of the infection requires not only expulsion of the worms but treatment of the anaemia.

Tetrachloroethylene is still the most widely used drug for hookworm infection. It is best administered in a suspension rather than in capsules so that effective action of the drug on the worms in the upper intestine can be assured. Alcohol and fatty foods should be avoided following treatment with tetrachloroethylene as they increase its absorption and therefore hepatotoxicity. Toxic effects are rare but occasionally nausea and headache or drowsiness may be experienced. It should be avoided in debilitated patients or young children.

Bephenium (section 5.5.2) is widely used and its side-effects are limited to occasional nausea and vomiting. A single dose of 2.5 g is given and repeated after 1–2 days. It is thought to be more effective against *Ancylostoma duodenale* than against *Necator americanus*. **Pyrantel** is very effective against hookworms and, like bephenium, has side-effects limited to occasional nausea and vomiting. A single dose of 10 mg/kg to a maximum of 1 g is given and repeated in 24–48 hours.

Bitoscanate is effective in a dosage of 100 mg at 12-hour intervals for 3 doses. Children of 10–14 years are given 2 doses of 100 mg and those 5–9 years 2 doses of 50 mg. Headache and giddiness are common side-effects along with gastro-intestinal symptoms. Alcohol and coffee appear to increase the frequency of side-effects and should be avoided at the time of treatment. Bitoscanate is slowly eliminated and the course of treatment with it should not be repeated for at least 2–3 weeks. In view of these limitations other drugs effective in hookworm infections are to be preferred.

Thiabendazole (section 5.5.1) and **tetramisole** may be used against hookworms but for good results rather longer courses are necessary than those required by bephenium, pyrantel, or tetrachloroethylene. **Mebendazole** (section 5.5.1) is also used against hookworms; the usual dose is 100 mg twice daily for 3 days.

5.5.5 Schistosomicides

(bilharziasis)

Adult *Schistosoma haematobium* worms live in the genito-urinary veins and adult *S. mansoni* in those of the colon and mesentery. *S. japonicum* is more widely distributed in veins of the alimentary tract and portal system.

Niridazole (Ambilhar®) is the drug of choice for *S. haematobium* infections. Toxic reactions including acute psychoses and/or convulsions may occur if venous anastomoses permit portal blood containing absorbed drug to by-pass the liver where it is normally conjugated. Liver damage is rare in children, who usually tolerate the drug well, but in adults with severe *S. mansoni* infections and liver damage, or in patients with *S. japonicum* infections in which liver damage is also common, the drug should be **avoided**. It is administered orally in doses of 25 mg/kg daily in divided doses morning and evening for 5–7 days.

Oxamniquine is the treatment of choice for *S. mansoni* infections; it is a quinoline compound given in doses of 20 mg/kg daily for 1–3 days. Toxicity is insignificant but activity against *S. haematobium* is low. **Metrifonate,** an organophosphorus compound, is given in doses of 7.5 mg/kg once every 2–4 weeks on 2–3 occasions. It is effective only against *S. haematobium.*

An alternative to niridazole is **stibocaptate** (Astiban®), usually given intramuscularly in doses of 8 mg/kg to a maximum dose of 500 mg. The dose is repeated daily for 5 days. **Hycanthone** (Etrenol®) is now rarely used because of unpredictable toxicity.

Antimony sodium tartrate and **sodium antimonylgluconate** (Triostam®) are occasionally used.

Lucanthone (Miracil D®, Nilodin®) is effective against *S. haematobium* infections and may be given orally but usually causes such severe nausea and giddiness that it is now seldom used.

5.5.6 Filaricides

Diethylcarbamazine (Banocide®) is highly effective against microfilariae and adults of *Loa loa* and of *Wuchereria bancrofti* and against the microfilariae of *Onchocerca volvulus*. It is less effective against adult *O. volvulus*. The destruction of the microfilariae is associated with release of antigens and a resulting allergic response. Headache, nausea, and sometimes vomiting are complained of and in onchocerciasis the filarial dermatitis may be temporarily aggravated and conjunctivitis and punctate keratitis temporarily increased. Antihistamines may be helpful in controlling these reactions but topical corticosteroids may be required for the skin irritation in severely affected patients.

With the object of limiting allergic responses in onchocerciasis, treatment is commenced with 250 micrograms/kg administered once or twice daily, then successive doses doubled until 3 mg/kg is given 3–4 times daily. This dosage is maintained for 21 days. Close medical supervision is necessary particularly in the early phase of treatment. **Diethylcarbamazine** is the treatment of choice for all patients with filarial infection; onchocerciasis is the most resistant of these but even heavily infected patients usually respond to 3–4 courses given at intervals of several months as required.

In very persistent cases **suramin** may be used for it is active against adult worms although it has little action on microfilariae. It is nephrotoxic and it is for this reason that its use is usually withheld except in chronically relapsing cases. When used, a preliminary test dose of 200 mg is administered intravenously and if well tolerated is followed by doses of 1 g dissolved in 10 ml of water for injections given intravenously at weekly intervals for 5–7 weeks. It is important to ensure that the urine is free from albumin and casts which if present contra-indicate further suramin treatment.

DIETHYLCARBAMAZINE CITRATE
Indications: filariasis
Cautions; Side-effects: see notes above
Dose: see notes above

Banocide® (Wellcome)
Tablets, scored, diethylcarbamazine citrate 50 mg. Price 20 tabs = **B**

5.5.7 Drugs for guinea worms
(dracontiasis)

Guinea worms, *Dracunculus medinensis*, may be killed and their removal from the tissues facilitated by a course of **niridazole** (Ambilhar®). Use of niridazole does not obviate the concomitant need for sterile dressing of the ulcer caused by a guinea worm and for its extraction, wherever possible, under sterile conditions.

5.5.8 Drugs for strongyloidiasis

Adult *Strongyloides stercoralis* live in the gut and produce larvae which penetrate the gut wall and invade the tissues, setting up a cycle of autoinfection. **Thiabendazole** (section 5.5.1) is the drug of choice, at a dosage of 25 mg/kg every 12 hours for 3 days.

6: Drugs used in the treatment of disorders of the ENDOCRINE SYSTEM

In this chapter, drug treatment is discussed under the following headings:

6.1 Drugs used in diabetes

Two groups of drugs are used in the treatment of diabetes, insulin and its preparations (section 6.1.1) and oral hypoglycaemic drugs (section 6.1.2).

The treatment of diabetic coma (section 6.1.3) and hypoglycaemia (section 6.1.4) is also discussed.

6.1.1 Insulin

Insulin plays a key role in the body's regulation of carbohydrate, fat, and protein metabolism. Diabetes mellitus is due to a deficiency in insulin synthesis and secretion, and the severity of the metabolic disturbance is directly related to the extent of the insulin deficiency. Patients with extreme deficiency require long-term replacement therapy with insulin, while those with a less marked deficiency may be able to maintain apparently normal health by dietary restriction of carbohydrate alone.

Insulin is a polypeptide hormone of complex structure; it is extracted from beef or pork pancreas and purified by crystallisation. Most insulin preparations contain a mixture of beef and pork insulins in variable proportions; although both are immunogenic in man, immunological resistance to insulin action is uncommon. When it does occur, antibodies are mainly directed against the beef component and may be overcome by changing to a pure pork preparation.

Insulin given by mouth is inactivated by gastro-intestinal enzymes, and it must therefore be given by injection; the subcutaneous route is ideal for most circumstances. When treating diabetic coma (section 6.1.3), insulin should be given by intravenous and/or intramuscular injection, since absorption from subcutaneous depots may be slow and erratic.

Minor allergic reactions at the sites of injections are still common during the first few weeks of treatment; they are usually transient and require no treatment. Lipo-atrophy is uncommon with highly-purified insulin preparations: if it does develop, it can sometimes be reversed by the use of injections of neutral pork insulin or monocomponent insulin.

About 25% of diabetics require insulin treatment; apart from those presenting in coma or precoma, insulin is needed by most of those who are underweight and ketotic at presentation. The majority of those who are of normal weight or obese can be managed by restriction of carbohydrate or energy intake alone or with the subsequent administration of oral hypoglycaemic drugs. Most children require insulin from the outset.

Since insulin secretion fluctuates from minute to minute in normal subjects, it is impossible to maintain normoglycaemia in the majority of diabetics by insulin injections once, twice, or even thrice daily. Symptoms are relieved rapidly as glycosuria is controlled. The aim of treatment is to achieve the best possible control of blood glucose, and close co-operation is needed between the patient and the medical team. To achieve control, mixtures of available insulin preparations may be required (such as Insulin Injection and Isophane Insulin Injection) and these combinations have to be worked out for the individual patient.

The energy and carbohydrate intake must be adequate to allow normal growth and development but obesity should be avoided. The carbohydrate intake is not restricted in non-obese patients on insulin but should be distributed throughout the day in such a way that it suits the type of insulin used. Fine control of blood glucose can be achieved by moving portions of carbohydrate from one meal to another without altering the total intake.

Insulin doses are best determined on an individual basis, by gradually increasing the dose to the maximum tolerated without troublesome hypoglycaemic reactions. Care should be taken to avoid inducing obesity by the administration of too much insulin.

There are three main types of insulin preparations:

1. those of **short** duration which have a relatively rapid action, for example Insulin Injection (Soluble);
2. those with an **intermediate** action, for example Isophane Insulin Injection and Insulin Zinc Suspension, Amorphous (Insulin Semilente); and
3. those whose action is slower in onset and lasts for **long** periods, for example Insulin Zinc Suspension (Insulin Lente) and Protamine Zinc Insulin.

The type of insulin used and its dose and frequency of administration depend on the particular needs of the patient. Patients with moderate to severe insulin deficiency are best started on Isophane Insulin Injection twice daily and a short-acting insulin can later be added to cover any hyperglycaemia which may follow breakfast or evening meal.

HIGHLY-PURIFIED INSULINS. Many highly-purified insulin preparations are now available; they have been subjected to more rigorous purification procedures to eliminate pro-insulin and other insulin precursors that are relatively more immunogenic than insulin. They are less immunogenic than the standard insulin preparations which are purified by recrystallisation.

The monospecies insulins are particularly helpful in cases of immunological resistance to conventional insulin and in patients with allergic reactions to the less highly purified preparations. Most diabetologists feel that all newly-diagnosed children and young adults should be treated with the highly-purified insulins from the outset. Production of antibodies to the highly-purified insulins is less than to the conventional insulins.

Care should be taken when changing a patient from conventional forms of soluble insulin to the highly-purified monospecies insulins since there is usually an immediate fall in insulin requirements and unless this is taken into consideration, hypoglycaemic reactions may be troublesome.

6.1.1.1 SHORT-ACTING INSULIN PREPARATIONS

Insulin Injection (soluble or regular insulin) is a clear solution of insulin of mixed beef and pork origin with an acid pH (about 3.2). When injected subcutaneously, its effect is maximal in 2–4 hours and lasts for up to 12 hours, although the duration of action is affected by the amount given. It is used chiefly in those patients with severe insulin deficiency whose insulin requirements may be large and change rapidly, as in acute infections or at the time of operations.

NEUTRAL INSULIN INJECTION. Several preparations of soluble insulin have the advantage of being neutral in reaction and are very similar in action to soluble insulin. The neutral solution allows more rapid absorption and reduces the incidence of discomfort at the site of injection. The highly purified monospecies insulins are of value in the patient who develops hypersensitivity to insulin from a particular species. These insulins are the only preparations from a specified animal, the others being of mixed animal origin. Occasionally, immunological resistance may develop to one species of insulin (usually beef) and this may usually be overcome by changing to the alternative species.

INSULIN INJECTION

(Soluble Insulin)

Indications: diabetes mellitus; diabetic coma (section 6.1.3)

Cautions: drug interactions: see Appendix 1

Side-effects: local reactions and lipo-atrophy at injection site; overdose causes hypoglycaemia

Dose: adjusted according to patient's requirements

Insulin Injection, 20 units/ml, price 10-ml vial = **D;** 40 units/ml, price 10-ml vial = **E;** 80 units/ml, price 10-ml vial = **F;** 320 units/ml, price 5-ml vial = **G**

NEUTRAL INSULIN INJECTION

(Neutral Insulin)

Indications: diabetes mellitus

Cautions; Side-effects; Dose: see under Insulin Injection

Actrapid MC® (Novo)
Injection, neutral insulin (porcine, highly purified) 40 units/ml, price 10-ml vial = **E;** 80 units/ml, price 10-ml vial = **F**

Hypurin Neutral® (Weddel)
Injection, neutral insulin (bovine, highly purified) 40 units/ml, price 10-ml vial = **E;** 80 units/ml, price 10-ml vial = **F**

Neusulin® (Wellcome)
Injection, neutral insulin (bovine, highly purified) 40 units/ml, price 10-ml vial = **E;** 80 units/ml, price 10-ml vial = **F**

Nuso® (Boots, Evans, Wellcome)
Injection, neutral insulin (bovine) 40 units/ml, price 10-ml vial = **E;** 80 units/ml, price 10-ml vial = **F**

Velosulin® (Nordisk)
Injection, neutral insulin (porcine, highly purified) 40 units/ml, price 10-ml vial = **E;** 80 units/ml, price 10-ml vial = **F**

6.1.1.2 INTERMEDIATE-ACTING INSULIN PREPARATIONS

Biphasic Insulin Injection (Rapitard MC®) is a mixture of beef insulin crystals in a solution of pork insulin; it is usually given twice daily.

Isophane Insulin Injection is of particular value for initiation of twice-daily insulin injections, producing much smoother blood glucose control than twice-daily soluble insulin. It can readily be combined with soluble insulin (pH 3 or 7) to produce a stable mixture retaining the properties of its two components. As a twice-daily regimen, it provides the most flexible replacement therapy available and is particularly useful during pregnancy. It is best to determine the ratio of soluble to isophane individually on the basis of frequent blood glucose readings (preferably made at home). Two ready-mixed preparations are available for those who cannot make their own (Mixtard 30/70® and Initard 50/50®).

BIPHASIC INSULIN INJECTION

Indications: diabetes mellitus

Cautions; Side-effects; Dose: see under Insulin Injection (section 6.1.1.1)

Rapitard MC® (Novo)
Injection, crystalline insulin (bovine, highly purified) 75%, neutral insulin (porcine, highly purified) 25%. 40 units/ml, price 10-ml vial = **E;** 80 units/ml, price 10-ml vial = **F**

GLOBIN ZINC INSULIN INJECTION

(Globin Insulin)
Indications: diabetes mellitus
Cautions; Side-effects; Dose: see under Insulin Injection (section 6.1.1.1); globin may cause allergic reactions

Globin Zinc Insulin Injection, 80 units/ml. Price 10-ml vial = **F**

INSULIN ZINC SUSPENSION (AMORPHOUS)

(Amorph. I.Z.S.)
Indications: diabetes mellitus
Cautions; Side-effects; Dose: see under Insulin Injection (section 6.1.1.1)

Insulin Zinc Suspension (Amorphous), Semilente, 40 units/ml, price 10-ml vial = **E;** 80 units/ml, price 10-ml vial = **F**
Semitard MC® (Novo)
Injection, insulin zinc suspension (amorphous) (porcine, highly purified) 40 units/ml, price 10-ml vial = **E;** 80 units/ml, price 10-ml vial = **F**

ISOPHANE INSULIN INJECTION

(Isophane Protamine Insulin Injection)
Indications: diabetes mellitus
Cautions; Side-effects; Dose: see under Insulin Injection (section 6.1.1.1); protamine may cause allergic reactions

Isophane Insulin Injection (NPH), 40 units/ml, price 10-ml vial = **E;** 80 units/ml, price 10-ml vial = **F**
Hypurin Isophane® (Weddel)
Injection, isophane insulin (bovine, highly purified) 40 units/ml, price 10-ml vial = **E;** 80 units/ml, price 10-ml vial = **F**
Initard 50/50® (Nordisk)
Injection, isophane insulin (porcine, highly purified) 50%, neutral insulin (porcine, highly purified) 50%. 40 units/ml, price 10-ml vial = **F;** 80 units/ml, price 10-ml vial = **G**
Insulatard® (Nordisk)
Injection, isophane insulin (porcine, highly purified) 40 units/ml, price 10-ml vial = **E;** 80 units/ml, price 10-ml vial = **G**
Mixtard 30/70® (Nordisk)
Injection, isophane insulin (porcine, highly purified) 70%, neutral insulin (porcine, highly purified) 30%. 40 units/ml, price 10-ml vial = **E;** 80 units/ml, price 10-ml vial = **G**
Neuphane® (Wellcome)
Injection, isophane insulin (bovine, highly purified) 40 units/ml, price 10-ml vial = **E;** 80 units/ml, price 10-ml vial = **F**

6.1.1.3 LONG-ACTING INSULIN PREPARATIONS

The amorphous form of **Insulin Zinc Suspension** (Semilente) has an intermediate action and the crystalline form (Ultralente) has a slow action. When the two preparations are mixed in different proportions, a wide range of action can be obtained. The aim in using a mixture of the suspensions is to control the diabetic condition with a single daily injection. A mixture containing 3 parts of amorphous and 7 parts of crystalline suspension is known as Insulin Zinc Suspension, Insulin Zinc Suspension (Mixed), or Lente insulin. Its peak activity occurs about 6 hours after injection and its action lasts up to 24 hours. Its main use is in moderately insulin-deficient patients who cannot be controlled adequately on diet and oral hypoglycaemic drugs. It is of only limited use in those with severe insulin deficiency.

If requirements for insulin zinc suspension exceed 40 units per day, diabetic control is usually easier on twice-daily insulin. It should not be used at dosage greater than 60 units per day. Neutral Insulin Injection, but not Insulin Injection (pH 3), can be mixed with insulin zinc suspension, to add a shorter-acting component.

Protamine Zinc Insulin, unlike Isophane Insulin, contains an excess of protamine and should not be mixed with soluble insulin as this leads to the formation of more protamine zinc insulin in the syringe and subcutaneous depot.

INSULIN ZINC SUSPENSION

(Insulin Zinc Suspension, Mixed; I.Z.S.)
Indications: diabetes mellitus
Cautions; Side-effects; Dose: see under Insulin Injection (section 6.1.1.1)

Insulin Zinc Suspension, Lente, 40 units/ml, price 10-ml vial = **E;** 80 units/ml, price 10-ml vial = **F**
Hypurin Lente® (Weddel)
Injection, insulin zinc suspension (bovine, highly purified) 40 units/ml, price 10-ml vial = **E;** 80 units/ml, price 10-ml vial = **F**
Lentard MC® (Novo)
Injection, insulin zinc suspension (bovine and porcine, highly purified) 40 units/ml, price 10-ml vial = **E;** 80 units/ml, price 10-ml vial = **F**
Monotard MC® (Novo)
Injection, insulin zinc suspension (porcine, highly purified) 40 units/ml, price 10-ml vial = **E;** 80 units/ml, price 10-ml vial = **F**
Neulente® (Wellcome)
Injection, insulin zinc suspension (bovine, highly purified) 40 units/ml, price 10-ml vial = **E;** 80 units/ml, price 10-ml vial = **F**

INSULIN ZINC SUSPENSION (CRYSTALLINE)

(Cryst. I.Z.S.)
Indications: diabetes mellitus

Cautions; Side-effects; Dose: see under Insulin Injection (section 6.1.1.1)

Insulin Zinc Suspension (Crystalline), Ultralente, 40 units/ml, price 10-ml vial = **E;** 80 units/ml, price 10-ml vial = **F**

Ultratard MC® (Novo)

Injection, insulin zinc suspension, crystalline (bovine, highly purified) 40 units/ml, price 10-ml vial = **E;** 80 units/ml, price 10-ml vial = **F**

PROTAMINE ZINC INSULIN INJECTION

Indications: diabetes mellitus

Cautions; Side-effects; Dose: see under Insulin Injection (section 6.1.1.1); protamine may cause allergic reactions; see also notes above

Protamine Zinc Insulin Injection, 40 units/ml, price 10-ml vial = **E;** 80 units/ml, price 10-ml vial = **F**

Hypurin Protamine Zinc® (Weddel)

Injection, protamine zinc insulin (bovine, highly purified) 40 units/ml, price 10-ml vial = **E;** 80 units/ml, price 10-ml vial = **F**

6.1.2 Oral hypoglycaemic drugs

6.1.2.1 Sulphonylureas
6.1.2.2 Biguanides

Oral hypoglycaemic drugs should not be used until patients have been shown not to respond adequately to a period of at least one month's restriction of energy and carbohydrate intake. They should be used to augment the effect of diet, and not to replace it.

6.1.2.1 SULPHONYLUREAS AND RELATED DRUGS

The sulphonylureas act mainly by augmenting insulin secretion and consequently are effective only when some residual pancreatic beta-cell activity is present.

Tolbutamide (Pramidex®, Rastinon®) has a short duration of action and is usually given twice daily; the total daily dose should not exceed 2 g. **Chlorpropamide** (Diabinese®, Melitase®) has a more prolonged action and need only be given once daily; the maximum effective dose is 500 mg daily. **Glibenclamide** (Daonil®, Euglucon®) has a duration of action intermediate between tolbutamide and chlorpropamide, but is usually given once daily within the dose range 2.5 to 20 mg.

Other sulphonylureas and related drugs include acetohexamide (Dimelor®), glibornuride (Glutril®), gliclazide (Diamicron®), glipizide (Glibenese®, Minodiab®), gliquidone (Glurenorm®), glymidine (Gondafon®), and tolazamide (Tolanase®).

All may lead to hypoglycaemia 4 hours or more after food but this is usually an indication of overdosage. Chlorpropamide may cause prolonged hypoglycaemia, particularly in the elderly and in those with renal disease; tolbutamide is preferable in the elderly. Chlorpropamide and tolbutamide may cause facial flushing after drinking alcohol; this effect is uncommon with glibenclamide. Sulphonylureas must be used with caution in patients with renal insufficiency.

Sulphonylureas are best avoided in obese patients unless their symptoms and diabetic control have not improved despite weight loss to within 15% of their ideal body weight.

ACETOHEXAMIDE

Indications: diabetes mellitus

Cautions; Contra-indications; Side-effects: see under Chlorpropamide

Dose: 0.25–1.5 g daily; up to 500 mg given as a single daily dose, higher doses divided

Dimelor® (Lilly)

Tablets, yellow, scored, acetohexamide 500 mg. Price 20 tabs = **C**

CHLORPROPAMIDE

Indications: diabetes mellitus (for use in diabetes insipidus, see section 6.5.2)

Cautions: see notes above. Drug interactions: see Appendix 1

Contra-indications: impaired adrenal, hepatic, renal, and thyroid function; pregnancy; diabetes complicated by surgery, severe infection, or coma

Side-effects: anorexia, nausea, vomiting, epigastric discomfort, weakness, paraesthesia; sensitivity reactions including fever, rashes, jaundice, eosinophilia, flushing with alcohol

Dose: up to 500 mg once daily, according to the patient's needs

Chlorpropamide Tablets, chlorpropamide 100 mg, price 20 tabs = **B;** 250 mg, price 20 tabs = **C**

Diabinese® (Pfizer)

Tablets, scored, chlorpropamide 100 mg. Price 20 tabs = **C**

Tablets, scored, chlorpropamide 250 mg. Price 20 tabs = **D**

Glymese® (DDSA)

Tablets, scored, chlorpropamide 250 mg. Price 20 tabs = **B**

Melitase® (Berk)

Tablets, scored, chlorpropamide 100 mg. Price 20 tabs = **B**

Tablets, scored, chlorpropamide 250 mg. Price 20 tabs = **C**

GLIBENCLAMIDE

Indications: diabetes mellitus

Cautions; Contra-indications: see under Chlorpropamide

Side-effects: see under Chlorpropamide (except facial flushing)

Dose: initially 5 mg daily; dose range 2.5–15 mg daily

Glibenclamide Tablets, glibenclamide 2.5 mg, price 20 tabs = **D**; 5 mg, price 20 tabs = **E**

Daonil® (Hoechst)
Tablets, scored, glibenclamide 5 mg. Price 20 tabs = **E**

Semi-Daonil® (Hoechst)
Tablets, scored, glibenclamide 2.5 mg. Price 20 tabs = **D**

Euglucon® (Roussel)
Tablets, glibenclamide 2.5 mg. Price 20 tabs = **D**
Tablets, scored, glibenclamide 5 mg. Price 20 tabs = **E**

GLIBORNURIDE

Indications: diabetes mellitus
Cautions; Contra-indications; Side-effects: see under Chlorpropamide
Dose: initially 12.5–25 mg daily; max. 75 mg daily

Glutril® (Roche)
Tablets, scored, glibornuride 25 mg. Price 20 tabs = **D**

GLICLAZIDE

Indications: diabetes mellitus
Cautions; Contra-indications: see under Chlorpropamide
Side-effects: gastro-intestinal disturbances, nausea, headache, rashes
Dose: initially, 40–80 mg daily

▼ **Diamicron®** (Servier)
Tablets, scored, gliclazide 80 mg. Price 20 tabs = **E**

GLIPIZIDE

Indications: diabetes mellitus
Cautions; Contra-indications; Side-effects: see under Chlorpropamide
Dose: initially 2.5–5 mg; max. 30 mg daily

Glipizide Tablets, glipizide 5 mg. Price 20 tabs = **C**

Glibenese® (Pfizer)
Tablets, scored, glipizide 5 mg. Price 20 tabs = **D**

Minodiab® (Farmitalia Carlo Erba)
Tablets, scored, glipizide 5 mg. Price 20 tabs = **C**

GLIQUIDONE

Indications: diabetes mellitus
Cautions: drug interactions: see Appendix 1
Contra-indications: severe hepatic or renal impairment, pregnancy, diabetes complicated by severe infection or surgery
Side-effects: gastro-intestinal disturbances, rashes
Dose: 45–60 mg daily in divided doses; max. 180 mg daily

▼ **Glurenorm®** (Winthrop)
Tablets, scored, gliquidone 30 mg. Price 20 tabs = **E**

GLYMIDINE

Indications: diabetes mellitus
Contra-indications: hepatic and renal impairment, pregnancy, surgery, severe infections
Side-effects: gastro-intestinal disturbances, allergic rashes; rarely leucopenia, thrombocytopenic purpura; intolerance to alcohol
Dose: initially 1.5 g with breakfast; max. 2 g daily

Gondafon® (Schering)
Tablets, scored, glymidine 500 mg. Price 20 tabs = **D**

TOLAZAMIDE

Indications: diabetes mellitus
Cautions; Contra-indications; Side-effects: see under Chlorpropamide
Dose: initially 100–250 mg with breakfast; max. 1 g daily

Tolanase® (Upjohn)
Tablets, scored, tolazamide 100 mg. Price 20 tabs = **B**
Tablets, scored, tolazamide 250 mg. Price 20 tabs = **D**

TOLBUTAMIDE

Indications: diabetes mellitus (for use in diabetes insipidus, see section 6.5.2)
Cautions; Contra-indications; Side-effects: see under Chlorpropamide
Dose: *by mouth,* 3 g on 1st day, 2 g on 2nd day, 1 g on 3rd day; maintenance dose 0.5–2 g daily
For diagnosis of diabetes mellitus, *by slow intravenous injection,* 1 g

Tolbutamide Tablets, tolbutamide 500 mg. Price 20 tabs = **B**

Pramidex® (Berk)
Tablets, scored, tolbutamide 500 mg. Price 20 tabs = **B**

Rastinon® (Hoechst)
Tablets, scored, tolbutamide 500 mg. Price 20 tabs = **C**
Injection, tolbutamide 50 mg (as sodium salt)/ml. Price 20-ml amp = **D**

6.1.2.2 BIGUANIDES

The biguanides **metformin** (Glucophage®) and **phenformin** (Dibotin®) act in a different way from the sulphonylureas. They are effective only in the presence of functioning pancreatic islet cells, and inhibit glucose absorption from the gut and glucose oxidation. They are most frequently used in overweight diabetics who will not, or cannot, lose weight. They should not be regarded as being interchangeable with the sulphonylureas.

Biguanides should not be used in the presence of renal or hepatic insufficiency.

Gastro-intestinal side-effects are uncommon with sustained-release preparations of phenformin. The duration of action of phenformin in the sustained-release form is 12 hours. The incidence of side-effects is low if the dose is not in excess of 50 mg twice daily. Metformin has an action lasting 8 to 12 hours; it is given in daily doses of 1 to 2 g.

Because of the real and unpredictable risk of lactic acidosis, the use of phenformin has declined and that of metformin increased. Metformin is not however, free from this hazard and patients not adequately controlled on diet and sulphonylureas alone should be considered as candidates for insulin therapy. The use of combinations of biguanides and sulphonylureas has declined as the incidence of adverse effects has become more widely recognised.

METFORMIN HYDROCHLORIDE

Indications: diabetes mellitus
Cautions: drug interactions: see Appendix 1
Contra-indications: renal or hepatic failure, congestive heart failure, severe infection, pregnancy, alcoholism
Side-effects: anorexia, nausea, vomiting, diarrhoea, lactic acidosis
Dose: 500 mg every 8 hours *or* 850 mg every 12 hours

Glucophage® (Rona)
Tablets, f/c, metformin hydrochloride 500 mg. Price 20 tabs = **B**
Tablets, f/c, metformin hydrochloride 850 mg. Price 20 tabs = **C**

PHENFORMIN HYDROCHLORIDE

Indications: diabetes mellitus
Cautions; Contra-indications; Side-effects: see under Metformin Hydrochloride; lactic acidosis more common with phenformin
Dose: initially, 25 mg twice daily; also see notes

Dibotin® (Winthrop)
Capsules, s/r, turquoise/clear enclosing white pellets, phenformin hydrochloride 25 mg. Price 20 caps = **B**
Capsules, s/r, blue/clear enclosing white pellets, phenformin hydrochloride 50 mg. Price 20 caps = **B**
Tablets, scored, phenformin hydrochloride 25 mg. Price 20 tabs = **A**

6.1.3 Treatment of diabetic coma

Soluble insulin is the only form of insulin that may be given intravenously and it should be used in the management of diabetic coma (hyperglycaemic coma). There is no unanimity on the best way to administer insulin to patients in diabetic coma or precoma; it is necessary to achieve and to maintain an adequate blood-insulin concentration until the metabolic disturbance is brought under control.

Absorption of insulin from intramuscular injections is usually rapid but may be impaired in those patients who are hypotensive or who have poor peripheral circulation. If a slow infusion pump is available, insulin is probably best given by the intravenous route; a single bolus (however large) will only achieve an adequate concentration for a short period of time. When given at a dose rate of 0.1 unit/kg/hour (7 units/hour in a 70-kg patient) plasma insulin is maintained at an adequate concentration so long as the infusion is continued.

Since insulin is liable to become adsorbed onto plastic syringes and infusion tubing, it is advisable to add human albumin to the syringe containing the insulin. A convenient method is to add 100 units of insulin to a 50-ml syringe filled with albumin solution; when infused at 3.5 ml/hour this achieves adequate blood-insulin concentrations in an average adult diabetic and leads to progressive reversal of the metabolic abnormalities in the majority of patients.

If the response is judged inadequate the infusion rate may be doubled or quadrupled. When blood glucose has fallen to 8 mmol/litre the rate of infusion can be dropped to about 0.02 unit/kg/hour (1.5 to 2 units/hour in a 70-kg patient) and continued until the patient is ready to take food by mouth.

If no slow infusion pump is available, insulin may be given by combined intravenous and intramuscular injection. The initial dose is 10 units intravenously and 10 units intramuscularly; hourly intramuscular injections of 5 units should be continued until the blood glucose has fallen to a satisfactory concentration.

In the presence of hypotension and poor tissue perfusion the intravenous route of insulin adminstration is preferable. Depots of insulin may build up during treatment and late hypoglycaemia should be watched for and treated appropriately.

6.1.4 Treatment of hypoglycaemia

Initially, dextrose or 3 or 4 lumps of sugar should be taken with a little water. If necessary, this may be repeated in 10 to 15 minutes.

If hypoglycaemic coma (insulin coma) occurs, up to 50 ml of 50% dextrose intravenous infusion should be given intravenously, or dextrose or sucrose may be given by stomach tube.

Glucagon can be given as an alternative to parenteral dextrose in hypoglycaemic coma or precoma. It is a polypeptide hormone produced by the alpha cells of the islets of Langerhans. Its action is to increase blood glucose concentration by mobilising glycogen stored in the liver.

Glucagon is used to treat acute hypoglycaemic reactions and it has the advantage that it can be injected by any route (intramuscular, subcutaneous, or intravenous) in a dose of 1 mg (1 unit) in circumstances when an intravenous injection of dextrose would be difficult or impossible to administer. Its use should be followed by the administration of dextrose by mouth as soon as the patient is conscious.

It may be issued to close relatives of insulin-treated patients for emergency use in hypoglycaemic attacks. It is often advisable to prescribe on an 'if necessary' basis to all hospitalised insulin-treated patients, so that it may be given rapidly by the nurses during an hypoglycaemic emergency. If not effective in 20 minutes the dose may be repeated.

Diazoxide (Eudemine®) is useful in the management of patients with chronic hypoglycaemia from excess endogenous insulin secretion, either from an islet cell tumour or islet cell hyperplasia. It has no place in the management of acute hypoglycaemia.

DIAZOXIDE

Indications: chronic hypoglycaemia (for use in hypertensive crisis see section 2.5.1)
Cautions: ischaemic heart disease, pregnancy, labour, impaired renal function. Drug interactions: see Appendix 1
Side-effects: anorexia, nausea, vomiting, hypertrichosis, hyperuricaemia, hypotension, oedema, tachycardia, arrhythmias, extrapyramidal effects
Dose: by mouth, initially 5 mg/kg daily in 2–3 divided doses

Eudemine® (A&H)
Tablets, s/c, diazoxide 50 mg. Price 20 tabs = **D**

GLUCAGON

Indications: acute hypoglycaemia
Cautions: severe hypertension may be provoked in phaeochromocytoma
Side-effects: nausea, vomiting, hypersensitivity reactions, hypokalaemia
Dose: by subcutaneous, intramuscular, or intravenous injection, 0.5–1 unit repeated after 20 minutes if necessary
Note: 1 unit of glucagon ≈ 1 mg of glucagon or glucagon hydrochloride

Glucagon Injection, powder for reconstitution, glucagon (as hydrochloride, with lactose). Price 1-unit vial = **E;** 10-unit vial = **J** (both with diluent)

6.2 Thyroid and antithyroid drugs

This section includes thyroid hormones (section 6.2.1) and antithyroid drugs (section 6.2.2).

6.2.1 Thyroid hormones

Thyroid hormones are used in hypothyroidism, and also in diffuse non-toxic goitre, lymphadenoid goitre, and thyroid carcinoma. Cretinism requires prompt treatment for normal development.

Thyroxine sodium (Eltroxin®) is the treatment of choice for maintenance therapy. The initial dose should not exceed 100 micrograms daily, or 25 micrograms in elderly patients or those with cardiac disease, increased at intervals of 2 to 4 weeks. The usual maintenance dose to relieve hypothyroidism is 100 to 300 micrograms daily.

In infants a daily dose of 50 micrograms should be given initially; subsequent therapy can be judged from plasma-thyroxine (T_4) measurements, clinical response, and skeletal maturation.

Liothyronine sodium (Tertroxin®) has a similar action to thyroxine but is more rapidly metabolised; 20 micrograms is equivalent to 100 micrograms of thyroxine. It may be used when a rapid response is desired, and for the investigation of certain thyroid disorders.

Liothyronine may be also used for the initiation of replacement therapy in patients with myxoedema and ischaemic heart disease since, if angina is precipitated the attack will be less prolonged than after thyroxine. The initial dose is 5 micrograms daily, increased at weekly intervals if angina is not precipitated. When a dose of 60 micrograms has been reached treatment can be changed to thyroxine.

Liothyronine injection is the treatment of choice in hypothyroid coma and may be given intravenously as an initial dose of 100 micrograms followed by 25 micrograms 6-hourly until improvement is noted. Adjunctive therapy includes intravenous fluids, hydrocortisone, and antibiotics; assisted ventilation is often required.

Dried **thyroid** should **not** be used as its effects are unpredictable.

LIOTHYRONINE SODIUM

(L-Tri-iodothyronine sodium)
Indications: hypothyroidism
Cautions: drug interactions: see Appendix 1
Contra-indications: angina, cardiovascular disorders
Side-effects: arrhythmias, anginal pain, tachycardia, cramps in skeletal muscles, headache, restlessness, excitability, flushing, sweating, diarrhoea, excessive weight loss
Dose: see notes above

Tertroxin® (Glaxo)
Tablets, scored, liothyronine sodium 20 micrograms. Price 20 tabs = **A**
Triiodothyronine (Glaxo)
Injection, powder for reconstitution, liothyronine sodium. Price 20-microgram amp = **F**

THYROXINE SODIUM

Indications: hypothyroidism
Cautions; Contra-indications; Side-effects: see under Liothyronine Sodium; has a delayed effect and cumulative action
Dose: see notes above

Thyroxine Tablets, thyroxine sodium 25, 50, and 100 micrograms. Price 20 tabs (all) = **A**

Eltroxin® (Glaxo)

Tablets, scored, thyroxine sodium 50 micrograms. Price 20 tabs = **A**

Tablets, thyroxine sodium 100 micrograms. Price 20 tabs = **A**

6.2.2 Antithyroid drugs

Carbimazole (Neo-Mercazole®) inhibits thyroxine synthesis. It should be given in an initial daily dose of 30 to 60 mg and maintained at this dose until the patient becomes euthyroid, usually 4 to 8 weeks; the dose may then be progressively reduced to a maintenance dose of between 5 and 15 mg daily. Rashes are common, and **propylthiouracil** may then be substituted, since cross-sensitivity between them is uncommon. Agranulocytosis is rare.

The dose of propylthiouracil is 300 to 450 mg daily. **Methylthiouracil** should **not** be used, as the incidence of side-effects is greater than with carbimazole or propylthiouracil.

It is no longer considered necessary to space doses of antithyroid drugs evenly throughout the 24 hours and the dose may be given once daily. Over-treatment with the rapid development of hypothyroidism is not uncommon and should be avoided particularly during pregnancy since it can cause foetal goitre.

Unless operation or use of radioactive iodine is planned, treatment should be for at least a year, and preferably two.

Potassium perchlorate (Peroidin®) blocks iodine uptake by the thyroid; it is used occasionally when toxic reactions appear with other antithyroid drugs, but may cause hypoplastic or aplastic anaemia and is now used infrequently.

Before partial thyroidectomy **iodine** should be given for about 2 weeks instead of carbimazole or propylthiouracil. Iodine should not be given to patients treated with potassium perchlorate since it leads to an exacerbation of thyrotoxicosis. Iodine can be prescribed as Aqueous Iodine Solution in a dose of 0.5 ml (65 mg total iodine) 3 times daily. Iodine should **not** be used for long-term treatment.

Radioactive sodium iodide (^{131}I and ^{125}I) solutions are used for the treatment of thyrotoxicosis, principally in patients over 45 years of age.

Propranolol (see section 2.4), 40 to 200 mg 6-hourly, is useful in patients whose symptoms can be partially relieved until full thyroid control is achieved. It is also used in doses of up to 5 mg intravenously in the treatment of thyrotoxic crises ('thyroid storm') in combination with sedation with chlorpromazine.

For the use of **protirelin** in the diagnosis of hyperthyroidism see section 6.7.2.

CARBIMAZOLE

Indications: thyrotoxicosis

Cautions: pregnancy

Contra-indications: tracheal obstruction, breast-feeding

Side-effects: nausea, headache, rashes, arthralgia; rarely alopecia, agranulocytosis

Dose: see notes above

Neo-Mercazole® (Nicholas)

Tablets, pink, scored, carbimazole 5 mg. Price 20 tabs = **B**

IODINE

Indications: pre-operative treatment of thyrotoxicosis

Cautions: pregnancy, children

Side-effects: hypersensitivity reactions including coryza-like symptoms, headache, lachrymation, conjunctivitis, pain in salivary glands, laryngitis, bronchitis, rashes; on prolonged treatment depression, insomnia, impotence, myxoedema; goitre in infants of mothers taking iodides

Aqueous Iodine Solution (Lugol's Solution), iodine 5%, potassium iodide 10% in purified water, freshly boiled and cooled, total iodine 130 mg/ml. Price 100 ml = **C**

Dose: 0.5 ml 3 times daily

POTASSIUM PERCHLORATE

Indications: thyrotoxicosis, but see notes

Contra-indications: large or retrosternal goitres

Side-effects: nausea, vomiting, rashes, fever, fatal aplastic anaemia, agranulocytosis, leucopenia, thrombocytopenia, pancytopenia, nephrotic syndrome

Dose: initially 200–250 mg every 6–8 hours; max. 1 g daily; reduce to 100–125 mg every 6–8 hours after 2–4 weeks

Peroidin® (Larkhall)

Tablets, potassium perchlorate 200 mg. Price 20 tabs = **C**

PROPYLTHIOURACIL

Indications: thyrotoxicosis

Cautions; Contra-indications; Side-effects: see under Carbimazole; also rarely tendency to haemorrhage

Dose: see notes above

Propylthiouracil Tablets, propylthiouracil 50 mg. Price 20 tabs = **B**

6.3 Corticosteroids

This section includes replacement therapy (section 6.3.1), suppression of disease processes (section 6.3.2), disadvantages of corticosteroids (section 6.3.3), and clinical management (section 6.3.4).

6.3.1 Replacement therapy

The adrenal cortex normally secretes the mainly glucocorticoid cortisone and hydrocortisone (cortisol) and the mineralocorticoids deoxycortone and aldosterone. Physiological replacement is achieved with hydrocortisone or cortisone acetate tablets. The salt-retaining action of these steroids requires reinforcement with **fludrocortisone** (Florinef®), which resembles aldosterone. **Prednisolone** or **prednisone** may also be used for replacement therapy in combination with fludrocortisone.

In Addison's disease or following adrenalectomy, **hydrocortisone** 20 to 30 mg or **cortisone acetate** 25 to 37.5 mg daily by mouth is usually required. This should be given in 2 doses, the larger in the morning and the smaller in the evening, mimicking the normal diurnal rhythm of cortisol secretion. The optimum daily dose should be determined for each individual on the basis of clinical response and also, if possible, by monitoring the plasma-cortisol concentration. Glucocorticoid therapy should be supplemented by fludrocortisone 50 to 200 micrograms daily.

In acute adrenocortical insufficiency, **hydrocortisone sodium succinate** is given intravenously in doses of 100 mg every 6 to 8 hours in sodium chloride intravenous infusion. **Prednisolone sodium phosphate** injection (Codelsol®) is an alternative preparation for intravenous or intramuscular use.

In hypopituitarism glucocorticoids should be given as in adrenocortical insufficiency, but since the production of aldosterone is also regulated by the renin-angiotensin system a mineralocorticoid is not often required. Additional replacement therapy with thyroxine and sex hormones should be given as indicated by the pattern of hormone deficiency that is present.

Cortisone acetate injection may be given intramuscularly but absorption is slower than by mouth and it has generally been **superseded** by hydrocortisone or prednisolone injections when parenteral treatment is indicated.

Corticosteroid cover for adrenalectomy, hypophysectomy or operations on patients on long-term treatment with corticosteroids is determined logically from the knowledge that in a normal person major stress will not lead to the secretion of more than 300 mg of cortisol in 24 hours. Once the stress is over, cortisol production rapidly returns to the usual 20 to 30 mg per 24 hours. A simple way of mimicking this is to administer hydrocortisone, initially parenterally but changing to oral therapy once this is possible.

On the day of operation hydrocortisone sodium succinate 100 mg is given intramuscularly with the premedication, and repeated 8-hourly. In the absence of any complications, the dose can be halved every 24 hours until a normal maintenance dose of 25 mg per 24 hours is reached on the 5th postoperative day. In the case of adrenalectomy it is not necessary to start mineralocorticoid therapy immediately and this can be withheld until the patient can take tablets. If there are post-operative complications, hydrocortisone may have to be continued at a slightly higher dose (50 to 75 mg per 24 hours) and a parenteral mineralocorticoid added.

Synthetic glucocorticoids of increased potency may be substituted for hydrocortisone but offer few advantages. They tend to have less mineralocorticoid activity than hydrocortisone; although this is often an advantage when they are used in the treatment of inflammatory and neoplastic diseases, it is rarely important in replacement therapy.

Dexamethasone and **betamethasone** have little if any mineralocorticoid action and because of their longer action are favoured for suppressing corticotrophin secretion in congenital adrenal hyperplasia. In common with all glucocorticoids their suppressive action on the hypothalamic-pituitary-adrenal axis is greatest and most prolonged when they are given at night. In normal subjects a single dose of 1 mg of dexamethasone at night is sufficient to inhibit corticotrophin secretion for 24 hours. This is the basis of the 'overnight dexamethasone suppression test' for diagnosing Cushing's syndrome.

Although most types of Cushing's syndrome are treated surgically, that which occasionally accompanies carcinoma of the bronchus is not usually amenable to surgery. **Metyrapone** (section 6.7.2), which interferes directly with steroid synthesis in the adrenal glands, has been found helpful in controlling the symptoms of the disease.

DEOXYCORTONE PIVALATE

Indications: adrenocortical insufficiency
Cautions; Contra-indications; Side-effects: section 6.3.3
Dose: *by intramuscular injection,* 50–100 mg every 2–4 weeks

Percorten M® (Ciba)
Injection, deoxycortone pivalate 25 mg/ml. Price 1-ml amp = **D**

FLUDROCORTISONE ACETATE

Indications: adrenocortical insufficiency, adrenal hyperplasia
Cautions; Contra-indications; Side-effects: section 6.3.3
Dose: adrenocortical insufficiency, 50–200 micrograms daily
Adrenal hyperplasia, 1–2 mg daily

Florinef® (Squibb)
Tablets, pink, scored, fludrocortisone acetate 100 micrograms. Price 20 tabs = **C**
Tablets, pink, scored, fludrocortisone acetate 1 mg. Price 20 tabs = **G**

For monographs on systemic glucocorticoids, see end of section 6.3.4

6.3.2 Suppression of disease processes

Betamethasone, dexamethasone, hydrocortisone, prednisolone, and prednisone are used for their anti-inflammatory effect; the table shows equivalent anti-inflammatory doses.

Table: Equivalent Doses of Glucocorticoids

Drug	Equivalent anti-inflammatory dose
Betamethasone	3 mg
Cortisone acetate	100 mg
Dexamethasone	3 mg
Hydrocortisone	80 mg
Methylprednisolone	16 mg
Prednisolone	20 mg
Prednisone	20 mg
Triamcinolone	16 mg

High potency is of no advantage, though the effect on water and electrolyte retention is important. **Prednisolone** is the glucocorticoid most commonly used by mouth for continued treatment. **Prednisone** is only active after conversion in the body to prednisolone. **Betamethasone** and **dexamethasone** are as satisfactory. All must be given in divided doses for a continuous effect. **Cortisone acetate** is not used for inflammatory disease suppression, as it causes fluid retention.

Hydrocortisone sodium succinate can be given by intravenous injection in *shock*. It begins to act within one hour, and since this use is temporary the dangers of high dosage do not apply. Cortisone acetate injections are only used intramuscularly for short periods when a patient cannot swallow; absorption is slower than by mouth. Injections of hydrocortisone and prednisolone can be used in the same way. Betamethasone and dexamethasone are used by mouth when water retention would be a disadvantage, as for example in treating traumatic *cerebral oedema.*

The action of corticosteroids in suppressing inflammatory reactions may be useful in conditions such as *rheumatoid arthritis, rheumatic fever, active chronic hepatitis,* and *ulcerative colitis*. The prognosis of serious conditions such as *systemic lupus erythematosus* and *polyarteritis nodosa* can be improved. The effects of the disease process may be suppressed and symptoms relieved, but the underlying condition is not cured, although it may ultimately burn itself out. If serious side-effects occur in response to the large doses of corticosteroids required to suppress the disease process, it is sometimes possible to reduce the dose of corticosteroid by giving a small dose of an immunosuppressive drug (see section 8.2.1).

Because corticosteroids reduce antibody formation, they may be used to suppress or modify *allergic reactions*. This may benefit some types of *asthma* and *skin diseases*. It may also lead to remissions of acquired *haemolytic anaemia,* the *nephrotic syndrome,* and some cases of *thrombocytopenic purpura*.

For the use of the corticosteroids in the treatment of *reticuloses* and some types of *leukaemia,* see section 8.2.2.

Corticosteroids are extensively used on the skin, and also as aerosols, eye-drops, enemas, and intra-articular injections. The formulation here is of the greatest importance and partly determines the choice of drug. A potent drug such as betamethasone valerate may be more effective than any strength of a weaker one such as hydrocortisone.

The use of corticosteroids in the treatment of many other disease processes is described elsewhere in the following sections:

colon and rectum, sections 1.5, 1.7.2 and 1.7.3
asthma, section 3.2
rheumatic diseases, section 10.1.2
eye, section 11.4
otitis externa, section 12.1.1
allergic rhinitis, section 12.2.1
aphthous ulcers, section 12.3.1
skin, section 13.4

6.3.3 Disadvantages of corticosteroids

Overdosage or prolonged use of corticosteroids may exaggerate some of the normal physiological actions of corticosteroids such as hypertension, sodium retention, potassium loss, muscle weakness, and diabetes. Osteoporosis is a danger, particularly in the elderly, as it may result in vertebral collapse. Mental disturbances may occur; a serious paranoid state or depression with risk of suicide may be induced, particularly in patients with a history of mental disorder. Euphoria is frequently observed. Peptic ulceration is a recognised complication which may result in haemorrhage or perforation.

In children, administration of corticosteroids may result in suppression of growth. Corticosteroids given during pregnancy may affect adrenal development in the child and cause cleft palate.

Modification of tissue reactions may result in spread of infection. Suppression of clinical signs may allow septicaemia or tuberculosis to reach an advanced stage before being recognised. Systemic corticosteroid therapy should be avoided in patients with psoriasis, as subsequent reduction in dose is commonly followed by a severe and persistent exacerbation.

ADRENAL SUPPRESSION. The administration of exogenous corticosteroids suppresses the secretion of corticotrophin and may lead to adrenal atrophy which can persist for years after stopping prolonged corticosteroid therapy; any illness or surgical emergency may then require further corticosteroid therapy to compensate for lack of sufficient adrenocortical response.

High doses of corticosteroids may cause Cushing's syndrome, with moon face, striae, and acne; it is usually reversible on withdrawal of treatment, but this must always be gradually tapered to avoid symptoms of acute adrenal insufficiency (see 'steroid card' below).

Several drugs reduce the effects of the corticosteroids; see Appendix 1.

6.3.4 Clinical management

Corticosteroids should not be used unless the benefits justify the hazards. Dosage varies widely in different diseases and in different patients.

In status asthmaticus, acute hypersensitivity reactions such as angioneurotic laryngeal oedema and anaphylactic shock, and other serious acute conditions, an immediate systemic corticosteroid effect is required. In such cases **hydrocortisone sodium succinate** given by intravenous injection in a dose of 100 to 300 mg can be life-saving. Doses of up to 500 mg of hydrocortisone intravenously have been used in severe shock, particularly when due to Gram-negative septicaemia. High doses should be given because the risk of complications is negligible with short-term therapy.

If the use of corticosteroids can save or prolong life, as in exfoliative dermatitis, pemphigus, or acute leukaemia, high doses must be given, as the complications of therapy are likely to be less serious than the effects of the disease itself.

When long-term corticosteroid therapy is used to relieve discomfort and disability in relatively benign chronic diseases such as rheumatoid arthritis the danger of treatment may become greater than the disabilities produced by the disease. To minimise side-effects the maintenance dose should be kept as low as possible, seldom exceeding the equivalent of 10 mg of prednisolone daily.

When treatment is to be discontinued, the dose should be reduced gradually over a period of several weeks or months depending on the dosage and duration of the therapy.

In an attempt to reduce pituitary-adrenal suppression in patients requiring long-term corticosteroid therapy, intermittent treatment has been used, either in short courses, or by giving the corticosteroid as a single dose on alternate days instead of daily. This is satisfactory in some cases and should be considered when prolonged treatment is necessary.

STEROID CARDS. Patients should carry cards giving details of their dosage and possible complications. These 'steroid cards' can be obtained from local Family Practitioner Committees or

DHSS Printing and Stationery Unit
Room 110
North Fylde Central Office
Norcross
Blackpool FY5 3TA

In Scotland 'steroid cards' are available from Health Boards.

Pharmacists may obtain these cards from the Pharmaceutical Society of Great Britain.

I am a patient on—

STEROID TREATMENT

which must not be stopped abruptly

and in the case of intercurrent illness may have to be increased

full details are available from the hospital or general practitioners shown overleaf →

STC1

INSTRUCTIONS

1. DO NOT STOP taking the steroid drug except on medical advice. Always have a supply in reserve.
2. In case of feverish illness, accident, operation (emergency or otherwise), diarrhoea or vomiting the steroid treatment MUST be continued. Your doctor may wish you to have a LARGER DOSE or an INJECTION at such times.
3. If the tablets cause indigestion consult your doctor AT ONCE.
4. Always carry this card while receiving steroid treatment and show it to any doctor, dentist, nurse or midwife whom you may consult.
5. After your treatment has finished you must still tell any new doctor, dentist, nurse or midwife that you have had steroid treatment.

ANAESTHESIA. Anaesthetists must know whether a patient is taking or has been taking corticosteroids as adrenal suppression may cause a precipitous fall in blood pressure during anaesthesia.

CHILDREN. In children the indications for corticosteroids are the same as for adults but risks are greater. The implications of starting these drugs are serious, and they should be used only when specifically indicated, in a minimal dosage, and for the shortest possible time. Prolonged or continuous treatment is rarely justified. Stunting of growth may be mitigated by giving corticotrophin, or by giving prednisolone as single doses on alternate days.

Stimulation of the adrenal cortex by **corticotrophin** or **tetracosactrin** has been used as an alternative to corticosteroids to control certain diseases, especially Crohn's disease (see section 1.5), severe asthma in children (section 6.5.1), and rheumatic diseases (section 10.1.2.1). There is no close relationship between the dose producing satisfactory clinical improvement and the equivalent dose of oral corticosteroid producing the same degree of improvement.

BETAMETHASONE

Indications: section 6.3.2
Cautions; Contra-indications; Side-effects: section 6.3.3
Dose: *by mouth,* 0.5–5 mg daily in divided doses
By intramuscular injection or intravenous injection or infusion, 4–20 mg, repeated up to 4 times in 24 hours

Betnelan® (Glaxo)
Tablets, scored, betamethasone 500 micrograms. Price 20 tabs = **C**

Betnesol® (Glaxo)
Tablets, pink, scored, soluble, betametnasone 500 micrograms (as sodium phosphate). Price 20 tabs = **C**
Injection, betamethasone 4 mg (as sodium phosphate)/ml. Price 1-ml amp = **C**

CORTISONE ACETATE

Indications: section 6.3.1
Cautions; Contra-indications; Side-effects: section 6.3.3
Dose: *by mouth,* 25–37.5 mg daily—see notes

Cortisone Tablets, cortisone acetate 5 mg, price 20 tabs = **A**; 25 mg, price 20 tabs = **B**

Cortelan® (Glaxo)
Tablets, scored, cortisone acetate 25 mg. Price 20 tabs = **C**

Cortistab® (Boots)
Tablets, scored, cortisone acetate 5 mg. Price 20 tabs = **A**
Tablets, scored, cortisone acetate 25 mg. Price 20 tabs = **B**
Injection (aqueous suspension), cortisone acetate 25 mg/ml. Price 10-ml vial = **C**

Cortisyl® (Roussel)
Tablets, scored, cortisone acetate 25 mg. Price 20 tabs = **C**

DEXAMETHASONE

Indications: sections 6.3.1 and 6.3.2
Cautions; Contra-indications; Side-effects: section 6.3.3
Dose: *by mouth,* 0.5–2 mg daily; up to 15 mg in severe disease
By intramuscular injection or intravenous injection or infusion, initially 0.5–20 mg of dexamethasone phosphate daily
Note: 1.3 mg dexamethasone sodium phosphate ≡ 1.2 mg dexamethasone phosphate ≡ 1 mg dexamethasone

Dexamethasone Tablets, dexamethasone 500 micrograms. Price 20 tabs = **C**

Decadron® (MSD)
Tablets, yellow, scored, dexamethasone 500 micrograms. Price 20 tabs = **C**
Tablets, blue, scored, dexamethasone 750 micrograms. Price 20 tabs = **D**
Injection, dexamethasone phosphate 4 mg (as sodium salt)/ml. Price 2-ml vial = **D**

Decadron Shock-Pak® (MSD)
Injection, dexamethasone 20 mg (as sodium phosphate)/ml. Price 5-ml vial = **J**

Dexacortisyl® (Roussel)
Tablets, scored, dexamethasone 500 micrograms. Price 20 tabs = **C**

Oradexon® (Organon)
Tablets, dexamethasone 500 micrograms. Price 20 tabs = **C**
Tablets, dexamethasone 2 mg. Price 20 tabs = **D**
Injection, dexamethasone sodium phosphate 5 mg/ml. Price 1-ml amp = **C**
Injection, dexamethasone 4 mg (as sodium phosphate)/ml. Price 2-ml vial = **D**

HYDROCORTISONE

Indications: section 6.3.1 and 6.3.2
Cautions; Contra-indications; Side-effects: section 6.3.3
Dose: *by mouth,* 20–30 mg daily—see notes
By intramuscular injection or intravenous injection or infusion, 100–500 mg (as sodium phosphate or succinate), repeated up to 4 times in 24 hours

Hydrocortisone Sodium Succinate Injection, powder for reconstitution, hydrocortisone (as sodium succinate). Price 100-mg vial (with diluent) = **C**; 500-mg vial = **E**

Efcortelan Soluble® (Glaxo)
Injection, powder for reconstitution, hydrocortisone (as sodium succinate). Price 100-mg vial (with diluent) = **C**

Efcortesol® (Glaxo)
Injection, hydrocortisone 100 mg (as sodium phosphate)/ml. Price 1-ml amp = **C**; 5-ml amp = **F**

Hydrocortistab® (Boots)
Tablets, scored, hydrocortisone 20 mg. Price 20 tabs = **B**
Hydrocortone® (MSD)
Tablets, scored, hydrocortisone 10 mg. Price 20 tabs = **B**
Tablets, scored, hydrocortisone 20 mg. Price 20 tabs = **C**
Solu-Cortef® (Upjohn)
Injection, powder for reconstitution, hydrocortisone (as sodium succinate). Price 100-mg vial (with diluent) = **C**

METHYLPREDNISOLONE

Indications: section 6.3.2
Cautions; Contra-indications; Side-effects: section 6.3.3
Dose: *by mouth,* in inflammatory disorders up to 16 mg daily; in allergic disorders, up to 40 mg daily, in divided doses
By intramuscular injection or intravenous injection or infusion, up to 120 mg

Depo-Medrone® (Upjohn)
Injection (aqueous suspension), methylprednisolone acetate 40 mg/ml. Price 1-ml vial = **E**; 2-ml vial or syringe = **F**; 5-ml vial = **H**
Medrone® (Upjohn)
Tablets, pink, scored, methylprednisolone 2 mg. Price 20 tabs = **D**
Tablets, scored, methylprednisolone 4 mg. Price 20 tabs = **E**
Tablets, scored, methylprednisolone 16 mg. Price 20 tabs = **H**
Solu-Medrone® (Upjohn)
Injection, powder for reconstitution, methylprednisolone (as sodium succinate). Price 40-mg mix-o-vial = **D**; 125-mg mix-o-vial = **F**; 0.5, 1-, and 2-g vial (all with solvent) = **J**

PREDNISOLONE

Indications: section 6.3.2
Cautions; Contra-indications; Side-effects: section 6.3.3
Dose: *by mouth,* initially up to 30 mg daily
By intravenous or intramuscular injection, up to 100 mg (as sodium phosphate)
By intramuscular injection, prednisolone acetate 25–100 mg

Prednisolone Tablets, prednisolone 1 and 5 mg. Price 20 tabs (both) = **A**
Codelcortone® (MSD)
Tablets, scored, prednisolone 5 mg. Price 20 tabs = **A**
Codelsol® (MSD)
Injection, prednisolone 16 mg (as sodium phosphate)/ml. Price 2-ml vial = **D**
Delta-Phoricol® (Wallace Mfg)
Tablets, prednisolone 5 mg. Price 20 tabs = **C**
Deltacortril Enteric® (Pfizer)
Tablets, brown, e/c, prednisolone 2.5 mg. Price 20 tabs = **B**
Tablets, red, e/c, prednisolone 5 mg. Price 20 tabs = **B**
Deltalone® (DDSA)
Tablets, prednisolone 1 mg. Price 20 tabs = **A**
Tablets, scored, prednisolone 5 mg. Price 20 tabs = **A**
Deltastab® (Boots)
Tablets, scored, prednisolone 1 mg. Price 20 tabs = **A**
Tablets, scored, prednisolone 5 mg. Price 20 tabs = **A**
Injection (aqueous suspension), prednisolone acetate 25 mg/ml. Price 5-ml vial = **B**
Precortisyl® (Roussel)
Tablets, prednisolone 1 mg. Price 20 tabs = **A**
Tablets, scored, prednisolone 5 mg. Price 20 tabs = **A**
Tablets, prednisolone 25 mg. Price 20 tabs = **D**
Prednesol® (Glaxo)
Tablets, pink, scored, soluble, prednisolone 5 mg (as sodium phosphate). Price 20 tabs = **D**
Sintisone® (Farmitalia Carlo Erba)
Tablets, scored, prednisolone steaglate 6.65 mg (≡ prednisolone 5 mg). Price 20 tabs = **D**

PREDNISONE

Indications: section 6.3.2
Cautions; Contra-indications; Side-effects: section 6.3.3
Dose: initially up to 30 mg daily

Prednisone Tablets, prednisone 1 and 5 mg. Price 20 tabs (both) = **A**
Decortisyl® (Roussel)
Tablets, prednisone 1 mg. Price 20 tabs = **A**
Tablets, scored, prednisone 5 mg. Price 20 tabs = **A**
Econosone® (DDSA)
Tablets, prednisone 1 mg. Price 20 tabs = **A**
Tablets, prednisone 5 mg. Price 20 tabs = **A**

TRIAMCINOLONE

Indications: section 6.3.2
Cautions; Contra-indications; Side-effects: section 6.3.3
Dose: *by mouth,* up to 24 mg daily in divided doses
By intramuscular injection, 40 mg of acetonide for depot effect, repeated at intervals according to the patient's response

Triamcinolone Tablets, triamcinolone 4 mg. Price 20 tabs = **D**
Adcortyl® (Squibb)
Tablets, scored, triamcinolone 4 mg. Price 20 tabs = **D**
Kenalog® (Squibb)
Injection (aqueous suspension), triamcinolone acetonide 40 mg/ml. Price 1-ml vial = **D**; 1-ml syringe = **E**; 2-ml syringe = **F**
Ledercort® (Lederle)
Tablets, blue, triamcinolone 2 mg. Price 20 tabs = **D**
Tablets, triamcinolone 4 mg. Price 20 tabs = **F**

6.4 Sex hormones

Sex hormones are described under the following section headings:

6.4.1 Female sex hormones
6.4.2 Male sex hormones and antagonists
6.4.3 Anabolic steroids

6.4.1 Female sex hormones

There are two groups of female sex hormones, the oestrogens (section 6.4.1.1) and progestogens (section 6.4.1.2). Combined hormone preparations for menopausal symptoms are listed in section 6.4.1.3 and for menstrual disorders in section 6.4.1.4. Combined and other preparations for use as contraceptives are in sections 7.3.1 and 7.3.2.

6.4.1.1 OESTROGENS

Oestrogens are necessary for the development of female secondary sexual characteristics; they stimulate myometrial hypertrophy, with endometrial hyperplasia which may lead to withdrawal bleeding when treatment is stopped, and they promote cornification of the vagina. They inhibit the production by the anterior pituitary of follicle-stimulating hormone (FSH), thereby suppressing ovulation.

Oestrogens are used in small doses over long periods to diminish the symptoms associated with the menopause; the development of postmenopausal osteoporosis is retarded. Hormone replacement is **not** indicated routinely in postmenopausal women. There is no evidence that 'natural' are in any way superior to 'synthetic' oestrogens and **ethinyloestradiol** is the drug of choice. If oestrogens are given on a long-term basis a low dose of progestogen should be added.

Sudden withdrawal of high-dose therapy causes menstrual bleeding and has been used to produce artificial menstruation in certain types of amenorrhoea. In spasmodic dysmenorrhoea, low doses of oestrogens combined with a progestogen, started early in the cycle, will inhibit ovulation and relieve the pain. Senile vaginitis and vulvitis are treated by oestrogens systemically or locally. Oestrogens are of benefit in some cases of breast cancer and cancer of the prostate (see section 8.3.1).

When oestrogens are used systemically there is an increased risk of thrombo-embolism and this must be borne in mind before they are prescribed. **Ethinyloestradiol** is about 25 times as potent as stilboestrol and is preferable in the treatment of menopausal symptoms, when 10 to 20 micrograms may be given daily.

Stilboestrol has been used for suppression of lactation. Its use has now been superseded by that of bromocriptine (section 6.7.1), an ergot derivative. Stilboestrol is used in the treatment of certain neoplastic conditions (see section 8.3.1).

ETHINYLOESTRADIOL

Indications: menopausal symptoms, amenorrhoea (for use in oral contraceptives, see section 7.3.1)
Cautions: pregnancy, diabetes, epilepsy, cardiac or renal disease, history of jaundice
Contra-indications: oestrogen-dependent carcinoma, history of thrombo-embolism, hepatic impairment, endometriosis, porphyria
Side-effects: nausea and vomiting, weight gain, breast enlargement and tenderness, withdrawal bleeding, sodium retention with oedema, changes in liver function, jaundice, rashes and chloasma, depression, headache, endometrial carcinoma in postmenopausal women
Dose: 10–50 micrograms thrice daily

Ethinyloestradiol Tablets, ethinyloestradiol 10 and 50 micrograms, price 20 tabs = **A**; 1 mg, price 20 tabs = **B**
Lynoral® (Organon)
Tablets, ethinyloestradiol 10 micrograms. Price 20 tabs = **A**
Tablets, ethinyloestradiol 1 mg. Price 20 tabs = **C**
Pabendrol® (P&B)
Tablets, ethinyloestradiol 10 micrograms. Price 20 tabs = **A**
Tablets, ethinyloestradiol 20 micrograms. Price 20 tabs = **A**
Tablets, ethinyloestradiol 50 micrograms. Price 20 tabs = **A**
Tablets, ethinyloestradiol 100 micrograms. Price 20 tabs = **A**
Tablets, ethinyloestradiol 1 mg. Price 20 tabs = **B**

CHLOROTRIANISENE

Indications: menopausal symptoms
Cautions; Contra-indications; Side-effects: see under Ethinyloestradiol
Dose: 12–24 mg daily for 30 days

Tace® (Merrell)
Tablets, scored, chlorotrianisene 24 mg. Price 20 tabs = **C**

DIENOESTROL

Indications: menopausal symptoms
Cautions; Contra-indications; Side-effects: see under Ethinyloestradiol
Dose: up to 5 mg daily

Dienoestrol Tablets, dienoestrol 300 micrograms, and 1 and 5 mg. Price 20 tabs (all) = **A**

OESTRADIOL

Indications: menopausal symptoms, amenorrhoea
Cautions; Contra-indications; Side-effects: see under Ethinyloestradiol

Dose: by mouth, oestradiol valerate 1–2 mg daily
By intramuscular injection, oestradiol benzoate 1–5 mg at 1–14 day intervals
By implantation, oestradiol 25–50 mg

Oestradiol Implants (Organon)
Implant, oestradiol 25 mg. Price each = **E**
Implant, oestradiol 50 mg. Price each = **G**
Implant, oestradiol 100 mg. Price each = **I**

Benztrone® (P&B)
Injection (oily), oestradiol benzoate 1 mg/ml. Price 1-ml amp = **B**
Injection (oily), oestradiol benzoate 5 mg/ml. Price 1- and 2-ml amp (both) = **B**

Progynova® (Schering)
Tablets, yellow, s/c, oestradiol valerate 1 mg. Price 21-tab calendar pack = **E**
Tablets, blue, s/c, oestradiol valerate 2 mg. Price 21-tab calendar pack = **E**

OESTRIOL

Indications: menopausal symptoms
Cautions; Contra-indications; Side-effects: see under Ethinyloestradiol
Dose: 250–500 micrograms daily

Hormonin® (Carnrick)
Tablets, pink, oestriol 270 micrograms, oestradiol 600 micrograms, oestrone 1.4 mg. Price 20 tabs = **C**
Dose: ½-2 tablets daily

Ovestin® (Organon)
Tablets, oestriol 250 micrograms. Price 20 tabs = **B**

OESTROGENS, CONJUGATED

Indications: menopausal symptoms, dysfunctional uterine bleeding
Cautions; Contra-indications; Side-effects: see under Ethinyloestradiol
Dose: 0.625–1.25 mg daily for 21 days, repeated after 7 days

Premarin® (Ayerst)
Tablets, maroon, s/c, conjugated oestrogens 625 micrograms. Price 20 tabs or 21-tab calendar pack = **C**
Tablets, yellow, s/c, conjugated oestrogens 1.25 mg. Price 20 tabs or 21-tab calendar pack = **D**
Tablets, purple, s/c, conjugated oestrogens 2.5 mg. Price 20 tabs = **E**

PIPERAZINE OESTRONE SULPHATE

Indications: menopausal symptoms
Cautions; Contra-indications; Side-effects: see under Ethinyloestradiol
Dose: 1.5–4.5 mg daily for 21–28 days, repeated after 5–7 days

Harmogen® (Abbott)
Tablets, peach, scored, piperazine oestrone sulphate 1.5 mg. Price 20 tabs = **D**

QUINESTRADOL

Indications: menopausal symptoms
Cautions; Contra-indications; Side-effects: see under Ethinyloestradiol
Dose: 500 micrograms 1–2 times daily

Pentovis® (Warner)
Capsules, green, quinestradol 250 micrograms. Price 20 caps = **D**

QUINESTROL

Indications: inhibition and suppression of lactation
Cautions; Contra-indications; Side-effects: see under Ethinyloestradiol
Dose: inhibition, 2 mg within 6 hours of delivery and a further 2 mg if symptoms persist
Suppression, 2 mg immediately and a further 2 mg after 48 hours if necessary

Estrovis® (Warner)
Tablets, pink, quinestrol 4 mg. Price 2 tabs = **D**

6.4.1.2 PROGESTOGENS

Progestogens modify some of the effects of oestrogens and act mainly on tissues sensitised by them; their effects are inhibited by excess of oestrogens. Synthetic progestogens are variably metabolised into testosterone and oestrogen; thus their side-effects vary with the preparation and dosage. There are two main groups of progestogens: *testosterone derivatives* such as norethisterone (Primolut N®) which also have some androgenic activity, and the naturally-occurring hormone *progesterone* and its *derivatives* such as hydroxyprogesterone.

Norethisterone is used in the treatment of endometriosis and dysfunctional uterine bleeding. Progestogens have been used in habitual abortion but their efficacy is in doubt. If they are used for this purpose they should be of the true progesterone-derivative type, e.g. **hydroxyprogesterone hexanoate** (Proluton Depot®) to avoid any masculinisation of a female foetus. This drug is also used in the treatment of carcinoma of the uterus (see section 8.3.2).

Combinations of oestrogens and progestogens are frequently used for premenstrual and menstrual disorders and as oral contraceptives (see section 7.3.1). In some preparations used in the management of menorrhagia, the dose of oestrogen is higher than in similar combinations used as oral contraceptives.

ALLYLOESTRENOL

Indications: habitual abortion
Cautions; Contra-indications; Side-effects: see under Norethisterone; but less virilising
Dose: 5–15 mg daily

Gestanin® (Organon)
Tablets, allyloestrenol 5 mg. Price 20 tabs = **E**

DYDROGESTERONE

Indications: amenorrhoea, endometriosis, dysfunctional uterine bleeding
Side-effects: rarely breakthrough bleeding (increase dose if it occurs)
Dose: 10 mg twice daily for 21 days, repeated after 7 days

Duphaston® (Duphar)
Tablets, scored, dydrogesterone 10 mg. Price 20 tabs = **F**

ETHISTERONE

Indications: menorrhagia
Cautions; Contra-indications; Side-effects: see under Norethisterone
Dose: 10–15 mg 3 times daily for 8 days prior to menstruation

Gestone-Oral® (P&B)
Tablets, ethisterone 10 mg. Price 20 tabs = **B**
Tablets, ethisterone 25 mg. Price 20 tabs = **C**

HYDROXYPROGESTERONE HEXANOATE

Indications: habitual abortion
Cautions; Contra-indications; Side-effects: see under Norethisterone; but less virilising
Dose: by intramuscular injection, 250–500 mg weekly

Proluton Depot® (Schering)
Injection, hydroxyprogesterone hexanoate 250 mg/ml. Price 1-ml amp = **E**; 1-ml syringe = **F**; 2-ml amp = **E**; 2-ml syringe = **G**

MEDROXYPROGESTERONE ACETATE

Indications: dysfunctional uterine bleeding, secondary amenorrhoea, endometriosis, habitual abortion (for use as a contraceptive, see section 7.3.2)
Cautions; Contra-indications; Side-effects: see under Norethisterone; but less virilising
Dose: by mouth, up to 40 mg daily
By intramuscular injection, 50 mg weekly or 100 mg every 2 weeks

Depo-Provera® (Upjohn)
Injection, medroxyprogesterone acetate 50 mg/ml. Price 1-ml vial = **D**; 3-ml vial = **F**; 5-ml vial = **G**
See also section 8.3.2

Provera® (Upjohn)
Tablets, scored, medroxyprogesterone acetate 5 mg. Price 20 tabs = **D**

NORETHISTERONE

Indications: dysfunctional uterine bleeding, amenorrhoea, endometriosis (for use as a contraceptive, see section 7.3.2)
Cautions: impaired cardiac or renal function, asthma, epilepsy
Contra-indications: undiagnosed vaginal bleeding, missed or incomplete abortion, impaired liver function
Side-effects: nausea, weight gain, headache, depression, changes in libido, gynaecomastia, altered menstrual cycles, virilisation of foetus, acne, urticaria
Dose: up to 25 mg daily

Primolut N® (Schering)
Tablets, norethisterone 5 mg. Price 20 tabs = **D**

Utovlan® (Syntex)
Tablets, scored, norethisterone 5 mg. Price 20 tabs = **D**

PROGESTERONE

Indications: dysfunctional uterine bleeding, habitual abortion
Cautions; Contra-indications; Side-effects: see under Norethisterone
Dose: by intramuscular injection, 5–10 mg daily or up to 20 mg 2–3 times weekly
By vagina or rectum, 200–400 mg daily

Cyclogest® (Collins)
Suppositories, progesterone 200 mg. Price 20 suppos = **G**
Suppositories, progesterone 400 mg. Price 20 suppos = **H**

Gestone® (P&B)
Injection, progesterone 10 mg/ml. Price 1-ml amp = **A**
Injection, progesterone 25 mg/ml. Price 1-ml amp = **A**
Injection, progesterone 50 mg/ml. Price 1- and 2-ml amp (both) = **B**

6.4.1.3 COMBINED PREPARATIONS FOR MENOPAUSAL SYMPTOMS

For ***Cautions; Contra-indications; Side-effects:*** see under Combined Oral Contraceptives, section 7.3.1.

Cyclo-Progynova 1 mg® (Schering)
Calendar pack, all s/c, 11 beige tablets, oestradiol valerate 1 mg; 10 brown tablets, oestradiol valerate 1 mg and levonorgestrel 250 micrograms. Price per pack = **E**
Dose: 1 beige tablet daily for 11 days, starting on 5th day of menstrual cycle or at any time if cycles have ceased or are infrequent, then 1 brown tablet daily for 10 days, followed by a 7-day interval

Cyclo-Progynova 2 mg® (Schering)
Calendar pack, all s/c, 11 white tablets, oestradiol valerate 2 mg; 10 orange tablets, oestradiol valerate 2 mg and levonorgestrel 500 micrograms. Price per pack = **E**
Dose: see above, but starting with 1 white tablet daily

Menophase® (Syntex)
Calendar pack, 5 pink tablets, mestranol 12.5

micrograms; 8 orange tablets, mestranol 25 micrograms; 2 yellow tablets, mestranol 50 micrograms; 3 green tablets, mestranol 25 micrograms and norethisterone 1 mg; 6 blue tablets, mestranol 30 micrograms and norethisterone 1.5 mg; 4 lavender tablets, mestranol 20 micrograms and norethisterone 750 micrograms. Price per pack = **E**
Dose: 1 pink tablet daily, starting on a Sunday, then 1 tablet daily in sequence

Mixogen® (Organon)
Tablets, ethinyloestradiol 4.4 micrograms, methyltestosterone 3.6 mg. Price 20 tabs = **B**
Dose: 1–2 tablets daily for 3 weeks, followed by a 7-day interval
Injection (oily), oestradiol benzoate 1 mg, oestradiol phenylpropionate 4 mg, testosterone propionate 20 mg, testosterone phenylpropionate 40 mg, and testosterone isohexanoate 40 mg/ml. Price 2-ml vial = **D**
Dose: by intramuscular injection, 1 ml every 3–4 weeks

Prempak 0.625® (Ayerst)
Calendar pack, all s/c, 21 maroon tablets, conjugated oestrogens 625 micrograms; 7 white tablets, norgestrel 500 micrograms. Price per pack = **D**
Dose: 1 maroon tablet daily for 14 days, then 1 white and 1 maroon tablet daily for 7 days, followed by a 7-day interval

Prempak 1.25® (Ayerst)
Calendar pack, all s/c, 21 yellow tablets, conjugated oestrogens 1.25 mg; 7 white tablets, norgestrel 500 micrograms. Price per pack = **E**
Dose: see above, but starting with 1 yellow tablet daily

Trisequens® (Organon)
Calendar pack, 12 blue tablets, oestradiol 2 mg, oestriol 1 mg; 10 white tablets, oestradiol 2 mg, oestriol 1 mg, norethisterone acetate 1 mg; 6 red tablets, oestradiol 1 mg, oestriol 500 micrograms. Price per pack = **E**
Dose: 1 blue tablet daily, starting on 5th day of menstrual cycle or at any time if cycles have ceased or are infrequent, then 1 tablet daily in sequence

6.4.1.4 COMBINED PREPARATIONS FOR MENSTRUAL DISORDERS

For ***Cautions; Contra-indications; Side-effects:*** see under Combined Oral Contraceptives, section 7.3.1.

Controvlar® (Schering)
Tablets, pink, s/c, norethisterone acetate 3 mg, ethinyloestradiol 50 micrograms. Price 21 tabs = **C**
Dose: 1 tablet daily for 21 days, starting on 5th day of menstrual cycle, followed by a 7-day interval

Enavid® (Searle)
Tablets, pink, scored, norethynodrel 5 mg, mestranol 75 micrograms. Price 20 tabs = **C**
Dose: up to 4 tablets daily

Metrulen® (Searle)
Tablets, ethynodiol diacetate 2 mg, mestranol 100 micrograms. Price 20 tabs = **C**
Dose: 1–3 tablets daily

Metrulen-M® (Searle)
Tablets, ethynodiol diacetate 1 mg, mestranol 100 micrograms. Price 20 tabs = **B**
Dose: 1 tablet daily from 5th to 25th day of cycle

Norlestrin® (P-D)
Tablets, pink, f/c, norethisterone acetate 2.5 mg, ethinyloestradiol 50 micrograms. Price 21-tab calendar pack = **C**
Dose: 1–2 tablets daily from 5th to 25th day of cycle

6.4.2 Male sex hormones and antagonists

Androgens cause masculinisation; they may be used as replacement therapy in castrated adults and in those who are hypogonadal due to either pituitary or testicular disease. In the normal male they depress spermatogenesis.

They are useless as a treatment of impotence unless it accompanies hypogonadism and should not be given until the hypogonadism has been properly investigated.

When given to patients with hypopituitarism they can lead to normal sexual development and potency but not fertility. If fertility is desired, the correct treatment is with chorionic gonadotrophin injection (HCG) and with menotrophin (FSH) (section 6.5.1) which will stimulate spermatogenesis as well as androgen production.

Caution should be used when androgens or chorionic gonadotrophin are used in treating boys with delayed puberty since the fusion of epiphyses is hastened and may result in short stature.

Androgens are sometimes effective in the treatment of disseminated carcinoma of the breast (see section 8.3.3) but their masculinising effects in the female have led to the preferential use of synthetic anabolic steroids (such as nandrolone) which cause less masculinisation.

Androgens, like oestrogens, have an anabolic action on protein metabolism, maintaining muscle mass and preventing osteoporosis; for these reasons gonadal hormonal replacement therapy may be indicated for reasons other than maintaining sexual activity.

Methyltestosterone and its synthetic analogues are only weakly active when given by mouth and not uncommonly cause cholestatic jaundice; for these reasons intramuscular depot preparations are preferable.

Testosterone propionate is effective for 1–2 weeks when given by intramuscular injection; the usual dose is 50 to 100 mg every 1–2 weeks. A mixture of testosterone esters in a depot form (Sustanon®) is satisfactory for replacement therapy which can usually be maintained with 250 mg once a month, although more frequent administration is sometimes needed. These preparations have superseded the implantation of testosterone pellets.

Cyproterone (Androcur®) is an anti-androgen used in the treatment of severe hypersexuality and sexual deviation in the male; it inhibits spermatogenesis and produces reversible infertility. Abnormal sperm forms are produced. Cyproterone is also used in the treatment of severe hirsutism in women. Hepatic tumours have been produced in *animal* studies. Careful consideration should be given to the risk/benefit ratio before commencing treatment.

CYPROTERONE ACETATE

Indications: see notes above
Cautions: chronic hepatic disease, adrenocortical function suppressed, diabetes mellitus, blood estimations required every 4–6 weeks, impaired ability to drive and operate machinery
Contra-indications: acute hepatic disease, malignant or wasting disease, severe depression, history of thrombo-embolic disorders, immature youths
Side-effects: gynaecomastia, galactorrhoea, benign breast nodules, sedation and depression, weight gain, changes in hair pattern
Dose: male hypersexuality, 50 mg twice daily

Androcur® (Schering)
Tablets, scored, cyproterone acetate 50 mg. Price 20 tabs = **I**

MESTEROLONE

Indications: hypogonadism
Cautions; Contra-indications; Side-effects: see under Testosterone
Dose: 25 mg 3–4 times daily

Pro-Viron® (Schering)
Tablets, scored, mesterolone 25 mg. Price 20 tabs = **E**

METHYLTESTOSTERONE

Indications: hypogonadism, but see notes above
Cautions; Contra-indications; Side-effects: see under Testosterone; also cholestatic jaundice
Dose: initially 30–50 mg daily, in divided doses

Methyltestosterone Tablets, methyltestosterone 5 mg, price 20 tabs = **B**; 10 mg, price 20 tabs = **C**; 25 mg, price 20 tabs = **D**; 50 mg, price 20 tabs = **E**

Plex-Hormone® (Consolidated)
Tablets, red, methyltestosterone 5 mg, deoxycortone acetate 500 micrograms, ethinyloestradiol 2 micrograms, tocopheryl acetate 5 mg. Price 20 tabs = **C**

Virormone-Oral® (P&B)
Tablets, methyltestosterone 5 mg. Price 20 tabs = **B**
Tablets, methyltestosterone 10 mg. Price 20 tabs = **B**
Tablets, methyltestosterone 25 mg. Price 20 tabs = **C**
Tablets, methyltestosterone 50 mg. Price 20 tabs = **D**

TESTOSTERONE

Indications: hypogonadism
Cautions: renal or hepatic impairment, circulatory failure, epilepsy, migraine
Contra-indications: breast cancer in men, prostatic carcinoma, pregnancy, nephrosis
Side-effects: oedema, increase in weight, hypercalcaemia, increased bone growth, premature closure of epiphyses if given in early puberty, high doses cause virilism in women, and suppress spermatogenesis
Dose: *sublingual administration,* 10–30 mg daily
By mouth, testosterone undecanoate 120–160 mg daily for 2–3 weeks, then 40–120 mg daily
By intramuscular injection, testosterone enanthate 250 mg every 2–3 weeks; testosterone propionate 10–50 mg 2–3 times weekly
By implantation, 100–600 mg; duration of effect 7–8 months

Testosterone Implants (Organon)
Implant, testosterone 100 mg. Price each = **E**
Implant, testosterone 200 mg. Price each = **G**

Plex-Hormone® (Consolidated)
Injection, testosterone propionate 20 mg, deoxycortone acetate 500 micrograms, oestradiol benzoate 100 micrograms, tocopheryl acetate 20 mg/ml. Price 1-ml amp = **B**

Primoteston Depot® (Schering)
Injection, testosterone enanthate 250 mg/ml. Price 1-ml amp = **F**

Restandol® (Organon)
Capsules, red-brown, testosterone undecanoate 40 mg in oily solution. Price 20 caps = **F**

Sustanon 100® (Organon)
Injection (oily), testosterone propionate 20 mg, testosterone phenylpropionate 40 mg, and testosterone isohexanoate 40 mg/ml. Price 1-ml amp = **D**
Dose: by intramuscular injection, 1 ml every 2 weeks

Sustanon 250® (Organon)
Injection (oily), testosterone propionate 30 mg, testosterone phenylpropionate 60 mg, testosterone isohexanoate 60 mg, and testosterone decanoate 100 mg/ml. Price 1-ml amp = **E**
Dose: by intramuscular injection, 1 ml every 4 weeks

Testoral Sublings® (Organon)
Sublingual tablets, testosterone 10 mg. Price 20 tabs = **C**

Virormone® (P&B)
Injection, testosterone propionate 10 mg/ml. Price 1-ml amp = **B**
Injection, testosterone propionate 25 mg/ml. Price 1-ml amp = **B**

Injection, testosterone propionate 50 mg/ml. Price 1- and 2-ml amp (both) = **B**

6.4.3 Anabolic steroids

All the anabolic steroids have some androgenic activity but they cause less virilisation than androgens in women. Their protein-building property led to the hope that they might be widely useful in medicine but this hope has not been realised. They have, for example, been given for osteoporosis in women and in cases of wasting. Their use as body builders or tonics is quite unjustified.

It is doubtful whether anabolic steroids should be used to increase height in children; apart from virilising properties, they may lead to premature closing of the epiphyses so that the eventual height is the same as or less than without treatment. Side-effects such as cholestatic jaundice may occur. They reduce the itching of chronic biliary obstruction but usually make the jaundice worse. Some anabolic steroids produce hepatic tumours in long-term use.

Anabolic steroids are also used in the treatment of some aplastic anaemias (see section 9.1.3), in the palliative treatment of breast cancer (see section 8.3.3) and to stimulate fibrinolysis. They are abused by some athletes although they have not been shown to have a beneficial effect.

ETHYLOESTRENOL

Indications: see notes above
Cautions; Contra-indications; Side-effects: see under Methandienone
Dose: 2–4 mg daily

Orabolin® (Organon)
Tablets, ethyloestrenol 2 mg. Price 20 tabs = **D**

METHANDIENONE

Indications: see notes above
Cautions: renal impairment, circulatory failure, diabetes, epilepsy, migraine. Drug interactions: see Appendix 1
Contra-indications: hepatic impairment, prostatic carcinoma, pregnancy
Side-effects: jaundice on prolonged treatment, virilism with high doses, acne, oedema
Dose: 5–10 mg daily

Dianabol® (Ciba)
Tablets, scored, methandienone 5 mg. Price 20 tabs = **C**

NANDROLONE

Indications: see notes above
Cautions; Contra-indications; Side-effects: see under Methandienone
Dose: by intramuscular injection, nandrolone decanoate 25–50 mg every 3 weeks; nandrolone phenylpropionate 25 mg weekly

Deca-Durabolin® (Organon)
Injection (oily), nandrolone decanoate 25 mg/ml. Price 1-ml amp or syringe = **D**
Injection (oily), nandrolone decanoate 50 mg/ml. Price 1-ml amp or syringe = **F**
Injection (oily), nandrolone decanoate 100 mg/ml. Price 1-ml amp = **G**

Durabolin® (Organon)
Injection (oily), nandrolone phenylpropionate 25 mg/ml. Price 1-ml amp or syringe = **C**
Injection (oily), nandrolone phenylpropionate 50 mg/ml. Price 1-ml syringe = **E**

NORETHANDROLONE

Indications: see notes above
Cautions; Contra-indications; Side-effects: see under Methandienone
Dose: 20–30 mg daily

Nilevar® (Searle)
Tablets, norethandrolone 10 mg. Price 20 tabs = **E**

OXYMETHOLONE

Indications: see notes above (for use in aplastic anaemia, see section 9.1.2)
Cautions; Contra-indications; Side-effects: see under Methandienone; jaundice and liver disturbances are common
Dose: for anabolic effect, 5–10 mg daily for 4–6 weeks, repeated after 10–15 days; CHILD 2.5–5 mg daily

Anapolon® (Syntex)
Tablets, oxymetholone 5 mg. Price 20 tabs = **D**

STANOZOLOL

Indications: see notes above (for use in aplastic anaemia, see section 9.1.2)
Cautions; Contra-indications; Side-effects: see under Methandienone
Dose: by mouth, 5 mg daily
By intramuscular injection, 50 mg every 2–3 weeks

Stromba® (Sterling Research)
Tablets, scored, stanozolol 5 mg. Price 20 tabs = **F**
Injection, stanozolol 50 mg/ml. Price 1-ml amp = **E**

6.5 Hypothalamic and pituitary hormones

This section includes hypothalamic and anterior pituitary hormones (section 6.5.1) and posterior pituitary hormones (section 6.5.2).

6.5.1 Hypothalamic and anterior pituitary hormones

Clomiphene (Clomid®) is an anti-oestrogen which is capable of stimulating gonadotrophin release by inhibiting the negative feed-back of gonadal steroids on the hypothalamus. It should only be administered under specialist supervision. Its main use is in inducing ovulation in patients with secondary amenorrhoea due to the Stein-Leventhal syndrome. In patients who produce a good oestrogen response to clomiphene but who show no biochemical evidence of corpus luteum formation, a single injection of **chorionic gonadotrophin** (HCG) 7 days after the clomiphene is sometimes of help.

Cyclofenil (Rehibin®) is used similarly to clomiphene in the treatment of anovulatory infertility, but may be less effective.

In women with proven hypopituitarism, ovulation and corpus luteum formation can be achieved with injections of **menotrophin** (human follicle-stimulating hormone, FSH) and **chorionic gonadotrophin;** this requires biochemical monitoring and cn only be undertaken in specialised centres.

Oligospermia due to a failure of gonadotrophin production can sometimes be successfully treated with injections of chorionic gonadotrophin and menotrophin. This treatment is useless in patients with either primary gonadal failure or mechanical blockage in the epididymis or vas deferens.

Gonadorelin (section 6.7.2) and **chorionic gonadotrophin** have both been used in the treatment of cryptorchidism and delayed puberty. Indiscriminate use should be **discouraged** since in the former condition it is of doubtful value and in the latter, detailed endocrinological investigation is required.

Corticotrophin and **tetracosactrin** have little therapeutic use in endocrinology and are used as diagnostic agents. They have been used to stimulate an adrenal cortex suppressed by chronic corticosteroid administration or following the removal of a unilateral adrenal cortical tumour but even in this role they are of limited use since suppression is often at the hypothalamic or pituitary level.

Corticotrophin and tetracosactrin are still occasionally used as an alternative to corticosteroids to control certain conditions, especially Crohn's disease and asthma in children, the alleged advantages being that there is no adrenocortical suppression and that linear growth may be inhibited to a lesser extent. Once a response has occurred, alternate-day therapy should be used if possible. The dose administered has to be judged by monitoring urinary 17-oxogenic steroid excretion since adrenal response is variable. **Tetracosactrin** is preferred as adrenal stimulation may last for up to 48 hours after each injection; allergic reactions may occur.

Growth hormone (somatotrophin, HGH) is effective in the treatment of short stature due to HGH deficiency. Only human growth hormone is active in man, and at present HGH preparations are only available at special centres. The daily replacement dose is in the range 0.5 to 1 unit by intramuscular injection.

The clinical uses of **protirelin,** the hypothalamic releasing hormone for thyrotrophin (thyrotrophin-releasing hormone, TRH) and **gonadorelin,** the releasing hormone for the gonadotrophins (gonadotrophin-releasing hormone, LH-RH) are not established and their main uses are as diagnostic agents (section 6.7.2).

CHORIONIC GONADOTROPHIN

HCG

Indications: see notes above

Cautions: cardiac or renal impairment, asthma, epilepsy, migraine, skin tests required if allergies exist

Side-effects: oedema, headache, tiredness, mood changes; sexual precocity with high doses; hyperstimulation may cause ovarian enlargement and possibility of multiple pregnancy

Dose: according to patient's requirements

Chorionic Gonadotrophin Injection, powder for reconstitution, chorionic gonadotrophin 500- and 1000-unit amp (both) = **C**; 5000-unit amp = **E** (all with solvent)

Gonadotraphon LH® (P&B)
Injection, powder for reconstitution, chorionic gonadotrophin. Price 500- and 1000-unit amp (both) = **C**; 5000-unit amp = **E** (all with solvent)

Pregnyl® (Organon)
Injection, powder for reconstitution, chorionic gonadotrophin. Price 500-unit amp = **C**; 1500-unit amp = **D**; 5000-unit amp = **E** (all with solvent)

Profasi® (Serono)
Injection, powder for reconstitution, chorionic gonadotrophin. Price 500- and 1000-unit amp (both) = **C**; 2000-unit amp = **D**; 5000-unit amp = **E** (all with solvent)

CLOMIPHENE CITRATE

Indications: anovulatory infertility—see notes above

Cautions: incidence of multiple births increased

Contra-indications: hepatic disease, ovarian cysts, endometrial carcinoma, pregnancy, abnormal uterine bleeding

Side-effects: hot flushes, abdominal discomfort, blurred vision, ovarian enlargement, nausea, vomiting, depression, insomnia, breast tenderness, weight gain

Dose: 50 mg daily for 5 days

Clomiphene Tablets, clomiphene citrate 50 mg. Price 20 tabs = **H**

Clomid® (Merrell)
Tablets, beige, scored, clomiphene citrate 50 mg. Price 20 tabs = **I**

Serophene® (Serono)
Tablets, scored, clomiphene citrate 50 mg. Price 20 tabs = **H**

CORTICOTROPHIN

ACTH

Indications: see notes above

Cautions; Contra-indications; Side-effects: see section 6.3.3; also caution in hypertension

Dose: according to patient's requirements

Acthar Gel® (Armour)

Injection, corticotrophin (with gelatin) 20 units/ml. Price 5-ml vial = **E**

Injection, corticotrophin (with gelatin) 40 units/ml. Price 2-ml vial = **E;** 5-ml vial = **G**

Injection, corticotrophin (with gelatin) 80 units/ml. Price 2.5-ml vial = **G**; 5-ml vial = **I**

ACTH/CMC (Ferring)

Injection, corticotrophin (with carboxymethylcellulose) 60 units/ml. Price 5-ml vial = **G**

CYCLOFENIL

Indications: anovulatory infertility—see notes above

Contra-indications: see under Clomiphene Citrate

Side-effects: hot flushes, abdominal discomfort, nausea; rarely cholestatic jaundice

Dose: initially, 100 mg twice daily for 3 cycles (or 3 months if cycles are irregular); if regular cycles are not established, 200 mg twice daily for 10 days starting on 3rd day of cycle, followed by 20 treatment-free days, repeated for at least 3 months

▼ **Rehibin®** (Thames)

Tablets, scored, cyclofenil 100 mg. Price 20 tabs = **F** (Hosp. only)

GROWTH HORMONE

Indications: short stature

Contra-indications: diabetes mellitus

Side-effects: antibody formation

Dose: see notes above

Crescormon® (KabiVitrum)

Injection, powder for reconstitution, human growth hormone. Price 4-unit vial (with diluent) = **J**

Nanormon® (Nordisk)

Injection, powder for reconstitution, human growth hormone. Price 4-unit vial (with diluent) = **G**

MENOTROPHIN

Indications: see notes above

Cautions: ovarian cysts, adrenal or thyroid disorders, intracranial lesions, exclude endocrine disorders

Side-effects: sensitivity reactions, ovarian enlargement, multiple pregnancy

Dose: according to patient's response

Gonadotraphon FSH® (P&B)

Injection, powder for reconstitution, serum gonadotrophin (from pregnant mares' serum). Price 1000-unit amp (with diluent) = **E**

Pergonal® (Serono)

Injection, powder for reconstitution, human follicle-stimulating hormone 75 units, human luteinising hormone 75 units, lactose. Price per amp (with solvent) = **G** (Hosp. only)

TETRACOSACTRIN

Indications: see notes above

Cautions; Contra-indications; Side-effects: see section 6.3.3

Dose: according to patient's requirements

Synacthen® (Ciba)

Injection, tetracosactrin 250 micrograms (as acetate)/ml. Price 1-ml amp = **C**

Synacthen Depot® (Ciba)

Injection, tetracosactrin 1 mg (as acetate)/ml, with zinc phosphate complex. Price 1-ml amp = **D;** 2-ml vial = **E**

Dose: initially 0.5–1 mg every 2–3 days

6.5.2 Posterior pituitary hormones

Vasopressin (antidiuretic hormone, ADH) is used in the treatment of diabetes insipidus of pituitary origin; it is of no value in the nephrogenic type. Vasopressin is given as **lypressin** (8-lysine vasopressin, Syntopressin®) or as the vasopressin analogue **desmopressin** (DDAVP®) which has a longer duration of action due to slower clearance from the circulation.

Desmopressin 2 to 4 micrograms by intramuscular injection produces an antidiuresis lasting 24 hours; 10 to 20 micrograms given intranasally produces antidiuresis for about 12 hours.

In diabetes insipidus of renal as well as of pituitary origin, some benefit may be obtained from the paradoxical antidiuretic effect of the **thiazide diuretics** (see section 2.2.1).

In diabetes insipidus of pituitary or hypothalamic origin **chlorpropamide** and **tolbutamide** (see section 6.1.2.1), but not other sulphonylureas, may reduce polyuria. They act by sensitising the renal tubules to the action of endogenous vasopressin and are useful only in mild cases. The dose of chlorpropamide should not exceed 350 mg daily in adults or 200 mg daily in children and great care should be taken to avoid hypoglycaemic reactions which can be particularly dangerous in patients with hypopituitarism. In diabetes insipidus following pituitary surgery or trauma, treatment may be required only for a limited period and it is particularly important to take precautions to avoid overdosage and unnecessary prolongation of therapy.

Carbamazepine (see section 4.8.1) has been shown to have an antidiuretic action. Although its exact mode of action is not yet known, it is probably similar to that of chlorpropamide. It is used in a dose of 200 mg once or twice daily.

DESMOPRESSIN

Indications: diabetes insipidus

Cautions: heart failure, asthma, epilepsy, migraine, pregnancy

Contra-indications: vascular disease, chronic nephritis
Dose: intranasally, 10–20 micrograms 1–2 times daily
By intramuscular or intravenous injection, 1–4 micrograms daily

DDAVP® (Ferring)
Intranasal solution, desmopressin 100 micrograms/ml. Price 2.5-ml dropper bottle and catheter = **H**
Injection, desmopressin 4 micrograms/ml. Price 1-ml amp = **C**

LYPRESSIN
Indications: diabetes insipidus
Cautions; Contra-indications: see under Desmopressin; also caution in hypertension
Side-effects: nausea, abdominal pain, urge to defaecate, nasal congestion with ulceration of mucosa
Dose: intranasally, 5–20 units 3–7 times daily

Syntopressin® (Sandoz)
Nasal spray, lypressin 50 units/ml, providing 2.5 units/squeeze. Price 5-ml spray bottle = **F**

PITUITARY (POSTERIOR LOBE)
Indications: diabetes insipidus
Cautions; Contra-indications: see under Desmopressin; also contra-indicated in hypertension
Side-effects: see under Vasopressin; also allergic rhinitis, asthma, alveolitis
Dose: by insufflation, 60–90 antidiuretic units daily in divided doses

Di-Sipidin® (P&B)
Insufflation capsules, pituitary (posterior lobe) 30 antidiuretic units. Price 25 caps and insufflator = **F**; 25 caps = **E**

VASOPRESSIN
Indications: diabetes insipidus
Cautions; Contra-indications: see under Desmopressin
Side-effects: nausea, cramp, desire to defaecate, uterine cramps in women, hypersensitivity reactions, constriction of coronary arteries (may cause anginal attacks and myocardial ischaemia)
Dose: by subcutaneous or intramuscular injection, 5–20 units at least twice daily

Pitressin® (P-D)
Injection, vasopressin 20 units/ml. Price 1-ml amp = **C** (Hosp. only)

6.6 Drugs for hypercalcaemia

This section includes calcitonin and salcatonin (section 6.6.1) and disodium etidronate (section 6.6.2).

Other drugs used in the treatment of hypercalcaemia include mithramycin (see section 8.1.2) and phosphorus compounds (see section 9.5.2).

6.6.1 Calcitonin and salcatonin

Calcitonin (Calcitare®) is involved with parathyroid hormone in the regulation of bone turnover and hence in the maintenance of calcium balance and homoeostasis. It is used to lower the serum-calcium concentration in some patients with hypercalcaemia (notably when associated with malignant disease) and in the treatment of severe Paget's disease of bone. The prolonged use of porcine calcitonin can lead to the production of neutralising antibodies. **Salcatonin** (Calsynar®, synthetic salmon calcitonin) is less immunogenic and thus more suitable for long-term therapy.

CALCITONIN AND SALCATONIN
Indications: see notes above
Cautions: avoid in pregnancy and lactation; porcine calcitonin may contain trace amounts of thyroid
Side-effects: nausea, vomiting, flushing, tingling of hands, unpleasant taste, inflammatory reactions at injection site
Dose: hypercalcaemia, *by subcutaneous or intramuscular injection,* calcitonin 4–8 units/kg daily, salcatonin 400 units every 6–8 hours
Paget's disease of bone, *by subcutaneous or intramuscular injection,* calcitonin 0.5–2 units/kg daily, salcatonin 50 units 3 days a week to 100 units daily

Calcitare® (Armour)
Injection, powder for reconstitution, porcine calcitonin. Price 160-unit vial (with gelatin diluent) = **H**

Calsynar® (Armour)
Injection, salcatonin 100 units/ml in saline/acetate. Price 1-ml amp = **H**
Injection, salcatonin 200 units/ml in saline/acetate. Price 2-ml vial = **J**

6.6.2 Disodium etidronate

Disodium etidronate (Didronel®) is adsorbed onto hydroxyapatite crystals, so slowing both their rate of growth and dissolution, and reduces the increased rate of bone turnover associated with Paget's disease (osteitis deformans). The initial dose is usually 5 mg/kg daily for up to 6 months, but 10 mg/kg daily may be used for up to 3 months if more rapid suppression of bone turnover is necessary. At least three months should elapse before retreatment.

DISODIUM ETIDRONATE
Indications: relief of pain in Paget's disease of bone
Cautions: enterocolitis, discontinue use if fractures occur

Contra-indications: impaired renal function
Side-effects: nausea, diarrhoea, increase in bone pain, increased risk of fractures with high doses
Dose: 5 mg/kg as a single daily dose for up to 6 months *or* 10 mg/kg for up to 3 months, avoiding food for 2 hours before and after treatment, particularly calcium and mineral containing products; see also notes above

▼ **Didronel®** (Brocades)
Tablets, disodium etidronate 200 mg. Price 20 tabs = **I**

6.7 Other endocrine drugs

This section includes bromocriptine (section 6.7.1), diagnostic agents (section 6.7.2), danazol (section 6.7.3), and trilostane (section 6.7.4).

6.7.1 Bromocriptine

Bromocriptine (Parlodel®) is a stimulant of dopaminergic receptors in the brain. It inhibits release of prolactin by the pituitary and is used to prevent and suppress lactation, and in the treatment of hypogonadism and galactorrhoea. It also inhibits the release of growth hormone and is used in acromegaly. For its use in the treatment of parkinsonism, see section 4.9.1.

BROMOCRIPTINE

Indications: see notes above
Cautions: monitor for pituitary enlargement, particularly during pregnancy; contraceptive advice if appropriate
Side-effects: nausea, vomiting, constipation, headache, dizziness, postural hypotension, drowsiness; with high doses, confusion, hallucinations, dyskinesia, dry mouth, leg cramps, pleural effusions (may necessitate withdrawal of treatment)
Dose: prevention/suppression of lactation, 2.5 mg on 1st day, then 2.5 mg twice daily for 14 days
Hypogonadism/galactorrhoea, initially 1.25–2.5 mg daily, increased gradually; usual dose 7.5 mg daily
Acromegaly, initially 1.25–2.5 mg daily, gradually increased; usual dose 20–60 mg daily

Parlodel® (Sandoz)
Tablets, ivory, scored, bromocriptine 2.5 mg (as mesylate). Price 20 tabs = **G**
Capsules, bromocriptine 10 mg (as mesylate). Price 20 caps = **J**

6.7.2 Diagnostic agents for endocrine disorders

Corticotrophin and **tetracosactrin** injections (section 6.5.1) are used to test adrenocortical function. The normal rise in plasma cortisol concentration which follows this administration does not occur in adrenocortical insufficiency.

Metyrapone (Metopirone®) by acting as a competitive inhibitor for 11β-hydroxylation, is capable of inhibiting cortisol production. In the presence of a normal functioning pituitary gland this results in an increase in ACTH production which in turn leads to increased synthesis and release of cortisol precursors from the adrenal cortex. These are measured in the urine as 17-oxogenic steroids. A normal response indicates adequate function of both pituitary and adrenal cortex; failure of response indicates malfunction of either or both endocrine glands. The function of the adrenal glands can be assessed independently with corticotrophin.

Protirelin (thyrotrophin-releasing hormone, TRH) is a useful diagnostic agent in difficult cases of hyperthyroidism; when injected intravenously into normal subjects it leads to a rapid rise in plasma thyrotrophin (TSH). Plasma thyrotrophin does not rise in patients with thyrotoxicosis because of feed-back inhibition of the pituitary by excess circulating thyroid hormone. Plasma thyrotrophin may not rise in patients with endocrine exophthalmos even when plasma thyroxine and triiodothyronine are within the normal range. Many patients with hypopituitarism show a reduced or delayed rise in thyrotrophin after protirelin. Protirelin also causes release of prolactin.

Gonadorelin (gonadotrophin-releasing hormone, LH-RH) when injected intravenously into normal subjects leads to a rapid rise in plasma-luteinising hormone (LH) and follicle-stimulating hormone (FSH) concentrations. It has not so far proved to be very helpful in differentiating hypothalamic from pituitary lesions.

Bovine **thyrotrophin** (thyroid stimulating hormone, TSH) is sometimes used to stimulate thyroidal activity. Its use is declining since alternative diagnostic tests are available and allergic side-effects from its use are common.

GONADORELIN

Indications: see notes above
Side-effects: nausea, headache, abdominal pain, increased menstrual bleeding
Dose: *by intravenous injection,* 100 micrograms

▼ **HRF** (Ayerst)
Injection, powder for reconstitution, gonadorelin. Price 100-microgram vial = **H**; 500-microgram vial = **J** (both with diluent)

▼ **Relefact LH-RH®** (Hoechst)
Injection, gonadorelin 100 micrograms/ml. Price 1-ml amp = **H**

▼ **Relefact LH-RH/TRH®** (Hoechst)
Injection, gonadorelin 100 micrograms, protirelin 200 micrograms/ml. Price 1-ml amp = **G**

METYRAPONE

Indications: see notes above
Cautions: gross hypopituitarism; many drugs interfere with estimation of steroids
Side-effects: nausea, vomiting
Dose: 750 mg every 4 hours for 6 doses

Metopirone® (Ciba)
Capsules, metyrapone 250 mg. Price 20 caps = **F**

PROTIRELIN
Indications: see notes above
Cautions: severe hypopituitarism, cardiac insufficiency, oral administration preferable in bronchial asthma and obstructive airways disease, early pregnancy
Side-effects: nausea; also after intravenous administration desire to micturate, flushing, dizziness, strange taste
Dose: by mouth, 40 mg
By intravenous injection, 200 micrograms

TRH (Roche)
Tablets, scored, protirelin 40 mg. Price 20 tabs = **J**
Injection, protirelin 100 micrograms/ml. Price 2-ml amp = **D**

THYROTROPHIN
Indications: see notes above
Cautions: angina, cardiac failure, hypopituitarism, patients receiving corticosteroids
Contra-indications: coronary thrombosis, adrenal insufficiency
Side-effects: nausea, vomiting, urticaria, transitory hypotension, thyroid swelling
Dose: by subcutaneous or intramuscular injection, 10 units

Thytropar® (Armour)
Injection, powder for reconstitution, thyrotrophin. Price 10-unit vial = **J**

6.7.3 Danazol

Danazol (Danol®) inhibits pituitary gonadotrophin secretion, and is used in the treatment of endometriosis. It has also been used for menorrhagia, mammary dysplasia, and gynaecomastia.

DANAZOL
Indications: see notes above
Cautions: cardiac, hepatic, or renal impairment, epilepsy, migraine; non-hormonal contraceptive methods should be used, if appropriate. Drug interactions: see Appendix 1
Contra-indications: pregnancy, ensure that patients with amenorrhoea are not pregnant
Side-effects: nausea, dizziness, rashes, backache, skeletal muscle spasm; mild androgenic effects including acne, oily skin, oedema, mild hirsutism, voice changes
Dose: 200–800 mg daily in 2–4 divided doses

Danol® (Winthrop)
Capsules, danazol 200 mg. Price 20 caps = **J**
Danol-½® (Winthrop)
Capsules, danazol 100 mg. Price 20 caps = **G**

6.7.4 Trilostane

Trilostane (Modrenal®) inhibits the synthesis of mineralocorticoids and glucocorticoids by the adrenal cortex, and its use is being evaluated for Cushing's syndrome and primary hyperaldosteronism.

TRILOSTANE
Indications: see notes above
Cautions: impaired liver and kidney function, monitor circulating corticosteroids and blood-electrolyte concentrations; non-hormonal contraceptive methods should be used, if appropriate. Drug interactions: see Appendix 1
Contra-indications: pregnancy
Dose: 60 mg 4 times daily for at least 3 days, then adjusted according to patient's response; usual dose range 120–480 mg daily in divided doses

▼**Modrenal®** (Sterling Research)
Capsules, pink/black, trilostane 60 mg. Price 20 caps = **G**

7: Drugs used in OBSTETRICS and GYNAECOLOGY

In this chapter, drugs are discussed under the following headings:

7.1 Drugs acting on uterine muscle
7.2 Treatment of vaginal and vulval conditions
7.3 Contraceptives

For hormonal therapy of gynaecological disorders see section 6.4.1.

7.1 Drugs acting on uterine muscle

This section includes myometrial stimulants (section 7.1.1) and relaxants (section 7.1.2).

7.1.1 Myometrial stimulants

Myometrial stimulants are used to induce abortion or induce or augment labour and to minimise blood loss from the placental site. They include oxytocin, ergometrine, and the prostaglandins.

INDUCTION OF ABORTION. The prostaglandins **dinoprost** (Prostin F2 alpha®) and **dinoprostone** (Prostin E2®) can be used for the induction of abortion, including missed abortion and hydatidiform mole.

The intravenous route is associated with a high incidence of side-effects, including phlebitis and intestinal colic, and its use is confined to cases of missed abortion and hydatidiform mole.

Extra- or intra-amniotic injection is preferable for the induction of late therapeutic abortion. Extra-amniotic administration of dinoprostone through a transcervical catheter can be by either intermittent or continuous instillation. Extra-amniotic dinoprostone is also of value as an adjunct in 'priming' the cervix prior to suction termination of pregnancy. The intra-amniotic route can only be used after about 14–16 weeks gestation. Dinoprost is given by a single injection of 40 mg which can be repeated if necessary.

Prostaglandin administration can be combined with an oxytocin infusion.

INDUCTION AND AUGMENTATION OF LABOUR. **Oxytocin** (Syntocinon®) is administered by slow intravenous infusion, preferably using an infusion pump, to induce or augment labour. Uterine activity must be monitored and hyperstimulation avoided. Large doses of oxytocin may result in excessive fluid retention. The absorption of oxytocin from buccal tablets is variable, so that the effect on uterine activity is not easily or accurately controllable.

Prostaglandins are not the drugs of choice for induction of labour at term because of the side-effects associated with intravenous administration and the risks to the foetus if hyperstimulation occurs after extra- or intra-amniotic administration. In the induction of preterm labour, if for example there is intrauterine foetal death or gross foetal malformation, prostaglandins may be more effective and can be combined with oxytocin infusion.

PREVENTION AND TREATMENT OF HAEMORRHAGE. Bleeding due to incomplete abortion can be controlled by **ergometrine** 125 to 250 micrograms by intravenous or intramuscular injection, depending on blood loss and the condition of the patient. Ergometrine is also used as a prophylactic measure at the time of surgical evacuation of the uterus.

For prophylaxis of postpartum haemorrhage ergometrine, with or without oxytocin is commonly used; either 5 units oxytocin and 500 micrograms ergometrine (Syntometrine®) by intramuscular injection at or after delivery of the anterior shoulder, or ergometrine 125 to 250 micrograms by intravenous injection at or after delivery of the anterior shoulder.

Atonic postpartum haemorrhage can be controlled by ergometrine 125 to 250 micrograms by intravenous injection, or oxytocin intravenous infusion.

DINOPROST

Indications: see notes above

Cautions: asthma, glaucoma, raised intra-ocular pressure, hypotension treated with pressor drugs

Contra-indications: predisposition to uterine rupture, severe toxaemia, previous pelvic infection; also cervicitis or vaginitis (for intra-amniotic use)

Side-effects: nausea, vomiting, diarrhoea, flushing, shivering, headache, dizziness, temporary pyrexia and raised white blood cell count; all dose-related and more common after intravenous administration; also local tissue reaction and erythema

Dose: *by intravenous infusion*, induction of labour, foetal intra-uterine death, 2.5 micrograms/minute for at least 30 minutes

Therapeutic termination of pregnancy, missed abortion, and hydatidiform mole, 25 micrograms/minute

Intra-amniotic injection, 40 mg

Prostin F2 alpha® (Upjohn)

Intravenous injection, dinoprost 5 mg (as trometamol salt)/ml. Price 1.5-ml amp = **F**; 5-ml amp = **J** (Hosp. only)

Intra-amniotic injection, dinoprost 5 mg (as trometamol salt)/ml. Price 4-ml amp = **J**; 8-ml amp = **J** (Hosp. only)

DINOPROSTONE

Indications: see notes above
Cautions; Contra-indications; Side-effects: see under Dinoprost; also local tissue irritation and erythema
Dose: by mouth, induction of labour, 500 micrograms, repeated at hourly intervals
By intravenous infusion, induction of labour, foetal intra-uterine death, 250 nanograms/minute for at least 30 minutes
Therapeutic termination of pregnancy, missed abortion, and hydatidiform mole, 2.5–5 micrograms/minute
Extra-amniotic instillation, 100 micrograms, repeated after 2 hours

Prostin E2® (Upjohn)
Tablets, dinoprostone 500 micrograms. Price 20 tabs = **I** (Hosp. only)
Intravenous injection, dinoprostone 1 mg/ml. Price 0.75-ml amp = **G** (Hosp. only)
Intravenous injection, dinoprostone 10 mg/ml. Price 0.5-ml amp = **I** (Hosp. only)
Extra-amniotic injection, dinoprostone 10 mg/ml. Price 0.5-ml amp (with diluent) = **I** (Hosp. only)

ERGOMETRINE MALEATE

Indications: see notes above
Cautions: toxaemia, hypertension, sepsis
Contra-indications: 1st and 2nd stages of labour, vascular disease, impaired hepatic and renal function
Side-effects: nausea, vomiting, transient hypertension
Dose: see notes above

Ergometrine Tablets, ergometrine maleate 250 and 500 micrograms, price 20 tabs (both) = **C**
Ergometrine Injection, ergometrine maleate 500 micrograms/ml. Price 1-ml amp = **A**
Syntometrine® (Sandoz)
Injection, ergometrine maleate 500 micrograms, oxytocin 5 units/ml. Price 1-ml amp = **A**
Dose: see notes above

OXYTOCIN

Indications: see notes above; also facilitation of lactation
Cautions: hypotension treated with pressor drugs, hypertonic uterine inertia, multiple pregnancy, high parity, previous Caesarean section
Contra-indications: see under Dinoprost
Side-effects: violent uterine contractions leading to rupture and foetal asphyxiation, hypertension and subarachnoid haemorrhage, foetal bradycardia and arrhythmias, excessive fluid retention
Dose: by slow intravenous infusion, as a solution containing 1 unit per litre, 2–5 milliunits per minute

Pitocin (P-D) *buccal tablets*, scored, oxytocin 200 units (as citrate). Price 20 tabs = **F**

Syntocinon® (Sandoz)
Injection, oxytocin 1 unit/ml. Price 2-ml amp = **A**
Injection, oxytocin 5 units/ml. Price 1-ml amp = **A**
Injection, oxytocin 10 units/ml. Price 1-ml amp = **A**; 5-ml amp = **C**
Nasal spray, oxytocin 40 units/ml. Price 5-ml bottle = **D**
Dose: 1 squeeze (about 2 units) into one or both nostrils 2–5 minutes before feeding infant

7.1.2 Myometrial relaxants

Beta$_2$-adrenoceptor stimulants (sympathomimetics) relax uterine muscle and may be used in selected cases in an attempt to inhibit premature labour. They may also be of value in reducing uterine tone in cases of acute foetal distress associated with excessive uterine activity, pending operative delivery; also in hypertonus induced by myometrial stimulants.

Sympathomimetics should not be used unless a clear benefit is likely to result from attempting to reduce uterine activity. Cardiovascular side-effects can be countered by administration of a beta-adrenoceptor blocking drug, e.g. propranolol (see section 2.4). Tachycardia is the commonest side-effect and may be extreme if atropine is also administered.

Prostaglandin inhibitors used to inhibit premature labour are suspected of causing premature closure of the ductus arteriosus.

Drugs used in the treatment of spasmodic dysmenorrhoea include prostaglandin-synthetase inhibitors such as **aspirin**, **mefenamic acid** and **naproxen sodium** (see section 4.7.1.1) and antispasmodics such as **hyoscine butylbromide** (Buscopan®).

ALVERINE CITRATE

Indications: spasmodic dysmenorrhoea
Side-effects: see section 1.2
Dose: 60–120 mg 1–3 times daily

Spasmonal® (Norgine)
Tablets, blue, alverine citrate 60 mg. Price 20 tabs = **D**

HYOSCINE BUTYLBROMIDE

Indications: spasmodic dysmenorrhoea
Cautions; Contra-indications; Side-effects: see section 1.2
Dose: by mouth, 20 mg 4 times daily, starting 2 days before expected date of menstruation and continuing for 3 days after commencement
By intramuscular or intravenous injection, 20 mg, repeated after 30 minutes if necessary

Buscopan® (Boehringer Ingelheim)
Tablets, s/c, hyoscine butylbromide 10 mg. Price 20 tabs = **C**
Injection, see section 1.2

ISOXSUPRINE HYDROCHLORIDE

Indications: premature labour
Contra-indications; Side-effects: see section 2.6.4
Dose: *by intravenous infusion*, 200–500 micrograms/minute until labour is arrested; subsequently *by intramuscular injection*, 10 mg every 3 hours for 24 hours, then every 4–6 hours for 48 hours; then *by mouth*, 20 mg every 6 hours for 48 hours

Duvadilan® (Duphar)
Tablets, pink, scored, isoxsuprine hydrochloride 20 mg. Price 20 tabs = **C**
Injection, isoxsuprine hydrochloride 5 mg/ml. Price 2-ml amp = **B**; 10-ml amp = **D**

ORCIPRENALINE SULPHATE

Indications: premature labour
Cautions; Side-effects: see under Ritodrine Hydrochloride
Dose: *by intravenous infusion*, 2.5 micrograms/minute for 5 minutes, increased until contractions are suppressed; max. 2.5 mg in 24 hours

Alupent Obstetric® (Boehringer Ingelheim)
Injection, orciprenaline sulphate 500 micrograms/ml. To be diluted before use. Price 10-ml amp = **C**

RITODRINE HYDROCHLORIDE

Indications: premature labour
Cautions: diabetes mellitus (frequent estimations of blood-sugar concentration required), treatment with corticosteroids, anaesthetics, potassium-depleting diuretics
Contra-indications: cardiac disorders, haemorrhage, hypertension, pre-eclampsia, cord compression, thyrotoxicosis, treatment with monoamine-oxidase inhibitors, tricyclic antidepressants, beta-adrenoceptor blocking drugs, antihypertensives
Side-effects: nausea, vomiting, flushing, sweating, tremor; tachycardia and hypotension with high doses
Dose: *by intravenous infusion*, initially 50 micrograms/minute, increased to 150–350 micrograms/minute and continued for 12–48 hours after contractions have ceased; or *by intramuscular injection*, 10 mg every 3–8 hours for 24–48 hours; then *by mouth*, 10 mg every 2 hours for 24 hours, followed by 10–20 mg every 4–6 hours

▼ Yutopar® (Duphar)
Tablets, yellow, scored, ritodrine hydrochloride 10 mg. Price 20 tabs = **F**
Injection, ritodrine hydrochloride 10 mg/ml. Price 1-ml amp = **B**; 5-ml amp = **D**

SALBUTAMOL

Indications: premature labour
Cautions; Contra-indications; Side-effects: see under Ritodrine Hydrochloride
Dose: *by intravenous infusion*, 10–45 micrograms/minute until contractions have ceased, then gradually reduced; subsequently *by mouth*, 4 mg every 6–8 hours

Ventolin® (A&H)
Solution for intravenous infusion, salbutamol 1 mg (as sulphate)/ml. Price 5-ml amp = **F**
Tablets, see section 3.1.1.1

TERBUTALINE SULPHATE

Indications: premature labour
Cautions; Contra-indications; Side-effects: see under Ritodrine Hydrochloride
Dose: *by intravenous infusion*, 10 micrograms/minute for 1 hour, gradually increased until contractions have ceased, then reduced; subsequently *by subcutaneous injection*, 250 micrograms every 6 hours for 3 days, and *by mouth*, 5 mg every 8 hours

Bricanyl® (Astra)
Injection, terbutaline sulphate 500 micrograms/ml. Price 1-ml amp = **A**
Tablets, see section 3.1.1.1

7.2 Treatment of vaginal and vulval conditions

Topical applications to the vulva and vagina include pessaries, dusting-powders, creams, and medicated tampons. Symptoms are likely to be primarily referable to the vulva, but infections almost invariably involve the vagina also, so that external applications to the vulva at best are likely to give only symptomatic relief and will not cure infections.

Creams are invariably preferable to ointments, which are not water permeable and adversely affect evaporation and dispersal of natural secretions. Aqueous medicated douches may disturb normal vagina acidity and bacterial flora.

Topical anaesthetic agents give only symptomatic relief and may cause sensitivity reactions. They are indicated only in cases of pruritus where specific local causes have been excluded.

Systemic drugs are required in the treatment of infections, especially those which are sexually transmitted, which, whilst manifest primarily by genital tract symptoms, may also affect other tissues.

7.2.1 Topical hormones
7.2.2 Anti-infective drugs

7.2.1 Topical hormones

When there is a lack of endogenous oestrogens (as in postmenopausal women) dienoestrol cream 0.01% may be used as an adjunct to other treatment of vaginal infections in order to improve the quality of the vaginal epithelium and increase natural resistance. Topical oestrogens are also used prior to vaginal surgery for prolapse when there is epithelial atrophy.

OESTROGENS, TOPICAL

Indications: see notes above
Cautions; Contra-indications; Side-effects: see under Ethinyloestradiol, section 6.4.1.1

Stilboestrol Pessaries, stilboestrol 500 micrograms. Price 12 pessaries = **D**
Insert 2 pessaries at night

Dienoestrol Cream (Ortho)
Cream, dienoestrol 0.01%. Price 78 g with applicator = **E**; 78 g = **D**
Insert 1–2 applicatorfuls daily for 1–2 weeks, then gradually reduced

Hormofemin® (Medo)
Cream, dienoestrol 0.025%. Price 40 g with applicator = **E**
Insert ½-1 applicatorful daily

Premarin® (Ayerst)
Vaginal cream, conjugated oestrogens 625 micrograms/g. Price 42.5 g with applicator = **E**
Insert 1–2 g daily for 3 weeks, followed by a 1-week interval

Tampovagan Stilboestrol and Lactic Acid® (Norgine)
Pessaries, stilboestrol 500 micrograms, lactic acid 5%. Price 10 pessaries = **D**
Insert 2 pessaries at night

7.2.2 Anti-infective drugs

Effective specific treatments are available for the common vaginal infections and the causal organism should be identified before instituting treatment.

Vaginal candidiasis is treated primarily by pessaries or cream which should be inserted high into the vagina, using a special applicator for the cream. Tampons coated with miconazole are also available. Candidal vulvitis is treated with cream but there is almost invariably associated vaginal infection which should also be treated.

Nystatin is a well established treatment. One pessary is inserted nightly for 14 to 28 nights, including the time of menstruation. It may be supplemented with cream for vulvitis and other superficial sites of infection. Imidazole drugs appear to be equally effective in shorter courses, for example **clotrimazole** and **econazole** for 3 days or **miconazole** for 5 or 7 days; **isoconazole** is given as a single dose. Vaginal applications may be supplemented with cream for vulvitis and other superficial sites of infection.

Recurrence is common if the full course of treatment has not been completed and also is particularly likely if there are predisposing factors such as antibiotic therapy, steroid contraceptive use, pregnancy, or diabetes mellitus. Possible reservoirs of infection may also lead to recontamination and should be treated. These include other skin sites such as the digits, nail beds, and umbilicus. Also, the partner may be the source of reinfection.

Trichomonal infections commonly involve the lower urinary tract as well as the genital system and require systemic treatment with either metronidazole or nimorazole. **Metronidazole** (see section 5.1.11.1) is given as a 200-mg tablet 3 times daily for 7 days or 800 mg in the morning and 1.2 g at night for 2 days. To achieve a high cure rate the course should be repeated after an interval of 7 days. The partner should be given the same course of treatment. Side-effects are more common with the short course of metronidazole and following the ingestion of alcohol.

Nimorazole (see section 5.4.3) is administered as a single oral dose of 2 g to each partner.

Bacterial infections of the lower genital tract may be caused by a wide range of organisms. The treatment of gonorrhoea and syphilis is described in section 5.1, Table 2. Infections with Gram-negative organisms are particularly common in association with gynaecological operations and trauma. Metronidazole is effective against certain Gram-negative organisms, especially *Bacteroides* spp. and may be used as a prophylactic measure in gynaecological surgery.

Antibacterial creams such as Sultrin® may be used in the treatment of mixed bacterial infections, for example, in infants. They are ineffective against *Candida* spp. and *Trichomonas vaginalis*.

GENITAL ANTIFUNGAL PREPARATIONS

Indications: vaginal and vulval candidiasis
Side-effects: local irritation, possibly including burning, oedema, erythema

Candeptin® (Pharmax)
Vaginal ointment, candicidin 3 mg/5-g application. Price 2 × 75 g with applicator = **F**
Vaginal tablets, buff, candicidin 3 mg. Price 28 tabs with applicator = **F**
Insert 3 mg night and morning for 14 days

Canesten® (Bayer)
Cream, clotrimazole 1%. Price 20 g = **D**; 50 g = **F**
Vaginal cream, clotrimazole 2%. Price 35 g (with 5-g applicators) = **F**
Insert 5 g twice daily for 3 days or once nightly for 6 nights
Vaginal tablets, clotrimazole 100 mg. Price 6 tabs with applicator = **E**
Vaginal tablets, clotrimazole 200 mg. Price 3 tabs with applicator = **E**
Insert 200 mg for 3 nights *or* 100 mg for 6 nights
Duopak, clotrimazole 100-mg vaginal tablets and cream as above. Price 6 tabs and 20 g cream = **F**

Ecostatin® (FAIR)
Cream, econazole nitrate 1%. Price 15 g = **D**; 30 g = **E**
Pessaries, econazole nitrate 150 mg. Price 3 pessaries with applicator = **F**
Insert 1 pessary for 3 nights
Twinpack, econazole nitrate pessaries and cream as above. Price 3 pessaries and 15 g cream = **G**

Fungilin® (Squibb)
Pessaries, yellow, amphotericin 50 mg. Price 15 pessaries = **D**
Insert 1-2 pessaries for 14 nights

Gyno-Daktarin® (Janssen)
Intravaginal cream, miconazole nitrate 2%. Price 78 g with applicator = **G**
Pessaries, miconazole nitrate 100 mg. Price 14 pessaries = **G**
Insert 200 mg for 7 nights *or* 100 mg night and morning for 7 days
Tampons, coated with miconazole nitrate 100 mg. Price 10 tampons = **F**
Insert 1 night and morning for 5 days
Combipack, miconazole nitrate pessaries and cream as above. Price 14 pessaries and 15 g cream = **G**

Gyno-Pevaryl® (Ortho)
Pessaries, econazole nitrate 150 mg. Price 3 pessaries = **F**
Insert 1 pessary for 3 nights
Combipack, econazole nitrate pessaries as above, econazole nitrate 1% cream. Price 3 pessaries and 15 g cream = **G**

Monistat® (Ortho)
Vaginal cream, miconazole nitrate 2%. Price 78 g with applicator = **G**
Pessaries, miconazole nitrate 100 mg. Price 14 pessaries = **G**
Insert 200 mg for 7 nights *or* 100 mg night and morning for 7 days

Nyspes® (DDSA)
Pessaries, buff, nystatin 100000 units. Price 15 pessaries = **C**
Insert 1-2 pessaries for at least 14 nights

Nystan® (Squibb)
Vaginal cream, nystatin 100000 units/4-g application. Price 60 g with applicator = **E**
Pessaries, yellow, nystatin 100000 units. Price 15 pessaries with applicator = **C**
Insert 100000-200000 units for at least 14 nights
Triple pack, nystatin tablets as above, nystatin gel 100000 units/g. Nystavescent® pessaries as below. Price 42 tablets + 28 pessaries + 30 g gel = **H**

Nystavescent® (Squibb)
Pessaries, yellow, effervescent, nystatin 100000 units. Price 15 pessaries with applicator = **D**
Insert as for Nystan® (above)

Pevaryl® (Ortho)
Cream, econazole nitrate 1%. Price 30 g = **E**
Lotion, econazole nitrate 1%. Price 30 ml = **E**

Pimafucin® (Brocades)
Cream, natamycin 2%. Price 25 g = **D**
Vaginal tablets (= pessaries), yellow, natamycin 25 mg. Price 21 tabs = **D**
Insert 1 pessary for 21 nights

▼ Travogyn® (Keymer)
Vaginal tablets (= pessaries), isoconazole nitrate 300 mg. Price 2 tabs = **F**
Insert 600 mg as a single dose preferably at night

SULPHONAMIDES, MIXED

Indications: bacterial vaginitis and cervicitis
Contra-indications: sulphonamide sensitivity, renal impairment
Dose: *by vagina*, 1 pessary or applicatorful of cream twice daily for 10 days

Sultrin® (Ortho)
Cream, sulphathiazole 3.42%, sulphacetamide 2.86%, sulphabenzamide 3.7%. Price 78 g with or without applicator = **E**
Vaginal tablets, sulphathiazole 172.5 mg, sulphacetamide 143.75 mg, sulphabenzamide 184 mg. Price 20 tabs with applicator = **E**

VAGINAL ANTISEPTIC PREPARATIONS

Aci-Jel® (Ortho)
Vaginal jelly, acetic acid 0.92%. Price 85 g with applicator = **E**; 85 g = **D**
To restore vaginal acidity insert 1 applicatorful twice daily

Betadine® (Napp)
Pessaries, brown, povidone-iodine 200 mg. Price 28 pessaries with applicator = **F**
Vaginal gel, brown, povidone-iodine 10%. Price 80 g with applicator = **E**
In vaginal infections insert 1 pessary or 1 applicatorful of gel twice daily for 2-4 weeks
VC kit, solution, povidone-iodine 10%. For dilution before use. Price 250 ml with measuring bottle and applicator = **E**
In vaginal infections douche daily for 14 days

Floraquin® (Searle)
Pessaries, cream, di-iodohydroxyquinoline 100 mg, boric acid, phosphoric acid. Price 25 pessaries with applicator = **D**
In vaginal infections insert 2 pessaries at night for 2 months

Penotrane® (WBP)
Pessaries, hydrargaphen 1.5 mg. Price 15 pessaries = **D**
Pessaries, hydrargaphen 5 mg. Price 15 pessaries = **D**
In vaginal infections insert 2 pessaries of 1.5 mg for 15 nights, repeated if necessary; use 2 pessaries of 5 mg similarly in severe infections

SVC® (M&B)
Vaginal tablets, effervescent, acetarsol 250 mg, boric acid. Price 25 tabs = **C**
In trichomonal infections insert 2-4 vaginal tablets twice daily until symptoms are relieved, then reduce dose

Tampovagan N® (Norgine)
Pessaries, neomycin sulphate 20 mg. Price 10 pessaries = **D**
In vaginitis insert 2 pessaries at night

7.3 Contraceptives

The criteria by which contraceptive methods should be judged are effectiveness, acceptability, and freedom from side-effects.

Hormonal contraception is the most effective method of fertility control, short of sterilisation, but has unwanted major and minor side-effects, especially for certain groups of women.

Intrauterine devices, usually made of inert plastic, have a high use-effectiveness but may produce undesirable side-effects, especially menorrhagia, or be otherwise unsuitable in a significant proportion of women. In order to minimise side-effects smaller devices with a copper coating have been introduced. Their contraceptive efficacy is as good as with the inert devices. They are particularly suitable for nulliparous women.

Barrier methods alone (condoms, diaphragms, and caps) are less effective but can be very reliable for well motivated couples if used in conjunction with a spermicide. Occasionally sensitivity reactions occur.

7.3.1 Combined oral contraceptives
7.3.2 Progestogen-only contraceptives
7.3.3 Chemical contraceptives

7.3.1 Combined oral contraceptives

Oral contraceptives containing an oestrogen and a progestogen are the most effective preparations for general use. The oestrogen content ranges from 20 to 50 micrograms (see Table below) and generally a preparation with the lowest oestrogen content which gives good cycle control in the individual patient is chosen. With low-oestrogen preparations the margin of safety is reduced and regularity of pill taking (even to time of day) becomes more critical.

Other critical factors which influence effectiveness are gastro-intestinal disturbances and some antibiotics, for example ampicillin, which interfere with absorption. Drugs which induce hepatic mono-oxidase activity (for example barbiturates, phenytoin, rifampicin, spironolactone) also increase the risk of failure (see Appendix 1).

The chemical nature and biological activity of the 4 progestogens in common use varies. In general, higher doses of progestogen reduce menstrual loss (even to the point of amenorrhoea in susceptible individuals) and induce greater weight gain.

The dosage regimen for combined oral contraceptives is usually 1 tablet daily for 21 days, followed by a 7-day interval. It is usually recommended that the first course is started on the 5th day of the cycle and ovulation may then not be inhibited during that cycle. Commencing on the 1st day of the cycle appears to give effective protection during that cycle.

Triphasic formulations (Logynon®, Trinordiol®) more closely mimic normal endogenous cyclical hormonal activity. The total dose of oestrogen is increased and the total dose of progesterone decreased over the cycle, compared with other combined preparations. They are recommended for a day 1 start.

Following childbirth oral contraception can be started at any time, but preferably not earlier than 2 weeks postpartum because of the increased risk of thrombosis. Established lactation is unaffected by oral contraceptives and there is no evidence that low-dose oral contraceptives have any adverse effect on the infant.

Combined oral contraceptives carry a small risk of thrombo-embolic and cardiovascular complications. This increases with oestrogen content, age, obesity, and cigarette smoking, and with predisposing conditions such as diabetes, hypertension, and familial hyperlipidaemia.

Hypertension may develop as the result of therapy but when it is due to contraceptive usage

Table. Hormone content of combined oral contraceptives

Preparation	Progestogen
Oestrogen: Ethinyloestradiol 20 micrograms	
Loestrin 20	Norethisterone acetate 1 mg
Oestrogen: Ethinyloestradiol 30 micrograms	
Conova 30	Ethynodiol diacetate 2 mg
Eugynon 30	Levonorgestrel 250 micrograms
Microgynon 30	Levonorgestrel 150 micrograms
Ovran 30	Levonorgestrel 250 micrograms
Ovranette	Levonorgestrel 150 micrograms
Oestrogen: Ethinyloestradiol 35 micrograms	
Brevinor	Norethisterone 500 micrograms
Norimin	Norethisterone 1 mg
Ovysmen	Norethisterone 500 micrograms
Oestrogen: Ethinyloestradiol 50 micrograms	
Anovlar 21	Norethisterone acetate 4 mg
Demulen 50	Ethynodiol diacetate 500 micrograms
Eugynon 50	Norgestrel 500 micrograms
Gynovlar 21	Norethisterone acetate 3 mg
Minilyn	Lynoestrenol 2.5 mg
Minovlar and **ED**	Norethisterone acetate 1 mg
Norlestrin	Norethisterone acetate 2.5 mg
Orlest 21	Norethisterone acetate 1 mg
Ovran	Levonorgestrel 250 micrograms
Ovulen 50	Ethynodiol diacetate 1 mg
Oestrogen: Mestranol 50 micrograms	
Norinyl-1	Norethisterone 1 mg
Norinyl-1/28	Norethisterone 1 mg
Ortho-Novin 1/50	Norethisterone 1 mg
Oestrogen: Sequential	
See under Triphasic formulations	

reversion to normotension occurs on cessation of treatment.

Oral contraceptives should be **avoided** in the month preceding elective surgery, providing an alternative reliable method of contraception is acceptable to the patient.

ORAL CONTRACEPTIVES (Combined)

Indications: contraception (for use of oestrogen–progestogen combinations to control menopausal and menstrual symptoms, see sections 6.4.1.3 and 6.4.1.4)

Cautions: diabetes, hypertension, cardiac or renal disease, migraine, epilepsy, depression, asthma, multiple sclerosis, wearing of contact lenses, cigarette-smokers, obesity. Drug interactions: see Appendix 1

Contra-indications: thrombosis and history of thrombo-embolic disease, recurrent jaundice, acute and chronic liver disease, Dubin–Johnson and Roter syndromes, sickle-cell anaemia, hyperlipidaemia, mammary or endometrial carcinoma, oestrogen-dependent tumours, severe migraine, undiagnosed vaginal bleeding, history of pruritus of pregnancy or herpes gestationis, deterioration of otosclerosis

Side-effects: nausea, vomiting, headache, breast tenderness, changes in body weight, changes in libido, depression, chloasma, hypertension, impairment of liver function, benign hepatic tumours, reduced menstrual loss, 'spotting' in early cycles, amenorrhoea

Dose: 1 tablet daily for 21 days starting on 5th day of cycle, and repeated after a 7-day interval (unless other instructions are given)

Anovlar 21® (Schering)
Tablets, green, s/c, norethisterone acetate 4 mg, ethinyloestradiol 50 micrograms. Price 21-tab calendar pack = **C**

Brevinor® (Syntex)
Tablets, norethisterone 500 micrograms, ethinyloestradiol 35 micrograms. Price 21-tab calendar pack = **B**

Conova 30® (Searle)
Tablets, f/c, ethynodiol diacetate 2 mg, ethinyloestradiol 30 micrograms. Price 21-tab calendar pack = **B**

Demulen 50® (Searle)
Tablets, ethynodiol diacetate 500 micrograms, ethinyloestradiol 50 micrograms. Price 21-tab calendar pack = **B**

Eugynon 30® (Schering)
Tablets, s/c, levonorgestrel 250 micrograms, ethinyloestradiol 30 micrograms. Price 21-tab calendar pack = **B**

Eugynon 50® (Schering)
Tablets, s/c, norgestrel 500 micrograms, ethinyloestradiol 50 micrograms. Price 21-tab calendar pack = **B**

Gynovlar 21® (Schering)
Tablets, pink, norethisterone acetate 3 mg, ethinyloestradiol 50 micrograms. Price 21-tab calendar pack = **C**

Loestrin 20® (P-D)
Tablets, blue, f/c, norethisterone acetate 1 mg, ethinyloestradiol 20 micrograms. Price 21-tab calendar pack = **C**

Microgynon 30® (Schering)
Tablets, beige, s/c, levonorgestrel 150 micrograms, ethinyloestradiol 30 micrograms. Price 21-tab calendar pack = **B**

Minilyn® (Organon)
Tablets, lynoestrenol 2.5 mg, ethinyloestradiol 50 micrograms. Price 22-tab calendar pack = **C**
Dose: 1 tablet daily for 22 days starting on 5th day of cycle, and repeated after a 6-day interval

Minovlar® (Schering)
Tablets, yellow, s/c, norethisterone acetate 1 mg, ethinyloestradiol 50 micrograms. Price 21-tab calendar pack = **B**

Minovlar ED® (Schering)
As for Minovlar and in addition 7 yellow lactose tablets. Price 28-tab calendar pack = **C**

Norimin® (Syntex)
Tablets, yellow, norethisterone 1 mg, ethinyloestradiol 35 micrograms. Price 21-tab calendar pack = **C**

Norinyl-1® (Syntex)
Tablets, norethisterone 1 mg, mestranol 50 micrograms. Price 21-tab calendar pack = **C**

Norinyl-1/28® (Syntex)
As for Norinyl-1 and in addition 7 orange lactose tablets. Price 28-tab calendar pack = **C**

Norlestrin® (P-D)
Tablets, pink, f/c, norethisterone acetate 2.5 mg, ethinyloestradiol 50 micrograms. Price 21-tab calendar pack = **C**

Orlest 21® (P-D)
Tablets, yellow, f/c, norethisterone acetate 1 mg, ethinyloestradiol 50 micrograms. Price 21-tab calendar pack = **B**

Ortho-Novin 1/50® (Ortho)
Tablets, norethisterone 1 mg, mestranol 50 micrograms. Price 21-tab calendar pack = **B**

Ovran® (Wyeth)
Tablets, levonorgestrel 250 micrograms, ethinyloestradiol 50 micrograms. Price 21-tab calendar pack = **B**

Ovran 30® (Wyeth)
Tablets, levonorgestrel 250 micrograms, ethinyloestradiol 30 micrograms. Price 21-tab calendar pack = **B**

Ovranette® (Wyeth)
Tablets, levonorgestrel 150 micrograms, ethinyloestradiol 30 micrograms. Price 21-tab calendar pack = **B**

Ovulen 50® (Searle)
Tablets, ethynodiol diacetate 1 mg, ethinyloestradiol 50 micrograms. Price 21-tab calendar pack = **B**

Ovysmen® (Ortho)
Tablets, norethisterone 500 micrograms, ethinyloestradiol 35 micrograms. Price 21-tab calendar pack = **B**

Triphasic formulations

Logynon® (Schering)

Calendar pack, all s/c, 6 brown tablets, levonorgestrel 50 micrograms, ethinyloestradiol 30 micrograms; 5 white tablets, levonorgestrel 75 micrograms, ethinyloestradiol 40 micrograms; 10 ochre tablets, levonorgestrel 125 micrograms, ethinyloestradiol 30 micrograms. Price 21 tabs = **C**

Dose: 1 tablet daily for 21 days, starting with tablet marked 1 on 1st day of cycle, and repeated after a 7-day interval

Logynon ED® (Schering)

As for Logynon and in addition 7 white placebo tablets. Price 28-tab calendar pack = **C**

Trinordiol® (Wyeth)

Calendar pack, all s/c, 6 brown tablets, levonorgestrel 50 micrograms, ethinyloestradiol 30 micrograms; 5 white tablets, levonorgestrel 75 micrograms, ethinyloestradiol 40 micrograms; 10 ochre tablets, levonorgestrel 125 micrograms, ethinyloestradiol 30 micrograms. Price 21 tabs = **C**

Dose: 1 tablet daily for 21 days, starting with tablet marked 1 on 1st day of cycle, and repeated after a 7-day interval

7.3.2 Progestogen-only contraceptives

When oestrogens are contra-indicated, progestogen-only preparations may offer a suitable alternative but have a higher failure rate than combined preparations. Menstrual irregularities (oligomenorrhoea, menorrhagia) are more common. Oral preparations are started on the 1st day of the cycle and taken every day.

Medroxyprogesterone acetate (Depo-Provera®) is a long-acting progestogen given by intramuscular injection. It is useful for short-term interim contraception, for example, before sterilisation or after rubella vaccination.

Progestogen-only preparations can be administered in the early puerperium without adverse effects.

Progesterone has been incorporated into an intra-uterine contraceptive device.

PROGESTOGEN-ONLY CONTRACEPTIVES

Indications: see notes above

Cautions; Contra-indications; Side-effects: see under Combined Oral Contraceptives, section 7.3.1; also irregular menstrual cycles

Dose: *by mouth*, 1 tablet daily starting on 1st day of cycle

Depo-Provera® (Upjohn)

Injection, medroxyprogesterone acetate 50 mg/ml. Price 3-ml vial = **F**. See also section 8.3.2

Dose: by intramuscular injection, 150 mg

Femulen® (Searle)

Tablets, ethynodiol diacetate 500 micrograms. Price 28-tab calendar pack = **C**

Micronor® (Ortho)

Tablets, norethisterone 350 micrograms. Price 42-tab calendar pack = **C**

▼ **Microval®** (Wyeth)

Tablets, levonorgestrel 30 micrograms. Price 35-tab calendar pack = **C**

Neogest® (Schering)

Tablets, brown, s/c, norgestrel 75 micrograms. Price 35-tab calendar pack = **C**

▼ **Norgeston®** (Schering)

Tablets, s/c, levonorgestrel 30 micrograms. Price 35-tab calendar pack = **C**

Noriday® (Syntex)

Tablets, yellow, norethisterone 350 micrograms. Price 28-tab calendar pack = **C**

7.3.3 Chemical contraceptives

Chemical contraceptives are useful additional safeguards but do not give adequate protection if used alone. They have two components: a spermicide and a vehicle which itself may have some inhibiting effect on sperm migration. They are formulated as pessaries, creams, pastes, gels, aerosol foams, and soluble films. The commonly used spermicides are all phenoxypolyethoxyethanol derivatives.

8: Drugs used in the treatment of MALIGNANT DISEASE and for IMMUNOSUPPRESSION

Dosage in malignant disease. Because of the complexity of dosage regimens in the treatment of malignant disease, dose statements have been omitted from some of the drug entries in this chapter. *In all cases detailed specialist literature should be consulted.*
In this chapter, drug treatment is discussed under the following headings:

Malignant disease may be treated by surgery, radiotherapy, and/or chemotherapy.

Certain tumours or auto-immune diseases are highly sensitive to chemotherapy but many are not, and inappropriate drug administration in these circumstances can only increase morbidity or mortality.

Cytotoxic drugs and corticosteroids are used as immunosuppressants and as therapy for malignant disease. The sex hormones are used to treat certain responsive tumours.

8.1 Cytotoxic drugs

Increasing numbers of cytotoxic drugs have become available in recent years and many more are at present under clinical trial.

Cytotoxic drugs are used in four main clinical settings. They are used to treat primary or metastatic malignant disease where previous experience has shown that a favourable response is likely. They are also used in patients with malignant disease rendered apparently disease-free by surgery or radiotherapy, but in whom previous experience has shown that relapse is a common problem. Some are used as immunosuppressants for a variety of auto-immune diseases (ulcerative colitis and Crohn's disease, see section 1.5; rheumatic disease, see section 10.1.3), and are also given to recipients of organ transplants where rejection may be a problem (section 8.2.1).

Cytotoxic drugs were initially used singly, but in recent years clear evidence has emerged that in many conditions combinations of drugs are more effective; for example the MVPP regimen used in Hodgkin's disease includes mustine, vinblastine, prednisolone, and procarbazine. The rationale for this is that drugs with different sites of action (for example an alkylating drug and a vinca alkaloid) will have at least an additive antitumour effect, and excessive toxicity can be avoided by ensuring that each drug in a combination has its predominant toxic effect at a different site.

The majority of these drugs act by interfering with cell division. No cytotoxic drug has yet been developed with complete tumour selectivity and most will damage all rapidly dividing cells, whether normal or neoplastic. All these drugs, with the exception of bleomycin, cause depression of bone-marrow function, resulting in reduced formation of erythrocytes, granulocytes, and platelets; anaemia and increased susceptibility to infections and haemorrhage are therefore potential toxic effects which may be severe and require intensive supportive therapy. Frequent haematological monitoring is required. Dosage may have to be reduced or omitted if marked bone-marrow depression occurs. The degree of this toxicity and its timing, however, varies markedly from drug to drug.

In addition, most drugs will cause gastro-intestinal disturbances, particularly nausea and vomiting, and a variable degree of alopecia, which in some cases may be total. These side-effects are usually short term and reversible. However, many of these drugs also have delayed or progressive toxicity which may severely limit their use, for example doxorubicin cardiotoxicity and bleomycin pulmonary toxicity. *Animal* studies have indicated the possibility of teratogenic effects of cytotoxic drugs.

Drug absorption, metabolism, and excretion vary widely among the different drugs in use. It is essential to be aware of sites of metabolism and excretion as damage to normal pathways may occur in malignant disease, resulting in drug retention and enhanced toxicity.

Many cytotoxic drugs are very expensive and all are potentially toxic. They are included, in various combinations, in many chemotherapy schedules, some of which are in regular use and others which are presently undergoing clinical trials. Administration of these toxic drugs should be undertaken or supervised only by clinicians experienced in their use.

8.1.1 Alkylating drugs

This group includes many of the commonly used chemotherapeutic drugs. They act by damaging DNA and interfering with cell replication.

In addition to the usual side-effects (section

8.1), there are two problems associated with their prolonged use. Firstly, gametogenesis is impaired, with resulting infertility during therapy. Although this may be reversible after short-term use, it may become permanent, particularly after long-term use in males. Secondly, a disturbing increase in the incidence of acute myeloid leukaemia has been noted when these drugs have been used continuously to treat certain tumours, such as ovarian carcinoma.

Busulphan (Myleran®) has a selective depressant action on bone marrow, and is used in the treatment of chronic myeloid leukaemia. Frequent blood counts are essential, as excessive myelosuppression may cause irreversible bone-marrow aplasia. Hyperpigmentation of the skin commonly occurs, and a rare but serious toxic effect is interstitial pulmonary fibrosis.

Chlorambucil (Leukeran®) is a useful alkylating drug and apart from reversible bone-marrow toxicity has minimal side-effects. It is commonly used to treat chronic lymphocytic leukaemia, certain of the non-Hodgkin lymphomas, and ovarian carcinoma.

Cyclophosphamide (Endoxana®) is a very commonly used drug which is inactive until metabolised by the liver. An increased fluid intake (3–4 litres/day) should be encouraged during administration to help avoid the haemorrhagic cystitis associated with high concentrations of urinary metabolites. Cyclophosphamide is used to treat a wide range of haematological malignancies, non-Hodgkin lymphomas, and solid tumours. **Ifosfamide** (Mitoxana®) is related to cyclophosphamide and has similar effects.

Lomustine (CCNU, CeeNU®) is a nitrosourea with high lipid solubility, and so crosses the blood-brain barrier. It is used alone in the treatment of malignant gliomas and other brain tumours, and in combination chemotherapy of Hodgkin's disease and some other solid tumours. Delayed bone-marrow suppression is a dose-limiting effect, and it is not usually given more frequently than every 6 weeks. **Carmustine** (BiCNU®) has similar activity.

Melphalan (Alkeran®) is used in the treatment of myelomatosis. Marrow toxicity is delayed and it is therefore usually administered at intervals of 4 to 6 weeks.

Mustine is one of the drugs included in the MVPP regimen for Hodgkin's disease. It should be used immediately after preparation and only be administered into a fast-running infusion. Local extravasation causes severe tissue necrosis. Severe vomiting is a common side-effect which has tended to limit its usefulness.

Estramustine (Estracyt®) is a stable combination of an oestrogen with mustine. It has been designed to treat tumours with oestrogen receptors, for example prostatic carcinoma, with the intention of carrying the alkylating drug component to tumour sites, increasing local effectiveness, and reducing systemic toxicity.

Uramustine (uracil mustard) is not widely used at present.

Ethoglucid (Epodyl®) has been used by intracavitary instillation in the treatment of non-invasive bladder carcinoma.

Thiotepa is mainly used by intracavitary instillation in the treatment of malignant effusions; it is also used in the treatment of bladder tumours and ovarian carcinoma.

Mitobronitol (Myelobromol®) is used in the treatment of chronic myeloid leukaemia.

Treosulfan is a bifunctional alkylating drug used for the management of ovarian carcinoma.

BUSULPHAN

Indications: chronic myeloid leukaemia
Cautions; Side-effects: see section 8.1 and notes above
Dose: induction of remission, 2–4 mg daily; maintenance, 0.5–2 mg daily

Myleran® (Wellcome)
Tablets, busulphan 500 micrograms. Price 20 tabs = **C**
Tablets, busulphan 2 mg. Price 20 tabs = **D**

CARMUSTINE

Indications: see notes above
Cautions; Side-effects: see section 8.1 and notes above

▼ **BiCNU®** (Mead Johnson)
Injection, powder for reconstitution, carmustine. Price 100-mg vial (with diluent) = **J** (Hosp. only)

CHLORAMBUCIL

Indications: see notes above (for use as an immunosuppressant see section 8.2.1)
Cautions; Side-effects: see section 8.1 and notes above
Dose: used alone, 5–10 mg daily for 3–6 weeks; maintenance, 2–4 mg daily

Leukeran® (Wellcome)
Tablets, yellow, chlorambucil 2 mg. Price 20 tabs = **E**
Tablets, yellow, chlorambucil 5 mg. Price 20 tabs = **F**

CYCLOPHOSPHAMIDE

Indications: see notes above (for use as an immunosuppressant, see section 8.2.1)
Cautions; Side-effects: see section 8.1 and notes above
Dose: *by mouth*, for immunosuppression, 50–100 mg daily

Cyclophosphamide Tablets, compression-coated or s/c, cyclophosphamide 50 mg. Price 20 tabs = **D**
Cyclophosphamide Injection, powder for reconstitution, cyclophosphamide, price 100-mg

vial = **C**; 200-mg vial = **D**; 500-mg vial = **E**; 1-g vial = **F**

Endoxana® (WBP)
Tablets, compression-coated, cyclophosphamide 10 mg. Price 20 tabs = **C**
Tablets, compression-coated, cyclophosphamide 50 mg. Price 20 tabs = **D**
Injection, powder for reconstitution, cyclophosphamide. Price 107-mg vial = **C**; 214-mg vial = **D**; 535-mg vial = **E**; 1.069-g vial = **F**

ESTRAMUSTINE PHOSPHATE

Indications: prostatic carcinoma
Cautions; Contra-indications; Side-effects: see section 8.1 and under Ethinyloestradiol, section 6.4.1.1
Dose: initially, 560 mg daily

▼ **Estracyt®** (Lundbeck)
Capsules, estramustine phosphate 140 mg (as sodium salt). Price 10 caps = **I**

ETHOGLUCID

Indications: non-invasive bladder carcinoma
Side-effects: frequency of micturition, dysuria, fall in leucocyte count
Dose: *by instillation*, 1% solution

Epodyl® (ICI)
Liquid, sterile ethoglucid. Plastic syringes should not be used. Price 1-ml amp = **E**

IFOSFAMIDE

Indications: see notes above
Cautions; Side-effects: see section 8.1 and notes under Cyclophosphamide

▼ **Mitoxana®** (WBP)
Injection, powder for reconstitution, ifosfamide. Price 500-mg vial = **G**; 1-g vial = **I**; 2-g vial = **J** (Hosp. only)

LOMUSTINE

Indications: see notes above
Cautions; Side-effects: see section 8.1 and notes above
Dose: used alone, 120–130 mg/m^2 body-surface every 4–6 weeks

Lomustine Capsules, lomustine 10 mg, price 20 caps = **H**; 40 mg, price 20 caps = **J**

▼ **CCNU®** (Lundbeck)
Capsules, blue/white, lomustine 10 mg. Price 20 caps = **H**
Capsules, blue, lomustine 40 mg. Price 20 caps = **J**

▼ **CeeNU®** (Mead Johnson)
Capsules, blue, lomustine 10 mg. Price 20 caps = **I**
Capsules, blue/green, lomustine 40 mg. Price 20 caps = **J**
Capsules, green, lomustine 100 mg. Price 20 caps = **J**

MELPHALAN

Indications: myelomatosis
Cautions; Side-effects: see section 8.1 and notes above; reduce dose in renal failure
Dose: *by mouth*, up to 10 mg daily for 7 days, repeated after 4–6 weeks

Alkeran® (Wellcome)
Tablets, pink, melphalan 2 mg. Price 20 tabs = **F**
Tablets, pink, melphalan 5 mg. Price 20 tabs = **G**
Injection, powder for reconstitution, melphalan. Price 100-mg vial (with solvent and diluent) = **J**

MITOBRONITOL

Indications: chronic myeloid leukaemia
Cautions; Side-effects: see section 8.1
Dose: initially 250 mg daily

Myelobromol® (Sinclair)
Tablets, mitobronitol 125 mg. Price 20 tabs = **H**

MUSTINE HYDROCHLORIDE

Indications: Hodgkin's disease—see notes above
Cautions; Side-effects: see section 8.1 and notes above; also caution in handling—vesicant and a nasal irritant

Mustine Hydrochloride (Boots)
Injection, powder for reconstitution, mustine hydrochloride. Price 10-mg vial = **C**

THIOTEPA

Indications: see notes above
Cautions; Side-effects: see section 8.1

Thiotepa (Lederle)
Injection, powder for reconstitution, thiotepa (with sodium chloride and bicarbonate). Price 15-mg vial = **G**

TREOSULFAN

Indications: see notes above
Cautions; Side-effects: see section 8.1
Dose: 1 g daily in 4 divided doses for 1 month followed by 1 month without treatment; repeated with dose adjusted if necessary

Treosulfan (Leo)
Capsules, treosulfan 250 mg. Price 20 caps = **G**

URAMUSTINE

Indications: see notes above
Cautions; Side-effects: see section 8.1

Uracil Mustard (Upjohn)
Capsules, yellow/blue, uramustine 1 mg. Price 20 caps = **E**

8.1.2 Cytotoxic antibiotics

Cytotoxic antibiotics interfere with DNA and RNA replication, and also protein synthesis. They have side-effects common to many anticancer drugs and many also have a tendency to increase tissue sensitivity to radiotherapy. Care should be taken when administering these drugs to patients who have received previous irradiation and they should preferably not be used simultaneously with radiotherapy.

Doxorubicin (Adriamycin®) is one of the most successful antitumour drugs. It commonly produces bone-marrow suppression and almost invariably causes alopecia which may be total. It should be given into a fast-running infusion as tissue extravasation causes severe local pain and necrosis.

The main problem with its use is cardiac toxicity. Supraventricular arrhythmias may occur immediately after administration. Moreover progressive myocardial damage may occur, which at high cumulative dosage produces an irreversible cardiomyopathy, and it is usual to limit total dosage to 550 mg/m^2 body-surface. Patients with pre-existing cardiac disease, or those who have received significant myocardial irradiation, should be given lower doses. Doxorubicin has been successfully used to treat the acute leukaemias, certain non-Hodgkin lymphomas, and many solid tumours.

Bleomycin is one of the few drugs not associated with clinically significant marrow toxicity. It may be given by subcutaneous, intramuscular, intravenous, or intracavitary injection.

The principal problem associated with its use is the occasional development of progressive pulmonary fibrosis. This is more common in older patients (particularly over 70 years) and those receiving a total dose of more than 300 mg. Bleomycin also commonly produces skin reactions. These may range from widespread pigmentation to the development of subcutaneous sclerotic plaques. A probable association with Raynaud's phenomenon has also been reported.

Bleomycin is one of the few drugs to show appreciable activity in squamous cell carcinoma. Its use is under study in head and neck tumours, non-Hodgkin lymphomas, and testicular teratomata.

Actinomycin D (Cosmegen Lyovac®) has been available for many years. It is given as an intravenous bolus. Particular care should be taken to avoid local tissue extravasation which may cause a severe reaction. Other toxic effects include bone-marrow suppression and stomatitis. Its main use is in childhood solid tumours, and in soft tissue sarcomata and testicular teratomata in adults.

Mithramycin (Mithracin®) is rarely used as a cytotoxic drug as it causes marked bone-marrow depression and thrombocytopenia, and a severe haemorrhagic diathesis due to multiple causes may occur. It has, however, found a place in the emergency therapy of severe hypercalcaemia associated with malignant disease.

Mitomycin has not found widespread use in this country because of bone-marrow toxicity. It has been used predominantly to treat gastro-intestinal tumours.

ACTINOMYCIN D

(Dactinomycin)

Indications: see notes above

Cautions; Side-effects: see section 8.1 and notes above

Cosmegen Lyovac® (MSD)

Injection, powder for reconstitution, actinomycin D (with mannitol). Price 500-microgram vial = **D**

BLEOMYCIN

Indications: squamous cell carcinoma—see notes above

Cautions; Side-effects: see section 8.1 and notes above; reduce dose in renal failure. Also caution in handling—irritant to skin

Bleomycin (Lundbeck)

Injection, powder for reconstitution, bleomycin (as sulphate). Price 5-mg amp = **G**; 15-mg amp = **J**

DOXORUBICIN HYDROCHLORIDE

Indications: see notes above

Cautions; Side-effects: see section 8.1 and notes above; also caution in handling—irritant to skin

Adriamycin® (Farmitalia Carlo Erba)

Injection, powder for reconstitution, doxorubicin hydrochloride (with lactose). Price 10-mg vial = **H**; 50-mg vial = **J**

MITHRAMYCIN

Indications: see notes above

Cautions; Side-effects: see section 8.1 and notes above

Mithracin® (Pfizer)

Injection, powder for reconstitution, mithramycin (with mannitol and sodium phosphate). Price 2.5-mg vial = **I**

MITOMYCIN

Indications: see notes above

Cautions; Side-effects: see section 8.1 and notes above; also irritant to tissues

Mitomycin C Injection, powder for reconstitution, mitomycin, price 2-mg vial = **E**; 10-mg vial = **H** (Hosp. only)

8.1.3 Antimetabolites

Antimetabolites act by incorporation into new nuclear material or by irreversible combination with vital cellular enzymes.

Methotrexate inhibits the enzyme dihydrofolate reductase, essential for the synthesis of purines and pyrimidines. It may be given orally, intramuscularly, intravenously, or intrathecally. Oral absorption becomes erratic above 30 mg/m^2 body-surface, while the maximum recommended intrathecal dose for adults is 12.5 mg.

The administration of massive doses of methotrexate followed by rescue with **folinic acid** is still under investigation and is of far from proven efficacy. Even in skilled hands, the procedure may produce major toxicity and should **not** be used outside specialist centres.

Methotrexate was first used to treat acute lymphatic leukaemia in children, but is now reserved for the management of CNS infiltration or for prophylaxis following the attainment of complete remission. Other uses include choriocarcinoma, and cancers of the breast, head and neck, and lung. It is also occasionally useful for some types of non-Hodgkin lymphoma.

Cytarabine (Cytosar®) acts by interfering with pyrimidine synthesis, and is used for induction or maintenance of remission in acute leukaemias. It is a potent bone-marrow suppressant and should only be used when facilities are available for frequent monitoring of blood counts.

Fluorouracil acts by blocking an enzyme essential for pyrimidine synthesis. It may be given orally or by infusion. It may be used in conjunction with other drugs in patients with breast cancer or alone in patients with gastro-intestinal cancers. Fluorouracil is also used topically for certain malignant skin lesions.

Mercaptopurine (Puri-Nethol®) is used as a remission-maintenance drug in acute leukaemias. Enhanced toxicity may occur if a patient is also receiving allopurinol because the enzyme xanthine oxidase is vital for its degradation.

Thioguanine (Lanvis®) is used solely for acute leukaemias.

Azathioprine is an antimetabolite, but is used as an immunosuppressant (section 8.2.1).

CYTARABINE

Indications: acute leukaemias
Cautions; Side-effects: see section 8.1 and notes above

Cytosar® (Upjohn)
Injection, powder for reconstitution, cytarabine. Price 100-mg vial (with diluent) = **F**

FLUOROURACIL

Indications: see notes above
Cautions; Side-effects: see section 8.1

Fluorouracil Capsules, fluorouracil 250 mg. Price 20 caps = **J**
Fluorouracil Injection, fluorouracil 25 mg (as sodium salt)/ml. Price 10-ml amp = **D**
▼ **Efudix®** (Roche)
Cream, fluorouracil 5%. Price 20 g = **E**

MERCAPTOPURINE

Indications: acute leukaemias
Cautions; Side-effects: see section 8.1 and notes above; reduce dose in renal failure
Dose: initially 2.5 mg/kg daily

Puri-Nethol® (Wellcome)
Tablets, fawn, scored, mercaptopurine 50 mg. Price 20 tabs = **G**

METHOTREXATE

Indications: see notes above
Cautions; Side-effects: see section 8.1 and notes above; reduce dose in renal failure. Drug interactions: see Appendix 1
Dose: *by mouth*, 10–25 mg weekly

Methotrexate Tablets, methotrexate 2.5 mg, price 20 tabs = **E**; 10 mg, price 20 tabs = **I**
Methotrexate Injection, methotrexate 2.5 mg (as sodium salt)/ml, price 1-ml amp = **C**, 2-ml amp = **D**; 25 mg/ml, price 1-ml amp = **E**, 2-ml amp = **F**, 10-ml amp = **J**; powder for reconstitution, price 50-mg vial = **G**, 500-mg vial = **J**, 1-g vial = **J**
Emtexate® (Nordic)
Injection, methotrexate 2.5 mg (as sodium salt)/ml. Price 2-ml amp = **D**
Injection, methotrexate 25 mg (as sodium salt)/ml. Price 2-ml amp = **F**
Injection, powder for reconstitution, methotrexate (as sodium salt). Price 500-mg vial = **J**; 1-g vial = **J**

THIOGUANINE

Indications: acute leukaemias
Cautions; Side-effects: see section 8.1 and notes above; reduce dose in renal failure
Dose: initially 2–2.5 mg/kg daily

Lanvis® (Wellcome)
Tablets, yellow, scored, thioguanine 40 mg. Price 20 tabs = **J**

8.1.4 Vinca alkaloids

These are plant alkaloids extracted from *Vinca rosea* which cause metaphase arrest by interfering with the assembly of microtubules. They have different but overlapping spectra of activity and toxicity.

Vincristine (Oncovin®) is a major drug in the management of the leukaemias and lymphomas, particularly for induction of remission, and also has activity against a variety of solid tumours. It is given intravenously and the maximum recommended dose is 2 mg (1 mg in elderly patients).

Vincristine is relatively marrow-sparing, its main toxicity being neuropathy which may take any form, but usually presents as a sensorimotor peripheral neuropathy, with paraesthesia, loss of tendon reflexes, and muscular weakness. Treatment should be withheld at the first sign of muscle weakness. Autonomic neuropathy causing constipation with ileus and abdominal pain is not uncommon. Occasionally a low-sodium state may occur.

Vinblastine (Velbe®) is often substituted for vincristine in the management of lymphomas. It is also used in the management of advanced malignant teratomata. It is more myelosuppressive but when used in recommended dosage causes neuropathy less commonly than vincristine.

Vindesine (Eldisine®) is a new vinca alkaloid at present on trial. It has both myelosuppressive and neuropathic effects, and its place in therapy is not yet established.

VINBLASTINE SULPHATE

Indications: see notes above
Cautions; Side-effects: see section 8.1 and notes above; also caution in handling—avoid contact with eyes

Velbe® (Lilly)
Injection, powder for reconstitution, vinblastine sulphate. Price 10-mg amp (with diluent) = **I**

VINCRISTINE SULPHATE

Indications: see notes above
Cautions; Side-effects: see section 8.1 and notes above

Oncovin® (Lilly)
Injection, powder for reconstitution, vincristine sulphate (with lactose). Price 1-mg vial = **I**; 2-mg vial = **J**; 5-mg vial = **J** (all with diluent)

VINDESINE SULPHATE

Indications: see notes above
Cautions; Side-effects: see section 8.1 and notes above

▼ Eldisine® (Lilly)
Injection, powder for reconstitution, vindesine sulphate (with mannitol). Price 5-mg vial (with diluent) = **J** (Hosp. only)

8.1.5 Other cytotoxic drugs

These are a miscellaneous collection of drugs with various modes of action.

Cisplatin (Neoplatin®) is a novel cytotoxic drug containing platinum, and is thought to act as an alkylating agent. It has been shown to have some activity against solid tumours, in particular malignant teratomata of testis. Potential toxicity includes deafness, peripheral neuropathy, and renal damage.

CISPLATIN

Indications: see notes above
Cautions; Side-effects: see section 8.1 and notes above

▼ Neoplatin® (Mead Johnson)
Injection, powder for reconstitution, cisplatin. Price 10-mg vial = **I**; 50-mg vial = **J** (Hosp. only)

A suspension of inactivated *Corynebacterium parvum* organisms is administered by intrapleural or intraperitoneal injection for the treatment of malignant pleural effusions and ascites. Side-effects include pyrexia. It is an immunostimulant. Treatment should be avoided within 10 days of chest surgery such as thoracotomy or lung resection as the incidence of side-effects is increased.

CORYNEBACTERIUM PARVUM VACCINE

Indications: see notes above
Side-effects: pyrexia, abdominal pain, nausea and vomiting

Coparvax® (Calmic)
Injection, powder for reconstitution, *Corynebacterium parvum* (inactivated). Price 7-mg vial = **J**

Dacarbazine (DTIC) may interfere with purine synthesis but its mode of action is largely unknown. It can occasionally produce short-term remission in advanced melanoma, and is used in second-line combinations in the treatment of Hodgkin's disease.

DACARBAZINE

Indications: see notes above
Cautions; Side-effects: see section 8.1; also caution in handling—irritant to skin and mucous membranes

DTIC-Dome (Dome)
Injection, powder for reconstitution, dacarbazine. Price 100-mg vial = **F**; 200-mg vial = **G**

Etoposide (Vepesid®) is related to podophyllotoxin. It may be given by mouth or by intravenous injection and is often used in conjunction with other drugs. It has shown antitumour activity in small cell lung carcinoma and resistant non-seminomatous testicular carcinoma.

Etoposide may be given as a single dose but there is some evidence that daily administration over a 5-day period may be more effective. A typical dosage regimen is 60–120 mg/m² body-surface daily by intravenous infusion for five consecutive days or double this dose by mouth, which may be repeated after not less than 21 days. Courses are generally repeated at 21-day intervals. Common toxicities are myelosuppression, nausea, vomiting, and alopecia.

ETOPOSIDE

Indications: see notes above

Cautions; Contra-indications; Side-effects: see section 8.1 and notes above

▼ Vepesid® (Mead Johnson)
Capsules, etoposide 100 mg. Price 1 cap = **I**
Injection, etoposide 20 mg/ml. To be diluted. Price 5-ml amp = **J**

Hydroxyurea (Hydrea®) is an orally active drug used mainly in chronic myeloid leukaemia refractory to busulphan. Close monitoring of blood counts is necessary.

HYDROXYUREA

Indications: see notes above
Cautions; Side-effects: see section 8.1 and notes above
Dose: 20–30 mg/kg daily *or* 80 mg/kg every 3rd day

Hydrea® (Squibb)
Capsules, pink/green, hydroxyurea 500 mg. Price 20 caps = **D**

Procarbazine (Natulan®) is used mainly in combination therapy for Hodgkin's disease. It is given orally and may cause gastro-intestinal upsets which tend to disappear after a few days. Procarbazine may cause inhibition of the oxidation of ethanol, resulting in a disulfiram-like reaction. Patients should therefore be advised not to take alcohol during treatment.

PROCARBAZINE

Indications: see notes above
Cautions; Side-effects: see section 8.1 and notes above; reduce dose in renal failure
Dose: initially 50 mg daily, gradually increased to 250–300 mg daily in divided doses

Natulan® (Roche)
Capsules, yellow, procarbazine 50 mg (as hydrochloride). Price 20 caps = **D**

Razoxane (Razoxin®) has been shown to have some effect in acute myeloid leukaemia and in non-Hodgkin lymphoma. There is some evidence that this drug may increase tumour response to radiotherapy.

RAZOXANE

Indications: see notes above
Cautions; Side-effects: see section 8.1
Dose: 125 mg twice daily, with radiotherapy

▼ Razoxin® (ICI)
Tablets, razoxane 125 mg. Price 20 tabs = **J**

Tamoxifen (Nolvadex®) is an anti-oestrogen which may act by blocking receptor sites in target organs, although other mechanisms are postulated. It is indicated for the palliative treatment of breast cancer and tends to produce less side-effects than the oestrogens, but those that occur are of a similar nature. Hypercalcaemia may be a problem.

TAMOXIFEN

Indications: see notes above
Cautions; Side-effects: see section 8.1 and notes above
Dose: breast cancer, initially 10 mg twice daily

Nolvadex® (ICI)
Tablets, tamoxifen 10 mg (as citrate). Price 20 tabs = **G**

8.2 Immunosuppressants

This section includes cytotoxic drugs used as immunosuppressants (section 8.2.1) and corticosteroids (section 8.2.2).

8.2.1 Cytotoxic immunosuppressants

Azathioprine (Imuran®) is the most commonly used cytotoxic immunosuppressant. It is used to prevent transplant rejection and also to treat a variety of auto-immune and collagen diseases (see section 10.1.3), usually when inadequate control is achieved with corticosteroids alone. It is converted to mercaptopurine in the liver and therefore requires an equivalent dose reduction when allopurinol is also prescribed. It is well tolerated, its predominant side-effect being bone-marrow suppression.

Cyclophosphamide and **chlorambucil** (section 8.1.1) are less commonly prescribed as immunosuppressants. Careful consideration should be given to the use of alternative therapy before these alkylating drugs are used in the auto-immune diseases as their chronic use may be associated with infertility, particularly in males, and an increased incidence of secondary malignancy. Cyclophosphamide should not be used as an immunosuppressant except in life-threatening situations.

Antilymphocyte immunoglobulin (Pressimmune®) is obtained from immunised horses. It has been used to prevent rejection of organ transplants and in auto-immune diseases, but in the absence of clear evidence of benefit from its use, it is not routinely employed for these purposes.

ANTILYMPHOCYTE IMMUNOGLOBULIN

Indications: see notes above
Cautions: test for hypersensitivity; acute infections
Side-effects: fever, shivering, nausea, hypotension, tachycardia; also anaphylactic reactions, urticaria, pruritus

Pressimmune® (Hoechst)
Injection, antilymphocyte immunoglobulin

(horse) 50 mg/ml. Price 5- and 10-ml amp (both) = **J** (Hosp. only)

AZATHIOPRINE

Indications: see notes above

Cautions; Side-effects: see section 8.1 and notes above; also rashes and muscle wasting. Reduce dose in severe renal failure

Dose: *by mouth*, 1–5 mg/kg daily

Imuran® (Wellcome)

Tablets, yellow, scored, azathioprine 50 mg. Price 20 tabs = **G**

Injection, powder for reconstitution, azathioprine (as sodium salt). Price 50-mg vial = **H**

8.2.2 Corticosteroids in malignant disease and immunosuppression

Prednisolone and **prednisone** are both used in malignant disease. Their major role is in the treatment of acute lymphoblastic leukaemia and non-Hodgkin lymphoma. They have a lympholytic action and are effective when included in chemotherapy combinations in these conditions.

Corticosteroids may also have a useful role in a proportion of patients with breast cancer and, in addition, they are commonly used for their euphoriant effect in the terminal stages of malignant disease.

The corticosteroids are also potent immunosuppressants. They are given prophylactically to transplant recipients where rejection is a problem, for example in renal transplantation, and are also used to treat rejection episodes. In addition they are used to treat a wide range of collagen and auto-immune diseases such as systemic lupus erythematosus, chronic active hepatitis, temporal arteritis, and auto-immune haemolytic anaemia.

It is important to embark on corticosteroid therapy only when there is clear evidence that it is likely to be effective. It is usual to commence therapy in these conditions at a relatively high dosage, such as 60 mg of prednisolone daily, and then to reduce the dose to the lowest maintenance dose commensurate with disease control.

For notes on the corticosteroids see section 6.3.

8.3 Sex hormones used in malignant disease

These drugs can be expected to produce feminising or virilising side-effects. They are best classified as oestrogens (section 8.3.1), progestogens (section 8.3.2), and androgens and anabolic steroids (section 8.3.3).

8.3.1 Oestrogens

Administration of these drugs may produce side-effects which include fluid retention and hypertension, gastro-intestinal disturbances, thrombo-embolic disease, hypercalcaemia, and feminising effects.

Stilboestrol is the most widely used oestrogen and is given by mouth. It provides good control in up to 80% of patients with metastatic prostatic carcinoma and is also of value in many postmenopausal patients with breast cancer. The most troublesome side-effects include nausea, vomiting, fluid retention, and in the case of males, loss of libido and gynaecomastia.

Fosfestrol (Honvan®) is activated by the enzyme acid phosphatase to produce stilboestrol. It can be given by mouth, or by intravenous injection. Perineal pain and pain in bony metastatic sites can occur following intravenous injection. There is no evidence that it is more effective than stilboestrol.

Ethinyloestradiol is the most potent oestrogen available. Unlike other oestrogens it is not metabolised in the liver. It is used in breast cancer and may be tolerated by patients who have severe gastro-intestinal side-effects from stilboestrol.

Polyestradiol (Estradurin®) is a long-acting oestrogen preparation.

ETHINYLOESTRADIOL

Indications: see notes above

Cautions; Contra-indications; Side-effects: see section 6.4.1.1 and notes above

Dose: 1–3 mg daily

Preparations

See section 6.4.1.1

CHLOROTRIANISENE

Indications: palliation of prostatic carcinoma

Cautions; Contra-indications; Side-effects: see under Ethinyloestradiol (section 6.4.1.1)

Dose: 24 mg daily

Preparations

See section 6.4.1.1

FOSFESTROL TETRASODIUM

Indications: see notes above

Cautions; Contra-indications; Side-effects: see under Ethinyloestradiol (section 6.4.1.1) and notes above

Dose: *by mouth*, 100–200 mg 3 times daily, reducing to once daily

By intravenous injection, 552–1104 mg daily for at least 5 days; maintenance 276–552 mg every 1–2 weeks

Honvan® (WBP)

Tablets, fosfestrol tetrasodium 100 mg. Price 20 tabs = **E**

Injection, fosfestrol tetrasodium 55.2 mg/ml. Price 5-ml amp = **C**

POLYESTRADIOL PHOSPHATE

Indications: prostatic carcinoma

Cautions; Contra-indications; Side-effects: see under Ethinyloestradiol (section 6.4.1.1) and notes above

Dose: by deep intramuscular injection, 80–160 mg every 4 weeks; maintenance 40–80 mg

Estradurin® (Lundbeck)
Injection, powder for reconstitution, polyestradiol phosphate (with mepivacaine and nicotinamide). Price 40-mg vial = **E**; 80-mg vial = **F** (both with diluent)

STILBOESTROL

Indications: see notes above
Cautions; Contra-indications; Side-effects: see under Ethinyloestradiol (section 6.4.1.1) and notes above
Dose: breast cancer, 10–20 mg daily
Prostatic cancer, 1–3 mg daily

Stilboestrol Tablets, stilboestrol 1 and 5 mg, price 20 tabs (both) = **A**; 25 mg, price 20 tabs = **B**; 100 mg, price 20 tabs = **C**

8.3.2 Progestogens

Side-effects are less common than with oestrogens, but include gastro-intestinal upsets and hepatotoxicity.

Norethisterone (Utovlan®) and esters of **gestronol** (Depostat®), **hydroxyprogesterone** (Proluton-Depot®), **medroxyprogesterone** (Provera®), and **norethisterone** (SH 420®) may all be useful in the management of endometrial carcinoma, breast cancer, refractory prostatic cancer, and rarely carcinoma of the kidney and testis.

GESTRONOL HEXANOATE

Indications: see notes above
Cautions; Contra-indications; Side-effects: see under Norethisterone (section 6.4.1.2) and notes above
Dose: *by intramuscular injection*, 200–400 mg every 5–7 days

Depostat® (Schering)
Injection (oily), gestronol hexanoate 100 mg/ml. Price 2-ml amp = **F**

HYDROXYPROGESTERONE HEXANOATE

Indications: see notes above
Cautions; Contra-indications; Side-effects: see under Norethisterone (section 6.4.1.2) and notes above
Dose: *by intramuscular injection*, 1 g one or more times weekly

Preparations
See section 6.4.1.2

MEDROXYPROGESTERONE ACETATE

Indications: see notes above
Cautions; Contra-indications; Side-effects: see under Norethisterone (section 6.4.1.2) and notes above
Dose: *by mouth*, 200–400 mg daily for up to 3 months

Depo-Provera® (Upjohn)
Injection, medroxyprogesterone acetate 150 mg/ml. Price 3-ml vial = **I**. See also section 6.4.1.2

Provera 100 mg® (Upjohn)
Tablets, scored, medroxyprogesterone acetate 100 mg. Price 20 tabs = **H**

NORETHISTERONE

Indications: see notes above
Cautions; Contra-indications; Side-effects: see section 6.4.1.2 and notes above
Dose: 40 mg daily, increased to 60 mg daily if required

Preparations
See section 6.4.1.2

NORETHISTERONE ACETATE

Indications: see notes above
Cautions; Contra-indications; Side-effects: see under Norethisterone (section 6.4.1.2) and notes above
Dose: 10 mg 3 times daily, increased to 60 mg daily if required

SH 420® (Schering)
Tablets, scored, norethisterone acetate 10 mg. Price 20 tabs = **F**

8.3.3 Androgens and anabolic steroids

These drugs are degraded in the liver. Side-effects include fluid retention; virilising and anabolic effects also occur.

Drostanolone (Masteril®) is an anabolic steroid with less virilising activity than testosterone. It is useful in the palliation of breast cancer, usually in premenopausal women.

Nandrolone phenylpropionate (Durabolin®) is also used for breast cancer in premenopausal women. It is given by weekly intramuscular injections as a depot preparation.

Nandrolone decanoate (Deca-Durabolin®) is used similarly, but injections are required only every 3 weeks.

DROSTANOLONE PROPIONATE

Indications: see notes above
Cautions; Contra-indications; Side-effects: see under Methandienone (section 6.4.3) and notes above
Dose: *by intramuscular injection*, 300 mg weekly

Masteril® (Syntex)
Injection, drostanolone propionate 100 mg/ml. Price 1-ml amp = **D**

NANDROLONE

Indications: see notes above

Cautions; Contra-indications; Side-effects: see under Methandienone (section 6.4.3) and notes above

Dose: *by intramuscular injection*, nandrolone decanoate 25–50 mg every 3 weeks; nandrolone phenylpropionate 25–50 mg weekly

Preparations

See section 6.4.3

9: Drugs affecting NUTRITION and BLOOD

This section includes drugs for the treatment of nutritional anaemias and foods, food supplements, vitamins, and electrolytes used in nutritional disorders. It does not include information on preparations of human blood or blood products which, in the United Kingdom, are supplied through the Department of Health and Social Security (England and Wales), the Scottish National Blood Transfusion Association (Scotland), and the Regional Transfusion Centre (Northern Ireland). Immunoglobulin injections are discussed in Chapter 14.

This chapter is arranged in the following sections:

9.1 Drugs used in anaemias

Before initiating treatment it is essential to determine which type of anaemia is present. Iron salts may be harmful if given alone to patients with folic acid or vitamin B_{12} deficiency.

Other than in the special cases indicated below, the only justification for iron treatment is the presence of a demonstrable iron-deficiency state. However, prophylaxis is justifiable in pregnancy, menorrhagia, after partial or total gastrectomy (where iron deficiency anaemia may be expected in up to 60% of patients), and in the management of low birth-weight infants such as premature babies, twins, and infants after Caesarean section. The National Blood Transfusion Service provides iron prophylaxis for female blood donors in some centres.

9.1.1.1 ORAL IRON THERAPY

Iron salts should be given by mouth unless there are good reasons for using another route. The commonly used ferrous salts show only marginal differences in efficiency of absorption of iron. Ferric salts are much less well absorbed than ferrous salts. Haemoglobin regeneration rate is little affected by the salt used, and in most patients the time factor is not critical. Choice of preparation is thus usually decided by incidence of side-effects.

The oral dose of elemental iron should be 100 to 200 mg daily. It is customary to start treatment with dried **ferrous sulphate**, 200 mg being given three times daily initially. It should be given after food to minimise gastric intolerance. If side-effects arise, dosage can be reduced or a change made to an alternative iron salt. It should be remembered, however, that an apparent improvement in tolerance on changing to another salt may be due to its lower content of elemental iron.

Table: Iron Salts

Iron salt	Amount	Content of ferrous iron
Ferrous fumarate	200 mg	65 mg
Ferrous gluconate	300 mg	35 mg
Ferrous glycine sulphate	225 mg	40 mg
Ferrous succinate	100 mg	35 mg
Ferrous sulphate	300 mg	60 mg
Ferrous sulphate, dried	200 mg	60 mg

THERAPEUTIC RESPONSE. The haemoglobin concentration should rise by about 100–200 mg per 100 ml per day. When the haemoglobin figure has risen to a normal level, treatment should be continued for a further six months in an attempt to replenish the iron stores. Epithelial tissue changes such as atrophic glossitis and koilonychia are usually improved although the response is often slow.

ADJUVANTS. Some oral preparations contain adjuvants such as ascorbic acid, or the iron is in the form of a chelate, which can be shown experimentally to produce a modest increase in absorption of iron. However, the therapeutic advantage is minimal. There can be neither theoretical nor clinical justification for the inclusion of other therapeutically active ingredients, especially the B group of vitamins, in orally administered preparations, except for folic acid in conjunction with an iron salt as prophylactic therapy for pregnant women (iron and folic acid preparations—see below).

SLOW-RELEASE CAPSULES AND TABLETS. These are designed to release iron gradually as the capsule or tablet passes along the gut so that a smaller amount of ionic iron is present in the lumen at any one time. It is claimed that each dose unit contains enough iron for 24 hours, thus giving simple once daily dosage.

These preparations are likely to carry the iron past the first part of the duodenum into an area of the gut where conditions for iron absorption are poor. The low incidence of side-effects may well be because of the small amounts of iron available under these conditions and so the preparations have no therapeutic advantage.

SIDE-EFFECTS. Because iron salts are astringent, gastro-intestinal irritation may occur, necessitating care in administration as described above. Nausea and epigastric pain may occur and are dose-related but the relationship between dose and altered bowel habit, giving rise to constipation or diarrhoea, is less clear. The incidence of side-effects due to ferrous sulphate is no greater than with other iron salts when compared on the basis of equivalent amounts of elemental iron.

FERROUS FUMARATE

Indications: iron-deficiency anaemia
Cautions; Side-effects; Dose: see under Ferrous Sulphate

Fersaday® (Glaxo)
Tablets, orange, f/c, ferrous fumarate 304 mg (100 mg iron). Price 28 tabs = **B**
Fersamal® (Glaxo)
Tablets, brown, ferrous fumarate 200 mg (65 mg iron). Price 20 tabs = **A**
Syrup (=mixture), brown, ferrous fumarate 140 mg (45 mg iron)/5 ml. Diluent syrup, life of diluted mixture 14 days. Price 200 ml = **D**
Galfer® (Galen)
Capsules, red/green, ferrous fumarate 290 mg (100 mg iron). Price 20 caps = **B**

FERROUS GLUCONATE

Indications: iron-deficiency anaemia
Cautions; Side-effects; Dose: see under Ferrous Sulphate

Ferrous Gluconate Tablets, red, s/c, ferrous gluconate 300 mg (35 mg iron). Price 20 tabs = **A**
Fergon® (Winthrop)
Tablets, red, s/c, ferrous gluconate 300 mg (35 mg iron). Price 20 tabs = **B**

FERROUS GLYCINE SULPHATE

Indications: iron-deficiency anaemia
Cautions; Side-effects; Dose: see under Ferrous Sulphate

Fe-Cap® (MCP)
Capsules, yellow/white, ferrous glycine sulphate 565 mg (100 mg iron). Price 30 caps = **C**
Ferrocontin Continus® (Napp)
Tablets, s/r, red, f/c, ferrous glycine sulphate 562.5 mg (100 mg iron). Price 20 tabs = **B**
Kelferon® (MCP)
Tablets, pink, s/c, ferrous glycine sulphate 225 mg (40 mg iron). Price 20 tabs = **C**
Plesmet® (Coates & Cooper)
Syrup (=elixir), ferrous glycine sulphate 141 mg (25 mg iron)/5 ml. Diluent syrup, life of diluted elixir 14 days. Price 100 ml = **C**

FERROUS SUCCINATE

Indications: iron-deficiency anaemia
Cautions; Side-effects; Dose: see under Ferrous Sulphate

Ferrous Succinate Tablets, orange, s/c, ferrous succinate 100 mg (35 mg iron). Price 20 tabs = **A**
Ferromyn® (Calmic)
Tablets, orange, s/c, ferrous succinate 100 mg (35 mg iron). Price 20 tabs = **B**
Elixir, brown, ferrous succinate 106 mg (37 mg iron)/5 ml. Diluent syrup, life of diluted elixir 14 days. Price 100 ml = **D**

FERROUS SULPHATE

Indications: iron-deficiency anaemia
Cautions: drug interactions: see Appendix 1
Side-effects: large doses often produce gastro-intestinal irritation, vomiting, diarrhoea; continued administration may result in constipation
Dose: ferrous iron, therapeutic, 120–180 mg daily in divided doses; prophylactic, 60 mg daily; CHILD, therapeutic, daily in divided doses, up to 1 year 36 mg, 1–5 years 72 mg, 6–12 years 120 mg

Ferrous Sulphate Tablets, f/c or s/c, dried ferrous sulphate 200 mg (60 mg iron) and 300 mg (90 mg iron). Price 20 tabs (both) = **A**
Ferrous Sulphate Mixture, Paediatric, ferrous sulphate 60 mg (12 mg iron)/5 ml (see Formulary). Price 100 ml = **A**
To be taken well diluted with water
Feospan® (SK&F)
Spansules® (=capsules s/r), clear/red, enclosing green and red pellets, dried ferrous sulphate 150 mg (45 mg iron). Price 20 caps = **B**
Ferro-Gradumet® (Abbott)
Filmtabs® (=tablets s/r), red, f/c, dried ferrous sulphate 325 mg (105 mg iron). Price 20 tabs = **B**
Ironorm® (Wallace Mfg)
Drops (=elixir), ferrous sulphate 116 mg (25 mg iron)/ml. Price 15 ml = **C**
Slow-Fe® (Ciba)
Tablets, s/r, dried ferrous sulphate 160 mg (48 mg iron). Price 20 tabs = **B**

IRON AND FOLIC ACID

Indications: prevention of iron and folic acid deficiencies in pregnancy
Cautions: the small doses of folic acid recommended for prophylaxis in the range 200–500 micrograms should not be used in the treatment of megaloblastic anaemias. Drug interactions: see Appendix 1
Side-effects: see under Ferrous Sulphate
Dose: prophylactic, the equivalent of approximately 100 mg of iron with 200–500 micrograms of folic acid, daily

Iron and Folic Acid Tablets, ferrous fumarate 304 mg (100 mg iron), folic acid 350 micrograms. Price 20 tabs = **B**
Co-Ferol® (Cox-Continental)
Tablets, red, s/c, ferrous fumarate 120 mg (40 mg

iron), folic acid 200 micrograms. Price 20 tabs = **A**

Fe-Cap Folic® (MCP)
Capsules, yellow/red, ferrous glycine sulphate 450 mg (80 mg iron), folic acid 350 micrograms. Price 30 caps = **C**

Fefol® (SK&F)
Spansules® (=capsules s/r), clear/green, enclosing red, yellow, and white pellets, dried ferrous sulphate 150 mg (45 mg iron), folic acid 500 micrograms. Price 20 caps = **B**

Feravol-F® (Carlton)
Tablets, ferrous gluconate 300 mg (35 mg iron), folic acid 3 mg. Price 20 tabs = **A**

Ferrocap-F 350® (Consolidated)
Capsules, s/r, pink, enclosing brown, white, and yellow granules, ferrous fumarate 330 mg (110 mg iron), folic acid 350 micrograms. Price 20 caps = **B**

Ferrocontin Folic Continus® (Napp)
Tablets, s/r, orange, f/c, ferrous glycine sulphate 526.5 mg (100 mg iron), folic acid 500 micrograms. Price 20 tabs = **B**

Ferrograd Folic® (Abbott)
Filmtabs® (=tablets s/r), red/yellow, f/c, dried ferrous sulphate 325 mg (105 mg iron), folic acid 350 micrograms. Price 20 tabs = **B**

Folex-350® (Rybar)
Tablets, pink, s/c, ferrous fumarate 308 mg (100 mg iron), folic acid 350 micrograms. Price 20 tabs = **B**

Folvron® (Lederle)
Tablets, red, s/c, dried ferrous sulphate 194 mg (57 mg iron), folic acid 1.7 mg. Price 20 tabs = **C**

Galfer FA® (Galen)
Capsules, red/yellow, ferrous fumarate 290 mg (100 mg iron), folic acid 350 micrograms. Price 20 caps = **B**

Kelfolate® (MCP)
Tablets, yellow, s/c, ferrous glycine sulphate 225 mg (40 mg iron), folic acid 150 micrograms. Price 20 tabs = **A**

Pregaday® (Glaxo)
Tablets, brown, f/c, ferrous fumarate 304 mg (100 mg iron), folic acid 350 micrograms. Price 28 tabs = **B**

Pregfol® (Wyeth)
Capsules, dark claret, dried ferrous sulphate 270 mg (81 mg iron), folic acid 500 micrograms. Price 20 caps = **B**

Slow-Fe Folic® (Ciba)
Tablets, s/r, cream, f/c, dried ferrous sulphate 160 mg (50 mg iron), folic acid 400 micrograms. Price 20 tabs = **B**

POLYSACCHARIDE-IRON COMPLEX

Indications: iron-deficiency anaemia
Cautions; Side-effects: see under Ferrous Sulphate
Dose: the equivalent of iron, prophylactic, 50 mg daily; therapeutic, 100 mg once or twice daily; CHILD, therapeutic, up to 1 year see below, 1–5 years 50 mg daily, 6–12 years 100 mg daily

Niferex® (Tillotts)
Tablets, brown, polysaccharide-iron complex equivalent to 50 mg of ferrous iron. Price 20 tabs = **B**
Elixir, brown, polysaccharide-iron complex equivalent to 100 mg of ferrous iron/5 ml. Diluent water for preparations or sorbitol solution, life of diluted elixir 14 days. Price 100 ml = **D**; 30-ml dropper bottle for paediatric use = **C**
Dose: by mouth, infant, 1 drop (approximately 0.04 ml) per pound body-weight 3 times daily

SODIUM IRONEDETATE

Indications: iron-deficiency anaemia
Cautions: drug interactions: see Appendix 1
Side-effects: see under Ferrous Sulphate
Dose: *by mouth*, the equivalent of iron, up to 55 mg 3 times daily; CHILD $\frac{1}{4}$–$\frac{1}{2}$ adult dose

Sytron® (P-D)
Elixir, sodium ironedetate equivalent to 27.5 mg of iron/5 ml. Diluent water for preparations, life of diluted elixir 14 days. Price 100 ml = **A**

COMPOUND PREPARATIONS

These preparations contain an iron salt and, usually, one or more vitamins or small amounts of substances intended to provide a 'mineral supplement'. There is no justification for prescribing such preparations, except for preparations of iron and folic acid for prophylactic use in pregnancy (see above).

Ferrous Sulphate Tablets, Compound, green, s/c, dried ferrous sulphate equivalent to 170 mg of $FeSO_4$, copper sulphate 2.5 mg, manganese sulphate 2.5 mg. Price 20 tabs = **A**

Anorvit® (Cox-Continental) *tablets*, acetomenaphthone, ascorbic acid, dried ferrous sulphate. Price 20 tabs = **A**

BC 500 with Iron® (Ayerst) *tablets*, red, f/c, calcium pantothenate, ferrous fumarate, nicotinamide, pyridoxine hydrochloride, riboflavine, sodium ascorbate, thiamine mononitrate. Price 20 tabs = **C**

FEAC® (Robins) *tablets*, s/r, red, f/c, ascorbic acid, dried ferrous sulphate, nicotinamide, pyridoxine hydrochloride, riboflavine, thiamine mononitrate. Price 20 tabs = **C**

Fe-Cap C® (MCP) *capsules*, yellow/orange, ascorbic acid, ferrous glycine sulphate. Price 30 caps = **C**

Fefol-Vit® (SK&F) *Spansules®* (=capsules s/r), clear/white, enclosing red, orange, yellow, and white pellets, ascorbic acid, calcium pantothenate, dried ferrous sulphate, folic acid, nicotinamide, pyridoxine hydrochloride, riboflavine, thiamine mononitrate. Price 20 caps = **C**

Feravol® (Carlton) *tablets*, ascorbic acid, dried ferrous sulphate, riboflavine, thiamine hydrochloride. Price 20 tabs = **A.** *Syrup* (=elixir), ascorbic acid, ferrous sulphate, riboflavine, thiamine hydrochloride. Price 100 ml = **A**

Feravol-G® (Carlton) *tablets*, ferrous gluconate, thiamine hydrochloride. Price 20 tabs = **A.** *Syrup* (=elixir), ingredients as for tablets. Price 100 ml = **A**

Ferfolic® (Sinclair) *tablets*, orange, s/c, ascorbic acid, ferrous gluconate, folic acid, nicotinamide, riboflavine, thiamine hydrochloride. Price 20 tabs = **B**

Ferfolic SV® (Sinclair) *tablets*, pink, s/c, ascorbic acid, ferrous gluconate, folic acid. Price 20 tabs = **B**

Fergluvite® (Sinclair) *tablets*, yellow, s/c, ascorbic acid, ferrous gluconate, nicotinamide, riboflavine, thiamine hydrochloride. Price 20 tabs = **B**

Ferraplex B® (Bencard) *tablets*, red, s/c, ascorbic acid, dried brewer's yeast, copper carbonate, dried ferrous sulphate, nicotinamide, riboflavine, thiamine hydrochloride. Price 20 tabs = **B**

Ferrlecit 100® (Wade) *tablets*, mauve, s/c, ascorbic acid, dried ferrous sulphate, sodium ferric citrate. Price 20 tabs = **B**

Ferrocap® (Consolidated) *capsules*, s/r, green/orange, enclosing brown and white granules, ferrous fumarate, thiamine hydrochloride. Price 20 caps = **B**

Ferrograd C® (Abbott) *tablets*, s/r, red, f/c, dried ferrous sulphate, sodium ascorbate. Price 30 tabs = **C**

Ferromyn B® (Calmic) *tablets*, brown, ferrous succinate, nicotinamide, riboflavine, thiamine hydrochloride. Price 20 tabs = **B**. *Elixir*, brown, 5 ml elixir = 1 tablet. Price 100 ml = **D**

Ferromyn S® (Calmic) *tablets*, orange, ferrous succinate, succinic acid. Price 20 tabs = **B**

Ferromyn S Folic® (Calmic) *tablets*, red, ingredients as for Ferromyn S tablets with folic acid. Price 20 tabs = **B**

Fesovit® (SK&F) *Spansules*® (=capsules s/r), colourless/yellow, enclosing red, orange, and white pellets, ascorbic acid, calcium pantothenate, dried ferrous sulphate, nicotinamide, pyridoxine hydrochloride, riboflavine, thiamine mononitrate. Price 20 caps = **B**

Folicin® (P&B) *tablets*, s/c, copper sulphate, dried ferrous sulphate, folic acid, manganese sulphate. Price 20 tabs = **A**

Forceval® (Unigreg) *capsules*, ascorbic acid, calcium hydrogen phosphate, calcium pantothenate, choline bitartrate, copper, cyanocobalamin, inositol, iodine, iron, lysine hydrochloride, magnesium, manganese, nicotinamide, phosphorus, potassium, pyridoxine hydrochloride, riboflavine, thiamine hydrochloride, vitamin A, vitamin D, vitamin E, zinc. Price 30 caps = **D**

Galfer-Vit® (Galen) *capsules*, maroon/orange, ferrous fumarate 305 mg (100 mg iron), thiamine mononitrate 2 mg, riboflavine 2 mg, pyridoxine hydrochloride 4 mg, nicotinamide 10 mg, sodium ascorbate 56 mg. Price 20 caps = **B**

Gastrovite® (MCP) *tablets*, pink, s/c, ascorbic acid, calciferol, calcium gluconate, ferrous glycine sulphate. Price 20 tabs = **B**

Gevral® (Lederle) *capsules*, brown, ascorbic acid, calciferol, calcium pantothenate, calcium phosphate, choline bitartrate, copper oxide, cyanocobalamin, ferrous fumarate, inositol, magnesium oxide, manganese dioxide, nicotinamide, potassium iodide, potassium sulphate, pyridoxine hydrochloride, riboflavine, thiamine mononitrate, d-α-tocopheryl acetate, vitamin A, yeast, zinc oxide. Price 30 caps = **D**

Givitol® (Galen) *capsules*, red/maroon, ferrous fumarate 305 mg (100 mg iron), folic acid 500 micrograms, thiamine mononitrate 2 mg, riboflavine 2 mg, pyridoxine hydrochloride 4 mg, nicotinamide 10 mg, sodium ascorbate 56 mg. Price 20 caps = **B**

Glykola® (Sinclair) *elixir*, caffeine, calcium glycerophosphate, chloroform spirit, ferric chloride solution, kola liquid extract. Price 100 ml = **C**. **Glykola Infans** *elixir, paediatric*, citric acid, ferric chloride solution, gentian compound infusion, kola liquid extract, manganese glycerophosphate. Price 100 ml = **C**

Iberet 500® (Abbott) *Filmtabs*® (=tablets, s/r), red, f/c, ascorbic acid, calcium pantothenate, dried ferrous sulphate, nicotinamide, pyridoxine hydrochloride, riboflavine, thiamine mononitrate. Price 20 tabs = **C**

Iberol® (Abbott) *Filmtabs*® (=tablets s/r), red, f/c, dried ferrous sulphate, liver fraction, nicotinamide, pyridoxine hydrochloride, riboflavine, sodium ascorbate, thiamine mononitrate. Price 20 tabs = **C**

Irofol C® (Abbott) *Filmtabs*® (=tablets s/r), red, f/c, dried ferrous sulphate, folic acid, sodium ascorbate. Price 20 tabs = **C**

Ironorm® (Wallace Mfg) *capsules*, ascorbic acid, cyanocobalamin, dried ferrous sulphate, folic acid, concentrated intrinsic factor, liver fraction II, nicotinamide, riboflavine, thiamine hydrochloride. Price 20 caps = **C**. *Tonic with iron* (=elixir), calcium pantothenate, cyanocobalamin, ferric ammonium citrate, glycerophosphates of calcium, manganese, sodium, and potassium, nicotinamide, proteolysed liver extract, pyridoxine hydrochloride, riboflavine, thiamine hydrochloride. Price 150 ml = **C**

Pregnavite Forte® (Bencard) *tablets*, scarlet, s/c, ascorbic acid, calcium phosphate, dried ferrous sulphate, nicotinamide, pyridoxine hydrochloride, riboflavine, thiamine hydrochloride, vitamin A, vitamin D. Price 20 tabs = **B**. **Pregnavite Forte F** *tablets*, lilac, s/c, ingredients as for Pregnavite Forte tablets, with folic acid. Price 20 tabs = **B**

Sidros® (Potter & Clarke) *tablets*, ascorbic acid, ferrous gluconate. Price 20 tabs = **A**

Tonivitan A & D® (Medo) *syrup* (=elixir), orange, calciferol, calcium glycerophosphate, copper sulphate, ferric ammonium citrate, manganese glycerophosphate, vitamin A. Price 100 ml = **B**

9.1.1.2 PARENTERAL IRON THERAPY

The only valid reason for administering iron preparations parenterally is failure of oral therapy. Such failure may be due to lack of patient co-operation with oral treatment, gastro-intestinal side-effects, continuing severe blood loss, and resistant malabsorption. Provided that the oral iron preparation is taken reliably and is absorbed, then with equivalent doses of iron the rate of haemoglobin response is not significantly faster when the intramuscular or intravenous instead of the oral route is used. The need for a rapid cure of the anaemia is therefore not met by intramuscular administration of iron.

For parenteral administration, it is customary to give a course of deep *intramuscular* injections lasting about 10 days. The manufacturer's dosage schedules should be consulted; these usually include a supplement for the reconstitution of the iron stores.

Iron dextran (Imferon® etc.) may also be administered as a single dose by slow intravenous infusion over 6 to 8 hours provided that there is no reaction within a few minutes of administration of a 1-ml test dose. Although the incidence of side-effects is low, disquieting adverse reactions may occur, especially in allergic subjects, and intravenous infusion is contra-indicated in asthmatic patients. Iron dextran should only be administered *intravenously* in selected cases where proper indications exist for its use, that is, when continuing blood loss is likely to be permanent and oral prophylaxis cannot keep pace, when a patient requiring parenteral iron has a small muscle mass or a haemostatic defect contra-indicating intramuscular injection or when reasons of psychological or social pressure make iron treatment by other means impracticable.

Preparations suitable for parenteral use contain iron either in the form of **Iron Dextran Injection**, containing a complex of ferric hydroxide with dextrans of high molecular weight, or as **Iron Sorbitol Injection** (Jectofer®), containing a complex of iron, sorbitol and citric acid. The latter preparation is **not** suitable for intravenous injection and, although the low mean molecular weight allows rapid absorption from the injection site, excretion in the saliva and substantial urinary losses from each dose also occur.

To prevent leakage along the needle track with subsequent staining of the skin, intramuscular injections should be deep for both preparations.

IRON DEXTRAN INJECTION

Contains 5% (50 mg/ml) of iron

Indications: iron deficiency anaemia (see notes above)

Cautions: when given by slow intravenous infusion patient should be under observation the whole time and for an hour afterwards. Antihistamines should be available. Caution in patients with a history of allergic conditions.

Contra-indications: severe liver disease, acute renal failure

Side-effects: staining of the skin if leakage along needle track occurs, transient nausea, vomiting, flushing, occasionally severe dyspnoea

Dose: by deep intramuscular injection, 1 ml initially on the first day, followed by 2 ml daily or at longer intervals according to the response; up to 5 ml may be given as a single dose

By slow intravenous infusion, diluted with dextrose intravenous infusion (5%) or sodium chloride intravenous infusion (0.9%), the required amount as a single large dose, over a period of 6–8 hours

Imferon® (Fisons)

Injection, iron dextran injection. Price 2-ml amp = **B**; 5-ml amp = **C**

Intravenous infusion, iron dextran injection. Price 20-ml amp = **F** (Hosp. only)

Ironorm® (Wallace Mfg)

Injection, iron dextran injection. Price 2-ml amp = **B**

IRON SORBITOL INJECTION

Contains 5% (50 mg/ml) of iron

Indications: iron-deficiency anaemia

Cautions: 24 hours should elapse between iron administered orally and start of therapy with iron sorbitol injection. When another injectable iron preparation has been used, a week should elapse between the last injection and the start of therapy with iron sorbitol

Contra-indications: liver disease, kidney disease (particularly pyelonephritis), untreated urinary-tract infections

Dose: by intramuscular injection, initially the equivalent of 1.5 mg of iron/kg for adults and children over 3.5 kg followed by suitable amounts according to response

Jectofer® (Astra)

Injection, iron sorbitol. Price 2-ml amp = **B**

9.1.2 Drugs used in megaloblastic anaemias

Most megaloblastic anaemias are due to lack of either **vitamin B_{12}** or **folic acid** and it is essential to establish, in every case, which deficiency is present and the underlying cause. In emergencies, where delay might be dangerous, it is sometimes necessary to administer both substances together while blood and serum assay results are awaited. Normally, however, appropriate treatment should be instituted only when the results of tests are available.

Vitamin B_{12} should be given prophylactically to patients who have undergone total gastrectomy or total ileal resection.

Hydroxocobalamin is now the form of vitamin B_{12} of choice. It is retained in the body longer than cyanocobalamin and thus for maintenance therapy need only be given at intervals of 2 to 3 months. Although a haematological response in vitamin-B_{12} deficiency may be obtained by small doses, it is customary to start treatment with 1 mg daily by intramuscular injection for 6 to 10 days to replenish the depleted body stores. Thereafter, maintenance treatment, which is usually for life, can be instituted. There is no evidence that larger doses provide any additional benefit in vitamin-B_{12} neuropathy.

Apart from the rare dietary deficiency, all other causes of vitamin-B_{12} deficiency are attributable to malabsorption and there is little place for the use of vitamin B_{12} orally or for vitamin B_{12} intrinsic factor complexes given by the same route.

Cyanocobalamin has been largely replaced by hydroxocobalamin.

Many causes of **folic acid** deficiency are self-limiting, or may yield to treatment, and there are thus few indications for long-term therapy. Even when untreated malabsorption is present, an oral dose of 5 to 10 mg daily of folic acid is usually sufficient to bring about a haematological response. However, treatment should continue for 3 to 4 months to replenish the body stores. Folic acid therapy should not be used indiscriminately in undiagnosed megaloblastic anaemia unless vitamin B_{12} is administered concurrently otherwise neuropathy may be precipitated. Caution should be exercised when administering folic acid to epileptic subjects and to patients who may have folate-dependent tumours.

Folic acid is widely used during pregnancy in the prevention of megaloblastic anaemia and can also be used prophylactically in chronic haemolytic states such as thalassaemia.

There is **no** justification for prescribing multiple-ingredient vitamin preparations containing these substances.

HYDROXOCOBALAMIN

Indications: Addisonian pernicious anaemia, subacute combined degeneration of the spinal cord, other causes of vitamin B_{12} deficiency
Cautions: should not be given before a diagnosis has been fully established
Dose: by intramuscular injection, initially 1 mg repeated 5 times at intervals of 2–3 days; maintenance dose 1 mg every 2 months; CHILD, dosage as for adult

Hydroxocobalamin Injection, hydroxocobalamin 250 micrograms/ml and 1 mg/ml. Price 1-ml amp (both) = **A**

Cobalin-H® (P&B)
Injection, hydroxocobalamin 250 micrograms/ml. Price 1-ml amp = **A**
Injection, hydroxocobalamin 1 mg/ml. Price 1-ml amp = **A**

Neo-Cytamen® (Glaxo)
Injection, hydroxocobalamin 250 micrograms/ml. Price 1-ml amp = **A**
Injection, hydroxocobalamin 1 mg/ml. Price 1-ml amp = **A**

CYANOCOBALAMIN

Indications; Cautions: see under Hydroxocobalamin and notes above
Dose: by intramuscular injection, initially 1 mg, repeated 10 times at intervals of 2–3 days; maintenance 250 micrograms every 4 weeks; CHILD, initially as for adult, subsequent dosage according to haematological response

Cyanocobalamin Injection, cyanocobalamin 1 mg/ml. Price 1 ml amp = **A**

Cobalin® (P&B)
Injection, cyanocobalamin 1 mg/ml. Price 1-ml amp = **A**

Cytacon® (Glaxo)
Tablets, f/c, cyanocobalamin 50 micrograms. Price 20 tabs = **A**
Liquid (=elixir), cyanocobalamin 35 micrograms/5 ml. Price 100 ml = **A**

Cytamen® (Glaxo)
Injection, cyanocobalamin 250 micrograms/ml. Price 1-ml amp = **A**
Injection, cyanocobalamin 1 mg/ml. Price 1-ml amp = **A**

Hepacon B_{12}® (Consolidated)
Injection, cyanocobalamin 100 micrograms and 1 mg/ml, price 1-ml amp (both) = **A**

Hepacon-B Forte® (Consolidated)
Injection, folic acid 2.5 mg, liver extract equivalent to vitamin B_{12} 15 micrograms, thiamine pyrophosphate 50 mg. Price 2-ml amp = **A**

FOLIC ACID

Indications: megaloblastic anaemias
Cautions: should never be given alone in the treatment of Addisonian pernicious anaemia and other vitamin B_{12}-deficiency states because it may precipitate the onset of subacute combined degeneration of the spinal cord; large and continuous doses of folic acid may lower the blood concentration of vitamin B_{12}
Dose: initially, 10–20 mg daily for 14 days or until a haematopoietic response has been obtained; maintenance, 5–10 mg daily; CHILD, initial 48 hours, daily, up to 1 year 500 micrograms/kg, 1–5 years 5 mg, 6–12 years 10 mg; maintenance, half the initial dose
In conjunction with iron salts, for prophylaxis in pregnancy: section 9.1.1.1

Folic Acid Tablets, folic acid 100 micrograms and 5 mg. Price 20 tabs (both) = **A**

FOLINIC ACID

Indications: antidote to folic acid antagonists; treatment of megaloblastic anaemias
Cautions: see under Folic Acid
Dose: as an antidote to folic acid antagonists, up to 120 mg in divided doses over 12 to 24 hours *by intramuscular or intravenous injection or infusion*, followed by 15 mg *by mouth* every 6 hours
In megaloblastic anaemias, 15 mg daily

Calcium Leucovorin (Lederle)
Tablets, scored, folinic acid 15 mg (as calcium salt). Price 10 tabs = **J**
Injection, folinic acid 3 mg (as calcium salt)/ml. Price 1-ml amp = **D**; 10-ml amp = **J**

9.1.3 Drugs used in hypoplastic and haemolytic anaemias

The anabolic steroids, pyridoxine hydrochloride, and various corticosteroids are used in hypoplastic and haemolytic anaemias.

The place of non-androgenic **anabolic steroids** in the therapy of aplastic anaemia remains somewhat controversial and their effectiveness is unclear. There is a wide geographical variation in the reported successful responses, possibly indicating a differing aetiology of the anaemia in various parts of the world. It is customary to prescribe high doses of oxymetholone, such as 50 mg 3 times daily, and to continue therapy for at least 3 to 6 months. At these dose levels, virilising side-effects may be expected in female patients and children.

It is unlikely that dietary deprivation of **pyridoxine hydrochloride** (section 9.6.2) produces haematological effects in man. However, certain forms of sideroblastic anaemia respond to pharmacological doses of pyridoxine, possibly reflecting its role as a co-enzyme during haemoglobin synthesis.

Since reversible sideroblastic anaemias respond to removal or treatment of the underlying cause, pyridoxine administration is only indicated in the idiopathic forms, both hereditary and acquired. Although complete cures have not been reported, some increase in haemoglobin level may occur. The dose required is usually high, up to 400 mg daily.

Corticosteroids (see section 6.3) have an important place in the management of a wide variety of haematological disorders. They include conditions with an immune basis such as auto-immune haemolytic anaemia, immune thrombocytopenias and neutropenias, and major transfusion reactions. They are also used in chemotherapy schedules for all forms of lymphoreticular malignancy, lymphoid leukaemias, and paraproteinaemias, including myelomatosis. Corticosteroids are used in aplastic anaemias, where their usefulness is more debatable.

It is possible that corticosteroids may also reduce the capillary fragility which occurs in the purpuric diseases, thus lessening bleeding.

Severe tissue iron overload may occur in aplastic and other refractory anaemias, mainly as the result of repeated blood transfusions. It is a particular problem in refractory anaemias with hyperplastic bone marrow, especially thalassaemia major, where excessive iron absorption from the gut and inappropriate iron therapy add to the tissue siderosis. Venesection therapy is obviously contra-indicated, but the long-term administration of iron chelaters such as **desferrioxamine mesylate** (page 22) is useful; a suitable regimen would consist of desferrioxamine mesylate, 0.5–1 g by intramuscular injection daily, supplemented by 2 g by intravenous injection at the time of blood transfusion. Iron output may be increased by combining desferrioxamine administration with large doses of ascorbic acid.

OXYMETHOLONE

Indications: aplastic anaemia; see also section 6.4.3, and notes above

Cautions; Contra-indications; Side-effects: see section 6.4.3 and notes above.

Dose: aplastic anaemia, 100–350 mg daily in divided doses; CHILD 2–4 mg/kg daily in divided doses

Anapolon 50® (Syntex)
Tablets, scored, oxymetholone 50 mg. Price 20 tabs = **I**

STANOZOLOL

Indications; Cautions; Contra-indications; Side-effects: see under Oxymetholone

Dose: by intramuscular injection, 50 mg every 2–3 weeks

Stromba® (Sterling Research)
Injection, stanozolol 50 mg/ml. Price 1-ml amp = **E**

9.2 Electrolyte and water replacement

9.2.1 Oral administration
9.2.2 Intravenous administration
9.2.3 Tables of electrolyte concentrations

9.2.1 Oral administration

9.2.1.1 Potassium supplements
9.2.1.2 Sodium chloride
9.2.1.3 Oral electrolyte replacement in diarrhoea

Electrolyte preparations may be administered orally to prevent or correct electrolyte deficits in certain chronic conditions such as potassium losses incurred with oral diuretic therapy (section 9.2.1.1 below) or sodium depletion in the salt wasting of chronic renal failure. Slow-release preparations are better tolerated and less liable to cause nausea or upper gastro-intestinal mucosal erosions.

9.2.1.1 POTASSIUM SUPPLEMENTS

Probably very few patients taking diuretics need potassium supplements. Patients receiving small doses of thiazides to reduce blood pressure seldom need them. The need for potassium supplements can be minimised by using the smallest dose of diuretic that controls the oedema, by intermittent use of the diuretics, and by keeping the patient's salt intake as low as possible without making food unpalatable.

Patients on potassium-losing thiazide or loop diuretics may need potassium supplements or one of the potassium-sparing diuretics (see section 2.2.3) if they:

1. have a poor intake of potassium, likely in the elderly on a poor diet;
2. are being treated with digoxin or other cardiac glycosides;
3. are receiving drugs which increase potassium loss (some corticosteroids or carbenoxolone);
4. have a high output of aldosterone, as is likely in cirrhosis with ascites, nephrosis, or very severe congestive heart failure; or,
5. are receiving very high doses of thiazide or loop diuretics.

Serum-potassium concentrations should be checked at intervals in patients taking diuretics and if below 3.5 mmol/litre, potassium supplements are needed. Doses in the range 10–50 mmol/day are usually required.

If a patient does have a low serum-potassium concentration it may be difficult to correct by using potassium supplements, and the combined diuretic and potassium preparations will certainly not be adequate. It may be more effective to use a potassium-sparing diuretic, which also conserves magnesium and zinc.

POTASSIUM SALTS

Indications: potassium depletion (see notes above)

Cautions: intestinal stricture, hiatus hernia (for sustained-release preparations)

Contra-indications: renal failure, serum potassium concentrations above 5 mmol/litre

Side-effects: nausea and vomiting (severe symp-

toms may indicate obstruction), oesophageal or small bowel ulceration
Dose: usual range 10–50 mmol K^+ daily

Potassium Tablets, Effervescent, potassium bicarbonate 500 mg, potassium acid tartrate 300 mg, each tablet providing 6.5 mmol of K^+. To be dissolved in water before administration. Price 20 tabs = **B**

Kay-Cee-L® (Geistlich)
Syrup (=elixir), red, potassium chloride (sugar-free) 1 mmol/ml. Price 100 ml = **B**

K-Contin Continus® (Napp)
Tablets, s/r, orange, s/c, potassium chloride 600 mg (8 mmol each of K^+ and Cl^-). Price 20 tabs = **A**

Kloref® (Cox-Continental)
Tablets, effervescent, betaine hydrochloride, potassium benzoate, bicarbonate, and chloride, equivalent to potassium chloride 500 mg (6.7 mmol each of K^+ and Cl^-). Price 20 tabs = **B**

Kloref-S® (Cox-Continental)
Granules, effervescent, betaine hydrochloride, potassium bicarbonate and chloride equivalent to potassium chloride 1.5 g (20 mmol each of K^+ and Cl^-)/sachet. Price 20 sachets = **D**

Leo K® (Leo)
Tablets, s/r, f/c, potassium chloride 600 mg (8 mmol each of K^+ and Cl^-). Price 20 tabs = **A**

Nu-K® (Consolidated)
Capsules, s/r, blue, potassium chloride 600 mg (8 mmol each of K^+ and Cl^-). Price 20 caps = **B**

Sando-K® (Sandoz)
Tablets, effervescent, potassium bicarbonate and chloride equivalent to potassium 470 mg (12 mmol of K^+) and chloride 285 mg (8 mmol of Cl^-). Price 20 tabs = **B**

Slow-K® (Ciba)
Tablets, s/r, orange, s/c, potassium chloride 600 mg (8 mmol each of K^+ and Cl^-). Price 20 tabs = **A**

HYPERKALAEMIA

POLYSTYRENE SULPHONATE RESINS

Indications: hyperkalaemia assocated with anuria or severe oliguria, and in dialysis patients
Contra-indications: avoid calcium-containing resin in hyperparathyroidism, multiple myeloma, sarcoidosis, or metastatic carcinoma, and sodium-containing resin in congestive heart failure
Dose: by mouth, 15 g 3–4 times daily in water (not fruit juice which has a high K^+ content)
By rectum, as an enema, 30 g in methylcellulose solution, retained for 9 hours
CHILD, any route, 0.5–1 g/kg daily

Calcium Resonium® (Winthrop)
Powder, brown, calcium polystyrene sulphonate. Price 300 g = **J**

Resonium A® (Winthrop)
Powder, buff, sodium polystyrene sulphonate. Price 454 g = **J**

9.2.1.2 SODIUM CHLORIDE

SODIUM CHLORIDE

Indications: electrolyte imbalance, also sections 9.2.1.3 and 9.2.2 below

Sodium Chloride Solution (Normal Saline), sodium chloride 0.9% (9 mg/ml) in purified water, freshly boiled and cooled. Price 100 ml = **A**
Note: this preparation must *not* be confused with 'normal sodium chloride solution' which is used as a chemical reagent and contains 5.85% of sodium chloride

Sodium Chloride Solution-tablets, sodium chloride 2.25 g, one solution-tablet dissolved in 250 ml of water for preparations provides a 0.9% solution. Price 20 tabs = **A**

Sodium Chloride Tablets, sodium chloride 300 mg. Price 20 tabs = **A**

Sodium Chloride Tablets, e/c, sodium chloride 450 mg. Price 20 tabs = **A**

Sodium Chloride and Dextrose Tablets, sodium chloride 450 mg, dextrose 200 mg. Price 20 tabs = **A**

Slow Sodium® (Ciba)
Tablets, s/r, sodium chloride 600 mg. Price 20 tabs = **A**

9.2.1.3 ORAL ELECTROLYTE REPLACEMENT IN DIARRHOEA

For severe diarrhoea the most important measures are to prevent or treat depletion of fluid and salts. This is particularly so for infants and frail or elderly patients who may become dangerously ill through dehydration alone in the course of a day.

A suitable preparation for replacement of lost fluid and salts in children is **Sodium Chloride and Dextrose Oral Powder, Compound**, available in containers for the preparation of 500 ml of solution (see Formulary). Sachets of **Sodium Chloride and Dextrose Oral Powder, Compound, Small Size**, contain the ingredients for preparing 200 ml of solution, that is, sufficient to fill the usual size feeding bottle. In either case the powder is dissolved in freshly boiled and cooled water and any unused solution should be discarded no later than 24 hours after preparation.

Electrosol® tablets are used for preparing a closely similar solution, but without the dextrose.

Sodium Chloride and Dextrose Oral Powder, Compound, Na^+ 35 mmol, K^+ 20 mmol, Cl^- 37 mmol, HCO_3^- 18 mmol, and dextrose 200 mmol/litre when reconstituted (see notes above and Formulary). Price 1 powder (22 g) = **A**

Sodium Chloride and Dextrose Oral Powder, Compound, Small Size, ingredients as above. Price 20 × 8.8-g powders = **B**

Dextrolyte® (Cow & Gate)

Oral solution, dextrose monohydrate, potassium chloride, sodium chloride, sodium lactate, providing Na^+ 35 mmol, K^+ 13.4 mmol, Cl^- 30.5 mmol, and dextrose 200 mmol/litre. Price 100 ml = **B** (Hosp. only)

Dioralyte® (Armour)

Oral Powder, sodium chloride and dextrose powder, compound, small size, 8.8-g sachets. Price 20 sachets = **E**

Electrosol® (Macarthys)

Tablets, effervescent, sodium chloride 200 mg, potassium chloride 160 mg, sodium bicarbonate 200 mg. 8 tablets dissolved in 1 litre of water provide a solution containing Na^+ 46.5 mmol, K^+ 17 mmol, Cl^- 44.5 mmol, and HCO_3^- 19 mmol. Price 20 tabs = **A**

9.2.2 Intravenous administration

Solutions are administered intravenously to meet normal fluid and electrolyte requirements or to replenish substantial deficits or continuing losses when the gastro-intestinal tract is incapable of handling the volumes of fluid required and the large electrolyte load.

All solutions are best infused slowly unless there is acute severe fluid or electrolyte depletion, or in certain situations of drug overdosage in which forced diuresis is advisable. Careful maintenance of the fluid volume is necessary in elderly patients, in those with impaired renal function, and in patients with established or incipient cardiac failure.

Total electrolyte care should take into account past and present losses, clinical assessment of fluid and electrolyte status, and biochemical measurements of blood or urine. It should be appreciated that, as well as sodium and potassium, other ions may also be required.

Isotonic solutions may be injected safely into peripheral veins. Strong dextrose solutions (containing 20% w/v or more of dextrose) may be used as an energy source for nutritional support, but must be given through a catheter inserted into a large central vein because they would otherwise cause thrombophlebitis.

Dextrose solutions may be used to provide water in a form iso-osmotic with plasma when there is no significant depletion of electrolytes. Dextrose intravenous infusion (5% w/v) is used to replenish major fluid losses or meet the daily water requirement of 1½–2½ litres. The energy content is so low that it makes only a minimal contribution to the body's requirements.

Sodium chloride and dextrose intravenous infusion provides water and some sodium ions particularly when the need for water replacement is greater than that for sodium, as in some cases of dehydration (particularly from vomiting), hyperosmotic diabetic coma, or other examples of water loss leading to excessive concentration of electrolyte.

Sodium chloride intravenous infusion provides water and sodium ions in physiologically comparable amounts when fluid losses are accompanied by sodium depletion of a similar order, for example in diabetic ketosis, severe diarrhoea, or losses from pancreatic or small bowel fistulae.

Potassium chloride and sodium chloride intravenous infusion and **potassium chloride and dextrose** intravenous infusion are used for potassium replacement. The second preparation is useful when potassium is required alone, the first when both potassium and sodium ions are to be provided.

Potassium ions should be infused at a rate not exceeding 20 mmol/hour and constant monitoring of plasma concentrations is necessary to prevent rises above the normal range, particularly in impaired renal function.

Sodium bicarbonate injection is used for correcting metabolic acidosis, a strong preparation being administered by slow intravenous injection and a weaker preparation by continuous infusion for forced alkaline diuresis, after cardiac arrest etc. The severity of acidosis must be assessed by measurement of pH, $P\text{CO}_2$, and plasma bicarbonate. Over-correction of bicarbonate losses is ill advised, and it is safer to restore a low pH to 7.2 initially and only cautiously raise it further, particularly in diabetic ketosis. It may be necessary to administer potassium ions concurrently, and monitoring of blood gases and concentrations of electrolytes is essential throughout.

Sodium lactate intravenous infusion is obsolete in metabolic acidosis, and carries the risk of producing lactic acidosis, particularly in seriously ill patients with poor tissue perfusion or impaired hepatic function.

DEXTROSE

Indications: fluid replacement, provision of energy

Side-effects: dextrose injections especially if hypertonic may have a low pH and irritate the venous intima so causing thrombophlebitis

Dose: by intravenous injection, a suitable volume of a preparation appropriate to the circumstances (see notes above)

Dextrose Intravenous Infusion, dextrose, usual strength 5% (50 mg/ml), but at other strengths up to 50%. 20% solution, price 20-ml amp = **C**; 25% solution, price 25-ml amp = **C**; 50% solution, price 20-ml amp = **C**; 25-ml amp = **C**; 50-ml amp = **D**

Other packs: see *note* following entry on sodium chloride and dextrose intravenous infusion

POTASSIUM CHLORIDE

Indications: electrolyte imbalance; also potassium supplements section 9.2.1.1

Cautions: for intravenous infusion, the concentration of solution should not exceed 3.2 g (43 mmol)/litre
Side-effects: rapid injection may be toxic to heart
Dose: by slow intravenous infusion, up to 6 g (80 mmol) daily

Potassium Chloride and Dextrose Intravenous Infusion, usual strength potassium chloride 0.3% (3 g, 40 mmol each of K^+ and Cl^-/litre) with 5% of anhydrous dextrose
Other packs: see *note* following entry on sodium chloride and dextrose intravenous infusion
Potassium Chloride and Sodium Chloride Intravenous Infusion, usual strength potassium chloride 0.3% (3 g/litre) and sodium chloride 0.9% (9 g/litre), containing 40 mmol of K^+, 150 mmol of Na^+, and 190 mmol of Cl^-/litre
Other packs: see *note* following entry on sodium chloride and dextrose intravenous infusion
Potassium Chloride, Sodium Chloride, and Dextrose Intravenous Infusion, sodium chloride 0.18% (1.8 g, 30 mmol of Na^+/litre) with 4% of anhydrous dextrose and usually sufficient potassium chloride to provide 10–40 mmol of K^+/litre (to be specified by the prescriber)
Other packs: see *note* following entry on sodium chloride and dextrose intravenous infusion
Potassium Chloride Solution, Strong (sterile), potassium chloride 15% (150 mg, approximately 2 mmol each of K^+ and Cl^-/ml). Must be diluted with not less than 50 times its volume of sodium chloride intravenous infusion or other suitable diluent. Price 10-ml amp = **B**
Solutions containing 10 and 20% of potassium chloride are also available in both 5- and 10-ml ampoules. Price per amp (all) = **B**

SODIUM BICARBONATE

Indications: metabolic acidosis.
Dose: by slow intravenous injection, a strong solution (up to 8.4%), or *by continuous intravenous infusion*, a weak solution (usually 1.4%), an amount appropriate to the body base deficit (see notes above)

Sodium Bicarbonate Intravenous Infusion, usual strength sodium bicarbonate 1.4% (14 g, 167 mmol each of Na^+ and HCO_3^-/litre).
5% solution available in 20- and 50-ml ampoules. Price 20-ml amp = **C**; 5-ml amp = **D**
Other packs: see *note* following entry on sodium chloride and dextrose intravenous infusion

SODIUM CHLORIDE

Indications: electrolyte imbalance, also sections 9.2.1.2 and 9.2.1.3
Cautions: restrict intake in impaired renal function, cardiac failure, hypertension, peripheral and pulmonary oedema, toxaemia of pregnancy
Side-effects: administration of large doses may give rise to salt accumulation and oedema

Potassium Chloride and Sodium Chloride Intravenous Infusion, and **Potassium Chloride, Sodium Chloride, and Dextrose Intravenous Infusion:** see above under Potassium Chloride
Ringer's Solution for Injection, calcium chloride (dihydrate) 322 micrograms, potassium chloride 300 micrograms, sodium chloride 8.6 mg/ml, providing the following ions (in mmol/litre), Ca^{++} 2.2, K^+ 4, Na^+ 147, Cl^- 156
Availability of other packs: see below following entry on sodium chloride and dextrose intravenous infusion
Sodium Chloride Intravenous Infusion, usual strength sodium chloride 0.9% (9 g, 150 mmol each of Na^+ and Cl^-/litre), this strength being supplied when normal saline for injection is requested. Price 2-ml amp = **A**; 5- and 10-ml amp (both) = **B**; 20-ml amp = **C**; 50-ml amp = **D**
Availability of other packs: see below
Sodium Chloride and Dextrose Intravenous Infusion, usual strength sodium chloride 0.18% (1.8 g, 30 mmol each of Na^+ and Cl^-/litre) and 4% of anhydrous dextrose
Other packs: see below
AVAILABILITY OF INFUSION SOLUTIONS. In the hospital service, water for injections, many solutions of dextrose, and electrolyte solutions for intravenous infusion are available in 500-ml and 1000-ml packs, and sometimes other sizes. For availability and price enquire locally.

SODIUM LACTATE

Indications: diabetic coma, diminished alkali reserve (but see notes above)

Sodium Lactate Intravenous Infusion, sodium lactate M/6, contains the following ions (in mmol/litre), Na^+167, HCO_3^- (as lactate) 167
Sodium Lactate Intravenous Infusion, Compound, (Hartmann's solution for injection), contains the following ions (in mmol/litre), Na^+ 131, K^+5, Ca^{++}2, HCO_3^- (as lactate) 29, Cl^- 111
Dose: 1000 ml or according to patient's needs
Other packs: see *note* following entry on sodium chloride and dextrose intravenous infusion

Water for Injections. Price 1-, 2-, and 5-ml amp (all) = **A**; 20-ml amp = **B**; 50-ml amp = **C**

DEXTRAN INTRAVENOUS INFUSIONS. Dextrans are polymers of glucose which are only slowly metabolised and are used to expand vascular volume in certain cases of shock such as burns, trauma, or Gram-negative septicaemia. They should **not** be used to replenish fluid loss from haemorrhage or dehydration for which blood, plasma protein, or electrolyte solutions should be used as appropriate.

Dextrans may interfere with blood group cross-matching or biochemical measurements, which should therefore be carried out **before** commencing infusion. **Dextran 70** intravenous infusion is used predominantly for volume expansion. **Dextran 40** intravenous infusion is used to improve peripheral blood flow in ischaemic disease of the limbs, peripheral thrombo-embolism, or occasionally fat embolism.

Gelatin and related injections are also sometimes used for temporary volume expansion.

DEXTRAN 40 INTRAVENOUS INFUSION, dextran '40' 10% in dextrose intravenous infusion (5%) or in sodium chloride intravenous infusion (0.9%)

Indications: conditions associated with peripheral local slowing of the blood flow; prophylaxis of post-surgical thromboembolic disease

Cautions: patients with congestive heart failure, renal impairment, polycythaemia; after blood and electrolyte replacement, rate of infusion to previously dehydrated patients not to exceed 500 ml/hour

Contra-indications: patients with thrombocytopenia, severe congestive heart failure, and renal failure

Side-effects: rarely anaphylactoid reactions, especially in patients with history of asthma

Dose: by intravenous infusion, initially 500–1000 ml, the first 500 ml being injected over a period of 30 minutes, followed by 1000–2000 ml daily by continuous infusion for 2 days, then 500–1000 ml daily for a further 3 days

Lomodex 40® (Fisons)
Intravenous infusion, dextran 40 intravenous infusion in dextrose intravenous infusion (5%) or in sodium chloride intravenous infusion (0.9%). Price 500-ml bottle (both) = **G**

Rheomacrodex® (Pharmacia)
Intravenous infusion, dextran 40 intravenous infusion in dextrose intravenous infusion (5%) or in sodium chloride intravenous infusion (0.9%). Price 500-ml bottle (both) = **F**

DEXTRAN 70 INTRAVENOUS INFUSION, dextran '70' 6% in dextrose intravenous infusion (5%) or in sodium chloride intravenous infusion (0.9%)

Indications: reduction in blood volume due to haemorrhage, shock etc; prophylaxis of post-surgical thromboembolic disease

Cautions; Contra-indications; Side-effects: see under Dextran 40 Intravenous Infusion

Dose: by intravenous infusion, after moderate to severe haemorrhage, 500–1000 ml rapidly initially followed by 500 ml later if necessary; in the treatment of severe burns, up to 3000 ml in the first few days with electrolytes

Lomodex 70® (Fisons)
Intravenous infusion, dextran 70 intravenous infusion in dextrose intravenous infusion (5%) or in sodium chloride intravenous infusion (0.9%). Price 500-ml bottle (both) = **E**

Macrodex® (Pharmacia)
Intravenous infusion, dextran 70 intravenous infusion in dextrose intravenous infusion (5%) or in sodium chloride intravenous infusion (0.9%). Price 500-ml bottle (both) = **E**

DEXTRAN 110 INTRAVENOUS INFUSION, dextran '110' 6% in dextrose intravenous infusion (5%) or in sodium chloride intravenous infusion (0.9%)

Indications: see under Dextran 70 Intravenous Infusion

Cautions: see under Dextran 40 Intravenous Infusion; blood samples for cross-matching to be taken before infusion

Contra-indications: haemorrhage associated with hypofibrinogenaemia

Side-effects: see under Dextran 40 Intravenous Infusion

Dose: by intravenous infusion, see under Dextran 70 Intravenous Infusion

Dextraven 110® (Fisons)
Intravenous infusion, dextran 110 intravenous infusion in dextrose intravenous infusion (5%) or in sodium chloride intravenous infusion. Price 500-ml bottle (both) = **E**

DEXTRAN 150 INTRAVENOUS INFUSION, dextran '150' 6% in dextrose intravenous infusion (5%) or in sodium choride intravenous infusion (0.9%)

Indications: reduction in blood volume due to haemorrhage, shock etc.

Cautions; Contra-indications: see under Dextran 110 Intravenous Infusion

Side-effects: see under Dextran 40 Intravenous Infusion

Dose: see under Dextran 70 Intravenous Infusion

Dextraven 150® (Fisons)
Intravenous infusion, dextran '150' 6% in dextrose intravenous infusion (5%) or in sodium chloride intravenous infusion. Price 500-ml bottle (both) = **E**

GELATIN

Indications: low blood volume

Dose: by intravenous infusion, 500–1000 ml of a 3.5–4% solution

Note: for this purpose the gelatin is partially degraded to give a product of molecular weight approximately 30 000; one form of degraded gelatin is called **polygeline**

Gelofusine® (Consolidated)
Injection, gelatin 4%, sodium chloride 0.9%. Price 500-ml bottle = **E**

Haemaccel® (Hoechst)
Injection, polygeline 35 g, Na^{+} 145 mmol, K^{+} 5.1 mmol, Ca^{++} 6.26 mmol, Cl^{-} 145 mmol/litre. Price 500-ml bottle = **F**

9.2.3 Tables of electrolyte concentrations

The concentrations of electrolytes in intravenous infusion fluids is generally given in millimoles (mmol)/litre. A millimole is the molecular weight of the ion in milligrams.

Table: Millimoles of each ion in 1 gram of salt

Electrolyte	mmol per g approx.
Ammonium chloride	18.7
Calcium chloride ($CaCl_2,2H_2O$)	Ca 6.8 Cl 13.6
Potassium bicarbonate	10
Potassium chloride	13.4
Sodium bicarbonate	11.9
Sodium chloride	17.1
Sodium lactate	8.9

Table: Electrolyte concentrations of intravenous fluids

Intravenous infusion	Millimoles per litre				
	Na^+	K^+	HCO_3^- equiv.	Cl^-	Ca^{++}
Normal Plasma Values	142	4.5	26	103	2.5
Citrated Plasma	150	12	—	55	—
Sodium Chloride 0.9%	150	—	—	150	—
Compound Sodium Lactate (Hartmann's)	131	5	29	111	2
Sodium Chloride 0.18% and Dextrose 4%	30	—	—	30	—
Potassium Chloride and Dextrose	—	40	—	40	—
Potassium Chloride and Sodium Chloride*	150	40	—	190	—
To correct metabolic acidosis					
Sodium Bicarbonate 1.4%	167	—	167	—	—
Sodium Bicarbonate 8.4% for cardiac arrest	1000	—	1000	—	—
Sodium Lactate (M/6)	167	—	167	—	—
To correct metabolic alkalosis					
Ammonium Chloride (M/6)	—	—	—	167	—

* Containing potassium chloride 0.3% and sodium chloride 0.9%.

Faeces, vomit, or aspiration should be saved and analysed where possible if abnormal losses are suspected; where this is impracticable the following approximations may be helpful in planning replacement therapy.

Table: Electrolyte content of gastro-intestinal secretions

Type of fluid	Millimoles per litre				
	H^+	Na^+	K^+	HCO_3^-	Cl^-
Gastric	40–60	20–80	5–20	—	100–150
Biliary	—	120–140	5–15	30–50	80–120
Pancreatic	—	120–140	5–15	70–110	40–80
Small bowel	—	120–140	5–15	20–40	90–130

9.3 Foods for special diets

These preparations are foods that have been modified in order to eliminate a particular constituent, or reduce its concentration, or are nutrient mixtures formulated as substitutes for foods which contain the unwanted ingredient. They are for patients who, because of genetically determined syndromes, either cannot tolerate or cannot metabolise certain common constituents of food. An example is the coeliac patient who cannot tolerate gluten which is present in products containing barley, oats, rye, and wheat. Such patients may be unable to tolerate even small amounts of gluten. In other cases, for example patients with phenylketonuria who cannot metabolise phenylalanine, a small amount of the material concerned, sufficient for tissue building and repair, must be incorporated in the formulation.

The reference 'ACBS' means that prescriptions issued in accordance with the advice of the Advisory Committee on Borderline Substances and endorsed 'ACBS' will not normally be investigated.

Corn oil (maize oil). Price 100 ml = **B**. ACBS: see Appendix 3

Fructose (laevulose). Price 500 g = **C**. ACBS: see Appendix 3

Glucose (dextrose monohydrate). Price 100 g = **A**. ACBS: see Appendix 3

Sunflower oil. Price 100 ml = **B**. ACBS: see Appendix 3

Aglutella Azeta® (GF Supplies)
Wafers, cream-filled, gluten-free, low potassium, low protein, low sodium. Price 168 g = **E**. ACBS: see Appendix 3

Aglutella Gentili® (GF Supplies)
Pasta, protein not more than 500 mg, carbohydrate 88.8 g, fat 500 mg/100 g, low Na^+ and K^+, gluten-free; macaroni, semolina, spaghetti, spaghetti rings. Price 250 g = **D**. ACBS: see Appendix 3

Albumaid® (Scientific Hospital Supplies)
Complete, powder, amino acids 89.4%, with vitamins, minerals, trace elements, free from carbohydrate and fat. Price 1 kg = **J**. ACBS: see Appendix 3
Methionine Low, powder, amino acids 40% with not more than 0.04% of methionine, carbohydrate 50%, with vitamins, minerals, and trace elements. Price 1 kg = **J**. ACBS: see Appendix 3

XP, powder, amino acids 40%, carbohydrate 50%, fat nil, phenylalanine not more than 10 mg per 100 g, with vitamins and minerals. Price 1 kg = **J**. ACBS: see Appendix 3

XP Concentrate, powder, amino acids 86%, carbohydrate and fat nil, phenylalanine not more than 25 mg per 100 g, with vitamins and minerals. Price 1 kg = **J**. ACBS: see Appendix 3

Alembicol D® (Alembic Products)

Fractionated coconut oil. Price 1 kg = **G**. ACBS: see Appendix 3

Aminogran® (A&H)

Food Supplement, powder, containing all essential amino acids except phenylalanine, for use with mineral mixture (see below). Price 500 g = **J**. ACBS: see Appendix 3

Mineral Mixture, powder, containing all appropriate minerals for use with the above food supplement and other synthetic diets. Price 250 g = **H**. ACBS: see Appendix 3

Aminutrin® (Geistlich)

Powder, amino acids for preparation with liquids for use as a protein source in oral or gastric-tube feeding, providing the equivalent of 11.7 g of protein/15-g sachet. Price per sachet = **D**. ACBS: see Appendix 3

Aproten® (Farmitalia Carlo Erba)

Various products, gluten-free, low protein, low Na^+ and K^+. Prices: anellini 250 g = **D**; biscuits 200 g (36) = **D**; crispbread 240 g = **D**; ditalini 250 g = **D**; flour 500 g = **C**; rigatini 250 g = **D**; tagliatelle 250 g = **D**. ACBS: see Appendix 3

Bi-Aglut® (Farmitalia Carlo Erba)

Biscuits, starch, sugar, eggs, skimmed milk solids, flavourings, gluten-free. Price 210 g (36) = **D**. ACBS: see Appendix 3

Calonutrin® (Geistlich)

Powder, polysaccharides 57 g, disaccharides 25 g, monosaccharides 18 g/100 g. For use as an energy source where there is no requirement to restrict Na^+ and K^+ intake. Price 100 g = **B**. ACBS: see Appendix 3

Caloreen® (Roussel)

Powder, water-soluble dextrins, predominantly polysaccharides containing an average of 5 glucose molecules, with less than 1.8 mmol of Na^+ and 0.3 mmol of K^+/100 g. For hypoglycaemia requiring a high energy, low fluid intake, whether or not Na^+ or K^+ restriction is essential. Price 100 g = **B**; 250 g = **C**. ACBS: see Appendix 3

Cantabread—see under Trufree®

Carobel® (Cow & Gate)

Powder, carob seed flour. Price 135 g = **E**. ACBS: see Appendix 3

Casilan® (Farley)

Powder, whole protein, containing all essential amino acids, 90% with less than 0.01% Na^+. Price 225 g = **E**. ACBS: see Appendix 3

Clinifeed® (Roussel)

Liquid feeds (sterilised) in cans of 375 ml in 5 formulations:

Clinifeed 400, protein 15 g, carbohydrate 55 g, fat 13.4 g, energy 1674 kJ (400 kcal)/375 ml with vitamins and minerals, vanilla flavour. Fructose-free. Price 375-ml can = **C**. Also available in chocolate flavour. ACBS: see Appendix 3

Clinifeed 500, protein 30 g, carbohydrate 70 g, fat 11 g, energy 500 kcal (2092 kJ)/375 ml with vitamins and minerals, vanilla flavour. Fructose-free. Price 375-ml can = **C**. ACBS: see Appendix 3

Clinifeed Iso, protein 10.5 g, carbohydrate 49 g, fat 15.4 g, energy 375 kcal (1575 kJ)/375 ml with vitamins and minerals, vanilla flavour. Fructose- and sucrose-free, low sodium. Price 375-ml can = **C**. ACBS: see Appendix 3

Clinifeed LLS, protein 22.5 g, carbohydrate 70 g, fat 15 g, energy 500 kcal (2092 kJ)/375 ml with vitamins and minerals, chicken flavour. Fructose- and lactose-free, low sodium. Price 375-ml can = **D**. ACBS: see Appendix 3

Comminuted Chicken Meat (Cow & Gate)

Suspension (aqueous). Price 110 g = **B**. ACBS: see Appendix 3

Cymogran® (A&H)

Powder, dried food low in phenylalanine (not more than 0.01%) containing the equivalent of 30% protein, carbohydrate 42.65%, fat 9%. Price 1 kg = **J**. ACBS: see Appendix 3

dp® (GF Supplies)

Biscuits, low-protein, chocolate-flavoured chip cookies. Price 170 g = **E**. ACBS: see Appendix 3

Edosol® (Cow & Gate)

Powder, protein 27.8%, carbohydrate 37.8%, fat 28.1%, mineral salts 4.5%, with not more than 0.03% of Na^+. For use as a 12.5% solution with additional vitamins to replace milk. Price 397 g = **F**. ACBS: see Appendix 3

Ensure® (Abbott)

Liquid, protein 14.5%, fat 32.5%, carbohydrate 53%, with minerals and vitamins, lactose-free. Price 235-ml bottle or can = **C**. ACBS: see Appendix 3

Flexical® (Mead Johnson)

Powder, corn syrup solids, hydrolysed casein, soya oil, modified tapioca starch, medium chain triglycerides, vitamins, and minerals, providing protein 9.9%, carbohydrate 66.9%, fat 15%. Gluten- and lactose-free. Price 454 g = **I**. ACBS: see Appendix 3

Forceval Protein® (Unigreg)

Powder, calcium caseinate 60%, carbohydrate 30%, with vitamins and minerals, providing not less than 55% protein, not more than 1% of fat, not more than 0.12% of Na^+. Price 300 g = **E**; 15 g-sachet = **A**. ACBS: see Appendix 3

Formula S® (Cow & Gate)

Powder, soya protein isolate, glucose syrup, vegetable oil, vitamins and minerals, providing carbohydrate 6.75%, fat 3%, and protein 2% when used as a 12.5% solution. Price 450 g = **D**. ACBS: see Appendix 3

Galactomin® (Cow & Gate)

Formula 17, powder, protein and fat 22.3 g each, carbohydrate 50.2 g, mineral salts 3 g/100 g. Used as a 12.5% solution with additional vitamins in place of milk. Price 454 g = **G**. ACBS: see Appendix 3

Formula 18, powder, modification of Formula 17 with reduced fat ('half-cream'—14.4%). Price 454 g = **G**. ACBS: see Appendix 3

Formula 19, powder, modification of Formula 17 with reduced fat (14.4%) and fructose as carbohydrate source. Price 454 g = **I**. ACBS: see Appendix 3

Glutenex® (Cow & Gate)

Biscuits, free from milk products, gluten-free. Price 18 × 14 g = **C**. ACBS: see Appendix 3

Gluten-free biscuits (Farley)

Biscuits. Price 200 g = **C**. ACBS: see Appendix 3

Gluten-free crackers (GF Supplies)

Biscuits. Price 100 g = **C**. ACBS: see Appendix 3

HF(2)® (Cow & Gate)

Powder, prepared from amino acids, liquid glucose, vegetable fat, and wheat starch, equivalent protein as amino acids histidine-free 25 g, carbohydrate 39.9 g, fat 26 g/100 g with vitamins and minerals. Used as a 12.5% solution. Price 454 g = **J**. ACBS: see Appendix 3

Hycal® (Beecham Foods)

Liquid, glucose syrup, protein-free, low-electrolyte, carbohydrate 49.5%. Flavours, blackcurrant, lemon, orange, raspberry. Price 171 ml (6 fl. oz.) = **B**. ACBS: see Appendix 3

Isocal® (Mead Johnson)

Liquid, maltodextrin, soya oil, caseinate solids, medium

chain triglycerides, soya protein isolate, vitamins, and minerals, providing protein 3.4%, carbohydrate 13.3%, fat 4.4%. Gluten- and lactose-free. Price 355 ml = **C**. ACBS: see Appendix 3

Juvela® (GF Supplies)

Juvela Gluten-free, bread/cake mix. Price 500 g = **E**. ACBS: see Appendix 3

Juvela Low Protein, bread/cake mix. Price 500 g = **E**. ACBS: see Appendix 3

Liquigen® (Scientific Hospital Supplies)

Emulsion, medium chain triglycerides 52%. Price 2 litres = **J**. ACBS: see Appendix 3

Locasol® (Cow & Gate)

Powder, protein 21.4 g, carbohydrate 51.6 g, fat 23.3 g, mineral salts 1.8 g, not more than 48 mg of Ca^{2+}/100 g. Used as a 12.5% solution with vitamin supplements in place of milk. Price 397 g = **G**. ACBS: see Appendix 3

Lofenalac® (Mead Johnson)

Powder, corn syrup solids, casein hydrolysate, corn oil, modified tapioca starch, vitamins, and minerals, protein 15%, carbohydrate 59.6%, fat 18%, phenylalanine not more than 0.1%. Gluten- and lactose-free. Price 2½ lb = **J**. ACBS: see Appendix 3

Maxijul® (Scientific Hospital Supplies)

Powder, polyglucose polymer, potassium 0.004%, sodium 0.046%. Gluten-, lactose-, and fructose-free. Price 100 g = **B**. Also available with lower concentrations of potassium and sodium as **Maxijul LE**. Price 100 g = **B**. ACBS: see Appendix 3

MCT Oil® (Mead Johnson)

Triglycerides from medium chain fatty acids. Price 950 ml = **H**. ACBS: see Appendix 3

MCT (1)® (Cow & Gate)

Powder, protein 25.6%, carbohydrate 40.6%, medium chain triglycerides 28%. Low in lactose and sucrose-free. Price 454 g = **F**. ACBS: see Appendix 3

Medium Chain Triglyceride (MCT) Oil® (Cow & Gate)

Triglycerides from medium chain fatty acids. Price 1000 ml = **H**. ACBS: see Appendix 3

Metabolic Mineral Mixture® (Scientific Hospital Supplies)

Powder, essential mineral salts. Price 250 g = **G**. ACBS: see Appendix 3

Minafen® (Cow & Gate)

Powder, equivalent of 12.5% protein, carbohydrate 48%, fat 31%, not more than 0.02% of phenylalanine. For use as 12.5% solution with additional vitamins. Price 454 g = **H**. ACBS: see Appendix 3

MSUD Aid® (Scientific Hospital Supplies)

Powder, containing full range of amino acids except isoleucine, leucine, and valine. Price 200 g = **J**. ACBS: see Appendix 3

Nestargel® (Nestlé)

Powder, carob seed flour 96.5%, calcium lactate 3.5%. Price 50 g = **D**. ACBS: see Appendix 3

Nutramigen® (Mead Johnson)

Powder, casein hydrolysate, corn oil, modified tapioca starch, sucrose, vitamins, and minerals, providing protein 15%, carbohydrate 59.6%, fat 18%. Gluten- and lactose-free. Price 454 g = **G**. ACBS: see Appendix 3

PK Aid 1® (Scientific Hospital Supplies)

Powder, containing essential amino acids except phenylalanine. Price 1 kg = **J**. ACBS: see Appendix 3

Portagen® (Mead Johnson)

Powder, corn syrup solids, medium chain triglycerides, sodium caseinate, sucrose, corn oil, vitamins, and minerals, providing protein 16.5%, carbohydrate 54.3%, fat 22.5%. Glucose- and lactose-free. Price 454 g = **G**. ACBS: see Appendix 3

Pregestimil® (Mead Johnson)

Powder, glucose syrup solids, casein hydrolysate, corn oil, modified tapioca starch, medium chain triglycerides, vitamins, and minerals, providing protein 12.8%, carbohydrate 61.6%, fat 18.3%. Gluten- and lactose-free. Price 454 g = **H**. ACBS: see Appendix 3

Prosobee® (Mead Johnson)

Liquid concentrate, prepared from soya protein isolate, soya oil, corn syrup solids, coconut oil, L-methionine, vitamins, and minerals, providing protein 4.1%, carbohydrate 13.8%, fat 7.2%. Gluten- and lactose-free. Price 385 ml = **D**

Powder, glucose syrup solids, soya protein isolate, corn oil, coconut oil, L-methionine, vitamins, and minerals, providing protein 15.6%, carbohydrate 51.4%, fat 27.9%. Gluten- and lactose-free. Price 394 g = **F**. ACBS: see Appendix 3

Prosparol® (DF)

Emulsion, arachis oil 50% in water. Price 500-ml = **E**. ACBS: see Appendix 3

Rite-Diet® (Welfare Foods)

Gluten-free. Sweet biscuits (without chocolate or sultanas). Price 150 g = **B**. Savoury biscuits. Price 125 g = **B**. Filled wafers. Price 150 g = **C**. Pasta (macaroni). Price 250 g = **B**. Bread (also low protein, with and without salt and with or without soya bran). Price 227 g = **C**. Bread mix. Price 500 g = **C**. Flour. Price 500 g = **C**. ACBS: see Appendix 3

Low protein. Sweet biscuits. Price 150 g = **B**. Filled wafers. Price 150 g = **C**. Pasta (macaroni). Price 250 g = **B**. Bread—see above. Flour mix (salt-free). Price 500 g = **C**. ACBS: see Appendix 3

Low sodium. Bread containing protein 8.5%, carbohydrate 53.8%, fat 5.5%, Na^+ 0.01%, K^+ 0.055%. Price 226 g = **C**. ACBS: see Appendix 3

Triosorbon® (BDH)

Powder, protein 19%, carbohydrate 56%, fat 19%, with vitamins and minerals. Gluten-free. Price 85-g sachet = **C**. ACBS: see Appendix 3

Tritamyl® (Procea)

Flour, self-raising (starch-based), gluten- and lactose-free. Price 2 kg = **D**. ACBS: see Appendix 3

Tritamyl PK® (Procea)

Flour, self-raising (starch-based), gluten-, lactose-, and protein-free. Price 2 kg = **D**. ACBS: see Appendix 3

Trufree® (Cantassium)

Bread mix, gluten-free, price 420 g = **D**; with rice bran, price 410 g = **D**. ACBS: see Appendix 3

Cantabread® bread mix, gluten- and grain-free. Price 280 g = **C**. ACBS: see Appendix 3

Flour, self-raising, gluten-free. Price 1 kg = **D**. ACBS: see Appendix 3

Velactin® (Wander)

Powder, protein 12%, methionine 0.3%, carbohydrate 62%, fat 19.5%, with added vitamins and minerals. Price 454 g = **E**. ACBS: see Appendix 3

Verkade® (GF Supplies)

Biscuits, gluten-free. Price 200 g (38) = **D**. ACBS: see Appendix 3

Vivonex® (Eaton)

Powder, amino acids 6.18 g, simple sugars 69 g, safflower oil 435 mg/80-g sachet, with added vitamins and minerals. For preparation with water before use. Price 80-g sachet = **D**; flavour sachets 60 × 2 g = **F**. **Vivonex HN**, powder, similar to Vivonex, amino acids 13.31 g, simple sugars 63.3 g, safflower oil 261 mg/80-g sachet. Price 80-g sachet = **D**. ACBS: see Appendix 3 (both)

Wysoy® (Wyeth)

Powder, soya protein isolate, sucrose, corn syrup solids, animal and vegetable oil, vitamins and minerals, providing carbohydrate 6.9%, fat 3.6%, and protein 2.1% when reconstituted. Price 500 g = **E**. ACBS: see Appendix 3

ASSOCIATED PRODUCTS

Ketovite® (P&B)

Tablets, yellow, ascorbic acid 16.6 mg, riboflavine 1 mg, thiamine hydrochloride 1 mg, pyridoxine hydrochloride 330 micrograms, nicotinamide 3.3 mg, calcium pantothenate 1.16 mg, alpha tocopheryl acetate 5 mg, inositol 50 mg, biotin 170 micrograms, folic acid 250 micrograms, acetomenaphthone 500 micrograms. Price 20 tabs = **B**

(Supplement) liquid, pink, vitamin A 2500 units, vitamin D 400 units, choline chloride 150 mg, cyanocobalamin 12.5 micrograms/5 ml. Price 100 ml = **C**

Dose: as a vitamin supplement with synthetic diets, 5 ml liquid daily and 1 tablet 3 times daily

Ruthmol® (Cantassium)

Salt substitute, potassium chloride 50%. Price 250 g = **D**

Selora® (Winthrop)

Salt substitute, potassium chloride 92.05%, potassium iodide 0.01%, hydrated calcium silicate 1%, glutamic acid 1.15%, potassium glutamate 5.79%. Price 227 g = **D**

9.4 Intravenous feeding

When feeding via the alimentary tract is not possible, nutrients may be given by intravenous infusion and complete nutrition achieved. This method is used in conditions such as extensive resection of the bowel, severe malabsorption as for example in Crohn's disease, prolonged ileus, major surgery, fistulas, multiple injuries, and severe burns.

Protein is given as mixtures of essential and non-essential synthetic L-amino acids, which have replaced the protein hydrolysate preparations formerly used. Ideally, all essential amino acids should be included with a wide variety of non-essential ones to provide sufficient nitrogen together with electrolytes (see also section 9.2.2). However, available solutions vary in composition. Most contain amino acids alone or with a partial energy source (see table) using combinations of glucose (dextrose), fructose (laevulose), sorbitol, and ethanol. Some are significantly deficient in electrolytes or particular amino acids.

Energy is provided in a ratio of 0.6–1.1 megajoules (150–250 kcals) per gram of protein nitrogen. The best energy source is **dextrose** (glucose). **Laevulose** (fructose), **sorbitol**, and **ethanol** are all less satisfactory although suitable for poorly nourished patients. Where more than 180 grams of carbohydrate as glucose is given per day, insulin may be necessary, particularly in traumatised or burned patients, or when sepsis is present. Dextrose in various strengths from 10–50% may be infused through a central venous catheter. Preparations are available with useful added ions and trace metals, for example Glucoplex®.

Fat emulsions may be used as an energy source with the advantages of a high energy to fluid volume ratio, neutral pH, and iso-osmolarity with plasma. They are however, less protein sparing than sugar solutions. In addition several days of adaptation are required to attain maximal utilisation.

Fat emulsions are contra-indicated in septic subjects and in hepatocellular jaundice. They may interfere with biochemical measurements such as those for blood gases and calcium. Daily blood checks are necessary to ensure adequate clearance from the blood stream.

Current opinion is that dextrose is a better energy source at less than one-fifth the cost. Fat is best reserved for use when high osmolar loads are unwise, to supply essential fatty acids. Dosage should be restricted to not more than 2 g/kg body-weight daily and should be such that it represents not more than 40% of the total energy given.

Fat is infused with amino acid solutions through a Y-connector in the giving set and not mixed prior to infusion. **Only compatible preparations such as Vitlipid® should be added to fat emulsions.** Reactions include occasional febrile episodes and rare anaphylactic responses. Available preparations are soya-bean oil emulsions (Intralipid®).

Total parenteral nutrition (TPN) requires the use of a solution containing amino acids, dextrose, insulin, electrolytes, trace metals, and vitamins. Fat is supplied as described above.

Before starting, the patient should be well oxygenated with a near normal circulating blood volume, renal function, and acid-base status. Appropriate biochemical tests should have been carried out beforehand and serious deficits corrected (section 9.2).

To minimise the possibility of infection, the principal fluids should be delivered via a central venous catheter. Only nutritional fluids should be given by this line. Nutritional and electrolyte status must be monitored continuously. Loading doses of vitamin B_{12} and folic acid are advised and other vitamins are given parenterally twice weekly. In prolonged feeding, weekly administration of fat emulsions by infusion will supply essential fatty acids.

OTHER SPECIAL FEEDING PREPARATIONS

Addamel® (KabiVitrum)

Injection, electrolytes and trace elements for addition to Vamin infusion solutions (see table), Ca^{2+} 5 mmol, Mg^{2+} 1.5 mmol, Cl^- 13.3 mmol/10 ml; traces of Fe^{3+}, Zn^{2+}, Mn^{2+}, Cu^{2+}, F^-, I^-. For adult use. Price 10-ml vial = **D**

Fosfor® (Consolidated)

Syrup (=elixir), phosphorylcolamine phosphate 5%. Price 100 ml = **B**

Injection, phosphorylcolamine phosphate sodium salt 25%. For use alone, or with dextrose intravenous infusion, or with other amino acids. Price 10-ml amp = **A**

Minamino® (Consolidated)

Syrup (=elixir), amino acids, copper sulphate, gastric mucosa extract, iron citrate, liver extract, manganese sulphate, spleen extract, vitamins B_1, B_2, B_6, B_{12}. Price 100 ml = **C**

Table: Proprietary Infusion Fluids for Parenteral Feeding

Preparation	Manufacturer	Nitrogen g/litre	Fat g/litre	Energy kJ/litre	Electrolytes mmol/litre					Other components/litre
					K^+	Mg^{2+}	Na^+	$Acet^-$	Cl^-	
Aminofusin L600 Price 1000 ml = **I**	BDH	7.6		2500	30	5	40	10	14	sorbitol 100 g, vitamins
Aminofusin L1000 Price 1000 ml = **I**	BDH	7.6		4200	30	5	40	10	14	ethanol 5.28%, sorbitol 100 g, vitamins
Aminofusin L Forte Price 500 ml = **I**	BDH	15.2		1700	30	5	40	10	27	vitamins
Aminoplex 5 Price 1000 ml = **I**	Geistlich	5.0		4200	28		35		43	ethanol 5%, sorbitol 125 g, malate 13.8 g
Aminoplex 12 Price 500 ml = **H**; 1000 ml = **J**	Geistlich	12.4		1400	30	2.5	35	5	67.2	
Aminoplex 14 Price 500 ml = **H**	Geistlich	13.4		1400	30		35		79	vitamins
Freamine II Price 500 ml = **H**	Boots	12.5		1400			10			$H_2PO_4^-$ 10
Glucoplex 1000 Price 500 ml = **E**; 1000 ml = **E**	Geistlich			4200	30	2.5	50		67	$H_2PO_4^-$ 18, Zn^{2+} 0.046, anhydrous dextrose 240 g
Glucoplex 1600 Price 500 ml = **E**; 1000 ml = **E**	Geistlich			6700	30	2.5	50		67	$H_2PO_4^-$ 18, Zn^{2+} 0.046, anhydrous dextrose 400 g
Intralipid 10% Price 100 ml = **F**; 500 ml = **H**	KabiVitrum		100	4600						glycerol 11 g
Intralipid 20% Price 100 ml = **G**; 500 ml = **I**	KabiVitrum		200	8400						glycerol 11 g
Laevuflex 20 Price 500 ml = **E**	Geistlich			3400						laevulose 200 g
Perifusin Price 1000 ml = **G**	BDH	5.0		550	30	5	40	10	9	malate 22.5

Plasma-Lyte 148 (water) Price 1000 ml = **D**	Travenol		84	5	1.5	140	27	98	gluconate 23
Plasma-Lyte 148 (dextrose) Price 1000 ml = **D**	Travenol		880	5	1.5	140	27	98	gluconate 23, dextrose
Plasma-Lyte M (dextrose) Price 1000 ml = **D**	Travenol		795	16	1.5	40	12	40	Ca^{2+} 2.5, lactate 12, dextrose
Pluritene Price 100 ml = **E**	Lipha	9.15	1900			15			sorbitol 40 g
Synthamin 9 Price 500 ml = **G**	Travenol	9.3	1000	60	5	73	100	70	$H_2PO_4^-$ 30
Synthamin 14 Price 500 ml = **H**	Travenol	14.3	1600	60	5	73	130	70	$H_2PO_4^-$ 30
Synthamin 14 without electrolytes Price 500 ml = **H**	Travenol	14.3	1600				68	34	
Synthamin 17 Price 500 ml = **H**	Travenol	16.9	1900	60	5	73	150	70	$H_2PO_4^-$ 30
Vamin fructose Price 500 ml = **H**	KabiVitrum	9.4	2700	20	1.5	50		55	Ca^{2+} 2.5, laevulose 100 g
Vamin glucose Price 100 ml = **F**; 500 ml = **H**; 1000 ml = **J**	KabiVitrum	9.4	2700	20	1.5	50		55	Ca^{2+} 2.5, anhydrous dextrose 100 g
Vamin N Price 500 ml = **H**	KabiVitrum	9.4	1000	20	1.5	50		55	Ca^{2+} 2.5

Note: 1000 kcal = 4.1868 MJ; 1 MJ (1000 kJ) = 238.8 kcal

Multibionta® (BDH)
Injection, ascorbic acid, dexpanthenol, nicotinamide, pyridoxine hydrochloride, riboflavine sodium phosphate, thiamine hydrochloride, tocopheryl acetate, vitamin A. Price 10-ml amp = **D**

Ped-El® (KabiVitrum)
Solution, sterile, Ca^{2+}, Cu^{2+}, Fe^{3+}, Mg^{2+}, Mn^{2+}, Zn^{2+}, Cl^-, F^-, I^-, P. for addition to Vamin amino acid solutions. For paediatric use. Price 20-ml vial = **D**

Proper-Myl® (Consolidated) *injection*, powder for reconstitution, freeze-dried yeast cells. Price per amp (with solvent) = **C**

Solivito® (KabiVitrum)
Injection, powder for reconstitution, biotin, cyanocobalamin, folic acid, glycine, nicotinamide, pyridoxine hydrochloride, riboflavine sodium phosphate, sodium ascorbate, sodium pantothenate, thiamine mononitrate. Dissolved in water for injections or dextrose intravenous infusion for adding to dextrose intravenous infusion. Price per vial = **D**

Vitlipid® (KabiVitrum)
Injection, adult, calciferol, phytomenadione, retinol palmitate. Emulsion for addition to Intralipid®. Price 10-ml vial = **D**
Injection, infant, ingredients as above. Price 10-ml vial = **D**

9.5 Calcium and phosphorus

9.5.1 Calcium
9.5.2 Phosphorus

9.5.1 Calcium

Supplements of **calcium** are seldom required and there is no good evidence that they are needed in osteoporosis. Calcium is of **no** value in the treatment of nail disorders or cramp. Calcium gluconate tablets may be of value in combination with high doses of vitamin D in the treatment of hypoparathyroidism (section 9.6.4).

In resuscitation after cardiac arrest, 10 ml of calcium gluconate injection may be given intravenously or by intracardiac injection. In tetany an initial injection of 10 ml is followed if necessary by continuous infusion.

CALCIUM SALTS

Indications: see notes (above); calcium deficiency
Side-effects: bradycardia, cardiac arrhythmias, and irritation after intravenous injection
Dose: *by mouth*, calcium gluconate or lactate 1–6 g (2.23–13.4 mmol of Ca) repeated as necessary
By intramuscular or slow intravenous injection, calcium gluconate 1–2 g (2.23–4.5 mmol of Ca)

Calcium Gluconate Tablets, calcium gluconate 600 mg. To be chewed before swallowing. Price 20 tabs = **B**

Calcium Gluconate Tablets, Effervescent, calcium gluconate 1 g. Price 20 tabs = **C**

Calcium Gluconate Injection, calcium gluconate 10%. Price 5- and 10-ml amp (both) = **B**

Calcium Lactate Tablets, calcium lactate 300 and 600 mg. Price 20 tabs = **A**

Calcium-Sandoz® (Sandoz)
Syrup (=elixir), calcium glubionate 3.27 g, calcium galactogluconate 2.17 g (325 mg of Ca^{++} or 8.1 mmol)/15 ml. Diluent syrup (without preservative), life of diluted elixir 14 days. Price 100 ml = **B**
Injection, calcium glubionate equivalent to 10% of calcium gluconate (93 mg of Ca^{++} or 2.32 mmol/10 ml). Price 10-ml amp = **B**

Sandocal® (Sandoz)
Tablets, effervescent, orange, calcium lactate gluconate 3.08 g, sodium bicarbonate, potassium bicarbonate, equivalent to Ca^{++} 400 mg (10 mmol), Na^+ 137 mg (6 mmol), K^+ 176 mg (4.5 mmol). Price 20 tabs = **D**

Ossopan® (Welbeck) *tablets*, hydroxyapatite 200 mg. Price 20 tabs = **C**. *Oral powder*, hydroxyapatite 820 mg/g. Price 50 g = **G**

HYPERCALCAEMIA

SODIUM CELLULOSE PHOSPHATE

Indications: hypercalcaemia, reduction of calcium absorption from food (in conjunction with low-calcium diet)
Contra-indications: congestive heart failure, renal impairment
Side-effects: diarrhoea
Dose: 5 g 3 times daily with meals; CHILD 10 g daily in 3 divided doses with meals

Calcisorb® (Riker)
Sachets, sodium cellulose phosphate 5 g. Price 10 sachets = **D**

TRISODIUM EDETATE

Indications: hypercalcaemia; removal of lime burns in the eye
Cautions: serum-calcium determinations required; caution in tuberculosis
Contra-indications: impaired renal function
Side-effects: nausea, diarrhoea, cramp; in overdosage renal damage
Dose: *by intravenous infusion* in sodium chloride intravenous infusion (0.9%) or dextrose intravenous infusion (5%), up to 70 mg/kg daily over 2–3 hours

Limclair® (Sinclair)
Injection, trisodium edetate 200 mg/ml. Price 5-ml amp = **D**
For topical use in the eye, dilute 1 ml to 50 ml with sterile purified water

9.5.2 Phosphorus

Oral treatment with sodium acid phosphate may be indicated in the control of hypercalcaemia, especially that due to metastatic carcinoma. The equivalent of 1 or 2 grams of elemental **phosphorus** is given daily (2–4 tablets of Phosphate-Sandoz®, see below) but it may cause diarrhoea and injudicious use can lead to impairment of renal function and soft tissue calcification. Certain forms of hypophosphataemic rickets may best be treated with oral phosphate combined with moderate doses of vitamin D.

Phosphate-Sandoz® (Sandoz)
Tablets, effervescent, anhydrous sodium acid phosphate 1.936 g, sodium bicarbonate, potassium bicarbonate, equivalent to phosphorus 500 mg, Na^+ 468.8 mg (20.4 mmol), K^+ 123 mg (3.1 mmol). Price 20 tabs = **C**

9.6 Vitamins

Vitamins are used for the prevention and treatment of specific deficiency states. Dietary deficiency of vitamins is rare in Britain except in people who exist for a long time on faddish or inadequate diets, but deficiency states may be seen in patients with gastro-intestinal or hepatic disease.

The use of vitamins to treat a large variety of conditions in which there is no evidence of vitamin deficiency is **not** justified. In the National Health Service, vitamins may be prescribed to prevent or treat vitamin deficiency but they are not regarded as medicines when prescribed as dietary supplements (see Appendix 3).

9.6.1 Vitamin A
9.6.2 Vitamin B group
9.6.3 Vitamin C
9.6.4 Vitamin D
9.6.5 Vitamin E
9.6.6 Vitamin K
9.6.7 Multivitamin preparations

9.6.1 Vitamin A

Deficiency of vitamin A (retinol) is rare in Britain even in disorders of fat absorption. If deficiency is diagnosed, treatment should be with one tablet of 50 000 units daily (Ro-A-Vit®). For prevention, 4000 units daily is adequate and is available in the combination preparation **vitamins A and D capsules** (4000 units of vitamin A per capsule) and in the multivitamin preparation **vitamins capsules** (2500 units of vitamin A per capsule, section 9.6.7).

Massive overdose can cause rough skin, dry hair, an enlarged liver, and a raised erythrocyte sedimentation rate and raised serum calcium and serum alkaline phosphatase concentrations.

Halibut-liver Oil Capsules, vitamin A 4000 units. Price 20 caps = **A**
Vitamins A and D Capsules, vitamin A 4000 units, vitamin D 400 units. Price 20 caps = **A**

Ro-A-Vit® (Roche)
Tablets, cream, s/c, vitamin A (retinol) 50 000 units (as acetate). Price 20 tabs = **B**
Injection (oily), vitamin A (retinol) 300 000 units (as palmitate)/ml. Price 1-ml amp = **C**
Dose: by deep intramuscular injection, 150 000–300 000 units monthly, frequency increased to weekly in acute deficiency states

9.6.2 Vitamin B group

Deficiency of the B vitamins, other than deficiency of vitamin B_{12} (section 9.1.2) is rare in Britain and is usually treated by preparations containing thiamine (B_1), riboflavine (B_2), and nicotinamide. Other members of the vitamin B complex such as aminobenzoic acid, biotin, choline, inositol, and pantothenic acid or panthenol may be included in vitamin B preparations but there is no evidence of their value. For folic acid preparations see sections 9.1.1.1 and 9.1.2.

Potassium aminobenzoate has been used in the treatment of various disorders associated with excessive fibrosis such as scleroderma but its therapeutic value is **doubtful**.

The addition of cyanocobalamin (B_{12}) to multiple-ingredient vitamin preparations for oral administration is futile.

Severe deficiency states and encephalopathy, associated with chronic alcoholism or debilitating disease, are best treated by intramuscular or intravenous administration of vitamins B and C injection (Pabrinex®, Parentrovite®). A pyridoxine (B_6) deficiency state may occur during isoniazid therapy.

Nicotinamide Tablets, nicotinamide 50 mg. Price 20 tabs = **A**
Nicotinic Acid Tablets, nicotinic acid, 25, 50, and 100 mg. Price 20 tabs (all) = **A**
Vitamins B and C Injection
Weak, for intramuscular use, ascorbic acid 500 mg, nicotinamide 160 mg, pyridoxine hydrochloride 50 mg, riboflavine 4 mg, thiamine hydrochloride 100 mg/4 ml. Price 4 ml (in 2 amps) = **B**
Strong, for intramuscular use, ascorbic acid 500 mg, nicotinamide 160 mg, pyridoxine hydrochloride 50 mg, riboflavine 4 mg, thiamine hydrochloride 250 mg/7 ml. Price 7 ml (in 2 amps) = **B**
Strong, for intravenous use, ascorbic acid 500 mg, anhydrous dextrose 1 g, nicotinamide 160 mg, pyridoxine hydrochloride 50 mg, riboflavine 4 mg, thiamine hydrochloride 250 mg/10 ml. Price 10 ml (in 2 amps) = **B**
Benerva® (Roche)
Tablets, thiamine hydrochloride 3, 10, 25 and 50 mg. Price 20 tabs (all) = **A**
Tablets, thiamine hydrochloride 100 mg. Price 20 tabs = **B**
Tablets, thiamine hydrochloride 300 mg. Price 20 tabs = **B**
Injection, thiamine hydrochloride 25 mg/ml. Price 1-ml amp = **A**

Injection, thiamine hydrochloride 100 mg/ml. Price 1-ml amp = **A**
Dose: by mouth or by intramuscular injection 10–100 mg daily; up to 600 mg daily in acute deficiency

Pabrinex® (P&B)
Intramuscular maintenance injection, vitamins B and C injection, weak, for intramuscular use. Price 4 ml (in 2 amps) = **B**
Intramuscular high potency injection, vitamins B and C injection, strong, for intramuscular use. Price 7 ml (in 2 amps) = **B**
Intravenous high potency injection, vitamins B and C injection, strong, for intravenous use. Price 10 ml (in 2 amps) = **B**

Parentrovite® (Bencard)
IMM Injection, vitamins B and C injection, weak, for intramuscular use. Price 4 ml (in 2 amps) = **B**
IMHP Injection, vitamins B and C injection, strong, for intramuscular use. Price 7 ml (in 2 amps) = **B**
IVHP Injection, vitamins B and C injection, strong, for intravenous use. Price 10 ml (in 2 amps) = **B**

Potaba® (Glenwood)
Capsules, red/white, potassium aminobenzoate 500 mg. Price 20 caps = **C**
Tablets, potassium aminobenzoate 500 mg. Price 20 tabs = **C**
Dose: Peyronie's disease, 12 g daily in divided doses after meals
Envules® (= powder in sachets), potassium aminobenzoate 3 g. Price 20 sachets = **F**

PYRIDOXINE HYDROCHLORIDE

(Vitamin B_6)
Indications: isoniazid-induced peripheral neuritis, idiopathic sideroblastic anaemia, deficiency states
Cautions: drug interactions: see Appendix 1
Dose: neuritis and deficiency states, 20–50 mg up to 3 times daily
Idiopathic sideroblastic anaemia, 100–400 mg daily in divided doses

Pyridoxine Tablets, pyridoxine hydrochloride 10, 20, and 50 mg. Price 20 tabs (all) = **B**

Benadon® (Roche)
Tablets, pyridoxine hydrochloride 20 mg. Price 20 tabs = **A**
Tablets, scored, pyridoxine hydrochloride 50 mg. Price 20 tabs = **B**

Complement Continus® (Napp)
Tablets, s/r, yellow, pyridoxine hydrochloride 100 mg. Price 28 tabs = **C**

VITAMIN B COMPLEX PREPARATIONS

These are preparations consisting mainly of various combinations of the B vitamins and vitamin C some of which also have other ingredients, all usually of minor importance. Multivitamin preparations with vitamins A and D are not in this list but in section 9.6.7

Vitamin B Tablets, Compound, nicotinamide 15 mg, riboflavine 1 mg, thiamine hydrochloride 1 mg. Price 20 tabs = **A**
Dose: prophylactic, 1–2 tablets daily

Vitamin B Tablets, Compound, Strong, brown, f/c or s/c, nicotinamide 20 mg, pyridoxine hydrochloride 2 mg, riboflavine 2 mg, thiamine hydrochloride 5 mg. Price 20 tabs = **A**
Dose: treatment of vitamin-B deficiency, 1–2 tablets 3 times daily

Allbee with C® (Robins) *capsules*, yellow/green, ascorbic acid, calcium pantothenate, nicotinamide, pyridoxine hydrochloride, riboflavine, thiamine mononitrate. Price 20 caps = **C**. *Elixir*, yellow, ascorbic acid, nicotinamide, pyridoxine hydrochloride, riboflavine phosphate sodium salt, thiamine mononitrate. Price 100 ml = **C**

Aluzyme® (Phillips Yeast) *tablets*, dried yeast, folic acid, nicotinic acid, riboflavine, thiamine hydrochloride. Price 20 tabs = **A**

Aneurone® (Philip Harris) *mixture*, caffeine, compound gentian infusion, sodium acid phosphate, strychnine hydrochloride, thiamine hydrochloride. Price 100 ml = **B**

BC 500® (Ayerst) *tablets*, orange, f/c, calcium pantothenate, cyanocobalamin, nicotinamide, pyridoxine hydrochloride, riboflavine, sodium ascorbate, thiamine mononitrate. Price 20 tabs = **C**

Becosym® (Roche) *tablets*, brown, f/c, vitamin B tablets, compound, strong. Price 20 tabs = **A. Forte** *tablets*, brown, f/c, nicotinamide 50 mg, pyridoxine hydrochloride 10 mg, riboflavine 15 mg, thiamine hydrochloride 15 mg. Price 20 tabs = **B**. *Syrup* (=elixir), orange, ingredients as for tablets, 5 ml being equivalent to 1 tablet. Price 100 ml = **C**

Benerva Compound® (Roche) *tablets*, yellow, vitamin B tablets, compound. Price 20 tabs = **A**

Bravit® (Galen) *tablets*, orange, s/c. ascorbic acid, nicotinamide, pyridoxine hydrochloride, riboflavine, thiamine hydrochloride. Price 20 tabs = **B**

Ce-Cobalin® (P&B) *syrup* (=elixir), ascorbic acid, cyanocobalamin. Price 100 ml = **B**

Effico® (Pharmax) *tonic* (=elixir), green, caffeine, compound gentian infusion, nicotinamide, thiamine hydrochloride. Price 100 ml = **A**

Hemoplex® (P&B) *injection*, liver extract crude, nicotinamide, pyridoxine hydrochloride, riboflavine, thiamine hydrochloride. Price 10-ml vial = **D**

Hepacon-Plex® (Consolidated) *injection*, calcium pantothenate, nicotinamide, vitamins B_1, B_2, B_6, B_{12}. Price 2-ml amp = **A**

Labiton® (LAB) *elixir*, brown, alcohol, aminobenzoic acid, caffeine, kola nut dried extract, thiamine hydrochloride. Price 100 ml = **B**

Lance B+C® (Kirby-Warrick) *tablets,* red, s/c, ascorbic acid, nicotinamide, pyridoxine hydrochloride, riboflavine, thiamine hydrochloride. Price 20 tabs = **B**

Lederplex® (Lederle) *elixir*, orange, choline, cyanocobalamin, inositol, soluble liver fraction, nicotinamide, pantothenic acid, pyridoxine hydrochloride, riboflavine, thiamine hydrochloride. Price 100 ml = **E**

Lipoflavonoid® (Lewis) *capsules*, pink/black, ascorbic acid, choline bitartrate, hydroxocobalamin, inositol, lemon bioflavonoid complex, methionine, nicotinamide, panthenol, pyridoxine hydrochloride, riboflavine, thiamine hydrochloride. Price 20 caps = **B**

Lipotriad® (Lewis) *capsules*, pink/clear, choline bitartrate, hydroxocobalamin, inositol, methionine, nicotinamide, panthenol, pyridoxine hydrochloride, riboflavine, thiamine hydrochloride. Price 20 caps = **B**. *Elixir*, ingredients as for capsules. Price 100 ml = **C**

Metatone® (P-D) *tonic*(= elixir), glycerophosphates of calcium, manganese, potassium, sodium, thiamine hydrochloride. Price 100 ml = **A**

Orovite® (Bencard) *tablets*, maroon, s/c, ascorbic acid, nicotinamide, pyridoxine hydrochloride, riboflavine, thiamine hydrochloride. Price 20 tabs = **C**. *Elixir*, ingredients as for tablets, 12.5 ml of elixir being equivalent to 1 tablet. Price 100 ml = **C**. Also **Orovite 7** see section 9.6.7

Potaba + 6® (Glenwood) *tablets*, potassium aminobenzoate, pyridoxine hydrochloride. Price 20 tabs = **C**

Surbex T® (Abbott) *tablets*, orange, nicotinamide, pyridoxine hydrochloride, riboflavine, sodium ascorbate, thiamine mononitrate. Price 20 tabs = **B**

Tonivitan B® (Medo) *syrup* (=elixir), red, calcium glycerophosphate, manganese glycerophosphate, nicotinamide, pyridoxine hydrochloride, riboflavine, strychnine glycerophosphate, thiamine hydrochloride. Price 100 ml = **A**. **Tonivitan A & D Syrup** section 9.1.3; **Tonivitan Capsules**, section 9.6.7

Vigranon B® (Wallace Mfg) *syrup* (=elixir), nicotinamide, panthenol, pyridoxine hydrochloride, riboflavine, thiamine hydrochloride. Price 150 ml = **C**

Villescon® (Boehringer Ingelheim) *tablets*, orange, s/c, ascorbic acid, nicotinamide, prolintane hydrochloride, pyridoxine hydrochloride, riboflavine, thiamine hydrochloride. Price 20 tabs = **C**. *Liquid* (=elixir), red, nicotinamide, prolintane hydrochloride, pyridoxine hydrochloride, riboflavine sodium phosphate, thiamine hydrochloride. Price 100 ml = **B**

Virvina® (MSD) *elixir*, nicotinamide, pyridoxine hydrochloride, riboflavine, thiamine hydrochloride, glycerophosphates of calcium, manganese, potassium, sodium. Price 100 ml = **A**

Wallachol® (Wallace Mfg) *tablets*, antitoxic principle from fresh liver, choline dihydrogen citrate, cyanocobalamin, inositol, dried liver, methionine, nicotinamide, pyridoxine hydrochloride, riboflavine, thiamine hydrochloride. Price 20 tabs = **B**. *Elixir*, ingredients similar to tablets. Price 100 ml = **C**

9.6.3 Vitamin C

(Ascorbic acid)

The only valid use of this vitamin is for the treatment of scurvy, a rare condition in Britain except in elderly people, usually living alone, who do not eat fruit or vegetables.

Claims that vitamin C ameliorates colds or promotes wound healing have not been proved.

ASCORBIC ACID

Indications: prevention and treatment of scurvy

Dose: prophylactic, 25–75 mg daily; therapeutic, not less than 250 mg daily in divided doses

Ascorbic Acid Tablets, ascorbic acid 25, 50, 100, and 200 mg, price 20 tabs (all) = **A**; 500 mg, price 20 tabs = **B**

Ascorbic Acid Injection, ascorbic acid 100 mg/ml. Price 5-ml amp = **B**

Roscorbic® (Roche)

Tablets, ascorbic acid 25, 50, or 200 mg, price 20 tabs (all) = **A**; 500 mg, price 20 tabs = **B**

Tablets, effervescent, ascorbic acid 1 g. Price 20 tabs = **C**

9.6.4 Vitamin D

(Cholecalciferol; Ergocalciferol)

Deficiency of vitamin D has been shown to occur in Asian subjects in Britain and vitamin D deficiency occurs in patients with malabsorption syndromes. In patients with severe renal disease, vitamin D is inadequately converted by the kidney into 1-α,25-dihydroxycholecalciferol, which is the active antirachitic factor, and rickets resistant to vitamin D may result.

Vitamin D deficiency can, in most cases be prevented and cured by doses of vitamin D ranging from 500 to 5000 units daily. This is best given as Calcium with Vitamin D Tablets (500 units of vitamin D per tablet) or Calciferol Solution (3000 units per ml).

In the treatment of resistant rickets and of hypoparathyroidism, very large doses of vitamin D are required, in the range 50 000 to 150 000 units per day. This is best given as High Strength Calciferol Tablets, (10 000 units per tablet). **Alfacalcidol** (1α-hydroxycholecalciferol, One-alpha®) or **calcitriol** (1α,25-dihydroxycholecalciferol, Rocaltrol®) is specifically indicated in certain cases of bone disease complicating renal failure and alphacalcidol may also be used in vitamin-D-dependent rickets and osteomalacia.

Dihydrotachysterol is used in certain cases of vitamin-D deficiency and resistant rickets. The initial dose in hypoparathyroidism is 1–2 mg and the maintenance dose is 0.5 to 2 mg.

Patients treated with large or potent doses of vitamin D preparations may develop hypercalcaemia and irreversible renal damage and so require frequent estimation of serum calcium.

Calciferol Tablets, High-strength, BP 1980, s/c, cholecalciferol or ergocalciferol 250 micrograms (10 000 units). Price 20 tabs = **B**
Note: it is essential to include the words 'high-strength' in the prescription

Calciferol Tablets, Strong, BP 1973, ergocalciferol 1.25 mg (50 000 units). Price 20 tabs = **B**
Note: it is essential to include the word 'strong' in the prescription

Calcium with Vitamin D Tablets, calcium sodium lactate 450 mg (or calcium lactate 300 mg), calcium phosphate 150 mg, ergocalciferol 12.5 micrograms (500 units). Price 20 tabs = **A**

Calciferol Solution, cholecalciferol or ergocalciferol 3000 units/ml in oil. Price 100 ml = **D**

Calciferol Injection, 300 000 units/ml in oil. Price 1- and 2-ml amp (both) = **B**

AT 10® (Sterling Research)

Solution, dihydrotachysterol 250 micrograms/ml. Price 15-ml dropper bottle = **I**

Chocovite® (Medo)

Tablets, buff, calciferol 15 micrograms (40 units/microgram), calcium gluconate 500 mg. Price 20 tabs = **B**

▼ **One-alpha**® (Leo)

Capsules, alfacalcidol 250 nanograms. Price 20 caps = **D**

Capsules, brown, alfacalcidol 1 microgram. Price 20 caps = **G**
Drops, alfacalcidol 5 micrograms/ml (250 nanograms/drop). Price 10 ml = **I**
Dose: ADULTS and CHILDREN over 20 kg, initially 1 microgram daily, adjusted according to the response; CHILD under 20 kg, 50 nanograms/kg daily
Maintenance 0.25–1 microgram

▼ **Rocaltrol**® (Roche)
Capsules, orange, calcitriol 250 nanograms. Price 20 caps = **F**
Capsules, orange, calcitriol 500 nanograms. Price 20 caps = **G**
Dose: initially 1–2 micrograms daily, gradually increased to 2–3 micrograms daily

Sterogyl-15® (Roussel)
Solution, for oral use, calciferol 400 000 units/ml. Price 1.5-ml amp = **B**

Tachyrol® (Duphar)
Tablets, scored, dihydrotachysterol 200 micrograms. Price 20 tabs = **E**

9.6.5 Vitamin E

(Tocopherols)

Despite claims for its efficacy in a variety of disorders there is no convincing evidence of its value.

ALPHA TOCOPHERYL ACETATE

Indications: vitamin-E deficiency
Dose: 3 to 15 mg daily
Note: the potency of *RRR*-α-tocopheryl acetate is about 1.36 units/mg and that of *all-rac*-α-tocopheryl acetate is about 1 unit/mg

Ephynal® (Roche) *tablets*, *all-rac*-α-tocopheryl acetate 3 mg, price 20 tabs = **A**; 10 mg, price 20 tabs = **A**; 50 mg, price 20 tabs = **B**; 200 mg, price 20 tabs = **C**

Vita-E® (Bioglan) *gels*® (=capsules), yellow, tocopheryl acetate 75 units, price 20 caps = **B**; 200 units, price 20 caps = **C**; red, 400 units, price 20 caps = **D**. *Gelucaps*® (=tablets), chewable, yellow, tocopheryl acetate 75 units. Price 20 tabs = **B**. *Succinate tablets*, tocopheryl succinate 50 units, price 20 tabs = **B**; 200 units, price 20 tabs = **D**

9.6.6 Vitamin K

Vitamin K is necessary for the production of blood clotting factors. In neonates deficiency of vitamin K may occur because the gut is sterile and there is no synthesis of the vitamin by *Escherichia coli.*

Because vitamin K is fat soluble, patients with fat malabsorption, especially if due to biliary obstruction or hepatic disease, may become deficient.

Oral anticoagulants act by interfering with vitamin K metabolism in the hepatic cells and their effects can be antagonised by giving vitamin K.

Vitamin-K deficiency in neonates may be treated with **phytomenadione** (vitamin K_1), 1 mg by intramuscular or intravenous injection. Synthetic analogues of vitamin K, such as menadiol sodium diphosphate, should be avoided because of the risk of kernicterus.

Haemorrhage associated with hypoprothrombinaemia caused by overdosage of anticoagulants may be treated with phytomenadione 2.5–20 mg by slow intravenous injection. Hypoprothrombinaemia due to anticoagulants, but without haemorrhage may be treated with phytomenadione 10–20 mg by mouth.

For the prevention of vitamin-K deficiency in malabsorption syndromes, a water-soluble preparation, **menadiol sodium diphosphate** must be used; the usual dose is about 10 mg daily by mouth or by injection.

After correction of hypoprothrombinaemia, resistance to oral anticoagulants persists for up to two weeks; patients with prosthetic valves who need to continue anticoagulant therapy but who bleed, should be treated with fresh plasma to elevate the prothrombin levels and the anticoagulant dose reduced.

MENADIOL SODIUM DIPHOSPHATE

Indications; Dose: see notes above

Synkavit® (Roche)
Tablets, scored, menadiol sodium diphosphate equivalent to 10 mg of menadiol phosphate. Price 20 tabs = **B**
Injection, menadiol sodium diphosphate equivalent to 10 mg of menadiol phosphate/ml. Price 1-ml amp = **A**
Injection, menadiol sodium diphosphate equivalent to 50 mg of menadiol phosphate/ml. Price 2-ml amp = **B**

PHYTOMENADIONE

Indications; Dose: see notes above
Cautions: intravenous injections should be given very slowly

Konakion® (Roche)
Tablets, s/c, phytomenadione 10 mg. Price 25 tabs = **F**
Injection, phytomenadione 2 mg/ml. Price 0.5-ml amp = **A**
Injection, phytomenadione 10 mg/ml. Price 1-ml amp = **B**

9.6.7 Multivitamin preparations

There are many preparations available. The proprietary preparations have no advantage over the non-proprietary preparations given separately and many are expensive. For other similar preparations, see sections 9.1.1.1 and 9.6.2.

Vitamins Capsules, ascorbic acid 15 mg, nicotinamide 7.5 mg, riboflavine 500 micrograms, thiamine hydrochloride 1 mg, vitamin A 2500 units, vitamin D 300 units. Price 20 caps = **A**

Abidec® (P-D) *capsules*, ascorbic acid, nicotinamide, pyridoxine hydrochloride, riboflavine, thiamine hydrochloride, vitamin A, vitamin D. Price 20 caps = **A**. *Drops*, ingredients as above, 0.6 ml approximately equivalent to 1 capsule. Price 2 × 25 ml (with dropper) = **D**

Calavite® (Carlton) *tablets*, ascorbic acid, calciferol, nicotinamide, pyridoxine hydrochloride, riboflavine, thiamine hydrochloride, vitamin A. Price 20 tabs = **A**

Calcimax® (Wallace Mfg) *syrup* (=elixir), brown, ascorbic acid, calciferol, calcium glycine hydrochloride, calcium pantothenate, cyanocobalamin, nicotinamide, pyridoxine hydrochloride, riboflavine, thiamine hydrochloride. Price 150 ml = **C**

Concavit® (Wallace Mfg) *capsules*, ascorbic acid, calciferol, cyanocobalamin, pyridoxine hydrochloride, riboflavine, thiamine hydrochloride, vitamin A, vitamin E. Price 20 caps = **C**. *Drops* and *syrup* (=elixir), ascorbic acid, calciferol, cyanocobalamin, dexpanthenol, nicotinamide, pyridoxine hydrochloride, riboflavine, thiamine hydrochloride, vitamin A. Price, drops 15 ml = **C**; syrup 150 ml = **C**

Dalivit® (P&B) *capsules*, red, ascorbic acid, calcium pantothenate, nicotinamide, pyridoxine hydrochloride, riboflavine, thiamine mononitrate, vitamin A, vitamin D. Price 20 caps = **A**. *Drops* and *syrup* (=elixir), ingredients as for capsules, 1.2 ml of drops or 10 ml of syrup approximately equivalent to 1 capsule. Prices, drops 15 ml = **B**; syrup 100 ml = **B**

Juvel® (Bencard) *tablets*, yellow, s/c, ascorbic acid, nicotinamide, pyridoxine hydrochloride, riboflavine, thiamine hydrochloride, vitamin A, vitamin D. Price 20 tabs = **B**. *Elixir*, ingredients as for capsules, 6.25 ml of elixir being equivalent to 1 capsule. Price 100 ml = **B**

Multivitamins (Evans) *tablets*, chocolate, s/c, ascorbic acid, nicotinamide, riboflavine, thiamine hydrochloride, vitamin A, vitamin D. Price 20 tabs = **A**

Multivite® (DF) *pellets*, brown, s/c, vitamin A, vitamin B, vitamin C, vitamin D. Price 20 pellets = **A**

Orovite 7® (Bencard) *granules*, orange, nicotinamide, riboflavine phosphate sodium salt, vitamin A palmitate, thiamine mononitrate, pyridoxine hydrochloride, vitamin C, vitamin D_2. Price 20 sachets = **D**

Polyvite® (Medo) *capsules*, red, ascorbic acid, calcium pantothenate, nicotinamide, pyridoxine hydrochloride, riboflavine, thiamine hydrochloride, vitamin A, vitamin D_2. Price 20 caps = **B**

Tonivitan® (Medo) *capsules*, chocolate, ascorbic acid, nicotinic acid, thiamine hydrochloride, vitamin A, vitamin D_2, dried yeast. Price 20 caps = **B**. Also Tonivitan A & D syrup section 9.1.1.1; Tonivitan B section 9.6.2

Verdiviton® (Squibb) *elixir*, cyanocobalamin, dexpanthenol, glycerophosphates of calcium, manganese, potassium and sodium, nicotinamide, pyridoxine hydrochloride, riboflavine, thiamine mononitrate. Price 240 ml = **D**

Vi-Daylin® (Abbott) *syrup* (=elixir), ascorbic acid, nicotinamide, pyridoxine hydrochloride, riboflavine, thiamine hydrochloride, vitamin A palmitate, vitamin D. Price 100 ml = **B**

Vitavel® (Bencard) *syrup* (=elixir), orange, ascorbic acid, thiamine hydrochloride, vitamin A, vitamin D_2. Price 100 ml = **B**

9.7 Bitters and tonics

Mixtures containing simple and aromatic bitters, such as gentian and alkali mixture, are traditional remedies for loss of appetite. All depend on suggestion and there is no advantage in prescribing the many exotically coloured and flavoured products which are available. Such preparations frequently contain, in addition to a bitter principle, various vitamins (section 9.6.2) or an iron salt (section 9.1.1.1).

Gentian Mixture, Alkaline (see Formulary). Price 100 ml = **A**

Neuro Phosphates® (SK&F) *elixir*, green, calcium and sodium glycerophosphates, strychnine alkaloid (in acid solution). Price 100 ml = **B**

10: Drugs used in the treatment of MUSCULOSKELETAL and JOINT DISEASES

In this chapter, drug treatment is discussed under the following headings:

10.1 Drugs used in rheumatic diseases and gout

Most rheumatic diseases are treated symptomatically by relieving pain and stiffness. Suitable drugs are described in section 10.1.1; those with a prominent anti-inflammatory effect are particularly useful.

In certain circumstances corticosteroids (section 10.1.2) may be used to suppress inflammation. Drugs are also available which may affect the disease process itself and favourably influence the outcome. For rheumatoid arthritis these include penicillamine, gold, hydroxychloroquine, chloroquine and immunosuppressants (section 10.1.3) and for gout the uricosuric agents and allopurinol (section 10.1.4).

For other analgesic preparations see section 4.7.

10.1.1 Anti-inflammatory analgesics

Anti-inflammatory analgesics have two separate actions. Taken in *single doses* they have analgesic activity comparable to that of paracetamol (section 4.7.1.1) or narcotic analgesics used in mild to moderate pain (section 4.7.1.2). Therefore they can be taken on demand for pain which is mild or intermittent or as a supplement to regular treatment.

Taken in *regular dosage* they have an anti-inflammatory effect. This combination of analgesic and anti-inflammatory properties makes these drugs particularly useful for treating conditions associated with pain and inflammation. Anti-inflammatory analgesics are therefore likely to be superior to paracetamol or narcotic analgesics such as dihydrocodeine in conditions such as rheumatoid arthritis, osteoarthritis, back pain, sprains, strains, traumatic conditions, frozen shoulder, fibrositis, other varieties of soft tissue rheumatism, and most types of arthritis.

Aspirin is a classic example of a compound with a dual role as an analgesic and anti-inflammatory drug. Certain of the anti-inflammatory analgesics included in section 10.1.1.2 have been particularly developed or promoted for their analgesic action. They include azapropazone, diflunisal, fenoprofen, ibuprofen, mefenamic acid, naproxen sodium, and zomepirac. As analgesics most of them are as effective as aspirin; zomepirac is more effective. Frequency of administration (4- to 6-hourly) is usually similar to aspirin but some of the longer-acting compounds, for example diflunisal, may be given 12-hourly. Most of them are, however, more expensive than aspirin or paracetamol.

Suitable analgesic doses, to be used when required, are indicated in section 4.7.1.1. Anti-inflammatory doses are given in sections 10.1.1.1 and 10.1.1.2 (below). The more recently introduced anti-inflammatory analgesics have certain advantages over aspirin, paracetamol, and the narcotic analgesics of section 4.7.1.2 in that they are safer in overdosage and do not cause the tolerance, dependence, and respiratory depression associated with narcotics.

Paracetamol and the **narcotic analgesics** (see section 4.7) have no demonstrable anti-inflammatory activity and are therefore **not included** in this section.

The differences in anti-inflammatory potency between drugs of this group are small but there is enormous variation in individual patient response. About 60% of patients will respond to any drug of this class and those who do not respond to one drug may well respond to another. It is therefore often necessary to try several drugs before one is found that suits a particular patient. Most of the drugs should produce an effect within a few days and should be changed if still ineffective after one week.

Dosage of anticoagulants may need to be adjusted when anti-inflammatory analgesics are used but the risk of haemorrhage is greatest with aspirin or other salicylates and phenylbutazone.

Aspirin is the traditional first choice as it is the oldest and least expensive drug of this group but many physicians prefer to start treatment with drugs such as those described in section 10.1.1.2 because they may be better tolerated.

10.1.1.1 ASPIRIN AND THE SALICYLATES

Aspirin is used as a simple analgesic as described in section 4.7.1.1. In regular high dosage it has about the same anti-inflammatory effect as indomethacin or phenylbutazone (section 10.1.1.2); 3.6 grams or more daily in divided doses is commonly used for active rheumatoid arthritis.

Doses below 2.4 grams of aspirin daily have few side-effects. Anti-inflammatory doses (3.6 grams or more daily) are associated with a much higher incidence of gastro-intestinal side-effects such as dyspepsia and gastric bleeding, or auditory side-effects, such as tinnitus, leading occasionally to deafness.

Gastro-intestinal side-effects may be minimised by taking the dose after meals. Numerous formulations are available which improve gastric tolerance and minimise occult bleeding. They include buffered aspirin preparations such as aloxiprin, micro-encapsulated aspirin, and enteric-coated aspirin. Some of these preparations have a slow onset of action and are therefore unsuitable for single-dose analgesic use.

Benorylate (Benoral®), an aspirin-paracetamol ester, is broken down after absorption from the gastro-intestinal tract. Doses need only be given twice daily and gastric tolerance is slightly better than with aspirin. As it is more slowly absorbed than paracetamol, hepatotoxicity in overdosage may be reduced.

ASPIRIN

Indications: pain and inflammation in rheumatic disease and other musculoskeletal disorders; see also section 4.7.1.1

Cautions: allergic disease, severe renal or hepatic impairment, dehydration, children (particularly under 1 year), pregnancy (particularly at term), breast-feeding, concurrent anticoagulant therapy. Drug interactions: see Appendix 1

Contra-indications: peptic ulceration

Side-effects: common with anti-inflammatory doses; gastro-intestinal discomfort, ulceration, bleeding, or nausea, hearing disturbances such as tinnitus (leading rarely to deafness), vertigo, mental confusion, hypersensitivity reactions (angioneurotic oedema, bronchospasm and rashes); rarely oedema, myocarditis, blood dyscrasias, particularly thrombocytopenia

Dose: 0.3–1 g every 4 hours; max. in acute conditions 8 g daily; CHILD up to 80 mg/kg daily in 5–6 divided doses, increased in acute conditions to 130 mg/kg. Doses should preferably be taken after meals

Aspirin Tablets, aspirin 300 mg. Price 20 tabs = **A**

Aspirin Tablets, Dispersible, aspirin 300 mg. Price 20 tabs = **A**

Aspirin Tablets, Dispersible, Paediatric, aspirin 75 mg. Price 20 tabs = **A**

Breoprin® (Sterling Research)
Tablets, scored, aspirin 648 mg (for intestinal release). Price 20 tabs = **C**
Dose: 1–2 tablets 3 times daily

Caprin® (Sinclair)
Tablets, pink, aspirin 324 mg (for intestinal release). Price 20 tabs = **B**

Claradin® (Nicholas)
Tablets, effervescent, scored, aspirin 300 mg. Price 20 tabs = **B**

Laboprin® (LAB)
Tablets, mottled white/brown, aspirin 300 mg, lysine 245 mg. Price 24 tabs = **B**

Levius® (Farmitalia Carlo Erba)
Tablets, s/r, aspirin 500 mg. Price 20 tabs = **B**

Nu-Seals Aspirin® (Lilly)
Tablets, red, e/c, aspirin 300 mg. Price 20 tabs = **B**
Tablets, red, e/c, aspirin 600 mg. Price 20 tabs = **B**

Palaprin Forte® (Nicholas)
Tablets, orange, scored, aloxiprin 600 mg (≡ aspirin 500 mg). To be taken dispersed in water, chewed, sucked, or swallowed whole. Price 20 tabs = **B**

Paynocil® (Beecham)
Tablets, scored, aspirin 600 mg, glycine 300 mg. To be dissolved on the tongue. Price 20 tabs = **B**

Solprin® (R&C)
Tablets (dispersible), aspirin 300 mg. Price 20 tabs = **A**

BENORYLATE

Aspirin-paracetamol ester

Indications: pain and inflammation in rheumatic disease (including Still's disease) and other musculoskeletal disorders; see also section 4.7.1.1

Cautions; Contra-indications: see under Aspirin (above) and Paracetamol (section 4.7.1.1)

Side-effects: see under Aspirin (above) and Paracetamol (section 4.7.1.1), but tolerance is slightly better than with aspirin and hepatotoxicity in overdosage may be lower than with paracetamol

Dose: 4–8 g daily divided into 2–4 doses; CHILD 3 months–1 year 25 mg/kg up to 4 times daily, 1–2 years 250 mg up to 4 times daily, 3–5 years 500 mg up to 3 times daily, 6–12 years 500 mg up to 4 times daily *or* for acute rheumatic conditions in children 1–12 years, initially 200 mg/kg daily, adjusted after 7 days to maintain a serum-salicylate concentration of 25–30 mg/100 ml. Doses should preferably be taken after meals

Benoral® (Winthrop)
Tablets, benorylate 750 mg. Price 20 tabs = **C**
Powder, benorylate 2-g sachet. Price 10 sachets = **D**

Suspension (= mixture), benorylate 2 g/5 ml. Diluent syrup, life of diluted mixture 14 days. Price 150 ml = **F**

CHOLINE MAGNESIUM TRISALICYLATE

Indications: pain and inflammation in rheumatic disease and other musculoskeletal disorders

Cautions; Contra-indications; Side-effects: see under Aspirin (above) but side-effects occur less frequently

Dose: 1–1.5 g of salicylate twice daily

▼ Trilisate® (Napp)

Tablets, orange, scored, choline magnesium trisalicylate ≡ salicylate 500 mg. Price 20 tabs = **D**

SALSALATE

Indications: pain and inflammation in mild rheumatic disease and other musculoskeletal disorders; see also section 4.7.1.1

Cautions; Contra-indications; Side-effects: see under Aspirin (above); side-effects may occur less frequently

Dose: 0.5–1 g 3–4 times daily preferably after meals

▼ Disalcid® (Riker)

Capsules, orange/grey, salsalate 500 mg. Price 20 caps = **D**

SODIUM SALICYLATE

Indications: pain and inflammation in rheumatic disease, particularly rheumatic fever; see also section 4.7.1.1

Cautions; Contra-indications; Side-effects: see under Aspirin (above). Caution in patients on low sodium diet and in congestive heart failure; avoid in acute renal disease

Dose: 0.5–2 g when necessary. In acute conditions 5–10 g daily in divided doses. Acute rheumatic fever, 1–1.5 g every 2 hours or 1.5–2 g every 3 hours, increasing intervals between doses to 4 and then 6 hours as symptoms abate; CHILD rheumatic fever 4–8 g daily in divided doses; max. 120 mg/kg daily

Sodium Salicylate Mixture, sodium salicylate 250 mg/5 ml (see Formulary). Price 100 ml = **A**

Sodium Salicylate Mixture, Strong, sodium salicylate 500 mg/5 ml (see Formulary). Price 100 ml = **A**

Entrosalyl® (Cox-Continental)

Tablets, gluten-coated, sodium salicylate 500 mg. Price 20 tabs = **B**

10.1.1.2 OTHER NON-STEROIDAL ANTI-INFLAMMATORY DRUGS

Many of these drugs are similar in efficacy to aspirin and some are as effective as indomethacin or phenylbutazone but they have the advantage of causing fewer and less severe side-effects. They are sometimes preferred to aspirin for the treatment of conditions such as mild rheumatoid arthritis, osteoarthritis, minor rheumatic conditions, sprains, strains, and sports injuries.

These drugs differ little from each other in efficacy though there is considerable variation in patient response, and the main differences between the drugs are in the incidence and type of side-effects (see below). Before treatment of a patient is started the prescriber should weigh efficacy against side-effects for each drug.

SIDE-EFFECTS AND CAUTIONS. Most of these drugs have similar side-effects and cautions. In general, they should be used with caution in gastric ulceration, allergic disorders (particularly asthma and hypersensitivity to salicylates), and renal and hepatic impairment. See also Drug interactions: Appendix 1.

Side-effects are generally mild and infrequent but include gastro-intestinal discomfort or occasionally bleeding, nausea, hypersensitivity reactions (particularly angioneurotic oedema, asthma, and rashes), headache, vertigo, and hearing disturbances such as tinnitus. Blood dyscrasias have occurred rarely with some of these anti-inflammatory drugs.

Naproxen (Naprosyn®) has emerged as one of the first choices as it combines good efficacy with a low incidence of side-effects and administration is only twice daily. However, there are other drugs which are just as effective and just as well tolerated. Some of the more recently introduced drugs, for example piroxicam, need only be given once daily. To suit a particular patient it may be necessary to try a number of different drugs.

Diflunisal (Dolobid®) and **sulindac** (Clinoril®) are similar in tolerance to naproxen. Although diflunisal is an aspirin derivative its clinical effect resembles more closely the propionic derivatives than its parent compound. Its long half-life allows twice-daily administration.

Fenoprofen (Fenopron®) is as effective as naproxen, and **flurbiprofen** (Froben®) may be slightly more effective. Both are associated with slightly more gastro-intestinal side-effects than ibuprofen or naproxen.

Ibuprofen (Brufen®) though associated with fewer side-effects than naproxen, has weaker anti-inflammatory properties. It is unsuitable for treating conditions where inflammation is prominent such as acute gout and ankylosing spondylitis.

Ketoprofen (Alrheumat®, Orudis®) has anti-inflammatory properties similar to ibuprofen and has more side-effects.

Azapropazone (Rheumox®) and **feprazone** (Methrazone®) are similar in effect to the propionic acid derivatives (fenoprofen, naproxen, etc., see above) and both have a tendency to cause rashes. Although chemically related to phenylbutazone, on present evidence azapropazone does not give rise to blood dyscrasias, but a few cases of thrombocytopenia and neutropenia have occurred with feprazone.

Newer drugs with similar clinical properties are benoxaprofen (Opren®), diclofenac (Voltarol®), fenbufen (Lederfen®), fenclofenac (Flenac®), piroxicam (Feldene®), tolmetin (Tolectin®), and zomepirac (Zomax®).

Benoxaprofen and **piroxicam** need only be given once daily. The side-effects of benoxaprofen differ somewhat from the other drugs; photosensitive rashes and onycholysis have been reported.

Tolmetin is similar to indomethacin in efficacy but has fewer of its side-effects. It is more effective than naproxen.

Both **fenbufen** and **fenclofenac** may have a particular tendency to cause rashes. Fenbufen is less likely to cause gastro-intestinal bleeding, and hypersensitivity reactions, headache, vertigo, and hearing disturbances are rare. Dosage adjustment is unnecessary in renal impairment.

Zomepirac may be more effective than aspirin as an analgesic but is not generally used to reduce inflammation.

Indomethacin, oxyphenbutazone, and phenylbutazone should only be used when the above non-steroidal anti-inflammatory drugs have proved ineffective.

Mefenamic acid (Ponstan®) and **flufenamic acid** (Meralen®) are related analgesics but their anti-inflammatory properties are minor and side-effects differ in that diarrhoea and occasionally haemolytic anaemia may occur which necessitates discontinuation of treatment.

Indomethacin (Indocid® etc.) is a potent anti-inflammatory drug which can be used in different ways. It can be used in acute gout and other self-limiting conditions starting with a high dose such as 50–100 mg, repeated after a few hours if necessary, and followed by reducing doses every 6 hours as the condition improves. Even higher doses are usually well tolerated for short periods of time and may be effective for the relief of night pain, sleep disturbance, and morning stiffness in inflammatory conditions when a large dose may be given at bedtime. Indomethacin suppositories or sustained-release capsules (Indocid-R®) administered at bedtime are particularly useful for early morning stiffness.

Indomethacin can also be given daily in divided doses but may give rise to headaches and gastro-intestinal side-effects.

Phenylbutazone (Butazolidin® etc.) is another potent anti-inflammatory drug but because of its dangerous side-effects it should be used only when other drugs have proved ineffective. It is particularly effective in acute gout and ankylosing spondylitis. Apart from the gastric side-effects it has two rare and dangerous side-effects. It causes fluid retention and in predisposed patients may precipitate cardiac failure. It also causes agranulocytosis (which may occur within the first few days of treatment) and aplastic anaemia. It is therefore wise to **avoid** the use of phenylbutazone except for short periods of treatment (up to one week), especially in elderly patients.

In ankylosing spondylitis prolonged administration may be necessary but it should not be used unless other drugs have been tried and have failed.

Oxyphenbutazone (Tanderil®) is similar to phenylbutazone and has no advantages.

AZAPROPAZONE

Indications: pain and inflammation in rheumatic disease and other musculoskeletal disorders; acute gout. See also section 4.7.1.1

Cautions; Side-effects: see notes above; photosensitivity has been reported. Avoid in hypersensitivity to phenylbutazone and related drugs

Dose: 1.2 g daily in 2 or 4 divided doses, preferably after meals; reduce for long-term therapy
Acute gout, 2.4 g in divided doses over 24 hours initially, then 1.8 g reducing to 1.2 g daily in divided doses

Rheumox® (Robins)

Capsules, orange, azapropazone 300 mg. Price 20 caps = **D**

Tablets, orange, f/c, scored, azapropazone 600 mg. Price 20 tabs = **F**

BENOXAPROFEN

Indications: pain and inflammation in rheumatic disease and other musculoskeletal disorders

Cautions; Side-effects: see notes above. Avoid prolonged direct exposure to sunlight as skin reactions may occur

Dose: 600 mg, as a single dose usually at bedtime *or* as 2 divided doses, preferably after meals

▼ Opren® (Dista)

Tablets, peach, benoxaprofen 300 mg. Price 20 tabs = **E**

DICLOFENAC SODIUM

Indications: pain and inflammation in rheumatic disease and other musculoskeletal disorders

Cautions; Side-effects: see notes above. Pain may occur at the injection site

Dose: *by mouth*, 25–50 mg 2-3 times daily, preferably after meals; reduce in long-term therapy
By intramuscular injection (in acute exacerbations), 75 mg 1–2 times daily
By rectum in suppositories, 100 mg, usually at night

▼ Voltarol® (Geigy)

Tablets, yellow, e/c, diclofenac sodium 25 mg. Price 20 tabs = **D**

Tablets, brown, e/c, diclofenac sodium 50 mg. Price 20 tabs = **F**

Injection, diclofenac sodium 25 mg/ml. Price 3-ml amp = **C**

Suppositories, diclofenac sodium 100 mg. Price 10 suppos = **E**

DIFLUNISAL

Indications: pain and inflammation in rheumatic disease and other musculoskeletal disorders; see also section 4.7.1.1

Cautions; Side-effects: see notes above

Dose: 250–500 mg twice daily preferably after meals

▼ **Dolobid®** (Morson)

Tablets, peach, f/c, diflunisal 250 mg. Price 20 tabs = **D**

Tablets, orange, f/c, diflunisal 500 mg. Price 20 tabs = **F**

FENBUFEN

Indications: pain and inflammation in rheumatic disease and other musculoskeletal disorders

Cautions; Side-effects: see notes above

Dose: 600 mg daily as a single dose, usually at bedtime *or* 600–900 mg daily in divided doses preferably after meals

▼ **Lederfen®** (Lederle)

Capsules, blue, fenbufen 300 mg. Price 20 caps = **F**

FENCLOFENAC

Indications: pain and inflammation in rheumatic disease and other musculoskeletal disorders

Cautions; Side-effects: see notes above; interferes with thyroid-function tests

Dose: 0.6–1.2 g daily, in 2 divided doses after meals; usual maintenance dose 900 mg daily

▼ **Flenac®** (R&C)

Tablets, fenclofenac 300 mg. Price 20 tabs = **E**

FENOPROFEN

Indications: pain and inflammation in rheumatic disease and other musculoskeletal disorders; see also section 4.7.1.1

Cautions; Side-effects: see notes above

Dose: 300–600 mg 3–4 times daily preferably after meals; max. 3 g daily

Fenopron® (Dista)

Tablets, orange, fenoprofen 300 mg (as calcium salt). Price 20 tabs = **D**

Tablets, orange, fenoprofen 600 mg (as calcium salt). Price 20 tabs = **E**

Fenopron D® (Dista)

Tablets (dispersible), fenoprofen 300 mg (as calcium salt). Price 20 tabs = **D**

Progesic

See section 4.7.1.1

FEPRAZONE

Indications: pain and inflammation in rheumatic disease and other musculoskeletal disorders

Cautions; Side-effects: see notes above. On prolonged therapy blood counts and surveillance for sodium and fluid retention are advisable

Contra-indications: cardiac disease likely to be aggravated by fluid retention, hepatic disease, and hypersensitivity to phenylbutazone and related drugs

Dose: 200–600 mg daily in divided doses preferably after meals

▼ **Methrazone®** (WBP)

Capsules, orange, feprazone 200 mg. Price 20 caps = **E**

FLUFENAMIC ACID

Indications: mild to moderate pain in rheumatoid arthritis, osteoarthritis, and related conditions

Cautions; Contra-indications; Side-effects: see under Mefenamic Acid

Dose: 200 mg 3 times daily after meals, reducing to 400 mg daily; not more than 10 mg/kg daily in patients less than 45 kg

Meralen® (Merrell)

Capsules, blue, flufenamic acid 100 mg. Price 20 caps = **D**

FLURBIPROFEN

Indications: pain and inflammation in rheumatic disease and other musculoskeletal disorders

Cautions; Side-effects: see notes above

Dose: 150–200 mg increased in acute conditions to 300 mg daily, divided into 3–4 doses, preferably after meals

▼ **Froben®** (Boots)

Tablets, yellow, s/c, flurbiprofen 50 mg. Price 20 tabs = **D**

Tablets, yellow, s/c, flurbiprofen 100 mg. Price 20 tabs = **F**

IBUPROFEN

Indications: pain and mild inflammation in rheumatic disease (including Still's disease) and other musculoskeletal disorders; see also section 4.7.1.1

Cautions; Side-effects: see notes above

Dose: 200–400 mg 4 times daily preferably after meals; max. 2.4 g daily in divided doses; CHILD 20 mg/kg daily, children under 30 kg max. in 24 hours 500 mg

Ibuprofen Tablets, f/c or s/c, ibuprofen 200 mg, price 20 tabs = **B**; 400 mg, price 20 tabs = **C**

Apsifen® (APS)

Tablets, pink, f/c or s/c, ibuprofen 200 mg. Price 20 tabs = **B**

Tablets, pink, f/c or s/c, ibuprofen 400 mg. Price 20 tabs = **C**

Brufen® (Boots)

Tablets, magenta, s/c, ibuprofen 200 mg. Price 20 tabs = **B**

Tablets, magenta, s/c, ibuprofen 400 mg. Price 20 tabs = **C**

Syrup (= elixir), orange, ibuprofen 100 mg/5 ml. Diluent syrup, life of diluted elixir 14 days. Price 100 ml = **B**

Ebufac® (DDSA)
Tablets, pink, s/c, ibuprofen 200 mg. Price 20 tabs = **B**
Tablets, pink, s/c, ibuprofen 400 mg. Price 20 tabs = **C**

▼ **Ibu-Slo®** (Rona)
Capsules, s/r, pink/clear, enclosing off-white pellets, ibuprofen 300 mg. Price 20 caps = **D**
Dose: 300–600 mg twice daily

INDOMETHACIN

Indications: pain and moderate to severe inflammation in rheumatic disease and other acute musculoskeletal disorders; acute gout

Cautions: may impair the ability to drive or operate machinery; allergic disease, particularly asthma; hepatic and renal impairment, epilepsy, parkinsonism, psychiatric disturbances, elderly patients. During prolonged therapy ophthalmic and blood examinations are advisable. Avoid rectal administration in proctitis and haemorrhoids. Drug interactions: see Appendix 1

Contra-indications: peptic ulceration, salicylate hypersensitivity

Side-effects: frequently headache, dizziness, and light-headedness (especially initially but reduce dose or discontinue if headache is persistent); gastro-intestinal discomfort, ulceration and bleeding (not always preceded by symptoms); rarely, drowsiness, mental confusion, depression, hypersensitivity reactions (bronchospasm, rashes, angioneurotic oedema), syncope, hearing disturbances, blood dyscrasias (particularly thrombocytopenia), hypertension, hyperglycaemia, blurred vision, corneal deposits, peripheral neuropathy. On rectal administration pruritus, discomfort, bleeding

Dose: *by mouth*, 25–50 mg 2–3 times daily, with milk or antacids, or after meals; max. 200 mg daily

Night pain or morning stiffness, 100 mg at bedtime

Treatment is usually for 5–14 days after which in rheumatic disease it may be reduced to a maintenance dose according to the patient's requirements

Acute gout and other acute self-limiting conditions, see notes above

By rectum in suppositories, 100 mg at night, repeated in the morning if required

Combined oral and rectal treatment, max. total daily dose 150–200 mg

Indomethacin Capsules, indomethacin 25 mg, price 20 caps = **C**; 50 mg, price 20 caps = **D**

Indomethacin Suppositories, indomethacin 100 mg. Price 10 suppos = **D**

Artracin® (DDSA)
Capsules, yellow, indomethacin 25 mg. Price 20 caps = **C**
Capsules, yellow, indomethacin 50 mg. Price 20 caps = **D**

Imbrilon® (Berk)
Capsules, yellow, indomethacin 25 mg. Price 20 caps = **C**
Capsules, yellow, indomethacin 50 mg. Price 20 caps = **D**
Suppositories, indomethacin 100 mg. Price 10 suppos = **D**

Indocid® (Morson)
Capsules, indomethacin 25 mg. Price 20 caps = **D**
Capsules, indomethacin 50 mg. Price 20 caps = **E**
Suspension (= mixture), indomethacin 25 mg/5 ml. Do not dilute. Price 100 ml = **D**
Suppositories, indomethacin 100 mg. Price 10 suppos = **E**

▼ **Indocid-R®** (Morson)
Capsules, s/r, yellow, indomethacin 75 mg. Price 20 caps = **F**
Dose: 1–2 capsules daily

Indoflex® (Unimed)
Capsules, indomethacin 25 mg. Price 20 caps = **C**

Mobilan® (Galen)
Capsules, purple/blue, indomethacin 25 mg. Price 20 caps = **C**
Capsules, purple/blue, indomethacin 50 mg. Price 20 caps = **D**

KETOPROFEN

Indications: pain and mild inflammation in rheumatic disease and other musculoskeletal disorders

Cautions; Side-effects: see notes above

Dose: *by mouth*, 50 mg 2–4 times daily preferably after meals

By rectum, 100 mg usually at bedtime

Ketoprofen Capsules, ketoprofen 50 mg. Price 20 caps = **D**

Ketoprofen Suppositories, ketoprofen 100 mg. Price 7 suppos = **E**

Alrheumat® (Bayer)
Capsules, cream, ketoprofen 50 mg. Price 20 caps = **D**
Suppositories, ketoprofen 100 mg. Price 10 suppos = **E**

Orudis® (M&B)
Capsules, green/purple, ketoprofen 50 mg. Price 20 caps = **D**
Capsules, pink, ketoprofen 100 mg. Price 20 caps = **E**
Suppositories, ketoprofen 100 mg. Price 7 suppos = **E**

MEFENAMIC ACID

Indications: mild to moderate pain in rheumatoid arthritis (including Still's disease), osteoarthritis, and related conditions

Cautions: allergic disease, particularly asthma; blood tests required during long-term treatment. Drug interactions: see Appendix 1

Contra-indications: inflammatory bowel disease, peptic ulceration, renal and hepatic impairment, pregnancy

Side-effects: drowsiness, dizziness, gastro-intestinal disturbances, bleeding, nausea, occasionally ulceration; severe diarrhoea, hypersensitivity, bronchospasm, rashes, cholestatic jaundice, rarely thrombocytopenia, haemolytic anaemia (withdraw treatment)
Dose: 500 mg 3 times daily after meals; CHILD over 6 months, 6.5 mg/kg 3–4 times daily for not longer than 7 days, except in juvenile chronic arthritis (Still's disease)

Ponstan® (P-D)
Capsules, ivory/blue, mefenamic acid 250 mg. Price 20 caps = **C**
Tablets forte, yellow, f/c, mefenamic acid 500 mg. Price 20 tabs = **D**
Paediatric suspension (= mixture), mefenamic acid 50 mg/5 ml. Diluent syrup, life of diluted mixture 14 days. Price 125 ml = **D**

NAPROXEN

Indications: pain and inflammation in rheumatic disease and other musculoskeletal disorders; acute gout; see also Naproxen Sodium, section 4.7.1.1
Cautions; Side-effects: see notes above
Dose: by mouth in rheumatic disease, 0.5–1 g daily in 2 divided doses; CHILD over 5 years 10 mg/kg daily in divided doses, preferably after meals
Acute gout, 750 mg initially, then 250 mg every 8 hours
By rectum in suppositories, 500 mg at bedtime
Combined oral and rectal treatment, max. total daily dose 1 g daily

Naprosyn® (Syntex)
Tablets, yellow, scored, naproxen 250 mg. Price 20 tabs = **D**
Tablets, yellow, scored, naproxen 500 mg. Price 20 tabs = **F**
Suspension (= mixture), yellow, naproxen 125 mg/5 ml. Diluent water for preparations or equal quantities of syrup and water for preparations, life of diluted mixture 14 days. Price 100 ml = **D**
Suppositories, naproxen 500 mg. Price 10 suppos = **E**
▼ **Synflex®** (Syntex)
Capsules, orange, naproxen sodium 275 mg (≡ naproxen 250 mg). Price 20 caps = **E**
For pain, see section 4.7.1.1

OXYPHENBUTAZONE

Indications: pain and severe inflammation in rheumatic disease and other acute musculoskeletal disorders including acute gout
Cautions; Contra-indications; Side-effects: see under Phenylbutazone
Dose: by mouth, 200 mg 2–3 times daily, with milk or antacids, or after meals, usually for 2 days, then reduced to 100 mg 2–3 times daily; max. in acute gout 800 mg daily; CHILD, 5–10 mg/kg daily in divided doses
By rectum, 250 mg at night, repeated in the morning if required
Combined oral and rectal treatment, max. total daily dose 650 mg

Tandacote® (Geigy)
Tablets, pink, e/c, s/c, oxyphenbutazone 100 mg. Price 20 tabs = **C**
Tanderil® (Geigy)
Tablets, beige, s/c, oxyphenbutazone 100 mg. Price 20 tabs = **C**
Suppositories, oxyphenbutazone 250 mg. Price 5 suppos = **C**

PHENYLBUTAZONE

Indications: pain and severe inflammation in rheumatic disease and other acute musculoskeletal disorders; acute gout
Cautions: where possible limit treatment to 7 days; elderly patients (reduce dose); breast feeding; avoid rectal administration in proctitis and haemorrhoids. Drug interactions: see Appendix 1
Contra-indications: cardiovascular disease, renal and hepatic disease, peptic ulceration, thyroid disease, hypersensitivity to phenylbutazone and related drugs
Side-effects: occur in 20–40% of patients, may require withdrawal in 10–15%; commonly gastro-intestinal discomfort, ulceration, bleeding, nausea, oedema, hypertension, vertigo, insomnia; rarely rashes (discontinue therapy), goitre, agranulocytosis, thrombocytopenia, aplastic anaemia (sometimes fatal), hepatitis. On injection, abscess formation and nerve damage
Dose: by mouth, 200 mg 2–3 times daily, with milk or antacids if necessary, or after meals, usually for 2 days, then reduced to 100 mg 2–3 times daily; CHILD, 5–10 mg/kg daily in divided doses
By rectum, 250 mg at night, repeated in the morning if required.
Combined oral and rectal treatment, max. total daily dose 650 mg
By deep intramuscular injection into the gluteal muscle, 600 mg (with lignocaine) every 2–3 days

Phenylbutazone Tablets, f/c or s/c, phenylbutazone 100 and 200 mg. Price 20 tabs (both) = **A**
Butacote® (Geigy)
Tablets, violet, e/c, s/c, phenylbutazone 100 mg. Price 20 tabs = **B**
Tablets, violet, e/c, s/c, phenylbutazone 200 mg. Price 20 tabs = **C**
Butazolidin® (Geigy)
Tablets, red, s/c, phenylbutazone 100 mg. Price 20 tabs = **B**
Tablets, s/c, phenylbutazone 200 mg. Price 20 tabs = **C**
Suppositories, phenylbutazone 250 mg. Price 5 suppos = **B**

Injection, phenylbutazone sodium 200 mg/ml with lignocaine 1%. Price 3-ml amp = **A**

Butazolidin Alka® (Geigy)

Tablets, phenylbutazone 100 mg, dried aluminium hydroxide gel 100 mg, magnesium trisilicate 150 mg. Price 20 tabs = **B**

Butazone® (DDSA)

Tablets, red, s/c, phenylbutazone 100 mg. Price 20 tabs = **A**

Tablets, s/c, phenylbutazone 200 mg. Price 20 tabs = A

PIROXICAM

Indications: pain and inflammation in rheumatic disease and other musculoskeletal disorders; acute gout

Cautions: see notes above

Side-effects: see notes above; also, rarely, oedema

Dose: 20 mg daily, increased in acute conditions to 40 mg daily

Acute gout, 40 mg initially, then 40 mg daily in single or divided doses for 4–6 days

▼ **Feldene®** (Pfizer)

Capsules, maroon/blue, piroxicam 10 mg. Price 20 caps = **E**

SULINDAC

Indications: pain and inflammation in rheumatic disease and other musculoskeletal disorders; acute gout

Cautions; Side-effects: see notes above

Dose: 100–200 mg twice daily after meals

Acute gout, 200 mg twice daily for 7–10 days

▼ **Clinoril®** (MSD)

Tablets, yellow, scored, sulindac 100 mg. Price 20 tabs = **E**

Tablets, yellow, scored, sulindac 200 mg. Price 20 tabs = **F**

TOLMETIN

Indications: pain and inflammation in rheumatic disease (including Still's disease) and other muscloskeletal disorders

Cautions; Side-effects: see notes above

Dose: 0.6–1.8 g daily in divided doses after meals; CHILD 20–25 mg/kg to a max. of 1.8 g daily in 3 or 4 divided doses

▼ **Tolectin®** (Ortho)

Tablets, scored, tolmetin 200 mg (as sodium salt). Price 20 tabs = **D**

▼ **Tolectin DS®** (Ortho)

Capsules, ivory/blue, tolmetin 400 mg (as sodium salt). Price 20 caps = **F**

ZOMEPIRAC

Indications: moderate pain in rheumatoid arthritis, osteoarthritis, and related conditions

Cautions; Side-effects: see notes above

Dose: 100 mg every 4–6 hours; max. 600 mg daily

▼ **Zomax®** (Ortho)

Tablets, yellow, scored, zomepirac 100 mg (as sodium salt dihydrate). Price 20 tabs = **E**

10.1.2 Corticosteroids and corticotrophin

Drugs in this group have been divided into systemic corticosteroids and corticotrophin (section 10.1.2.1) and local corticosteroid injections (section 10.1.2.2)

10.1.2.1 SYSTEMIC CORTICOSTEROIDS AND CORTICOTROPHIN

The general actions and uses of the corticosteroids are described in section 6.3. Treatment with corticosteroids in rheumatic diseases should be reserved for specific indications when other anti-inflammatory agents have proved unsuccessful.

An initial dose of corticosteroid is given to induce remission and the dose then gradually reduced to the lowest maintenance dose that will control the disease, or if possible discontinued altogether. A major problem is that relapse may occur as dosage reduction is made, particularly if this is carried out too rapidly. The tendency is therefore to increase and maintain dosage and consequently the patient becomes dependent on corticosteroids.

Prednisolone is used for most purposes although equivalent doses of most other corticosteroids can be used (see section 6.3.2 for table of equivalents). **Cortisone acetate** and **hydrocortisone** are unsuitable for antirheumatic treatment because they have a greater sodium-retaining effect. Corticosteroid-analgesic combination preparations are no longer used because the dosage of the components needs to be adjusted independently.

Corticosteroids should preferably be **avoided** in children as they prevent growth by suppressing the hypothalamic-pituitary-adrenal axis and corticotrophin (see section 6.5.1) may be used instead. Alternate day treatment is preferred, especially with corticosteroids; it is also preferred with corticotrophin after the initial treatment has controlled disease activity. Corticotrophin is also sometimes used in resistant cases of frozen shoulder.

Polymyalgia rheumatica and **temporal (giant cell) arteritis** are always treated with corticosteroids. The usual initial dose of prednisolone in polymyalgia rheumatica is 10 to 15 mg daily and in temporal arteritis 40 to 60 mg daily (the higher dose being used if visual symptoms occur). Treatment should be continued until remission occurs and doses then gradually reduced. Relapse is common if therapy is stopped within 3 years but most patients can discontinue treatment after approximately 3 to 6 years after which recurrences become rare.

Polyarteritis nodosa and **polymyositis** are usually treated with corticosteroids. An initial dose of 60 mg of prednisolone daily is often used and reduced to a maintenance dose of 10 to 15 mg daily.

Systemic lupus erythematosus is treated with corticosteroids when necessary using a similar dosage regimen to that for polyarteritis nodosa and polymyositis (above). Patients with pleurisy, pericarditis, or other systemic manifestations will respond to corticosteroids which can be reduced to alternate-day treatment and then gradually withdrawn. In some mild cases corticosteroid treatment may be stopped after a few months. Many mild cases of systemic lupus erythematosus do not require corticosteroid treatment.

Systemic corticosteroids should **not** be used to suppress symptoms of **rheumatoid arthritis** since effective doses may cause Cushing's syndrome. However, when alternative anti-inflammatory drugs have proved unsuccessful, small doses of corticosteroids such as prednisolone 5 to 7.5 mg daily, gradually reduced, may be useful in elderly patients whose symptoms respond particularly well; similar doses may be used at night to relieve morning stiffness.

Ankylosing spondylitis should **not** be treated with corticosteroids. Corticotrophin is sometimes used in patients with acute **gout** who do not respond to the usual drugs (section 10.1.4).

See section 6.3.4 for systemic corticosteroids and their preparations. Dosage in rheumatic diseases should be calculated from the doses for prednisolone given in the notes (above).

10.1.2.2 LOCAL CORTICOSTEROID INJECTIONS

Corticosteroids are injected locally for anti-inflammatory effect. In inflammatory conditions of the joints, particularly in rheumatoid arthritis, they are given by *intra-articular injection* to relieve pain, increase mobility, and reduce deformity in one or a few joints. Full aseptic precautions are essential. Infected areas and unstable joints should be avoided. On repeated injection joint damage has occurred (especially with the synthetic corticosteroids).

Smaller amounts of corticosteroids may also be injected directly into soft tissues for the relief of inflammation in conditions such as **tennis elbow** or **compression neuropathies.** In **tendinitis**, injections should be made into the tendon sheath and not directly into the tendon.

Cortisone acetate is **not** effective for local injection and hydrocortisone acetate or one of the synthetic analogues such as triamcinolone hexacetonide is generally used. The risk of necrosis and muscle wasting may be slightly increased.

Corticosteroid injections are also injected into soft tissues for the treatment of skin lesions (see section 13.4).

DEXAMETHASONE SODIUM PHOSPHATE

Indications: local inflammation of joints and soft tissues

Cautions; Contra-indications; Side-effects: see notes above and section 6.3.3

Dose: *by intra-articular injection*, large joints 2–4 mg, small joints 0.8–1 mg

By intralesional injection, 0.2–6 mg, according to the amount of soft tissue, at intervals of 3–21 days according to response

Note: 1.3 mg dexamethasone sodium phosphate ≡ 1.2 mg dexamethasone phosphate ≡ 1 mg dexamethasone

Decadron® (MSD)

Injection, dexamethasone phosphate 4 mg/ml (as sodium salt) (≈ 4.4 mg/ml dexamethasone sodium phosphate). Price 2-ml vial = **D**

Oradexon® (Organon)

Injection, dexamethasone sodium phosphate 5 mg/ml. Price 1-ml amp = **C**

Injection, dexamethasone 4 mg/ml (as sodium phosphate) (≈ 5.2 mg/ml dexamethasone sodium phosphate). Price 2-ml vial = **D**

HYDROCORTISONE ACETATE

Indications: local inflammation of joints and soft tissues

Cautions; Contra-indications; Side-effects: see notes above and section 6.3.3

Dose: *by intra-articular or intralesional injection*, 5–50 mg, according to joint size or amount of soft tissue; not more than 3 joints should be treated in 1 day

Hydrocortisone Acetate Injection (aqueous suspension), hydrocortisone acetate 25 mg/ml. Price 1-ml amp = **A**

Hydrocortistab® (Boots)

Injection (aqueous suspension), hydrocortisone acetate 25 mg/ml. Price 5-ml vial = **B**

METHYLPREDNISOLONE ACETATE

Indications: local inflammation of joints and soft tissues

Cautions; Contra-indications; Side-effects: see notes above and section 6.3.3

Dose: *by intra-articular or intralesional injection*, 4–80 mg, according to joint size or amount of soft tissue, repeated every 1–5 weeks according to the response

Depo-Medrone® (Upjohn)

Injection (aqueous suspension), methylprednisolone acetate 40 mg/ml. Price 1-ml vial = **E**; 2-ml vial or syringe = **F**; 5-ml vial = **H**

▼ **Depo-Medrone with Lignocaine**® (Upjohn)

Injection (aqueous suspension), methylprednisolone acetate 40 mg, lignocaine hydrochloride 10 mg/ml. Price 2-ml vial = **F**

PREDNISOLONE ACETATE

Indications: local inflammation of joints and soft tissues

Cautions; Contra-indications; Side-effects: see notes above and section 6.3.3

Dose: by intra-articular or intralesional injection, 5–25 mg according to joint size or amount of soft tissue; not more than 3 joints should be treated daily

Deltastab® (Boots)

Injection (aqueous suspension), prednisolone acetate 25 mg/ml. Price 5-ml vial = **B**

PREDNISOLONE PIVALATE

Indications: local inflammation of joints and soft tissues

Cautions; Contra-indications; Side-effects: see notes above and section 6.3.3

Dose: by intra-articular or intralesional injection, 10–50 mg, according to joint size or amount of soft tissue

Ultracortenol® (Ciba)

Injection (aqueous suspension), prednisolone pivalate 50 mg/ml. Price 1-ml amp = **D**

PREDNISOLONE SODIUM PHOSPHATE

Indications: local inflammation of joints and soft tissues

Cautions; Contra-indications; Side-effects: see notes above and section 6.3.3

Dose: by intra-articular or intralesional injection, prednisolone 1.6–24 mg, according to joint size or amount of soft tissue

Codelsol® (MSD)

Injection, prednisolone 16 mg/ml (as prednisolone sodium phosphate). Price 2-ml vial = **D**

TRIAMCINOLONE ACETONIDE

Indications: local inflammation of joints and soft tissues

Cautions; Contra-indications; Side-effects: see notes above and section 6.3.3

Dose: by intra-articular injection, 2.5–40 mg according to joint size

By intralesional injection, 2–3 mg; max. 30 mg (5 mg at any one site). Doses are repeated every 1–2 weeks according to the response

Adcortyl Intra-articular/Intradermal® (Squibb)

Injection (aqueous suspension), triamcinolone acetonide 10 mg/ml. Price 1-ml amp = **C**; 5-ml vial = **F**

Kenalog Intra-articular/Intramuscular® (Squibb)

Injection (aqueous suspension), triamcinolone acetonide 40 mg/ml. Price 1-ml vial = **D**

TRIAMCINOLONE HEXACETONIDE

Indications: local inflammation of joints and soft tissues

Cautions; Contra-indications; Side-effects: see notes above and section 6.3.3

Dose: by intra-articular or intralesional injection, 2–30 mg, according to joint size or area of soft tissue, repeated at intervals of not less than 3–4 weeks according to the response

By intracutaneous injection, up to 500 micrograms/square inch of affected skin

Lederspan® (Lederle)

Injection (aqueous suspension), triamcinolone hexacetonide 5 mg/ml. Price 5-ml vial = **E**

Injection (aqueous suspension), triamcinolone hexacetonide 20 mg/ml. Price 1-ml vial = **E**; 5-ml vial = **H**

10.1.3 Drugs which may affect the rheumatic disease process

Certain drugs such as **gold** (sodium aurothiomalate), **penicillamine**, **hydroxychloroquine**, **chloroquine**, and **immunosuppressants** are considered disease-specific in that they are said to affect the disease process in rheumatoid arthritis and related conditions but do not affect other types of inflammatory arthritis. They differ from the anti-inflammatory drugs in a number of ways. They do not produce an immediate therapeutic effect but reach a full response after 4 to 6 months of treatment; they improve not only the signs and symptoms of joint disease but also the extra-articular manifestations of rheumatoid arthritis such as nodules; they also reduce erythrocyte sedimentation rate and rheumatoid factor. Some, for example penicillamine, may retard the radiological progression of the disease.

These drugs are mainly used in rheumatoid arthritis where treatment with anti-inflammatory drugs has been unsuccessful or where there is evidence of disease progression such as the development of deformities or worsening radiological changes. Since, in the first few months, the course of rheumatoid arthritis is unpredictable, it is usual to delay treatment for about 6 months depending on the progress of the disease, but treatment should be initiated before joint damage becomes irreversible.

Penicillamine and related drugs are also sometimes used in rheumatoid arthritis where there are troublesome extra-articular features such as vasculitis, and in patients who are taking excessive doses of corticosteroids. Where the response is satisfactory there is often a striking reduction in requirements of both corticosteroids and other drugs. Gold, penicillamine and related drugs may also be used to treat juvenile chronic arthritis (Still's disease) when indications are similar.

Gold and **penicillamine** are effective in palindromic rheumatism and **chloroquine** is sometimes used to treat systemic lupus erythematosus and discoid lupus erythematosus.

Gold (as **sodium aurothiomalate**) must be given by intramuscular injection. It is usual to begin treatment with doses of 1, 5 and 10 mg at intervals of 1 week to test the patient's tolerance; thereafter doses of 50 mg are given at weekly intervals until a response is obtained. Benefit is not to be expected until about 8 doses have been given. The interval between injections is then gradually increased to 2 and then to 4 weeks but intervals of 6 weeks may be suitable in some patients.

If relapse occurs dosage should be immediately increased to 50 mg weekly and only once control is obtained should a reduction in dosage again be instituted. It is important to avoid complete relapse since second courses of gold are not usually effective. Treatment should be continued indefinitely.

Gold therapy should be discontinued in the presence of blood dyscrasias or proteinuria which is above 30 mg/100 ml and has no incidental cause such as urinary-tract infection (associated with immune complex nephritis). Patients should therefore undergo blood counts, including platelets, and urine examinations before each injection. Rashes often occur after 2 to 6 months and necessitate discontinuation of treatment.

SODIUM AUROTHIOMALATE

Indications: severe active or progressive rheumatoid arthritis, palindromic rheumatism, juvenile chronic arthritis

Cautions: see notes above. Patients should report any untoward symptoms (fever, sore throat, malaise, bruising). Caution in renal and hepatic impairment, elderly patients, eczema, treatment with drugs which can cause blood dyscrasias, for example phenylbutazone

Contra-indications: see notes above. Also exfoliative dermatitis, disseminated lupus erythematosus, pregnancy, nursing mothers, patients recently subjected to irradiation

Side-effects: severe reactions (occasionally fatal) in up to 5% of patients; mouth ulcers, skin reactions, oedema, proteinuria, blood dyscrasias (sometimes sudden and fatal); rarely colitis, peripheral neuritis, pulmonary fibrosis

Dose: administered on expert advice, ADULT, see notes above; CHILD, *by intramuscular injection*, slowly increased to the following maximum weekly doses: under 25 kg 10 mg, 25–50 kg 20 mg, over 50 kg 50 mg

Myocrisin® (M&B)

Injection 1 mg, sodium aurothiomalate 2 mg/ml. Price 0.5-ml amp = **B**

Injection 5 mg, sodium aurothiomalate 10 mg/ml. Price 0.5-ml amp = **B**

Injection 10 mg, sodium aurothiomalate 20 mg/ml. Price 0.5-ml amp = **C**

Injection 20 mg, sodium aurothiomalate 40 mg/ml. Price 0.5-ml amp = **C**

Injection 50 mg, sodium aurothiomalate 100 mg/ml. Price 0.5-ml amp = **D**

Penicillamine has a similar action to gold. It appears to have a greater effect on radiological progression, and more patients are able to continue treatment than with gold but side-effects occur frequently. An initial dose of 125 to 250 mg daily is given, increased after 4 to 6 weeks to 250 to 500 mg daily; some patients respond to doses as small as 250 mg daily and others may require 1 g daily.

Patients should be warned not to expect improvement for at least 6 to 12 weeks after treatment is initiated. Blood counts, including platelets, and urine examinations should be carried out every 4 weeks to detect blood dyscrasias and proteinuria. A reduction in platelet count indicates that treatment with penicillamine should be stopped, subsequently re-introduced at a lower dosage level and then, if possible, gradually increased. Proteinuria, associated with immune complex nephritis, occurs in 10 to 15% of patients, but treatment may be continued provided that renal function tests remain normal, oedema is absent, and the 24-hour urinary excretion of protein does not exceed 2 g.

Penicillamine is usually avoided in patients with hepatic impairment because of its hepatotoxicity. Its use is however justified in conditions such as Wilson's disease when it is used for the elimination of copper ions.

Nausea may occur but is not usually a problem provided that penicillamine is taken with food and that low initial doses are used and only gradually increased. Loss of taste may occur about 6 weeks after treatment is started but usually returns 6 weeks later irrespective of whether or not treatment is discontinued. Rashes are a common side-effect. Those which occur in the first few months of treatment disappear when the drug is stopped and treatment may then be re-introduced at a lower dose level and gradually increased. Late rashes are more resistant and often necessitate discontinuation of treatment.

PENICILLAMINE

Indications: severe active or progressive rheumatoid arthritis, palindromic rheumatism, juvenile chronic arthritis, Wilson's disease, chronic active hepatitis, primary biliary cirrhosis, cystinuria

Cautions: see notes above. Also caution in renal or hepatic impairment; avoid concurrent gold, chloroquine, hydroxychloroquine or immunosuppressive treatment. Drug interactions: see Appendix 1

Contra-indications: see notes above

Side-effects: hypersensitivity reactions (may necessitate discontinuation of treatment); nausea, anorexia, taste loss, mouth ulcers, muscle weakness, skin reactions (see notes above—sometimes severe), extravasation of blood into the skin, oedema, proteinuria, blood dyscrasias (sometimes fatal), rarely myasthenia, febrile reactions, systemic lupus erythematosus

Dose: rheumatoid arthritis, administered on expert advice, ADULT, see notes above; CHILD initial dose, under 20 kg 25 mg twice daily; over

20 kg 50 mg twice daily slowly increased over several weeks according to the response
Wilson's disease, 0.5–2 g daily in divided doses; CHILD up to 20 mg/kg daily in divided doses on an empty stomach
Chronic active hepatitis (after disease is controlled), 500 mg daily in divided doses slowly increased over 3 months; usual maintenance dose 1.25 g
Primary biliary cirrhosis, 250 mg daily, increasing weekly to a maintenance dose of 0.75-1 g daily in divided doses, then reduced as liver copper concentrations return to normal
Cystinuria, 0.5–4 g (usually 1–2 g) daily in divided doses; CHILD 30 mg/kg daily in divided doses; maintain adequate fluid intake

Penicillamine Tablets, f/c, penicillamine 125 mg, price 20 tabs = **D**; 250 mg, price 20 tabs = **F**

Cuprimine® (MSD)
Capsules, yellow, penicillamine 250 mg. Price 20 caps = **E**

Distamine® (Dista)
Tablets, scored, f/c, penicillamine 50 mg. Price 20 tabs = **C**
Tablets, f/c, penicillamine 125 mg. Price 20 tabs = **D**
Tablets, f/c, penicillamine 250 mg. Price 20 tabs = **F**

Pendramine® (BDH)
Tablets, scored, f/c, penicillamine 125 mg. Price 20 tabs = **D**
Tablets, scored, f/c, penicillamine 250 mg. Price 20 tabs = **F**

Chloroquine and **hydroxychloroquine** have a similar action to gold and are better tolerated than either gold or penicillamine but their use is limited by their ocular toxicity. However, retinopathy is rare provided the doses given below are not exceeded. Nevertheless all patients should have a full ophthalmic examination before starting treatment and then subsequently at 3-monthly intervals. Ocular toxicity is also reduced if the drug is not given continuously for longer than 1 year and some physicians advise their patients to stop treatment for 2 months of each year.

These drugs are best **avoided** in elderly patients as it is difficult to distinguish ageing changes from drug-induced retinopathy.

CHLOROQUINE

Indications: active rheumatoid arthritis, systemic lupus erythematosus, discoid lupus erythematosus
Cautions: renal and hepatic impairment, pregnancy, porphyria, psoriasis, elderly patients; regular ophthalmic examinations required (see notes above)
Contra-indications: hypersensitivity to quinine, concurrent therapy with hepatotoxic drugs or sodium aurothiomalate
Side-effects: gastro-intestinal disturbances, headache, visual disturbances, irreversible retinal damage, corneal opacities, depigmentation or loss of hair, skin reactions (sometimes severe—may necessitate discontinuation of treatment), hearing disturbances such as tinnitus, leading rarely to deafness; rarely neuromyopathy, myopathy, psychiatric disturbances, photosensitisation, and blood dyscrasias (usually thrombocytopenia)
Dose: administered with expert advice, initially chloroquine 150–300 mg daily after meals; maintenance chloroquine 150 mg
Note: 150 mg chloroquine ≡ 200 mg chloroquine sulphate ≡ 250 mg chloroquine phosphate (approx.)

Preparations
See section 5.4.1

HYDROXYCHLOROQUINE SULPHATE

Indications: active rheumatoid arthritis, systemic lupus erythematosus, discoid lupus erythematosus
Cautions; Contra-indications; Side-effects: see under Chloroquine and notes (above)
Dose: administered with expert advice, initially 400–600 mg daily in divided doses after meals; maintenance 200–400 mg daily

Plaquenil® (Winthrop)
Tablets, orange, s/c, hydroxychloroquine sulphate 200 mg. Price 20 tabs = **F**

When used in rheumatoid arthritis **immunosuppressants** have a similar action to gold and are useful alternatives in cases that have failed to respond to gold, penicillamine, chloroquine, or hydroxychloroquine.

Azathioprine is usually chosen and is given in a dose of 1.5 to 2.5 mg per kilogram body-weight daily in divided doses. Blood counts should be carried out every 4 to 6 weeks to detect possible neutropenia which is usually resolved by reducing the dose. Nausea, vomiting, and diarrhoea may occur, usually starting early during the course of treatment, and may necessitate withdrawal of the drug. *Herpes zoster* infection may also occur during treatment.

Chlorambucil is another immunosuppressant which is used in rheumatoid arthritis; a dose of 5 mg daily is usually given. Regular blood counts including platelets should be carried out. **Cyclophosphamide** is too toxic for use in rheumatoid arthritis.

Immunosuppressants are also used in the management of severe cases of systemic lupus erythematosus and other connective tissue disorders. They are often given in conjunction with corticosteroids for patients with severe or progressive renal disease though the evidence for their benefit is doubtful. They may be used in cases of polymyositis which are resistant to corticosteroids. They are used for their corticosteroid-sparing effect in patients whose corticosteroid requirements are excessive. **Azathioprine** is usually used but **chlorambucil** is an alternative and **methotrexate** has been used in polymyositis.

Azathioprine and methotrexate are used in the treatment of psoriatic arthropathy for severe or progressive cases which are not controlled with anti-inflammatory drugs. There is an impression that **azathioprine** is the more effective for psoriatic arthritis and that **methotrexate** is the more effective for skin manifestations. Methotrexate is usually given in a dose of 25 mg weekly by mouth. Regular blood counts should be carried out.

See sections 8.1.3 and 8.2.1 for antimetabolites and immunosuppressant drugs and preparations.

10.1.4 Drugs used in the treatment of gout

It is important to distinguish drugs used for the treatment of acute attacks of gout from those used in the long-term control of the disease. The latter exacerbate and prolong the acute manifestations if given during an attack.

Acute attacks of gout are most often treated with **anti-inflammatory analgesics** such as naproxen, indomethacin, and phenylbutazone (section 10.1.1.2). Colchicine is an alternative. Aspirin is contra-indicated in acute gout.

Indomethacin is often chosen in acute attacks. High doses are usually well tolerated for short periods (50 to 100 mg repeated after a few hours if necessary and followed by reducing doses every 6 hours as the patient improves). If courses of treatment last for less than one week side-effects are unusual despite the high doses used.

Colchicine is probably not as effective as indomethacin or phenylbutazone and its use is limited by its toxicity.

In resistant cases of acute gout **corticotrophin** is very effective and is given in a dose of 80 units by intramuscular injection repeated after a day or two if necessary.

There are two possible approaches to the **long-term control of gout.** The formation of uric acid from purines may be reduced with the **xanthine-oxidase inhibitor** allopurinol, or the **uricosuric drugs** probenecid or sulphinpyrazone may be used to increase the excretion of uric acid in the urine. Treatment should be continued indefinitely.

Allopurinol (Zyloric®) is a convenient well tolerated drug which is now widely used. It is especially useful in patients with renal impairment or urate stones where uricosuric drugs cannot be used. It is usually given once daily, as the active metabolite of allopurinol has a long half-life, but amounts over 300 mg daily should be given in divided doses. Allopurinol treatment should not be started within 3 weeks of an acute attack of gout, as further attacks may be precipitated. It is well tolerated in most patients but may occasionally cause rashes.

The uricosuric drugs include **probenecid** (Benemid®) and **sulphinpyrazone** (Anturan®). They can be used instead of treatment with allopurinol, or in conjunction with it in cases that are resistant to treatment.

Salicylates antagonise the uricosuric drugs but they do not antagonise the action of allopurinol. Crystallisation of urate in the urine may occur with the uricosuric drugs and it is important to ensure that there is an adequate urine output especially in the first few weeks of treatment. As an additional precaution the urine may be rendered alkaline.

The number of acute gout attacks may be increased in the first few months of treatment with allopurinol or the uricosuric drugs. It is therefore necessary to give some prophylaxis during this time and colchicine or anti-inflammatory analgesics can also be used for this purpose.

The anti-inflammatory analgesics are described in section 10.1.1.

ALLOPURINOL

Indications: gout prophylaxis, hyperuricaemia

Cautions: administer prophylactic colchicine during initial therapy; ensure adequate fluid intake (2 litres/day); render urine alkaline if uric acid overload is high; reduce dose in renal and hepatic impairment (in renal failure adjustment of dosage is necessary during dialysis). In neoplastic conditions treatment with allopurinol (if required) should be commenced before cytotoxic drugs are given. Drug interactions: see Appendix 1

Contra-indications: acute gout attack and 3 weeks after

Side-effects: most common are rashes, sometimes with fever (may be sign of impending hypersensitivity reaction—withdraw therapy but when rash is mild re-introduce cautiously; discontinue immediately on recurrence); gastro-intestinal disorders. drowsiness. Rarely malaise, headache, vertigo, taste disturbances, hypertension, symptomless xanthine deposits in muscle, alopecia, hepatitis

Dose: initially 100 mg daily as a single dose, after meals, gradually increased over 1–3 weeks according to the serum or urinary uric acid concentration to about 300 mg daily; usual maintenance dose 200–600 mg, rarely 900 mg daily; CHILD 10–20 mg/kg daily

Allopurinol Tablets, allopurinol 100 mg, price 20 tabs = **E**; 300 mg, price 20 tabs = **G**

Caplenal® (Berk)
Tablets, scored, allopurinol 100 mg. Price 20 tabs = **E**

Zyloric® (Calmic)
Tablets, scored, allopurinol 100 mg. Price 20 tabs = **E**
Tablets, scored, allopurinol 300 mg. Price 28 tabs = **I**

COLCHICINE

Indications: acute gout, short-term prophylaxis

during initial therapy with allopurinol and uricosuric drugs
Cautions: elderly and debilitated patients, cardiac, gastro-intestinal, or renal disease, pregnancy and lactation
Side-effects: most common are nausea, vomiting, and abdominal pain; large doses may also cause profuse diarrhoea, gastro-intestinal haemorrhage, rashes, and renal damage. Rarely peripheral neuritis, alopecia, and with prolonged treatment blood dyscrasias
Dose: 1 mg initially, followed by 500 micrograms every 2–3 hours until relief of pain is obtained or vomiting or diarrhoea occurs, or until a total dose of 10 mg has been reached. The course should not be repeated within 3 days. Prevention of attacks during initial treatment with allopurinol or uricosuric drugs, 500 micrograms 2–3 times daily

Colchicine Tablets, colchicine 250 micrograms, price 20 tabs = **A**; 500 micrograms, price 20 tabs = **B**

PROBENECID

Indications: gout prophylaxis, hyperuricaemia; reduction of tubular excretion of penicillins and certain cephalosporins
Cautions: during initial gout therapy administer prophylactic colchicine, ensure adequate fluid intake (about 2 litres daily), render urine alkaline if uric acid overload is high; peptic ulceration, ineffective in renal failure. Drug interactions: see Appendix 1
Contra-indications: concurrent salicylate therapy, blood dyscrasias, nephrolithiasis, acute gout attack and 3 weeks after
Side-effects: infrequent; occasionally nausea and vomiting, urinary frequency, headache, flushing, dizziness, rashes; rarely hypersensitivity, nephrotic syndrome, hepatic necrosis, aplastic anaemia
Dose: uricosuric therapy, initially 250 mg twice daily preferably after meals, increased after a week to 500 mg twice daily then up to 2 g daily in 2–4 divided doses according to serum-uric acid concentration
Penicillin and cephalosporin therapy, 2 g daily; CHILD daily, over 2 years initially 25 mg/kg (700 mg/m^2) then 40 mg/kg (1.2 g/m^2) daily; over 50 kg, adult dose

Benemid® (MSD)
Tablets, scored, probenecid 500 mg. Price 20 tabs = **B**

SULPHINPYRAZONE

Indications: gout prophylaxis, hyperuricaemia
Cautions; Contra-indications: see under Probenecid. Regular blood counts are advisable. Avoid in hypersensitivity to phenylbutazone and related drugs. Drug interactions: see Appendix 1
Side-effects: gastro-intestinal disorders, occasionally hypersensitivity reactions; rarely blood dyscrasias
Dose: 100–200 mg daily in divided doses, with milk or after meals, increasing over 2–3 weeks according to the serum-uric acid concentration to about 600–800 mg daily in divided doses and reducing for maintenance

Anturan® (Geigy)
Tablets, yellow, s/c, sulphinpyrazone 100 mg. Price 20 tabs = **C**
▼ *Tablets*, yellow, s/c, sulphinpyrazone 200 mg. Price 20 tabs = **D**

10.2 Drugs used in other musculoskeletal disorders

Drugs in this section have been divided into those which enhance neuromuscular transmission (section 10.2.1) and muscle relaxants (section 10.2.2)

10.2.1 Drugs which enhance neuromuscular transmission

Anticholinesterase drugs are used to enhance neuromuscular transmission in voluntary and involuntary muscle in conditions such as myasthenia gravis. They prolong the action of acetylcholine by inhibiting the action of the enzyme acetylcholinesterase. Excessive dosage of these drugs may reduce neuromusuclar transmission and precipitate the so-called 'cholinergic crises' by causing a depolarising block. This may be difficult to distinguish from a worsening myasthenic state.

Side-effects of anticholinesterases are due to their parasympathomimetic action. Muscarinic effects include increased sweating, salivary, and gastric secretion, also increased gastro-intestinal and uterine motility, and bradycardia. These effects may be antagonised by atropine.

Edrophonium (Tensilon®) has a very brief action and is therefore used only for the diagnosis of myasthenia gravis. A single test-dose will cause a dramatic but transient improvement in muscle power in patients with the disease.

It can also be used to determine whether a patient with myasthenia is receiving inadequate or excessive treatment with cholinergic drugs; if treatment is excessive an injection of edrophonium would either have no effect or intensify symptoms (cholinergic crisis).

Neostigmine (Prostigmin®) has a longer duration of action than edrophonium and produces a therapeutic effect for up to 4 hours. Its pronounced muscarinic action is a disadvantage, and simultaneous administration of an anticholinergic drug such as atropine or propantheline may be required to prevent colic or excessive salivation. In severe disease neostigmine may be given every 2 hours and the effect may be lost overnight.

Pyridostigmine (Mestinon®) is less powerful and slower in action than neostigmine but it has a longer duration of action. It is preferred in patients whose muscles are weak on wakening. It has a comparatively mild gastro-intestinal effect. Pyridostigmine would therefore appear to have some advantages over neostigmine in the treatment of myasthenia gravis.

Ambenonium (Mytelase®) has a slightly longer duration of action than pyridostigmine.

Distigmine (Ubretid®) has the most protracted action but the danger of a cholinergic crisis caused by accumulation of the drug is greater than with shorter-acting drugs. **Physostigmine** is now mainly used as a miotic (see section 11.6).

Corticosteroids and **immunosuppressants** are also used to improve neuromuscular transmission in myasthenia gravis. Plasmapheresis may also be used.

The anticholinesterases neostigmine and edrophonium are used at the end of anaesthesia to reverse the actions of the non-depolarising muscle relaxants (see section 15.1.6).

AMBENONIUM CHLORIDE

Indications: myasthenia gravis

Cautions; Contra-indications; Side-effects: see under Neostigmine. Atropine should not be given concurrently as it may mask signs of overdosage

Dose: 5–25 mg 3–4 times daily adjusted according to the response; doses above 200 mg daily require careful supervision

Mytelase® (Sterling Research)

Tablets, f/c, ambenonium chloride 10 mg. Price 20 tabs = **D**

DISTIGMINE BROMIDE

Indications: myasthenia gravis

Cautions; Contra-indications; Side-effects: see under Neostigmine

Dose: initially 5 mg daily half an hour before breakfast, increased, according to the response, at intervals of 3–4 days; max. 20 mg daily; CHILD up to 10 mg daily according to age

Ubretid® (Berk)

Tablets, scored, distigmine bromide 5 mg. Price 20 tabs = **I**

EDROPHONIUM CHLORIDE

Indications: diagnosis of myasthenia gravis, detection of under or overdosage with cholinergic drugs (see notes above)

Cautions; Contra-indications; Side-effects: see under Neostigmine

Dose: diagnosis of myasthenia gravis, *by intravenous injection*, 2 mg followed after 30 seconds (if no adverse reaction has occurred) by 8 mg; in adults without suitable veins *by intramuscular injection* 10 mg

Detection of over or underdosage of cholinergic drugs, *by intravenous injection*, 2 mg one hour after the last dose of cholinergic drug

Tensilon® (Roche)

Injection, edrophonium chloride 10 mg/ml. Price 1-ml amp = **B**

NEOSTIGMINE

Indications: treatment and diagnosis of myasthenia gravis

Cautions: asthma, bradycardia, recent myocardial infarction, epilepsy, hypotension, parkinsonism, vagotonia. Atropine or other antidote to muscarinic effects may be necessary, particularly when given by injection

Contra-indications: intestinal or urinary obstruction

Side-effects: nausea, vomiting, increased salivation, diarrhoea, abdominal cramps. Signs of overdosage are increased gastro-intestinal discomfort, bronchial secretions, and sweating, involuntary defaecation and micturition, miosis, nystagmus, bradycardia, hypotension, agitation, excessive dreaming, and weakness eventually leading to paralysis

Dose: by mouth, neostigmine bromide 75–300 mg or more, daily in divided doses at suitable intervals; CHILD, neonate 1–5 mg every 4 hours, older children 15–60 mg daily in divided doses

By subcutaneous, intramuscular, or intravenous injection, neostigmine methylsulphate 1–2.5 mg at suitable intervals; CHILD, neonate 50–250 micrograms every 4 hours, older children 200–500 micrograms daily in divided doses

By intramuscular injection, diagnosis, neostigmine methylsulphate 1–1.5 mg with atropine sulphate 600 micrograms

Prostigmin® (Roche)

Tablets, scored, neostigmine bromide 15 mg. Price 20 tabs = **B**

Injection, neostigmine methylsulphate 500 micrograms/ml. Price 1-ml amp = **A**

Injection, neostigmine methylsulphate 2.5 mg/ml. Price 1-ml amp = **A**

PYRIDOSTIGMINE BROMIDE

Indications: myasthenia gravis

Cautions; Contra-indications; Side-effects: see under Neostigmine; weaker muscarinic action

Dose: by mouth, 0.3-1.2 g daily in divided doses at suitable intervals; CHILD, neonate 5–10 mg every 4 hours, older children 10 mg initially, increased by 5-mg amounts according to response

By subcutaneous, intramuscular or intravenous injection, 2–5 mg daily in divided doses; CHILD, neonate 200–400 micrograms every 4 hours, older children initially 0.25–1 mg, increasing according to response

Mestinon® (Roche)

Tablets, scored, pyridostigmine bromide 60 mg. Price 20 tabs = **C**

Injection, pyridostigmine bromide 1 mg/ml. Price 1-ml amp = **A**

10.2.2 Muscle relaxants

Skeletal muscle relaxant drugs described in this section are used for the relief of muscle spasm or spasticity. They act principally on the central nervous system with the exception of dantrolene which has a peripheral site of action. They differ in action from the muscle relaxants used in anaesthesia (section 15.1.5) which block transmission of impulses at the neuromuscular junction.

A treatable neurological cause for spasticity should be excluded before treatment is begun but the choice of drug is not influenced by the type of spasticity. The major disadvantage of treatment with these drugs is that reduction in muscle tone can cause a loss of splinting action of the spastic leg and trunk muscles which sometimes leads to an increase in disability.

Diazepam is the drug of first choice. Sedation and, occasionally, extensor hypotonus are disadvantages associated with its use. Other benzodiazepines also have muscle-relaxant properties, particularly **chlordiazepoxide**, **ketazolam**, **medazepam**, and **clorazepate**. Muscle-relaxant doses are similar to the anxiolytic doses (section 4.1.2).

Baclofen (Lioresal®) produces a clinical effect similar to diazepam. It acts at spinal level to reduce muscle tone. The dose should be increased slowly to avoid sedation and hypotonia.

Dantrolene (Dantrium®) acts directly on skeletal muscle but nevertheless produces central adverse effects. As with baclofen the dose should be increased slowly.

The clinical efficacy of **carisoprodol**, **chlormezanone**, **meprobamate**, **methocarbamol**, and **orphenadrine citrate** as muscle relaxants is **not** well established. These compounds are often included in compound analgesic preparations (section 4.7.1.3). Tigloidine (Tiglyssin®) has been superseded by more effective drugs for the treatment of muscular rigidity and spasticity.

Quinine is effective in relieving nocturnal leg cramps.

DIAZEPAM

Indications: muscle spasm of varied aetiology
Cautions; Side-effects: see section 4.1.2. Hypotonia may occur. Special precautions are necessary when diazepam is given by intravenous injection
Dose: *by mouth*, 2–15 mg daily in divided doses, increased if necessary to 60 mg according to response
Spasticity with minimal brain damage, CHILD 2–40 mg daily in divided doses
By intramuscular or slow intravenous injection, in acute muscle spasm, 10 mg repeated if necessary after 4 hours; CHILD, 100–200 micrograms/kg, repeated if necessary
By intravenous injection, tetanus, 100–300 micrograms/kg repeated every 1–4 hours

Preparations
See section 4.1.2

BACLOFEN

Indications: muscle spasm in spastic conditions
Cautions: psychiatric illness, cerebrovascular disease, renal impairment, epilepsy; avoid abrupt withdrawal
Side-effects: nausea, vomiting, drowsiness, confusion, fatigue, muscle hypotonia, hypotension
Dose: 5 mg 3 times daily, preferably after meals, gradually increased; max. 100 mg daily; CHILD up to 8 years 5–10 mg daily in 3–4 divided doses, gradually increased to a max. of 40 mg daily; over 8 years 10 mg daily in divded doses, gradually increased to a max. of 60 mg daily

Lioresal® (Ciba)
Tablets, scored, baclofen 10 mg. Price 20 tabs = **E**

CARISOPRODOL

Indications: muscle spasm (see notes above)
Cautions; Side-effects: see under Meprobamate, section 4.1.2. Drowsiness is common
Dose: 350 mg 3–4 times daily

Carisoma® (Pharmax) *tablets*, carisoprodol 125 and 350 mg. Price 20 tabs (both) = **B**
Carisoma Co— see section 4.7.1.3

CHLORMEZANONE

Indications: muscle spasm (see notes above)
Cautions; Side-effects: see under Diazepam (section 4.2.1)
Dose: 200 mg 3 times daily or 400 mg at bedtime; max. 800 mg daily

Trancopal® (Sterling Research) *tablets*, yellow, chlormezanone 200 mg. Price 20 tabs = **D**
Lobak—see section 4.7.1.3
Trancoprin—see section 4.7.1.3

DANTROLENE SODIUM

Indications: muscle spasm in spastic conditions
Cautions: impaired cardiac, pulmonary, and hepatic function; test liver function before and 6 weeks after initiating therapy. Therapeutic effect may take a few weeks to develop but if treatment is ineffective it should be discontinued after 45 days. Patients should not drive or operate machinery until therapy is stabilised. Avoid in children or when spasticity is useful, for example, locomotion. May enhance effects of CNS depressants
Side-effects: transient drowsiness, dizziness, weakness, malaise, fatigue, diarrhoea (reduce dose if necessary), occasionally urinary or musculoskeletal disturbances, rashes, and, rarely, jaundice
Dose: initially 25 mg daily, gradually increased over 7 weeks to a max. of 100 mg 4 times daily

▼ **Dantrium®** (Eaton)
Capsules, orange/cream, dantrolene sodium 25 mg. Price 20 caps = **E**
Capsules, orange/cream, dantrolene sodium 100 mg. Price 20 caps = **H**

MEPROBAMATE

See section 4.1.2

METHOCARBAMOL

Indications: muscle spasm, usually in muscle injury (see notes above)

Cautions: may enhance action of CNS depressants. Avoid injection in renal impairment

Contra-indications: coma or pre-coma states, brain damage, epilepsy, tachycardia, glaucoma, prostatic hypertrophy, bladder neck obstruction

Side-effects: lassitude, light headedness, dizziness, restlessness, anxiety, confusion, drowsiness, nausea, allergy, convulsions

Dose: *by mouth*, 1.5 g 4 times daily

By intramuscular or slow intravenous injection or infusion, 1–3 g daily in divided doses; max. 3 g daily for 3 days, except in treatment of tetanus

Robaxin 750® (Robins) *tablets*, scored, methocarbamol 750 mg. Price 20 tabs = **D.** *Injection*, methocarbamol 100 mg/ml in aqueous macrogol 300. Price 10-ml amp = **C**

Robaxisal Forte—see section 4.7.1.3

ORPHENADRINE CITRATE

Indications: mild muscle spasm, usually in muscle injury (see notes above)

Cautions; Contra-indications; Side-effects: see under Benzhexol, section 4.9.2. Avoid in children. Anticholinergic effects are infrequent

Dose: *by mouth*, 200–300 mg daily in divided doses (given as slow-release tablets night and morning)

By intramuscular or slow intravenous injection, 60 mg repeated after 12 hours if necessary

Norflex® (Riker) *tablets*, s/r, orphenadrine citrate 100 mg. Price 20 tabs = **C.** *Injection*, orphenadrine citrate 30 mg/ml. Price 2-ml amp = **C**

Norgesic—see section 4.7.1.3

QUININE

Indications: nocturnal leg cramps

Cautions: cardiac disease

Contra-indications: pregnancy, particularly near term, optic neuritis

Side-effects: repeated high doses cause hearing disturbances (tinnitus, deafness), visual disturbances, rarely hypersensitivity

Dose: quinine bisulphate, dihydrochloride, hydrochloride, or sulphate 200–300 mg at bedtime

Preparations

See section 5.4.1

TIGLOIDINE HYDROBROMIDE

Indications: muscle spasm in spasticity (see notes above)

Cautions; Side-effects: see under Benzhexol, section 4.9.2; anticholinergic effects are rare but caution in glaucoma

Dose: 1–2 g daily in 3 divided doses after meals

Tiglyssin® (DF) *tablets*, tigloidine hydrobromide 250 mg. Price 20 tabs = **E**

10.3 Drugs for the relief of soft-tissue inflammation

10.3.1 Enzymes

The enzymes in this section have fibrinolytic or proteolytic activity. Their therapeutic effectiveness is **doubtful**. They are claimed to relieve inflammation, bruising, swelling, and other soft-tissue trauma by removing coagulated blood, exudate, and necrotic tissue. They include **bromelains, chymotrypsin, deoxyribonuclease, streptokinase-streptodornase**, and **trypsin**. Some are also used to facilitate expectoration by liquefaction of bronchial secretions. See section 2.10 for streptokinase and urokinase, which also have fibrinolytic activity, and section 13.13 for desloughing agents used in ulcer treatment.

Hyaluronidase (Hyalase®) is used to render the tissues more easily permeable to injected fluids.

BROMELAINS

Indications: adjunctive treatment of soft tissue inflammation and oedema

Cautions; Side-effects: see under Chymotrypsin

Ananase Forte® (Rorer)

Tablets, orange, e/c, bromelains 100 000 Rorer units. Price 20 tabs = **D**

Dose: 1 tablet 4 times daily

CHYMOTRYPSIN

Indications: adjunctive treatment of soft-tissue inflammation and oedema

Cautions: severe hepatic and renal impairment, anticoagulant therapy; test for sensitivity before intramuscular injection

Side-effects: nausea, vomiting, diarrhoea, rarely severe hypersensitivity, rash

Dose: *by mouth*, alpha-chymotrypsin 100 000 USP units 4 times daily, half an hour before meals

By intramuscular injection, alpha-chymotrypsin 5000 USP units 1–3 times daily

Chymar® (Armour)

Injection, powder for reconstitution, alpha-chymotrypsin 5000 USP units. Price vial (with diluent) = **C**

Chymoral® (Armour)

Tablets, red, e/c, trypsin, alpha-chymotrypsin, providing 50 000 USP units. Price 20 tabs = **D**

Tablets forte, pink, e/c, twice strength of Chymoral Tablets. Price 20 tabs = **E**

Deanase DC® (Consolidated)

Tablets, e/c, delta-chymotrypsin 10 mg. Price 20 tabs = **D**

Dose: 2 tablets twice daily for 3 days then 1 twice daily

DEOXYRIBONUCLEASE

Indications: removal of tissue exudate and coagulated blood

Side-effects: irritation on local application and hypersensitivity on prolonged use; bronchospasm and irritation of the respiratory tract on inhalation of an aerosol

Dose: *by aerosol inhalation*, 250 000 units in 10 ml sterile water twice daily

By intramuscular injection (every 2 days as required) or *by intravenous injection*, (for immediate effect) 1 mega-unit

Local injection, 1 mega-unit in 2–3 ml of sodium chloride intravenous infusion 0.9%

For bladder irrigation, 1 mega-unit in 50 ml sterile water

Deanase® (Consolidated)

Powder, deoxyribonuclease (pancreatic) 250 000 units and 1 mega-unit (stated to be synergised with magnesium ions). For preparation of injections or solutions for inhalation or instillation. Price 250 000-unit vial = **D**; 1 mega-unit vial = **F**

HYALURONIDASE

Indications: to enhance permeation of subcutaneous or intramuscular injections, local anaesthetics, and subcutaneous infusions; soft-tissue inflammation

Contra-indications: intravenous injection, bites or stings, infection or malignancy at injection site

Side-effects: hypersensitivity

Dose: to enhance tissue permeability, *by subcutaneous or intramuscular injection*, usually 1500 units, either mixed with the injection fluid or injected into the site, before injection is administered

By subcutaneous infusion, 500–1500 units mixed with 500–1000 ml infusion fluid

Hyalase® (Fisons)

Injection, powder for reconstitution, hyaluronidase (ovine). Price 1500-unit amp = **B**

STREPTOKINASE-STREPTODORNASE

Indications: removal of tissue exudates and coagulated blood

Cautions: disturbances of blood-clotting mechanisms, history of collagen disease

Contra-indications: haemorrhage, reduced plasminogen or fibrinogen concentrations

Side-effects: rarely allergic reactions

Varidase® (Lederle)

Tablets, peach, streptokinase 10 000 units, streptodornase 2500 units. Price 12 tabs = **G**

Dose: 1 tablet 4 times daily for 4–6 days

Topical (= powder), streptokinase 100 000 units, streptodornase 25 000 units. For preparing solutions for topical use. Price per vial = **G**

TRYPSIN

Indications: removal of tissue exudates, necrotic tissue, and coagulated blood in body cavities

Cautions; Side-effects: see under Chymotrypsin; avoid bleeding areas, ulcerating carcinomas, and aerosol inhalation in asthmatics or oral or nasal lesions; local application may cause severe burning

Trypure® (Novo)

Powder, trypsin 45 000 USP units/g (approx.). Price 50-mg vial (with diluent) = **C**

For use in body cavities

Dispersible powder, trypsin 1% for topical application. Price 5-g sprinkler bottle with 45 ml wetting solution containing lignocaine hydrochloride 2% = **D**

Spray pack, trypsin 1% for topical applications. Price 25-g aerosol container with 45 ml wetting solution containing lignocaine hydrochloride 2% = **G**

10.3.2 Rubefacients

These preparations act by counter-irritation. Pain, whether superficial or deep-seated, is relieved by any method which itself produces irritation of the skin, for example, heat or mustard oil. There is little evidence that the blood supply to the viscera is improved by stimulation of the skin.

Counter-irritation is comforting in painful lesions of the muscles, tendons, and joints, and in non-articular rheumatism. An unnecessarily large number of substances have been, and still are, used as counter-irritants. They probably all act through the same essential mechanism and differ mainly in intensity and duration of action.

There is no satisfactory evidence that preparations of adrenaline or aspirin, applied topically are of value in the relief of deep-seated pain.

Liniments and **ointments** should be applied with gentle massage 2–3 times daily avoiding broken or inflamed skin.

Adrenaline Cream (Drug Tariff Formula), adrenaline solution 20 ml, chlorocresol 100 mg, emulsifying ointment 30 g, dilute hydrochloric acid 0.04 ml, sodium metabisulphite 40 mg/100 g, in purified water, freshly boiled and cooled (contains adrenaline 1 in 5000). Price 50 g = **A**

Kaolin Poultice, heavy kaolin 52.7%, thymol 0.05%, boric acid 4.5%, peppermint oil 0.05%, methyl salicylate 0.2%, glycerol 42.5%. Price 200 g = **B**. Warm and apply directly or between layers of muslin; avoid application of overheated poultice

Kaolin Poultice K/L Pack® (K/L Pharmaceuticals)

Kaolin poultice. Price 4 × 100-g pouches = **E**

Immerse one pouch in boiling water for up to 40 seconds, remove cover, and apply

Methyl Salicylate Liniment, methyl salicylate 25% see Formulary. Price 100 ml = **B**

Methyl Salicylate Ointment, methyl salicylate 50%, white beeswax 25%, hydrous wool fat 25%. Price 100 g = **C**

Turpentine Liniment, turpentine oil 65%, camphor 5%, soft soap 7.5%, water 22.5%. Price 100 ml = **B**

White Liniment, turpentine oil 25%, ammonium chloride 1.25%, dilute ammonia solution 4.5%, oleic acid 8.5%, water 62.5%. Price 100 ml = **A**

Algesal® (Nicholas) *cream*, diethylamine salicylate. Price 40 g = **B**

Algipan® (Wyeth) *balm* (= cream), methyl nicotinate, capsicum oleoresin, glycol salicylate, histamine dihydrochloride. Price 40 g = **B**

Aradolene® (Rorer) *cream*, diethylamine salicylate, 'capsicin water-soluble', menthol, rectified camphor oil. Price 40 g = **B**

Aspellin® (Rorer) *liniment*, ammonium salicylate, camphor, menthol, ethyl and methyl salicylates. Price 100 ml = **B**. *Spray*, same ingredients as liniment. Price 130 ml = **C**

Balmosa® (Pharmax) *cream*, camphor, capsicum oleoresin, menthol, methyl salicylate. Price 20 and 40 g (both) = **B**

Bayolin® (Bayer) *cream*, benzyl nicotinate, glycol salicylate, heparinoid. Price 35 g = **C**

Bengué's Balsam® (Bengué) *balsam* (= ointment), menthol, methyl salicylate. Price 25 g = **B**

Bengué's Balsam SG® (Bengué) *balsam* (=cream), menthol, methyl salicylate. Price 25 g = **B**

Cremalgex® (Norton) *cream*, capsicum oleoresin, glycol salicylate, histamine hydrochloride, methyl nicotinate. Price 30 g = **B**

Cremalgin® (Berk) *cream*, capsicum oleoresin, glycol salicylate, histamine hydrochloride, methyl nicotinate. Price 50 g = **C**

Cremathurm® (Sinclair) *cream*, capsicum oleoresin, ethyl nicotinate, histamine acid phosphate, methyl salicylate. Price 25 g = **B**

▼ Difflam® (Carnegie) *cream*, benzydamine hydrochloride 3%. Price 30 g = **E**

Dubam® (Norma) *aerosol* (= application), glycol salicylate, methyl nicotinate, methyl salicylate. Price 113-g aerosol spray = **C**

Finalgon® (Boehringer Ingelheim) *ointment*, butoxyethyl nicotinate, vanillylnonanamide. Price 20 g (with applicator) = **B**

Intralgin® (Riker) *gel*, salicylamide, benzocaine. Price 50 g = **C**

Movelat® (Luitpold-Werk) *cream*, corticosteroids, a heparinoid, salicylic acid. Price 50 g = **D**. *Gel*, same constituents as cream in water-miscible basis. Price 50 g = **D**

P.R. Spray® (Crookes Products) *aerosol spray* (= application), dichlorodifluoromethane, trichlorofluoromethane. Price 200-g spray = **B**

Skefron® (SK&F) *aerosol jet* (= application), dichlorodifluoromethane, trichlorofluoromethane. Price 200-g spray = **C**

Transvasin® (R&C) *cream*, benzocaine, ethyl nicotinate, hexyl nicotinate, tetrahydrofurfuryl salicylate. Price 30 g = **B**

11: Drugs acting on the
EYE

In this chapter, drug treatment is discussed under the following headings:

The entries in this chapter generally relate only to local eye treatment. Systemic indications and side-effects of many of the drugs are given elsewhere (see index).

11.1 Administration of drugs to the eye

EYE-DROPS AND EYE OINTMENTS. When administered in the form of eye-drops, drugs penetrate the eyeball, probably through the cornea. However, systemic effects, which are usually undesirable, may well arise from absorption of drugs into the general circulation via conjunctival vessels or from the nasal mucosa after the excess of the preparation has drained down through the tear ducts. For example, timolol maleate (a beta$_1$-adrenoceptor blocking drug), administered as eye-drops reduces pulse rate.

Eye ointments are often applied to lid margins for blepharitis. They may also be used in the conjunctival sac for other conditions especially where a prolonged action is required.

EYE LOTIONS. These are solutions for the irrigation of the conjuctival sac. They act mechanically to flush out irritants or foreign bodies or to remove infected discharges. **Sodium Chloride Eye Lotion** (section 11.8.2) is widely used. However, the lotion, which is sterile, should be used once only from a previously unopened container for first aid, while for treatment it should be used for no longer than 24 hours after the container is first opened. A convenient alternative is **Sodium Chloride Intravenous Infusion** 0.9% which is identical in composition to the eye lotion. In emergency, tap water drawn freshly from the main (not stored water) will suffice.

OTHER PREPARATIONS. Subconjunctival injection may be used to administer anti-infective drugs, mydriatics, or corticosteroids. The drug diffuses through the sclera to the anterior and posterior chambers and vitreous humour in higher concentration than can be achieved by absorption from eye-drops. However, because the dose-volume is limited (usually not more than 1 ml), this route is suitable only for drugs which are readily soluble.

Drugs such as antibiotics and corticosteroids may be administered systemically to treat an eye condition.

Suitable plastic devices which gradually release a specified amount of drug over a period of, say, 1 week are also used (for example Ocuserts®).

11.2 Control of microbial contamination

Preparations for the eye should be sterile when issued. For routine domiciliary use they are supplied in multiple-application containers for individual use. They contain a suitable preservative and provided that contamination is avoided they may be used for about one month after which a new container should be opened (if treatment is to be continued) and the old one discarded.

In eye surgery it is wise to use single-application containers. Preparations used during intra-ocular procedures and others that may penetrate into the anterior chamber must be isotonic and without preservatives and buffered if necessary to a neutral pH. Large volume intravenous infusion preparations are not suitable for this purpose. For all surgical procedures, a previously unopened container is used for each patient.

11.3 Anti-infective preparations

11.3.1 Topical preparations

Lachrymation quickly dilutes or eliminates aqueous solutions. Ideally, therefore, eye-drops should therefore be instilled (after an initial loading with drops every 10 minutes for half an hour) hourly for the first day or so. It may be worth advising that the upper eyelid be lifted, the patient being recumbent, and 1 or 2 drops directed into the upper fornix.

A reasonable alternative for night-time use is an eye ointment because of its longer action. In addition it will soften crusts which cause the lids and eye lashes to adhere together when the patient is asleep. A small quantity of eye ointment is applied to the eye or lid margin as appropriate.

Dibromopropamidine isethionate eye ointment (Brolene®) is suitable for the treament of **blepharitis** and acute and chronic **conjunctivitis. Propamidine isethionate** is used similarly in the form of eye-drops. The use of **mercuric oxide eye ointment,** even for short periods, is **not recommended**.

When prescribing antibiotics, in general, it is preferable to use topically in the eye antibiotics that are seldom or never used for systemic infections. However, the possibility of systemic absorption (see above under 11.1) must be taken into consideration. Examples of antibiotics with a wide spectrum of activity are **chloramphenicol, framycetin, neomycin,** and **polymyxin B**. **Gentamicin** is effective for treating infections due to *Pseudomonas aeruginosa.* Another antibacterial drug is **sulphacetamide** used at strengths of 10 to 30% in eye-drops and as a 2.5 or 6% eye ointment.

Many antibiotic preparations also incorporate a corticosteroid but such mixtures should **not** be used unless a patient is under close specialist supervision (section 11.4). A 'red eye' is sometimes caused by the *Herpes simplex* virus which produces a dendritic ulcer. This may be difficult to diagnose. Treatment with corticosteroids with or without antibiotics will aggravate the condition with a significant chance of loss of vision or even loss of the eye.

Herpes simplex infections producing, for example, dendritic corneal ulcer can be treated with **idoxuridine**. Eye-drops containing 0.1% are applied every hour during the day and every 2 hours at night; eye ointment containing 0.5% is applied every 4 hours. Alternatively **vidarabine** (Vira-A®) may be applied as a 3% eye ointment 5 times a day. **Acyclovir** (Zovirax®) is a new drug that is activated within herpes-infected cells. For the treatment of *Herpes simplex* infections a 3% eye ointment is applied 5 times a day.

For mass **antitrachomal** treatment, the WHO recommends **tetracycline hydrochloride** eye ointment (Achromycin®); **chlortetracycline** eye ointment is also used. It is applied to both eyes twice daily for 5 days in each month for 6 months. Chloramphenicol is not as effective.

ACYCLOVIR

Indications: see notes above

▼Zovirax® (Wellcome)
Eye ointment, acyclovir 3%. Price 4.5 g = **G**

CHLORAMPHENICOL

Indications: local treatment of infections (see notes above)
Apply eye-drops or eye ointment every 3 hours

Chloramphenicol Eye-drops, chloramphenicol 0.5%. Price 10 ml = **B**

Chloromycetin® (P-D)
Ophthalmic ointment (= eye ointment), chloramphenicol 1%. Price 4 g = **C**
Redidrops (= eye-drops), chloramphenicol 0.5%. Price 5 ml = **C**; 10 ml = **D**

Minims Chloramphenicol® (S&N Pharm.)
Eye-drops, chloramphenicol 0.5%. Price 20 × 0.5 ml = **F**

Opulets Chloramphenicol® (Alcon)
Eye-drops, chloramphenicol 0.5%. Price 20 × 0.25 ml = **F**

Sno-Phenicol® (S&N Pharm.)
Eye-drops, chloramphenicol 0.5%, in a viscous vehicle. Price 10 ml = **C**

CHLORTETRACYCLINE HYDROCHLORIDE

Indications: local treatment of infections, including trachoma (see notes above)
Apply eye ointment every 2 hours (acute infections)

Aureomycin® (Lederle)
Ophthalmic ointment (= eye ointment), chlortetracycline hydrochloride 1%. Price 3.5 g = **C**

DIBROMOPROPAMIDINE ISETHIONATE

Indications: local treatment of infections (see notes above)
Apply eye ointment 2–3 times daily

Brolene® (M&B)
Eye ointment, dibromopropamidine isethionate 0.15%. Price 5 g = **C**

FRAMYCETIN SULPHATE

Indications: local treatment of infections (see notes above)
Apply eye-drops or eye ointment 3–4 times daily

Framycetin Sulphate Eye-drops, framycetin sulphate 0.5%. Price 5 ml = **D**; 8 ml = **E**

Framycetin Sulphate Eye Ointment, framycetin sulphate 0.5%. Price 3.5 and 5 g (both) = **C**

Framygen® (Fisons)
Drops (for ear or eye), framycetin sulphate 0.5%. Price 5 ml = **D**
Eye ointment, framycetin sulphate 0.5%. Price 3.5 g = **C**

Soframycin® (Roussel)
Eye-drops, framycetin sulphate 0.5%. Price 8 ml = **E**
Eye ointment, framycetin sulphate 0.5%. Price 5 g = **C**
Ophthalmic powder, framycetin sulphate (sterile) for preparing subconjunctival injections. Price 500-mg vial = **E**

GENTAMICIN

Indications: local treatment of infection (see notes above)
Apply eye-drops 3–6 times daily

Gentamicin Eye-drops, gentamicin 0.3% (as sulphate). Price 5 and 10 ml (both) = **D**

Alcomicin® (Alcon)
Eye-drops, gentamicin 0.3% (as sulphate). Price 5 ml = **D**

Genticin® (Nicholas)
Eye-drops, gentamicin 0.3% (as sulphate). Price 10 ml = **D**

IDOXURIDINE

Indications: local treatment of *Herpes simplex* infections (see notes above)

Idoxuridine Eye-drops, idoxuridine 0.1%. Price 10 ml = **D**; 15 ml = **E**

Idoxuridine Eye Ointment, idoxuridine 0.5%. Price 3 g = **C**; 5 g = **F**

Dendrid® (Alcon)
Eye-drops, idoxuridine 0.1%. Price 15 ml = **D**

Idoxene® (Spodefell)
Eye ointment, idoxuridine 0.5%. Price 3 g = **C**

Kerecid® (SK&F)
Eye-drops, idoxuridine 0.1%. Price 15 ml = **F**
Eye ointment, idoxuridine 0.5%. Price 5 g = **F**

Ophthalmadine® (SAS)
Eye-drops, idoxuridine 0.1%. Price 10 ml = **D**
Eye ointment, idoxuridine 0.5%. Price 3 g = **D**

MAFENIDE PROPIONATE

Indications: local treatment of infections
Apply eye-drops 3–4 times daily

Sulfomyl® (Winthrop)
Eye-drops, mafenide propionate 5%. Price 10 ml = **C**

MERCURIC OXIDE

Indications: local treatment of infections (see notes above)

Mercuric Oxide Eye Ointment, mercuric oxide 1%. Price 3 g = **A**

NEOMYCIN SULPHATE

Indications: local treatment of infections (see notes above)
Apply eye-drops or eye ointment 3–4 times daily

Neomycin Sulphate Eye-drops, neomycin sulphate 0.5%. Price 10 ml = **C**

Graneodin® (Squibb)
Ophthalmic ointment (= eye ointment), gramicidin 0.025%, neomycin sulphate 0.25%. Price 3.6 g = **B**

Minims Neomycin Sulphate® (S&N Pharm.)
Eye-drops, neomycin sulphate 0.5%. Price 20 × 0.5 ml = **F**

Myciguent® (Upjohn)
Eye ointment, neomycin sulphate 0.5%. Price 3.9 g = **B**

Neosporin® (Calmic)
Eye-drops, gramicidin 25 units, neomycin sulphate 1700 units, polymyxin B sulphate 5000 units/ml. Price 5 ml = **D**

Nivemycin® (Boots)
Eye-drops, neomycin sulphate 0.5%. Price 10 ml = **B**

POLYMYXIN B SULPHATE

Indications: local treatment of infections (see notes above)

Polyfax® (Calmic)
Ophthalmic ointment (= eye ointment), polymyxin B sulphate 10000 units, bacitracin zinc 500 units/g. Price 4 g = **C**
Apply twice daily

Terramycin with Polymyxin B Sulphate® (Pfizer)
Ophthalmic ointment (= eye ointment), oxytetracycline 5 mg (as hydrochloride), polymyxin B sulphate 10 000 units/g. Price 3.5 g = **B**
Apply 4–6 times daily

PROPAMIDINE ISETHIONATE

Indications: local treatment of infections (see notes above)

Brolene® (M&B)
Eye-drops, propamidine isethionate 0.1%. Price 10 ml = **C**
Apply 4 times daily

SULPHACETAMIDE SODIUM

Indications: local treatment of infections (see notes above)
Apply eye-drops or eye ointment every 2–12 hours

Sulphacetamide Eye-drops, sulphacetamide sodium 10 and 30%. Price 10 ml (both) = **C**
Note: when Weak Sulphacetamide Eye-drops are prescribed a 10% solution is supplied; when Strong Sulphacetamide Eye-drops are prescribed a 30% solution is supplied

Albucid® (Nicholas)
Eye-drops, sulphacetamide sodium 10, 20, and 30%. Price 10 ml (all) = **C**
Eye ointment, sulphacetamide sodium 2.5 and 6%, greasy basis. Price 4 g (both) = **C**
Eye ointment, sulphacetamide sodium 10%, water-miscible basis. Price 4 g = **C**

Bleph-10 Liquifilm® (Allergan)
Eye-drops, sulphacetamide sodium 10%. Price 5 ml = **B**

Isopto Cetamide® (Alcon)
Eye-drops, sulphacetamide sodium 15%, hypromellose 0.5%. Price 15 ml = **D**

Minims Sulphacetamide Sodium® (S&N Pharm.)
Eye-drops, sulphacetamide sodium 10%. Price 20 × 0.5 ml = **F**

Ocusol® (Boots)
Eye-drops, sulphacetamide sodium 5%, zinc sulphate 0.1%. Price 10 ml = **B**

TETRACYCLINE HYDROCHLORIDE

Indications: local treatment of infections, including trachoma (see notes above)
Apply eye-drops or eye ointment every 2–12 hours

Achromycin® (Lederle)
Ophthalmic oil suspension (= eye-drops), tetracycline hydrochloride 1%, in sesame oil vehicle. Price 6 ml = **D**

Ointment (for ear or eye), tetracycline hydrochloride 1%. Price 3.5 g = **C**

VIDARABINE

Indications: local treatment of *Herpes simplex* infections (see notes above)

▼ **Vira-A®** (P-D)
Eye ointment, vidarabine 3%. Price 3.5 g = **G**

FUNGAL INFECTIONS OF THE EYE

Fungal infections of the cornea tend to occur after agricultural injuries, especially in hot and humid climates. Orbital mycosis is rare, and when it occurs is usually due to direct spread of infection from the paranasal sinuses. It may be advisable to administer natamycin eye-drops 5–10% or eye ointment 1% prophylactically. Increasing age, debility, or immunosuppression by drugs, for example, following renal transplantation, may encourage fungal proliferation in many parts of the body. The spread of infection via the blood-stream occasionally produces a metastatic endophthalmitis.

As with bacteria and viruses, a wide range of fungi have been incriminated in human diseases. Increasing numbers of specific agents are being evolved for intensive therapy followed, as necessary, by long-term treatment. Unfortunately, precise identification is often a slow process. However, the presence on a slide of both yeast forms and filaments suggests *Candida*, especially *C. albicans*, which is common. Intensive treatment with flucytosine eye-drops 1.5% or alternatively clotrimazole 1% or miconazole 1–2% is effective. Flucytosine may also be given by mouth (see section 5.2).

Filaments alone indicate the need for treatment with econazole, at least initially; infections with *Aspergillus* species are commonest in this group. Mycotic keratitis due to *Fusarium solani* (the organism responsible for potato wilt) is becoming more common; it may be treated with econazole or thiabendazole. For *Penicillium* species, econazole or miconazole is used but some isolates are sensitive only to thiabendazole. Amphotericin is best avoided because of toxicity to the epithelium.

AVAILABILITY OF ANTIFUNGAL PREPARATIONS. It should be noted that the drugs mentioned in this section are not generally available as eye-drop formulations in the United Kingdom. Treatment will normally be carried out at specialist centres, but requests for information about supplies of preparations not available commercially should be addressed to the Area Pharmaceutical Officer (or equivalent in Scotland or Northern Ireland) or to Moorfields Eye Hospital, City Road, London EC1V 2PD (01-253 3411).

11.3.2 Systemic preparations

In severe infections, systemic treatment is given in addition to topical therapy as, for example, in gonococcal conjunctivitis in the newborn and infective endophthalmitis. The blood-aqueous barrier usually breaks down in the latter case allowing intra-ocular penetration of systemically administered drugs unless the intra-ocular pressure is raised. Subconjunctival injection of a suitable drug may also help to achieve a high intra-ocular concentration.

Pyrimethamine (see section 5.4.1) administered systemically, is appropriate for treatment of toxoplasma choroidoretinitis; clindamycin, and sulphadiazine are other possibilities.

Other drugs suitable for the systemic treatment of eye infections are included in chapter 5.

11.4 Corticosteroids and other anti-inflammatory preparations

Corticosteroids administered topically, by subconjunctival injection, and systemically have an important place in treating scleritis, iridocyclitis, and some other eye conditions such as iritis which can be usefully treated with corticosteroids on an alternate-day basis. There are two main dangers. The first is aggravation of dendritic corneal ulceration, due to misdiagnosis already referred to (section 11.3.1), when the corticosteroid is administered in eye-drops. Secondly, again arising from the use of eye-drop formulations, a steroid glaucoma may be produced, after a few weeks treatment, in patients predisposed to chronic simple glaucoma, especially with dexamethasone and prednisolone.

Oxyphenbutazone eye ointment (Tanderil®) does not have the disadvantages of corticosteroids and can be used in the treatment of iridocyclitis and episcleritis.

Topical preparations of antihistamines such as eye-drops containing antazoline sulphate and xylometazoline hydrochloride (Otrivine-Antistin®, below) may be used for allergic conjunctivitis.

Mast cell stabilisation by use of sodium cromoglycate eye-drops (Opticrom®) may be useful for vernal catarrh and other allergic forms of conjunctivitis as an alternative to corticosteroids.

ANTAZOLINE SULPHATE

Indications: allergic conjunctivitis

Otrivine-Antistin® (Ciba)
Eye-drops, antazoline sulphate 0.5%, xylometazoline hydrochloride 0.05%. Price 10 ml = **C**
Apply 2–3 times daily

BETAMETHASONE SODIUM PHOSPHATE

Indications: local treatment of inflammation
Cautions; Side-effects: see notes above
Apply eye-drops every 1–2 hours or eye ointment 2–4 times daily

Betnesol® (Glaxo)
Drops (for ear, eye, or nose), betamethasone sodium phosphate 0.1%. Price 5 ml = **C**
Eye ointment, betamethasone sodium phosphate 0.1%. Price 3 g = **C**
Betnesol-N® (Glaxo)
Drops (for ear, eye, or nose), see section 12.1.1.
Eye ointment, betamethasone sodium phosphate 0.1%, neomycin sulphate 0.5%. Price 3 g = **C**

CLOBETASONE BUTYRATE

Indications: local treatment of inflammation
Cautions; Side-effects: see notes above; reduced tendency to raise intra-ocular pressure
Apply eye-drops every 1–6 hours

Eumovate® (Glaxo)
Eye-drops, clobetasone butyrate 0.1%. Price 5 ml = **D**; 10 ml = **F**
Eumovate-N® (Glaxo)
Eye-drops, clobetasone butyrate 0.1%, neomycin sulphate 0.5%. Price 5 ml = **D**; 10 ml = **F**

DEXAMETHASONE

Indications: local treatment of inflammation
Cautions; Side-effects: see notes above
Apply eye-drops every 1–4 hours

Maxidex® (Alcon)
Eye-drops, dexamethasone 0.1%, hypromellose 0.5%. Price 5 ml = **D**; 15 ml = **E**
Maxitrol® (Alcon)
Eye-drops, dexamethasone 0.1%, hypromellose 0.5%, neomycin 0.35% (as sulphate), polymyxin B sulphate 6000 units/ml. Price 5 ml = **D**
Eye ointment, dexamethasone 0.1%, neomycin 0.35% (as sulphate), polymyxin B sulphate 6000 units/g. Price 3.5 g = **D**
Sofradex® (Roussel)
Drops and *ointment* (for ear or eye), see section 12.1.1

FLUOROMETHOLONE

Indications: local treatment of inflammation
Cautions; Side-effects: see notes above
Apply eye-drops every 1–4 hours or eye ointment every 3–4 hours

FML Liquifilm® (Allergan)
Ophthalmic suspension (= eye-drops), fluorometholone 0.1%. Price 5 ml = **D**; 10 ml = **F**

HYDROCORTISONE ACETATE

Indications: local treatment of inflammation
Cautions; Side-effects: see notes above

Chloromycetin Hydrocortisone® (P-D)
Eye ointment, chloramphenicol 1%, hydrocortisone acetate 0.5%. Price 4 g = **C**
Cortucid® (Nicholas)
Eye drop cream (= eye ointment), hydrocortisone acetate 0.5%, sulphacetamide sodium 10%. Price 3 g = **C**
Framycort® (Fisons)
Drops (for ear or eye), framycetin sulphate 0.5%, hydrocortisone acetate 0.5%. Price 5 ml = **D**
Eye ointment, framycetin sulphate 0.5%, hydrocortisone acetate 0.5%. Price 3.5 g = **D**

Hydrocortistab® (Boots)
Eye-drops, hydrocortisone acetate 1%. Price 10 ml = **B**
Eye ointment, hydrocortisone acetate 2.5%. Price 3 g = **B**
Neo-Cortef® (Upjohn)
Drops and *ointment* (for ear or eye), see section 12.1.1

OXYPHENBUTAZONE

Indications: local treatment of inflammation
Apply eye ointment 2–5 times daily

Tanderil® (Geigy)
Eye ointment, oxyphenbutazone 10%. Price 5 g = **C**
Tanderil Chloramphenicol® (Geigy)
Eye ointment, chloramphenicol 1%, oxyphenbutazone 10%. Price 5 g = **C**

PREDNISOLONE SODIUM PHOSPHATE

Indications: local treatment of inflammation
Cautions; Side-effects: see notes above
Apply eye-drops every 1–2 hours

Minims Prednisolone® (S&N Pharm)
Eye-drops, prednisolone sodium phosphate 0.5%. Price 20 × 0.5 ml = **F**
Predsol® (Glaxo)
Drops (for ear or eye), prednisolone sodium phosphate 0.5%. Price 5 ml = **C**; 10 ml = **D**
Predsol-N® (Glaxo) *drops* (for ear or eye), see section 12.1.1
Sulfapred® (Wallace Mfg)
Eye-drops, prednisolone sodium phosphate 0.5%, sulphacetamide sodium 10%. Price 5 ml = **C**

SODIUM CROMOGLYCATE

Indications: allergic conjunctivitis
Apply eye-drops 4 times daily

Opticrom® (Fisons)
Eye-drops, sodium cromoglycate 2%. Price 10 ml = **F**

11.5 Mydriatics and cycloplegics

The two properties of dilatation of the pupil and paralysis of the ciliary muscle are usually possessed equally by anticholinergic drugs applied topically but they vary in potency. Short-acting, relatively weak mydriatics which paralyse the sphincter pupillae are used by the ophthalmologist to allow a better view of the fundus of the eye. The relative potencies and durations of action of the principal drugs, in ascending order are tropicamide (3 hours), lachesine (mydriatic effect 6 hours, cycloplegic effect midway between homatropine and atropine), cyclopentolate, hyoscine, and homatropine (all 24 hours), and atropine (7 days or longer).

Homatropine or **atropine** are preferable for producing cycloplegia for refraction in young children; atropine is the less suitable because of its long duration of action. It is used for the treatment of iridocyclitis mainly to prevent posterior synechiae.

Contact dermatitis is not uncommon with all of the above mydriatic drugs, especially atropine, and toxic systemic reactions to this drug may occur in the very young and the very old.

Mydriasis may be achieved for a few hours by the use of **neutral adrenaline eye-drops** (Eppy® etc.) or **phenylephrine eye-drops**, which stimulate the dilator pupillae muscle. Mydriasis may precipitate acute closed-angle ('congestive') glaucoma in a few patients, usually aged over 60 years, who are predisposed to the condition because of a small eyeball with a shallow anterior chamber and small diameter cornea. A family history is significant. Mydriatics should be avoided in such patients. Alternatively, one pupil only should be dilated at each visit and pilocarpine eye-drops used to re-establish miosis.

ATROPINE SULPHATE

Indications: refraction procedures in young children; see also notes above
Cautions: action persistent, may precipitate glaucoma; see also notes above

Atropine Eye-drops, atropine sulphate 1%. Price 10 ml = **B**
Isopto Atropine® (Alcon)
Eye-drops, atropine sulphate 1%, hypromellose 0.5%. Price 5 ml = **C**
Minims Atropine Sulphate® (S&N Pharm.)
Eye-drops, atropine sulphate 1 and 2%. Price 20 × 0.5 ml (both) = **F**
Opulets Atropine Sulphate® (Alcon)
Eye-drops, atropine 1%. Price 20 × 0.25 ml = **F**

CYCLOPENTOLATE HYDROCHLORIDE

Indications: see notes above
Cautions: patients with raised intra-ocular pressure; see notes above

Minims Cyclopentolate Hydrochloride® (S&N Pharm.)
Eye-drops, cyclopentolate hydrochloride 0.5 and 1%. Price 20 × 0.5 ml (both) = **F**
Mydrilate® (WBP)
Eye-drops, cyclopentolate hydrochloride 0.5 and 1%. Price 5 ml (both) = **C**
Opulets Cyclopentolate Hydrochloride® (Alcon)
Eye-drops, cyclopentolate hydrochloride 1%. Price 20 × 0.25 ml = **F**

HOMATROPINE HYDROBROMIDE

Indications; Cautions: see notes above

Homatropine Eye-drops, homatropine hydrobromide 1 and 2%. Price 10 ml (both) = **C**
Minims Homatropine Hydrobromide® (S&N Pharm.)
Eye-drops, homatropine hydrobromide 2%. Price 20 × 0.5 ml = **F**

HYOSCINE HYDROBROMIDE

Indications; Cautions: see notes above

Hyoscine Eye-drops, usual strength hyoscine hydrobromide 0.25%. Price 10 ml = **B**
Minims Hyoscine Hydrobromide® (S&N Pharm.)
Eye-drops, hyoscine hydrobromide 0.2%. Price 20 × 0.5 ml = **F**

LACHESINE CHLORIDE

Indications: see notes above; useful in patients hypersensitive to other mydriatics
Cautions: see notes above

Lachesine Eye-drops, lachesine chloride 1%. Price 10 ml = **D**

PHENYLEPHRINE HYDROCHLORIDE

Indications; Cautions: see notes above

Phenylephrine Eye-drops, phenylephrine hydrochloride 10%. Price 10 ml = **C**
Isopto Frin® (Alcon)
Eye-drops, phenylephrine hydrochloride 0.12%, hypromellose 0.5%. Price 15 ml = **D**
Minims Phenylephrine Hydrochloride® (S&N Pharm.)
Eye-drops, phenylephrine hydrochloride 10%. Price 20 × 0.5 ml = **F**
Prefrin® (Allergan)
Eye-drops, phenylephrine hydrochloride 0.12%. Price 15 ml = **D**
Zincfrin® (Alcon)
Eye-drops, phenylephrine hydrochloride 0.12%, zinc sulphate 0.25%. Price 15 ml = **D**

TROPICAMIDE

Indications; Cautions: see notes above

Minims Tropicamide® (S&N Pharm.)
Eye-drops, tropicamide 0.5 and 1%. Price 20 × 0.5 ml (both) = **F**
Mydriacyl® (Alcon)
Eye-drops, tropicamide 0.5 and 1%. Price 5 ml (both) = **D**

11.6 Treatment of glaucoma

An abnormally high intra-ocular pressure, glaucoma, may result in blindness associated with pressure-excavation of the optic disk ('glaucomatous cupping'). In virtually all cases, rise in pressure is due to reduced outflow of aqueous humour, the inflow remaining constant. Probably the commonest condition is *chronic simple glaucoma* where the obstruction is in the trabecular meshwork.

Glaucoma may be treated by the application of eye-drops containing miotics, adrenaline, guanethidine, or beta-adrenoceptor blocking drugs such as timolol. Other drugs such as acetazolamide and dichlorphenamide are given by mouth and, in emergency or before surgery, mannitol may be given by intravenous infusion.

MIOTICS. The small pupil is an unfortunate side-effect of these drugs (except when **pilocarpine** is used temporarily while patients await operation for *closed-angle glaucoma)*. The key factor is the opening up of the inefficient drainage channels in the trabecular meshwork resulting from contraction or spasm of the ciliary muscle. This unfortunately also produces accommodation spasm, which is especially disadvantageous in patients under 40 years of age. Pilocarpine has a duration of action of 3 to 4 hours. **Physostigmine** is more potent. It is still used in **physostigmine and pilocarpine eye-drops** but is not usually used now on its own. **Carbachol** is sometimes used to lower intra-ocular pressure, usually in conjunction with other miotics such as physostigmine. In severe cases **ecothiopate iodide** (Phospholine Iodide®) produces a more prolonged potent effect but the risk of cataract and other side-effects has to be weighed against the benefit.

ADRENALINE. This probably acts both by reducing the rate of production of aqueous humour and increasing the outflow through the trabecular meshwork. It is contra-indicated in closed-angle glaucoma because it is a mydriatic, unless an iridectomy has been carried out.

Guanethidine (Ganda®, Ismelin®) enhances and prolongs the effects of adrenaline. It is also used alone and produces an initial mydriasis together with an increased aqueous outflow followed by a miosis and reduced aqueous secretion.

BETA-ADRENOCEPTOR BLOCKING DRUGS. **Timolol maleate** (Timoptol®) a $beta_1$ blocking drug used as 0.25 and 0.5% eye-drops reduces intra-ocular pressure very effectively in chronic simple glaucoma, probably by reducing the rate of production of aqueous humour. Like many other beta-adrenoceptor blocking drugs such as propranolol, it also reduces intra-ocular pressure when administered systemically. Absorption of timolol occurs following topical application. Caution is therefore necessary in patients with asthma, bradycardia, or heart failure.

SYSTEMIC DRUGS. The side-effects of beta-adrenoceptor blocking drugs are probably sufficient to prevent their being prescribed by the ophthalmologist for administration by mouth. Hence **acetazolamide** (Diamox® etc.) will retain a significant place in treatment. It inhibits carbonic anhydrase, hence reducing the bicarbonate in aqueous humour and the water secreted with it, resulting in a fall in the intra-ocular pressure. **Dichlorphenamide** (Daranide®) has a similar but more prolonged action. Both these drugs have a moderate incidence of side-effects, giving rise, especially in the elderly, to parasthesia, lack of appetite, and depression. Intravenous hypertonic **mannitol,** or **glycerol** by mouth, are useful short-term ocular hypotensive drugs. Acetazolamide by intramuscular or intravenous injection is also useful in the pre-operative treatment of closed-angle glaucoma.

ACETAZOLAMIDE

Indications; Side-effects: see notes above
Cautions: drug interactions: see Appendix 1
Dose: *by mouth or by intravenous injection,* initially 500 mg, subsequent doses 250 mg every 6 hours

Acetazolamide Tablets, acetazolamide 250 mg. Price 20 tabs = **B**

Diamox® (Lederle)
Sustets® (= capsules s/r), orange, acetazolamide 500 mg. Price 20 caps = **F**
Dose: 1 capsule twice daily
Tablets, acetazolamide 250 mg. Price 20 tabs = **D**
Sodium Parenteral (= injection), powder for reconstitution, acetazolamide (as sodium salt). Price 500-mg vial = **I**

ADRENALINE

Indications; Contra-indications: see notes above
Apply eye-drops 1–2 times daily

Epifrin® (Allergan)
Eye-drops, adrenaline 1% (as hydrochloride). Price 10 ml = **D**
Eye-drops, adrenaline 2% (as hydrochloride). Price 10 ml = **D**

Eppy® (S&N Pharm.)
Eye-drops, adrenaline 1%. Price 7.5 ml = **D**

Isopto Epinal® (Alcon)
Eye-drops, adrenaline 0.5 and 1% (as borate complex) and hypromellose 0.5%. Price 7.5 ml (both) = **D**

Simplene® (S&N Pharm.)
Eye-drops, adrenaline 0.5 and 1%, in a viscous vehicle. Price 7.5 ml (both) = **E**

CARBACHOL

Indications: see notes above
Apply eye-drops 3 times daily

Isopto Carbachol® (Alcon)
Eye-drops, carbachol 3%, hypromellose 1%. Price 15 ml = **D**

DEMECARIUM BROMIDE®

Indications: glaucoma
Apply eye-drops 1–2 times daily

Tosmilen® (Sinclair)
Eye-drops, demecarium bromide 0.25%. Price 5 ml = **F**
Eye-drops, demecarium bromide 0.5%. Price 5 ml = **G**

DICHLORPHENAMIDE

Indications; Side-effects: see notes above
Dose: initially 100–200 mg, then 100 mg every 12 hours, adjusted according to the patient's response

Daranide® (MSD)
Tablets, yellow, scored, dichlorphenamide 50 mg. Price 20 tabs = **C**
Oratrol® (Alcon)
Tablets, scored, dichlorphenamide 50 mg. Price 20 tabs = **C**

ECOTHIOPATE IODIDE

Indications; Side-effects: see notes above
Apply eye-drops 1–2 times daily

Phospholine Iodide® (Ayerst)
Eye-drops, ecothiopate iodide 0.03% when reconstituted. Price 5 ml = **E**
Eye-drops, ecothiopate iodide 0.06, 0.125, and 0.25% when reconstituted. Price 5 ml (all) = **E**

GUANETHIDINE MONOSULPHATE

Indications: see notes above
Apply eye-drops 1–2 times daily

▼ Ganda® (S&N Pharm.)
Eye-drops '1 + 0.2', guanethidine monosulphate 1%, adrenaline 0.2% in a viscous vehicle. Price 7.5 ml = **E**
Eye-drops '3 + 0.5', guanethidine monosulphate 3%, adrenaline 0.5% in a viscous vehicle. Price 7.5 ml = **F**
Eye-drops '5 + 0.5', guanethidine monosulphate 5%, adrenaline 0.5% in a viscous vehicle. Price 7.5 ml = **F**
Eye-drops '5 + 1', guanethidine monosulphate 5%, adrenaline 1% in a viscous vehicle. Price 7.5 ml = **F**
Ismelin® (Ciba)
Eye-drops, guanethidine monosulphate 5%. Price 5 ml = **D**

PHYSOSTIGMINE SULPHATE

Indications; Side-effects: see notes above
Apply eye-drops 2–6 times daily

Physostigmine Eye-drops, physostigmine sulphate 0.25 and 0.5%. Price 10 ml (both) = **C**
Physostigmine and Pilocarpine Eye-drops, usual strengths physostigmine sulphate 0.25% with pilocarpine hydrochloride 2% or 4% or physostigmine sulphate 0.5% with pilocarpine hydrochloride 4%. Price 10 ml (0.25% with 2%) = **B**; 10 ml (0.25% with 4%) = **C**; 10 ml (0.5% with 4%) = **B**

PILOCARPINE HYDROCHLORIDE

Indications; Side-effects: see notes above
Apply eye-drops 3–6 times daily

Pilocarpine Eye-drops, pilocarpine hydrochloride 0.5, 1, 2, 3, and 4%. Price 10 ml (up to 1%) = **B**; 10 ml (2, 3, and 4%) = **C**
Isopto Carpine® (Alcon)
Eye-drops, pilocarpine hydrochloride 0.5, 1, 2, and 3%, all with hypromellose 0.5%. Price 10 ml (all) = **C**
Eye-drops, pilocarpine hydrochloride 4% or 6% and hypromellose 0.5%. Price 15 ml (both) = **D**
▼ Ocusert® (M&B)
Pilo-20 ocular insert, s/r, pilocarpine 20 micrograms released per hour for 1 week. Price per insert = **E**
Pilo-40 ocular insert, s/r, pilocarpine 40 micrograms released per hour for 1 week. Price per insert = **E**
Sno-Pilo® (S&N Pharm.)
Eye-drops, pilocarpine hydrochloride 0.5, 1, 2, 3, and 4% in a viscous vehicle. Price 10 ml (all) = **C**

PILOCARPINE NITRATE

Indications; Side-effects: see notes above
Apply eye-drops 3–6 times daily

Minims Pilocarpine Nitrate® (S&N Pharm.)
Eye-drops, pilocarpine nitrate 1, 2, 3, and 4%. Price 20 × 0.5 ml (all) = **F**

TIMOLOL MALEATE

Indications; Side-effects: see notes above
Apply eye-drops twice daily

▼ Timoptol® (MSD)
Eye-drops, timolol maleate 0.25 and 0.5%, in Ocumeter® metered-dose unit. Price per unit (both) = **G**

11.7 Local anaesthetics

Oxybuprocaine and amethocaine are probably the most widely used topical local anaesthetics. Proxymetacaine (Ophthaine®) causes less initial stinging and is useful for children. Cocaine, by potentiating noradrenaline, produces useful vasoconstriction, but is now much less used in surgery. Oxybuprocaine or a combined preparation of lignocaine and fluorescein is used for tonometry. Lignocaine, with or without adrenaline, is injected into the eyelids for minor surgery, while a retrobulbar injection may be used for major eye surgery.

AMETHOCAINE HYDROCHLORIDE

Indications: local anaesthetic

Amethocaine Eye-drops, amethocaine hydrochloride 0.5 and 1%. Price 10 ml (0.5%) = **B**; 10 ml (1%) = **C**
Minims Amethocaine Hydrochloride® (S&N Pharm.)
Eye-drops, amethocaine hydrochloride 0.5 and 1%. Price 20 × 0.5 ml (both) = **F**

COCAINE HYDROCHLORIDE
Indications: local anaesthetic

CD **Cocaine Eye-drops,** cocaine hydrochloride 4%. Price 10 ml = **E**
CD **Cocaine and Homatropine Eye-drops,** cocaine hydrochloride 2%, homatropine hydrobromide 2%. Price 10 ml = **D**

LIGNOCAINE HYDROCHLORIDE
Indications: local anaesthetic
Minims Lignocaine and Fluorescein® (S&N Pharm.)
Eye-drops, lignocaine hydrochloride 4%, fluorescein sodium 0.25%. Price 20 × 0.5 ml = **F**
Xylocaine® (Astra)
Eye-drops, lignocaine hydrochloride 4%. Price 4 ml = **D**

OXYBUPROCAINE HYDROCHLORIDE
Indications: local anaesthetic

Minims Benoxinate (Oxybuprocaine) Hydrochloride® (S&N Pharm.)
Eye-drops, oxybuprocaine hydrochloride 0.4%. Price 20 × 0.5 ml = **F**
Opulets Benoxinate (Oxybuprocaine) Hydrochloride® (Alcon)
Eye-drops, oxybuprocaine hydrochloride 0.4%. Price 20 × 0.25 ml = **F**

PROXYMETACAINE HYDROCHLORIDE
Indications: local anaesthetic

Ophthaine® (Squibb)
Eye-drops, proxymetacaine hydrochloride 0.5%. Price 15 ml = **E**

11.8 Miscellaneous ophthalmic preparations

11.8.1 Preparations for tear deficiency

Chronically sore eyes associated with reduced tear secretion, usually in cases of rheumatoid arthritis (Sjögren's syndrome), often respond to hypromellose eye-drops and other similar viscous preparations.

HYPROMELLOSE ETC.
Indications: tear deficiency

Hypromellose Eye-drops, hypromellose 4000 (or 4500 or 5000) 0.3%. Price 10 ml = **B**
Adsorbotear® (Alcon)
Eye-drops, hydroxyethylcellulose 0.44%, macrogol 0.2%, povidone 1.5%. Price 10 ml = **E**
Isopto Alkaline® (Alcon)
Eye-drops, hypromellose 1%. Price 15 ml = **C**
Isopto Plain® (Alcon)
Eye-drops, hypromellose 0.5%. Price 15 ml = **C**
Tears Naturale® (Alcon)
Eye-drops, dextran '70' 0.1%, hypromellose 0.3%. Price 15 ml = **D**

POLYVINYL ALCOHOL
Indications: tear deficiency

Liquifilm Tears® (Allergan)
Eye-drops, polyvinyl alcohol 1.4%. Price 15 ml = **D**

11.8.2 Other preparations

Zinc sulphate is a traditional so-called astringent which has been used in eye-drops for treatment of excessive lachrymation. Zinc sulphate and adrenaline eye-drops is also used but there is a risk in patients predisposed to closed-angle glaucoma. Simple eye ointment is a bland sterile preparation which may be used to remove crusts in blepharitis. Sodium chloride eye lotion has already been mentioned (section 11.1).

Fluorescein sodium and rose bengal are used in diagnostic procedures and for locating damaged areas of the cornea due to injury or disease.

ACETYLCHOLINE CHLORIDE
Indications: cataract surgery, penetrating keratoplasty, iridectomy, and other anterior segment surgery requiring rapid miosis

Miochol® (CooperVision)
Solution for intra-ocular irrigation, acetylcholine chloride 1%, mannitol 3% when reconstituted. Price 2 ml = **F**

CASTOR OIL

Minims Castor Oil® (S&N Pharm.)
Eye-drops, castor oil. Price 20 × 0.5 ml = **F**

CHYMOTRYPSIN
Indications: zonulolysis in intracapsular cataract extraction

Chymar-Zon® (Armour)
Injection, powder for reconstitution, alphachymotrypsin 750 USP units. Price per vial (with diluent) = **J**
Zonulysin® (Henleys)
Injection, powder for reconstitution, alphachymotrypsin 300 USP units (≡ 1.5 microkatals). Price per vial (with diluent) = **E**

FLUORESCEIN SODIUM
Indications: detection of lesions and foreign bodies

Fluorescein Eye-drops, fluorescein sodium 1%. Price 10 ml = **C**

Minims Fluorescein Sodium® (S&N Pharm.) *Eye-drops,* fluorescein sodium 1% or 2%. Price 20 × 0.5 ml (both) = **F**

Opulets Fluorescein Sodium® (Alcon) *Eye-drops,* fluorescein sodium 1%. Price 20 × 0.25 ml = **F**

PARAFFIN, YELLOW, SOFT

Indications: see notes above

Simple Eye Ointment, liquid paraffin 10%, wool fat 10%, in yellow soft paraffin. Price 3 g = **B**

ROSE BENGAL

Indications: detection of lesions

Minims Rose Bengal® (S&N Pharm.) *Eye-drops,* rose bengal 1%. Price 20 × 0.5 ml = **F**

SODIUM CHLORIDE

Indications: irrigation, including first-aid removal of harmful substances

Sodium Chloride Eye Lotion, sodium chloride 0.9%. Price 200 ml = **C**

Minims Sodium Chloride® (S&N Pharm.) *Eye-drops,* sodium chloride 0.9%. Price 20 × 0.5 ml = **F**

Opulets Sodium Chloride® (Alcon) *Eye-drops,* sodium chloride 0.9%. Price 20 × 0.25 ml = **F**

ZINC SULPHATE

Indications; Cautions: see notes above

Zinc Sulphate Eye-drops, zinc sulphate 0.25%. Price 10 ml = **C**

Zinc Sulphate and Adrenaline Eye-drops, zinc sulphate 0.25%, adrenaline acid tartrate 0.09% (equivalent to 1 in 2000 adrenaline). Price 10 ml = **C**

11.9 Contact lenses

Many patients wear these lenses and special care is required in prescribing eye preparations for them. Unless medically indicated the lens should not be worn during intensive courses of treatment for infections. If the patient is wearing hard lenses the use of eye-drops containing anti-inflammatory drugs over long periods of time is to be deprecated. Some drugs can spoil hydrophilic plastic lenses. Therefore unless eye-drops are specifically indicated as safe to use with hydrophilic contact lenses, the lenses should be removed before instillation and not worn during the period of treatment.

Hydrophilic plastic used for many soft contact lenses will selectively bind certain preservatives and could then be a source of irritation. Thiomersal is usually satisfactory. Chlorhexidine acetate is satisfactory in some cases, while phenylmercuric acetate or nitrate is usually satisfactory but is not recommended for long-term treatment. Benzalkonium chloride is unsuitable in all cases.

Sodium chloride solution 0.9% (sterile) can be used to store soft hydrophilic lenses provided that the case with lens and solution are regularly subjected to a heat treatment to reduce microbial contamination (such as 80°C for 40 minutes).

12: Drugs used in the treatment of diseases of the EAR, NOSE, and OROPHARYNX

In this chapter, drug treatment is discussed under the following headings:

12.1 Drugs acting on the ear

12.1.1 Otitis externa

Otitis externa may be due to primary infection with bacteria or fungi, sometimes caused by discharge from the middle ear but frequently due to eczema which may or may not be secondarily infected.

Otitis externa may be treated by local application of ear-drops or ointment. Insufflations may also be used.

Aluminium acetate has a local astringent action and is used in the form of ear-drops (usually on quarter-inch gauze) to reduce pain and swelling. Aluminium acetate ear-drops (8%) must be prepared freshly but is usually preferred to aluminium acetate ear-drops (13%).

If otitis externa is caused by eczema **corticosteroid** ear-drops are suitable. If there is secondary infection with pain and purulent discharge, drops containing corticosteroids and antibiotics may be used, but for a short time only.

In infection the most important treatment is regular and careful cleansing of the ear and removal of discharge. The routine use of local anti-infective preparations should be avoided as far as possible because of sensitivity reactions to the anti-infective and also to certain vehicles such as propylene glycol. Moreover, resistance to the antibacterial may develop, fungal infection may develop, and many antibacterials are ototoxic. However, they may be useful in the short term in conjunction with regular skilled cleansing.

A number of **antibacterial** preparations are available, many also containing corticosteroids. **Clioquinol** (in Locorten-Vioform®) is useful for mild infections. Ear-drops containing chlorhexidine, polymyxins, or aminoglycosides (framycetin, gentamicin, or neomycin) should be **avoided** when the tympanic membrane is perforated for this may lead to permanent deafness. **Chloramphenicol** ear-drops should be **avoided** as they cause a high incidence of hypersensitivity skin reactions (10% of patients) as do **nitrofurazone** ear-drops.

Fungal infections such as aspergillosis are often the result of prolonged use of antibacterial ear-drops. They are often difficult to eradicate and expert advice is required. Even after apparent cure supervision over several months is advised for there may be a recurrence.

There are a number of **compound preparations** containing two or more anti-ineffective drugs, some with corticosteroids; their use has no great advantage over simpler preparations.

Ear-drops or **ointment** should be **applied** using 3–4 drops of a liquid preparation or a similar quantity of ointment warmed if necessary, inserted into the affected ear. If discharge is profuse, ear-drops applied directly may be washed away; in these circumstances the ear canal should be carefully cleaned and a quarter-inch gauze wick impregnated with the ear-drops should be introduced into it.

ASTRINGENT PREPARATIONS

ALUMINIUM ACETATE

Indications: inflammation in otitis externa

Aluminium Acetate Ear-drops (13%), consists of aluminium acetate solution (BPC). Price 20 ml = **A**
Insert into the meatus or apply on a gauze wick which should be kept saturated with the ear-drops

Aluminium Acetate Ear-drops (8%), prepared by diluting 8 parts of aluminium acetate solution (BPC) with 5 parts of purified water, freshly boiled and cooled. It must be freshly prepared. Price 20 ml = **A**
Directions as above

ANTI-INFLAMMATORY PREPARATIONS

BETAMETHASONE SODIUM PHOSPHATE

Indications: eczematous inflammation in otitis externa
Cautions: avoid prolonged use
Contra-indications: untreated infection

Betnesol® (Glaxo)
Drops (for ear, eye, or nose), betamethasone sodium phosphate 0.1%. Price 5 ml = **C**; 10 ml = **D**
Apply every 2–3 hours; reduce frequency of application when relief is obtained

PREDNISOLONE SODIUM PHOSPHATE

Indications: eczematous inflammation in otitis externa
Cautions: avoid prolonged use
Contra-indications: untreated infection

Predsol® (Glaxo)
Drops (for ear or eye), prednisolone sodium phosphate 0.5%. Price 5 ml = **C**; 10 ml = **D**
Apply every 2–3 hours; reduce frequency of application when relief is obtained

ANTI-INFECTIVE PREPARATIONS

CHLORAMPHENICOL

Indications: bacterial infection in otitis externa
Cautions; Contra-indications: see under Framycetin Sulphate
Side-effects: high incidence of sensitivity reactions

Chloramphenicol Ear-drops 5% and **10%,** chloramphenicol in propylene glycol. Price 10 ml (5%) = **A**; 5 ml (10%) = **B**; 10 ml (10%) = **D**
Apply 2–3 times daily

Chloromycetin® (P-D)
Ear-drops, chloramphenicol 10% in propylene glycol. Price 5 ml = **B**

Otopred® (Typharm)
Ear-drops, chloramphenicol 1%, prednisolone 0.25%. Price 3 ml = **C**
Apply 4 times daily; reduce frequency of application to twice daily when relief is obtained

CLIOQUINOL

Indications: mild bacterial or fungal infections in otitis externa
Cautions; Contra-indications: see under Framycetin Sulphate
Side-effects: local sensitivity; stains skin and clothing

Locorten-Vioform® (Ciba)
Ear-drops, clioquinol 1%, flumethasone pivalate 0.02%. Price 7.5 ml = **C**
Apply 2 or more times daily

FRAMYCETIN SULPHATE

Indications: bacterial infection in otitis externa
Cautions: avoid prolonged use; see also notes above
Contra-indications: perforated ear-drum
Side-effects: local sensitivity; ototoxicity (see notes above)

Framycort® (Fisons)
Drops (for ear or eye), framycetin sulphate 0.5%, hydrocortisone acetate 0.5%. Price 5 ml = **E**
Apply 3–4 times daily

Framygen® (Fisons)
Drops (for ear or eye), framycetin sulphate 0.5%. Price 5 ml = **D**
Apply 3–4 times daily

GENTAMICIN

Indications; Cautions; Contra-indications; Side-effects: see under Framycetin Sulphate

Genticin® (Nicholas)
Drops (for ear or eye), gentamicin 0.3% (as sulphate). Price 10 ml = **D**
Apply 3–4 times daily

Gentisone HC® (Nicholas)
Ear-drops, gentamicin 0.3% (as sulphate), hydrocortisone acetate 1%. Price 10 ml = **E**
Apply 3–4 times daily

HALQUINOL

Indications: mild bacterial or fungal infections in otitis externa
Cautions; Contra-indications: see under Framycetin Sulphate
Side-effects: local sensitivity; stains skin and clothing

Remotic® (Squibb)
Ear-drops, halquinol 0.75%, triamcinolone acetonide 0.025% in oil, 0.3-ml yellow single-application capsule. Price 15 caps = **C**
Apply 2–3 times daily

NEOMYCIN SULPHATE

Indications; Cautions; Contra-indications; Side-effects: see under Framycetin Sulphate
Apply ear-drops every 2–3 hours or ear ointments 2–4 times daily. Reduce frequency of application when relief is obtained

Betnesol-N® (Glaxo)
Drops (for ear, eye, or nose), betamethasone sodium phosphate 0.1%, neomycin sulphate 0.5%. Price 5 ml = **C**; 10 ml = **D**

Neo-Cortef® (Upjohn)
Drops (for ear or eye), hydrocortisone acetate 1.5%, neomycin sulphate 0.5%. Price 5 ml = **D**; 10 ml = **E**
Ointment (for ear or eye), hydrocortisone acetate 1.5%, neomycin sulphate 0.5%. Price 3.9 g = **D**

Predsol-N® (Glaxo)
Drops (for ear or eye), neomycin sulphate 0.5%, prednisolone sodium phosphate 0.5%. Price 5 ml = **C**; 10 ml = **D**

NEOMYCIN UNDECENOATE

Indications: bacterial or fungal infections in otitis externa
Cautions; Contra-indications; Side-effects: see under Framycetin Sulphate

Audicort® (Lederle)
Ear-drops, neomycin 0.35%, undecenoic acid 0.7% (as neomycin undecenoate), triamcinolone acetonide 0.1%, benzocaine 5%. Price 5 ml = **E**; 10 ml = **F**
Apply 3–4 times daily

NITROFURAZONE

Indications: bacterial infection in mild otitis externa
Cautions; Contra-indications: see under Framycetin Sulphate

Side-effects: high incidence of sensitivity reactions

Furacin® (Eaton)
Soluble ointment, nitrofurazone 0.2%. Price 25 g = **B**
Solution (= ear-drops), nitrofurazone 0.2%. Price 10 ml = **A**
Apply 3–4 times daily

TETRACYCLINE HYDROCHLORIDE

Indications: susceptible bacterial infection in otitis externa
Cautions; Contra-indications: see under Framycetin Sulphate
Side-effects: local sensitivity; stains skin and clothing

Achromycin® (Lederle)
Ointment (for ear or eye), tetracycline hydrochloride 1%. Price 3.5 g = **C**
Apply every 2 hours

COMPOUND ANTI-INFECTIVE PREPARATIONS

Otoseptil® (Napp)
Ear-drops, hydrocortisone 1 mg, neomycin 670 micrograms (as undecenoate), tyrothricin 1 mg, ethylene oxide-polyoxypropylene glycol condensate 10 mg/ml. Price 8 ml = **D**
Otosporin® (Calmic)
Ear-drops, hydrocortisone 10 mg, neomycin sulphate 3400 units, polymyxin B sulphate 10000 units/ml. Price 5 ml = **E**; 10 ml = **F**
Ototrips® (Consolidated)
Ear-drops, bacitracin 20000 units, polymyxin B sulphate 16000 units, trypsin 25000 USP units, gelatin 15 mg, sodium chloride 27 mg/3 ml when reconstituted. Price 3 ml = **E**
Sofradex® (Roussel)
Drops (for ear or eye), dexamethasone sodium metasulphobenzoate 500 micrograms, framycetin sulphate 5 mg, gramicidin 50 micrograms/ml. Price 8 ml = **E**.
Ointment (for ear or eye), dexamethasone 500 micrograms, framycetin sulphate 5 mg, gramicidin 50 micrograms/g. Price 5 g = **E**
Terra-Cortril® (Pfizer)
Ear suspension (= ear-drops), hydrocortisone acetate 15 mg, oxytetracycline 5 mg (as hydrochloride), polymyxin B sulphate 10000 units/ml. Price 5 ml = **D**
Tri-Adcortyl Otic® (Squibb)
Ear ointment, gramicidin 0.025%, neomycin 0.25% (as sulphate), nystatin 100000 units, triamcinolone acetonide 0.1% in Plastibase®. Price 10 g = **C**

OTHER AURAL PREPARATIONS

Spirit ear-drops and phenol ear-drops are rarely used now: they were used in ears with a perforated drum and discharge, or after mastoid operations to reduce secondary infection. Hydrogen peroxide ear-drops are also obsolete. Choline salicylate and phenazone are mild analgesics but of doubtful value when applied topically. There is no place for the use of local anaesthetics in ear-drops.

Audax® (Napp)
Ear-drops, choline salicylate 20%, ethylene oxide-polyoxypropylene glycol condensate 1.25%. Price 8 ml = **C**
Auralgicin® (Fisons)
Ear-drops, benzocaine 1.4%, chlorbutol 1%, ephedrine hydrochloride 1%, phenazone 5.5%, potassium hydroxyquinoline sulphate 0.1% in glycerol. Price 12.5 ml = **D**
Auraltone® (Rorer)
Ear-drops, benzocaine 1%, phenazone 5% in glycerol. Price 15 ml = **C**
Norgotin® (Norgine)
Ear-drops, amethocaine hydrochloride 1%, chlorhexidine acetate 0.1%, ephedrine hydrochloride 1%, in propylene glycol. Price 16 ml = **C**
Sedonan® (Napp)
Ear-drops, chlorbutol 1%, phenazone 5% in glycerol. Price 8 ml = **B**

12.1.2 Otitis media

Otitis media is a frequent complication of upper respiratory tract infections, especially in children 5–7 years old.

Local treatment is ineffective. Mild attacks may resolve spontaneously but acute attacks should be treated systemically (for suitable antibacterial treatment see section 5.1, table 1). Identification of the infecting organism by bacteriological examination of the discharge, if present, is helpful in selecting the appropriate treatment. Analgesics, such as **aspirin** given by mouth, are used to relieve pain.

Decongestants and mucolytics (see sections 3.7 and 3.10) are of unproved value in relieving "glue ear" in otitis media.

12.1.3 Removal of ear wax

Softening agents are used to facilitate removal of wax. The most effective and least harmful are **sodium bicarbonate ear-drops**, warm **olive oil**, and **glycerol**. Dioctyl sodium sulphosuccinate is also used but is more expensive.

The use of organic solvent preparations to dissolve ear wax should be **avoided**. They are rarely effective and they may cause irritation.

Softening agents should be introduced into the meatus on a cotton-wool plug and left for several hours or overnight. After 3 nights of such treatment the ear is syringed gently with warm water.

Glycerol. Price 10 ml = **A**
Olive Oil (warm before use). Price 10 ml = **A**
Sodium Bicarbonate Ear-drops (see Formulary). Price 10 ml = **A**
Audinorm® (Carlton)
Ear-drops, dioctyl sodium sulphosuccinate 5%, glycerol 10%. Price 12 ml = **B**
Molcer® (Wallace Mfg)
Ear-drops, dioctyl sodium sulphosuccinate 5%. Price 15 ml = **B**
Soliwax® (Concept)
Ear capsules (= ear-drops), dioctyl sodium sulphosuccinate 5% in oil, red, single-application capsules. Price 10 caps = **B**

Waxsol® (Norgine)
Ear-drops, dioctyl sodium sulphosuccinate 5%. Price 16 ml = **C**

Organic solvent preparations for removal of wax

Cerumol® (LAB)
Ear-drops, chlorbutol 5%, paradichlorobenzene 2%, turpentine oil 10%. Price 11 ml = **A**

Xerumenex® (Napp)
Ear-drops, chlorbutol 5%, triethanolamine polypeptide oleate condensate 10%, in propylene glycol. Price 8 ml = **B**

12.2 Drugs acting on the nose

Nasal conditions are frequently treated by local application of nasal drops. As drops impair ciliary function the smallest effective amount should be applied as infrequently as possible. Preservatives in many nasal drops may cause a transient burning sensation within the nose.

12.2.1 Drugs used in nasal allergy
12.2.2 Topical nasal decongestants
12.2.3 Oral nasal decongestants
12.2.4 Anti-infective nasal preparations

12.2.1 Drugs used in nasal allergy

The running nose, sneezing, and nasal obstruction of hay fever and nasal allergy (allergic rhinitis) may be only a minor symptom requiring no therapy, may be a nuisance or, occasionally, may be very disabling and justify systemic **corticosteroid** therapy for short periods, for example with students taking an important examination.

The oral **antihistamines** (see section 3.4.1) are useful for they reduce the rhinorrhoea and sneezing, but usually have less effect on nasal congestion especially in seasonal allergies. A serious disadvantage is that they cause drowsiness in many patients and may impair ability to drive or operate machinery.

Sodium cromoglycate may be effective in preventing both nasal allergies and nonallergic rhinitis. Treatment may be continued for many months in responsive patients. There are no serious side-effects. Local **corticosteroid** preparations applied to the nose by metered-dose spray may be effective.

Oral and intramuscular (depot) corticosteroid preparations (see section 6.3.4) are highly effective in the treatment of nasal allergy, but their use should be reserved for very severe cases. They should be used for as short a period as possible as they impair pituitary-adrenal function.

BECLOMETHASONE DIPROPIONATE

Indications: allergic rhinitis
Cautions: untreated nasal infection, prolonged use, previous treatment with corticosteroids by mouth
Side-effects: sneezing after administration
Dose: *by nasal inhalation*, adults and children over 6 years, 100 micrograms (2 puffs) into each nostril twice daily

Beconase® (A&H)
Nasal spray (= aerosol inhalation), beclomethasone dipropionate 50 micrograms/metered inhalation, 200-dose unit with nasal adapter. Price complete unit = **G**

BETAMETHASONE SODIUM PHOSPHATE

Indications; Cautions; Side-effects: see under Beclomethasone Dipropionate
Dose: *by nasal instillation*, 2–3 drops of 0.1% solution into each nostril 2–3 times daily

Betnesol® (Glaxo)
Drops (for ear, eye, or nose), betamethasone sodium phosphate 0.1%. Price 5 ml = **C**; 10 ml = **D**

FLUNISOLIDE

Indications; Cautions; Side-effects: see under Beclomethasone Dipropionate
Dose: *by nasal inhalation*, 50 micrograms into each nostril 2–3 times daily; CHILD over 5 years 25 micrograms into each nostril, max. 3 times daily

▼ **Syntaris**® (Syntex)
Nasal spray, flunisolide 25 micrograms/0.1 ml metered spray. Price 24 ml with pump and applicator = **G**

HYDROCORTISONE ACETATE

Indications; Cautions; Side-effects: see under Beclomethasone Dipropionate
Dose: *by nasal insufflation*, 15 mg daily in divided doses

Pabracort® (P&B)
Nasal insufflation, capsule, hydrocortisone acetate 15 mg for use with insufflator. Price 10 caps = **C**; 10 caps with insufflator = **E**; 25 caps = **D**

SODIUM CROMOGLYCATE

Indications: prophylaxis of allergic and non-allergic rhinitis (see notes above)
Side-effects: local irritation, particularly during initial treatment with insufflations

Lomusol® (Fisons)
Nasal spray, sodium cromoglycate inhalation 2.6 mg (0.13 ml)/metered spray. Price 2 × 9.5 ml with pump and spray = **G**; 2 × 9.5 ml refill = **G**
Dose: by nasal application, adults and children, 2.6 mg into each nostril 6 times daily

Rynacrom® (Fisons)
Nasal insufflation, cartridges, pink, sodium cromoglycate 10 mg for use with insufflator. Price 20 cartridges = **C**; insufflator = **D**

Dose: by nasal insufflation, adults and children, 10 mg in each nostril up to 4 times daily
Nasal drops, sodium cromoglycate 2%. Price 15 ml = **F**
Dose: by nasal instillation, adults and children, 2 drops into each nostril 6 times daily
Nasal spray, sodium cromoglycate 2%. Price 17.5 ml = **G**
Dose: by nasal application, adults and children, 2 sprays in each nostril 6 times daily

12.2.2 Topical nasal decongestants

Sodium chloride 0.9% given as nasal drops often relieves nasal congestion for it helps to liquefy mucous secretions. Preparations containing **sympathomimetic** drugs produce vasoconstriction of mucosal blood vessels and a decrease in the thickness of the swollen nasal mucosa giving relief to the nasal obstruction. Unfortunately if treatment is prolonged a rebound secondary vasodilatation occurs with recurrence of nasal congestion: further applications of the sympathomimetic preparations result eventually in the development of tolerance, diminished therapeutic effect, and damage to the nasal cilia.

Ephedrine Nasal Drops (0.5 and 1.0%) is the safest preparation, is effective within 1 minute, and last for several hours. Tolerance develops rapidly. It may be useful in infants with feeding difficulty because of nasal congestion. The nostril should be cleaned with cotton wool pledgets soaked in the ephedrine nasal drops just before feeding.

Naphazoline, oxymetazoline, phenylephrine, and **xylometazoline** are more potent than ephedrine, have a longer action, and are more likely to cause rebound nasal congestion. Xylometazoline (Otrivine®) and oxymetazoline (Afrazine®, Iliadin-Mini®) are less liable to induce tolerance than naphazoline and phenylephrine.

Antihistamines applied topically are ineffective.

EPHEDRINE HYDROCHLORIDE

Indications: nasal congestion
Cautions: avoid excessive use; caution in infants under 3 months. Drug interactions: see Appendix 1
Side-effects: local irritation; after excessive use tolerance with diminished effect, rebound congestion

Ephedrine Nasal Drops, ephedrine hydrochloride 0.5% (see Formulary). Price 10 ml = **A**
Instil 1–2 drops into each nostril when required
Ephedrine Nasal Drops 1%, ephedrine hydrochloride 1% (see Formulary). Price 10 ml = **A**
Directions as above

OXYMETAZOLINE HYDROCHLORIDE

Indications: nasal congestion
Cautions; Side-effects: see under Ephedrine Hydrochloride

Afrazine® (Kirby-Warrick)
Nasal drops, oxymetazoline hydrochloride 0.05%. Price 15 ml = **B**
Instil 2–3 drops into each nostril every 8–12 hours when required
Paediatric nasal drops, oxymetazoline hydrochloride 0.025%. Price 15 ml = **B**
CHILD 2–5 years: instil 2–3 drops into each nostril when required
Nasal spray, oxymetazoline hydrochloride 0.05%. Price 15 ml = **B**
2–3 applications to each nostril every 8–12 hours when required
Iliadin Mini® (Merck)
Nasal drops, oxymetazoline hydrochloride 0.05% in 0.3-ml single-application containers. Price 10 units = **C**
Instil half contents of single-application container into each nostril every 8–12 hours when required
Iliadin-Mini Paediatric® (Merck)
Nasal drops, oxymetazoline hydrochloride 0.025% in 0.3-ml single-application containers. Price 10 units = **C**
CHILD under 6 years: instil half contents of single-application container into each nostril every 8–12 hours when required

XYLOMETAZOLINE HYDROCHLORIDE

Indications: nasal congestion
Cautions; Side-effects: see under Ephedrine Hydrochloride

Otrivine® (Ciba)
Nasal drops, xylometazoline hydrochloride 0.1%. Price 14 ml = **B**
Instil 2–3 drops into each nostril every 8–12 hours when required
Paediatric nasal drops, xylometazoline hydrochloride 0.05%. Price 10 ml = **B**
CHILD: instil 1–2 drops into each nostril every 8–12 hours when required
Nasal spray, xylometazoline hydrochloride 0.1%. Price 14 ml = **B**
1–2 applications to each nostril every 8–12 hours when required

OTHER NASAL DECONGESTANT PREPARATIONS

Antistin-Privine® (Ciba)
Nasal drops and *spray*, antazoline sulphate 0.5%, naphazoline nitrate 0.025%. Price 14 ml (both) = **B**
Hayphryn® (Winthrop)
Nasal spray, phenylephrine hydrochloride 0.5%, thenyldiamine hydrochloride 0.1%. Price 15 ml = **B**
Neophryn® (Winthrop)
Nasal drops and *spray*, phenylephrine hydrochloride 0.25%. Price 15 ml (both) = **C**
Otrivine-Antistin® (Ciba)
Nasal drops and *spray*, antazoline sulphate 0.5%, xylometazoline hydrochloride 0.05%. Price 14 ml (both) = **B**

12.2.3 Oral nasal decongestants

These preparations are of doubtful value. Most of them contain antihistamines (which may cause drowsiness affecting the ability to drive or operate machinery), and sympathomimetics (so that they should be avoided in patients taking monoamine-oxidase inhibitor antidepressive drugs, or those suffering from hypertension, hyperthyroidism, or diabetes).

Preparations of this type are included in sections 3.4.1 and 3.10.

12.2.4 Anti-infective nasal preparations

A chlorhexidine and neomycin cream (Naseptin®) is effective in eradicating a staphylococcal carrier state from the nasal vestibule. Otherwise it is doubtful whether there is any place for anti-infective nasal preparations as they are unlikely to affect the course of colds or upper respiratory tract infections and they may cause ciliary damage. Systemic treatment (see section 5.1, table 1) should be used when necessary. Nasal drops contining mild silver protein are rarely used because of the risk of argyria.

Argotone® (Rona)
Nasal drops, ephedrine hydrochloride 0.9%, mild silver protein 1%. Price 20 ml = **B**.
Nasal spray, ephedrine hydrochloride 0.9%, mild silver protein 1%. Price 15 ml = **B**

Betnesol-N® (Glaxo)
Drops (for ear, eye, and nose), betamethasone sodium phosphate 0.1%, neomycin sulphate 0.5%. Price 5 ml = **C**; 10 ml = **D**

Biomydrin® (Warner)
Nasal spray, gramicidin 0.005%, neomycin sulphate 0.1%, thonzylamine hydrochloride 1%, phenylephrine hydrochloride 0.25%. Price 15 ml = **B**

Dexa-Rhinaspray® (Boehringer Ingelheim)
Nasal inhalation, dexamethasone 21-isonicotinate 20 micrograms, neomycin sulphate 100 micrograms, tramazoline hydrochloride 120 micrograms/metered inhalation. Price 125-dose unit = **E**

Locabiotal® (Servier)
Nasal inhalation, fusafungine 125 micrograms/metered inhalation. Price 200-dose unit = **D**

Naseptin® (ICI)
Cream, chlorhexidine hydrochloride 0.1%, neomycin sulphate 0.5%. Do not dilute. Price 5 g = **B**
For treatment of staphylococcal infections apply to nostrils 4 times daily for 10 days; for preventing nasal carriage of staphylococcal infections apply to nostrils twice daily. Avoid contact with eyes and ears

Rhinamid® (Bengué)
Nasal drops, butacaine sulphate 0.026%, ephedrine hydrochloride 1%, sulphanilamide 0.4%. Price 30 ml = **B**

Soframycin® (Roussel)
Nebuliser, framycetin sulphate 12.5 mg, gramicidin 50 micrograms, phenylephrine hydrochloride 2.5 mg/ml. Price 15 ml = **D**

Vibrocil® (Zyma)
Nasal drops, dimethindene maleate 250 micrograms, neomycin sulphate 3.5 mg, phenylephrine 2.5 mg/ml. Price 15 ml = **B**.
Nasal gel, dimethindene maleate 250 micrograms, neomycin sulphate 3.5 mg, phenylephrine 2.5 mg/g. Price 12 g = **B**.
Nasal spray, dimethindene maleate 250 micrograms, neomycin sulphate 3.5 mg, phenylephrine 2.5 mg/ml. Price 10 ml = **B**

12.3 Drugs acting on the oropharynx

12.3.1 Drugs used in non-specific mouth ulceration (aphthous ulcers)

Recurrent single or multiple aphthous ulcers are often a nuisance and occasionally are extremely painful. Local treatment aims at protecting the ulcerated area and enabling healing to occur, and at relieving pain or reducing inflammation, but it is difficult to retain the drug in contact with the lesion. A **carboxymethylcellulose gelatin paste** (Orabase®) or **powder** (Orahesive®) has a mechanical protective effect. **Corticosteroids** in lozenges (Corlan®) or in paste (Adcortyl in Orabase®) are the most effective. **Carbenoxolone sodium gel** (Bioral®) and **tetracycline mouth-bath** may be of value. **Choline salicylate paste** (Bonjela®, Teejel®) may relieve the pain of minor aphthous ulcers. **Benzydamine hydrochloride** (Difflam®) is used as an analgesic mouth-wash for oral ulceration and other painful conditions. Local anaesthetics as in compound benzocaine lozenges also provide pain relief but may cause sensitisation with sore inflamed lips and tongue.

Local application of sticks of **toughened silver nitrate** and **alum** may relieve pain for a short time but cause **tissue damage** and delay healing.

BENZYDAMINE HYDROCHLORIDE

Indications: painful inflammatory conditions of oropharynx
Side-effects: occasional numbness or stinging

▼ Difflam Oral Rinse® (Carnegie)
Solution, green, benzydamine hydrochloride 0.15%. Price 200 ml = **E**
Rinse or gargle, using 15 ml, diluted if necessary, every 1½–3 hours as required for not more than 7 days.

CARBENOXOLONE SODIUM

Indications: mild oral and perioral lesions

Bioral Gel® (Winthrop)
Oral paste, carbenoxolone sodium 2% in adhesive basis. Price 5 g = **C**
Apply after meals and at bedtime

CORTICOSTEROIDS

Indications: oral and perioral lesions
Contra-indications: untreated oral infection

Adcortyl in Orabase® (Squibb)
Oral paste, triamcinolone acetonide 0.1% in adhesive basis. Price 10 g = **C**
Apply a thin layer 2–4 times daily

Corlan® (Glaxo)
Pellets (= lozenges), hydrocortisone 2.5 mg (as sodium succinate). Price 20 lozenges = **D**
Dissolve one lozenge slowly in the mouth in close contact with the lesion 2–4 times daily

LOCAL ANAESTHETICS

Indications: relief of pain in oral lesions
Cautions: avoid prolonged use; hypersensitivity may occur

Benzocaine Lozenges, Compound, benzocaine 100 mg, menthol 3 mg. Price 20 lozenges = **A**
Dissolve one slowly in the mouth when necessary

Medilave® (Martindale)
Gel, benzocaine 1%, cetylpyridinium chloride 0.01%. Price 10 g = **B**
Adults and children over 6 months, apply a thin layer 3–4 times daily

Oral-B® (Cooper)
Oral gel, lignocaine 0.6%, cetylpyridinium chloride 0.02%, cineole 0.1%, menthol 0.06%. Price 15 g = **B**
Apply every 3 hours when required

SALICYLATES

Indications: mild oral and perioral lesions
Cautions: frequent application, especially in children, may give rise to salicylate poisoning

Choline Salicylate Paste (Choline salicylate dental paste DPF), choline salicylate 8.7% in a flavoured gel basis. Price 10 g = **B**
Apply every 3–4 hours with gentle massage before meals and at bedtime

Bonjela® (R&C)
Oral gel, choline salicylate dental paste. Price 10 g = **B**

Teejel® (Napp)
Oral gel, choline salicylate dental paste. Price 10 g = **B**

Peralvex® (Norgine)
Oral paint, anthraquinone glycosides 5%, salicylic acid 1%. Price 16 ml = **C**
Apply 3–4 times daily

SODIUM CARBOXYMETHYLCELLULOSE

Indications: mechanical protection of oral and perioral lesions

Orabase® (Squibb)
Oral gel, sodium carboxymethylcellulose 16.58%, pectin 16.58%, gelatin 16.58%, in Plastibase.® Price 30 g = **C**; 100 g = **D**
Apply a thin layer when necessary after meals

Orahesive® (Squibb)
Powder (with adhesive properties), sodium carboxymethylcellulose, pectin, gelatin, equal parts. Price 25 g = **C**
Sprinkle on the affected area

TETRACYCLINE

Indications: severe recurrent aphthous ulceration
Side-effects: fungal superinfection

Tetracycline Mouth-bath, consists of Tetracycline Mixture, tetracycline ≡ tetracycline hydrochloride 125 mg/5 ml, see section 5.1.3
10 ml to be held in the mouth for 2–3 minutes 3 times daily for not longer than 3 days followed by a period of at least 3 days before treatment is recommenced

12.3.2 Oropharyngeal anti-infective drugs

The commonest cause of a sore throat is a viral infection which does not benefit from antibacterial treatment. Streptococcal sore throats require systemic **penicillin** therapy (see section 5.1.1). Vincent's angina (acute ulcerative gingivitis) responds to systemic **metronidazole** (see section 5.1.11.1) or **nimorazole** (see section 5.4.3).

Candida infections cause thrush and stomatitis. They are sometimes a sequel to the use of broad-spectrum antibiotics or antineoplastics, and withdrawing the drug may lead to rapid resolution. Otherwise, **nystatin** suspension or **amphotericin** lozenges may be effective; **polynoxylin** and **dequalinium** are less effective. **Miconazole** should be reserved for use when other antifungal drugs are ineffective. **Crystal violet** paint (see section 13.11) is effective but causes unsightly staining. It still has a place in the treatment of infants.

Herpes infections of the mouth, if they require treatment, which is usually not the case, respond to **tetracycline** mouth-bath (section 12.3.1). **Idoxuridine** is seldom needed for herpetic mouth infections.

AMPHOTERICIN

Indications: oral and perioral fungal infections

Fungilin® (Squibb)
Lozenges, yellow, amphotericin 10 mg. Price 20 lozenges = **C**
Dissolve 1 lozenge slowly in the mouth 4 times daily increased to 8 times daily when necessary
Suspension, orange, amphotericin 100 mg/ml. Price 12 ml with pipette = **D**
Place 1 ml in the mouth and retain near lesions 4 times daily for 14 days

Fungilin in Orabase® (Squibb)
Oral paste, amphotericin 2% (in orabase). Price 10 g = **C**
Apply a thin layer 2–4 times daily for 14 days

DEQUALINIUM CHLORIDE

Indications: mild oral fungal infections

Dequadin® (Farley)
Lozenges, orange, dequalinium chloride 250 micrograms. Price 20 lozenges = **B**
Dissolve 1 lozenge slowly in the mouth when required
Labosept® (LAB)
Pastilles, red, dequalinium chloride 250 micrograms. Price 20 pastilles = **B**
Suck 1 pastille slowly when required

IDOXURIDINE

Indications: oral and perioral herpetic lesions (see notes above)

Idoxuridine Paint, idoxuridine 0.1% in purified water. Identical in composition with idoxuridine eye-drops (see section 11.3.1). It should **not** be confused with a paint containing idoxuridine 5% in dimethyl sulphoxide used in dermatology (see section 13.10.3)
Apply to lesions up to 5 times daily

MICONAZOLE

Indications: oral fungal infections

Daktarin® (Janssen)
Oral gel, miconazole 25 mg/ml. Price 40 g = **E**
Place 5–10 ml in the mouth and retain near lesions before swallowing, 4 times daily

NATAMYCIN

Indications: oral fungal infections

Pimafucin® (Brocades)
Oral suspension, natamycin 10 mg/ml. Price 5-ml dropper bottle = **C**
Place 10 drops in the mouth after meals and retain near lesions; INFANTS 4 drops

NYSTATIN

Indications: oral and perioral fungal infections

Nystatin Mixture, nystatin 100 000 units/ml. Do not dilute. Price 30 ml = **D**
Place 1 ml in the mouth and retain near lesions 4 times daily, continued for 48 hours after lesions have resolved
Nystan® (Squibb)
Suspension, yellow, nystatin 100 000 units/ml. Price 30 ml with pipette = **E**
Note: Nystan Pessaries (see section 7.2.2) may be used as lozenges
Nystatin-Dome® (Dome)
Suspension, yellow, nystatin 100 000 units/ml. Price 30 ml with 1-ml spoon = **E**

POLYNOXYLIN

Indications: mild oral fungal infections

Anaflex® (Geistlich)
Lozenges, polynoxylin 30 mg. Price 50 lozenges = **E**
Suck 1 lozenge slowly 6–10 times daily

TETRACYCLINE

Section 12.3.1

12.3.3 Antiseptic lozenges and sprays

There is no convincing evidence that antiseptic lozenges and sprays have a beneficial action and they sometimes irritate and cause sore tongue and sore lips.

Benzalkonium Lozenges, benzalkonium chloride 500 micrograms. Price 20 lozenges = **B**
AAA® (Armour)
Mouth and throat spray, benzocaine 1.5%, cetalkonium chloride 0.0413%. Price 60-dose unit = **D**
Bradosol® (Ciba)
Lozenges, domiphen bromide 500 micrograms. Price 24 lozenges = **A**
Eludril® (Concept)
Aerosol spray, amethocaine hydrochloride 0.015%, chlorhexidine gluconate 0.05%. Price 55 ml = **D**
Faringets® (Winthrop)
Lozenges, brown, miristalkonium chloride iodine adduct 4 mg. Price 20 lozenges = **B**
Hibitane® (ICI)
Lozenges, benzocaine 2 mg, chlorhexidine hydrochloride 5 mg. Price 20 lozenges = **B**
Locabiotal® (Servier)
Aerosol spray, fusafungine, 125 micrograms/metered inhalation. Price 200-dose unit with nasal and oral adapter = **D**
Merocaine® (Merrell)
Lozenges, benzocaine 10 mg, cetylpyridinium chloride 1.4 mg. Price 24 lozenges = **B**
Merocets® (Merrell)
Lozenges, yellow, cetylpyridinium chloride 0.66%. Price 24 lozenges = **B**
Oralcer® (Vitabiotics)
Lozenges, ascorbic acid 6 mg, clioquinol 35 mg. Price 20 lozenges = **B**
Strepsils® (Crookes Products)
Lozenges, amylmetacresol 600 micrograms, 2,4-dichlorobenzyl alcohol 1.2 mg. Price 24 lozenges = **B**
Tyrosolven® (Warner)
Lozenges, yellow, benzocaine 5 mg, cetylpyridinium chloride 1 mg, tyrothricin 1 mg. Price 20 lozenges = **B**
Tyrozets® (MSD)
Lozenges, pink, benzocaine 5 mg, tyrothricin 1 mg. Price 12 lozenges = **A**

12.3.4 Mouth-washes, gargles, and dentifrices

Mouth-washes have a mechanical cleansing action and freshen the mouth. Warm **compound sodium chloride mouth-wash** or **compound thymol glycerin** is as useful as any.

Hydrogen peroxide mouth-wash has a mechanical cleansing effect due to frothing when in contact with oral debris. **Sodium perborate** (Bocasan®) is similar in effect to hydrogen peroxide.

There is recent evidence that **chlorhexidine** has a specific effect in inhibiting the formation of plaque on teeth.

There is no convincing evidence that gargles are effective.

ACETARSOL

Indications: gingivitis, pyorrhoea, stomatitis

Pyorex® (Bengué)
Dentifrice, acetarsol 0.45% (as lithium salt), aminacrine hydrochloride 0.006%, sodium ricinoleate 0.76%. Price 50 g = **B**

CETYLPYRIDINIUM CHLORIDE

Indications: oral hygiene

Merocet® (Merrell)
Solution (= mouth-wash or gargle), cetylpyridinium chloride 0.05%. Price 200 ml = **B**
To be used undiluted or diluted with an equal volume of warm water

CHLORHEXIDINE GLUCONATE

Indications: oral hygiene; inhibition of plaque formation (0.2% and 1% preparations)

Corsodyl® (ICI)
Dental gel, red, chlorhexidine gluconate 1%. Price 50 g = **C**
Brush on the teeth once or twice daily
Mouth-wash, pink, chlorhexidine gluconate 0.2%. Price 250 ml = **C**
Rinse the mouth with 10 ml for about 1 minute twice daily

Eludril® (Concept)
Mouth-wash, red, chlorhexidine gluconate 0.1%, chlorbutol 0.1%, chloroform 0.5%. Price 90 ml = **C**
Use 10 ml in ½ a tumblerful of warm water 3–4 times daily

HEXETIDINE

Indications: oral hygiene

Oraldene® (Warner)
Mouth-wash or *gargle*, hexetidine 0.1%. Price 100 ml = **B**
Use 15 ml undiluted 2–3 times daily

HYDROGEN PEROXIDE

Indications: oral hygiene, see notes above

Hydrogen Peroxide Mouth-wash, consists of hydrogen peroxide solution (6%). Price 100 ml = **A**
Rinse the mouth for 2–3 minutes with 15 ml in half a tumblerful of warm water.

PHENOL

Indications: oral hygiene

Phenol Gargle, phenol glycerin 5% (see Formulary). Price 100 ml = **A**
To be diluted with an equal volume of warm water

Chloraseptic® (Eaton)
Throat spray or *gargle*, phenol 1.4%. Price 120 ml with spray = **C**
Use undiluted as a throat spray, undiluted or diluted with an equal volume of water as a mouth-wash or gargle

POVIDONE-IODINE

Indications: oral hygiene

Betadine® (Napp)
Mouth-wash or *gargle*, povidone-iodine 1%. Price 250 ml = **C**
To be used undiluted or diluted with an equal volume of warm water

SODIUM CHLORIDE

Indications: oral hygiene, see notes above

Sodium Chloride Mouth-wash, Compound, sodium chloride 1.5% (see Formulary). Price 100 ml = **A**
To be diluted with an equal volume of warm water

SODIUM PERBORATE

Indications: oral hygiene, see notes above

Bocasan® (Cooper)
Mouth-wash, sodium perborate 70%. Price 8 × 1.7-g sachets = **B**
Use 1 sachet in 30 ml of water

THYMOL

Indications: oral hygiene, see notes above

Mouth-wash Solution-tablets, thymol 0.81 mg, sodium benzoate 32.4 mg, with colouring and flavouring in effervescent basis. Price 20 solution-tablets = **A**
Dissolve 1 tablet in a tumblerful of warm water

Thymol Glycerin, Compound, glycerol 10%, thymol 0.05% with colouring and flavouring. Price 100 ml = **A**
To be used undiluted or diluted with 3 volumes of warm water

13: Drugs acting on the SKIN

The skin is particularly amenable to treatment by local application as there is intimate contact between the drug and the target tissue with a minimum of systemic effects. However when a substance is used topically there may be difficulty in regulating the total quantity applied to the area concerned and lack of patient compliance may be a problem.

In this chapter, drug treatment is discussed under the following headings:

13.1 Vehicles and diluents

VEHICLE. Both the vehicle and the active ingredients are important in the treatment of skin conditions and it is being increasingly recognised that the vehicle alone may have a greater therapeutic value than a mere placebo effect. The vehicle affects the degree of hydration of the skin, and the penetration of active drug in the preparation.

The vehicle, the indication for which the drug is prescribed, solubility, cosmetic and general acceptability to the patient, and the safety and stability of the final preparation should all be considered.

DILUTION. Because of the complexity of many formulations, dilution is undesirable except where a particular diluent is known to be suitable. Suitable diluents for individual preparations are given in the relevant entries. Inappropriate diluents may impair the activity or stability of the preparation, even though no physical change is apparent. Diluted creams are generally given a life of 2 weeks.

QUANTITY. Suitable quantities of dermatological preparations to be prescribed for specific areas of the body are given under Prescription Writing.

CHOICE OF VEHICLE

The vehicle may take the form of a cream, ointment, lotion, paste, dusting-powder, application, collodion, liniment, or paint base. The properties of the various forms are described below but it should be noted that there are some preparations having intermediate properties, for example ointments with some properties of a cream.

CREAMS are either water-miscible and readily washed off, or oily and not so easily washed off. They usually contain a preservative to minimise microbial growth. Generally, creams moisten the skin more than ointments, and are usually cosmetically more acceptable to the patient.

Aqueous Cream, emulsifying ointment 30%, phenoxyethanol 1%, in freshly boiled and cooled purified water. Price 100 g = **B**

Buffered Cream, emulsifying ointment 30%, citric acid monohydrate 0.5%, sodium phosphate 2.5%, chlorocresol 0.1%, in freshly boiled and cooled purified water. Price 100 g = **B**

Cetomacrogol Cream, *Formula A*, cetomacrogol emulsifying ointment 30%, chlorocresol 0.1%, in freshly boiled and cooled purified water. Price 100 g = **E**
Formula B, cetomacrogol emulsifying ointment 30%, propyl hydroxybenzoate 0.08%, methyl hydroxybenzoate 0.15%, benzyl alcohol 1.5%, in freshly boiled and cooled purified water. Price 100 g = **D**

Ultrabase® (Schering)
Cream, liquid paraffin 10%, white soft paraffin 10%, stearyl alcohol 8%. Price 50 g = **C**; 500 g = **G**

OINTMENTS are greasy preparations which are normally anhydrous and insoluble in water. The most commonly used ointment bases consist of soft paraffin or a combination of soft paraffin with liquid paraffin and hard paraffin. Modern ointment bases may have occlusive properties on the skin surface, encourage hydration and be miscible with water. Water-soluble ointments contain macrogols which are freely soluble in water and are therefore readily washed off. They have a limited but useful application in circumstances where ready washability is needed. Ointments are suitable for chronic, dry lesions. Contact sensitivity to lanolin and wool alcohols may occur and ointments containing these substances must be avoided in sensitised patients.

Cetomacrogol Emulsifying Ointment, cetomacrogol emulsifying wax 30%, liquid paraffin 20%, white soft paraffin 50%. Price 100 g = **B**

Emulsifying Ointment, emulsifying wax 30%, white soft paraffin 50%, liquid paraffin 20%. Price 100 g = **B**

Hydrous Ointment (oily cream), dried magnesium sulphate 0.5%, phenoxyethanol 1%, water for preparations 48.5%, in wool alcohols ointment. Price 100 g = **B**

Hydrous Wool Fat, wool fat 70% in freshly boiled and cooled purified water. Price 100 g = **B**

Hydrous Wool Fat Ointment, hydrous wool fat 50%, yellow soft paraffin 50%. Price 100 g = **B**

Macrogol Ointment, macrogol '4000' 35%, macrogol '300' 65%. Price 100 g = **B**

Paraffin, white soft (white petroleum jelly). Price 100 g = **B**

Paraffin, yellow soft (yellow petroleum jelly). Price 100 g = **B**

Paraffin Ointment, (see Formulary). Price 100 g = **B**

Simple Ointment, cetostearyl alcohol 5%, hard paraffin 5%, wool fat 5% in yellow or white soft paraffin. Price 100 g = **B**

Wool Alcohols Ointment, wool alcohols 6%, yellow or white soft paraffin 10%, hard paraffin 24% in liquid paraffin. Price 100 g = **B**

Unguentum Merck® (Merck)

Cream, cetostearyl alcohol 9%, glyceryl monostearate 3%, saturated neutral oil 2%, liquid paraffin 3%, white soft paraffin 32%, propylene glycol 5%, polysorbate '40' 6%, silicic acid 0.1%, sorbic acid 0.2%. Price 50 g = **D**; 100 g = **E**

LOTIONS are usually aqueous solutions or suspensions which cool diffusely inflamed unbroken skin. They cool by evaporation and should be reapplied frequently. Volatile solvents increase the cooling effect but are liable to cause stinging. Astringent drugs, such as potassium permanganate and aluminium acetate, precipitate protein. This may assist in sealing an exuding surface, especially on the hands and feet.

SHAKE LOTIONS containing an insoluble powder are applied to less acute, scabbed and dry lesions. In addition to cooling they leave a deposit of inert powder on the skin surface.

PASTES are stiff preparations containing a high proportion of finely powdered solids such as zinc oxide and starch. The standard example is Compound Zinc Paste to which other active ingredients may be added (e.g. dithranol). Pastes are used for circumscribed lesions such as those which occur in lichen simplex, chronic eczema, or psoriasis. They are less occlusive than ointments and can be used to protect sub-acute, lichenified or excoriated skin.

Zinc Paste, Compound, zinc oxide 25%, starch 25%, white soft paraffin 50%. Price 25 g = **A**

DUSTING-POWDERS are used in folds where friction may occur between opposing skin surfaces. They should not be applied in areas that are very moist as they tend to cake and abrade the skin. **Talc** acts as a lubricant powder but does not absorb moisture whereas **starch** is less lubricant but absorbs water. Other inert powders such as kaolin or zinc oxide may also be used in the formulation of dusting-powders.

For preparations, see section 13.2.3.

APPLICATIONS are usually viscous solutions, emulsions, or suspensions for application to the skin.

COLLODIONS are painted on the skin and allowed to dry to leave a flexible film over the site of application. They may be used to seal minor cuts and wounds or as a means of holding a dissolved drug in contact with the skin for a long period.

Collodion, Flexible, castor oil 2.5%, colophony 2.5% in a collodion basis, prepared by dissolving pyroxylin (10%) in a mixture of 3 volumes of ether and 1 volume of alcohol (90%). Price 10 ml = **A**

Caution: highly inflammable

LINIMENTS are liquid preparations which are intended for external application and may contain substances possessing analgesic, rubefacient, soothing, or stimulating properties. They should not be applied to broken skin.

For preparations see section 10.3.2.

PAINTS are liquid preparations intended for application with a brush to the skin or mucous surfaces.

13.2 Emollient and barrier preparations

13.2.1 Emollients and barrier creams

Emollients soothe, smooth and hydrate the skin and are indicated for all dry scaling disorders (such as ichthyosis). Their effects are short-lived and they should be applied frequently even after improvement occurs. They are useful in dry eczematous disorders, and to a lesser extent in psoriasis (section 13.5). Simple preparations such as **aqueous cream** are often as effective as the more complex proprietary formulations; sprays offer little advantage but, in general, the choice depends on patient preference. Some ingredients may cause sensitisation, notably hydrous wool fat (lanolin) or antibacterials and this should be suspected if an eczematous reaction occurs at the site of application.

Camphor, menthol, and phenol have a mild antipruritic effect when used in emollient preparations. Calamine and zinc oxide may also be included as they slightly enhance therapeutic efficacy; they are particularly useful in dry eczema. Zinc and titanium preparations have mild astringent properties. Thickening agents such as talc and kaolin may also be included. Preparations containing antibacterial drugs should be avoided unless infection is present (section 13.10).

Urea is employed as a hydrating agent. It is used in scaling conditions and may be useful in elderly patients and infantile eczemas. It is often used with other topical agents such as corticosteroids to enhance penetration.

Barrier creams often contain water-repellent substances such as **dimethicone** or other silicones. They are used to give protection against irritation or repeated hydration (nappy rash, areas around stomata, sore areas in the elderly, bedsores, etc.).

Whatever is applied is no substitute for adequate nursing care, and it is doubtful if these water-repellent creams are any more effective than the traditional compound zinc ointments.

Aqueous Cream—section 13.1

Dimethicone Cream, dimethicone '350' 10%, cetostearyl alcohol 5%, cetrimide 0.5%, chlorocresol 0.1%, liquid paraffin 40%, freshly boiled and cooled purified water 44.4%. Price 50 g = **B**

Hydrous Ointment—section 13.1

Titanlum Dioxide Paste, titanium dioxide 20%, chlorocresol 0.1%, red ferric oxide 2%, glycerol 15%, light kaolin 10%, zinc oxide 25%, in water for preparations. Price 25 g = **A**

Zinc Cream, zinc oxide 32%, arachis oil 32%, calcium hydroxide 0.045%, oleic acid 0.5%, wool fat 8%, in freshly boiled and cooled purified water. Price 50 g = **B**

Zinc Ointment, zinc oxide 15%, in simple ointment. Price 25 g = **A**

Zinc and Castor Oil Ointment, zinc oxide 7.5%, castor oil 50%, arachis oil 30.5%, beeswax, white 10%, cetostearyl alcohol 2%. Price 25 g = **A**

Aquadrate® (Eaton)
Cream, urea 10%, in a powder-in-cream basis. Price 30 g = **D**; 100 g = **F**

Calmurid® (Pharmacia)
Cream, urea 10%, in a water-miscible basis. Diluent aqueous cream, life of diluted cream 14 days. Price 50 g = **D**; 100 g = **E**; 300 g = **H**

Dermalex® (Dermalex)
Skin lotion, allantoin, hexachlorophane, squalane. Price 30 ml = **B**; 100 ml = **D**

E45® (Crookes Products)
Cream, methyl hydroxybenzoate, wool fat, triethanolamine, stearic acid, self-emulsifying monostearin, light liquid paraffin, white soft paraffin. Price 50 g = **B**; 500 g = **D**

Eczederm® (Quinoderm)
Cream, calamine 20.88%, starch 2.09% in an emollient basis. Price 25 g = **C**

Emulsiderm® (Dermal)
Emulsion (= cream), benzalkonium chloride, isopropyl myristate, liquid paraffin. Price 250 ml = **E**

Massé Breast Cream® (Ortho)
Cream, arachis oil, cetyl alcohol, glycerol, glyceryl monostearate, lanolin, polysorbate 60, potassium hydroxide, sorbitan monostearate, stearic acid. Price 28 g = **B**

Metanium® (Bengué)
Ointment, titanium dioxide, peroxide, salicylate, and tannate. Price 13 g = **A**; 35 g = **C**

Natuderm® (Burgess)
Cream, glycerides, glycerol, polysorbate 60, sorbitan monostearate, squalane, squalene, free sterols, sterol esters, waxes. Price 40 g = **C**; 100 g = **D**; 450 g = **G**

Noratex® (Norton)
Cream, cod-liver oil, light kaolin, talc, wool fat, zinc oxide. Price 500 g = **D**

Nutraderm® (Alcon)
Cream, liquid paraffin in a water-miscible basis. Price 75 ml = **D**.
Lotion, liquid paraffin in a water-miscible basis. Price 150 ml = **D**

Oilatum® (Stiefel)
Cream, arachis oil, povidone, in a water-miscible basis. Price 40 g = **D**

Prehensol® (Dermal)
Cream, zinc salicylate 2%, lecithin 0.5%. Price 50 g = **E**. For detergent dermatitis

Rikospray Silicone® (Riker)
Application, aldioxa, cetylpyridinium chloride, dimethicone 1000 (pressurised aerosol pack). Price 200-g unit = **E**

Septex® (Norton)
No. 1 cream, cetrimide, oleic acid, zinc oxide. Price 50 g = **A**.

Siopel® (ICI)
Cream, cetrimide, dimethicone. Price 50 g = **B**; 500 g = **E**

Sprilon® (Pharmacia)
Spray application, dimethicone 200, dimethicone 350, zinc oxide, in ointment basis. Price 200-g unit = **E**

Stuart Silicone Protective® (Stuart)
Spray application, dimethicone (pressurised aerosol spray). Price 200 g = **C**

Sudocrem® (Tosara)
Cream, benzyl alcohol, benzyl benzoate, benzyl cinnamate, lanolin, zinc oxide. Price 65 g = **B**; 125 g = **B**; 325 g = **C**

Syl® (R&C)
Cream, benzalkonium chloride, dimethicone 350, cellulose nitrate. Price 100 g = **B**

Thovaline® (Ilon)
Aerosol (= application), cod-liver oil, light kaolin, talc, wool fat, zinc oxide (pressurised aerosol pack). Price 142 g = **D**.
Ointment, ingredients as for aerosol. Price 15 g = **A**; 40 and 60 g (both) = **B**; 90 and 125 g (both) = C; 500 g = **D**

Ultrabase—section 13.1

Unguentum Merck—section 13.1

Vasogen® (Pharmax)
Cream, calamine, dimethicone, zinc oxide. Price 20 g = **B**; 40 g = **B**; 100 g = **C**

13.2.2 Emollient bath additives

Emulsifying Ointment—see section 13.1
Aveeno Colloidal® (Cooper)
Bath additive, oat protein fraction. Price 6 × 50-g sachet = **D**
Aveeno Oilated® (Cooper)
Bath additive, oat protein fraction, liquid paraffin. Price 6 × 30-g sachet = **D**
Emulsiderm—section 13.2.1
Ollatum Emollient® (Stiefel)
Solution, acetylated wool alcohols, liquid paraffin. Price 150 ml = **D**; 350 ml = **F**
Polytar® (Stiefel)
Emollient (= bath additive), arachis oil extract of crude coal tar, cade oil, coal tar solution, liquid paraffin, tar. Price 250 ml = **E**. ACBS: see Appendix 3

13.2.3 Dusting-powders

For notes on use see section 13.1.

Talc Dusting-powder, starch 10% in sterilised purified talc. Price 100 g = **B**
Zinc, Starch and Talc Dusting-powder, zinc oxide 25%, starch 25%, sterilised purified talc 50%. Price 50 g = **A**
Cordocel® (Pharm. Mfg Co.) *dusting-powder*, alum and zinc, paediatric. For application to the umbilical cord. Price 10 × 2-g sachet = **B**
Cordocel-H® (Pharm. Mfg Co.) *dusting-powder*, alum and zinc, paediatric, with hexachlorophane. For application to the umbilical cord. Price 10 × 2-g sachet = **B**
Madecassol® (Rona) *dusting-powder*, centella. Price 2 g = **C**
Zeasorb® (Stiefel) *dusting-powder*, aldioxa, chloroxylenol, pulverised maize core. Price 30 g = **D**

13.3 Local anaesthetic and antipruritic preparations

Pruritus may be caused by systemic disease (such as drug hypersensitivity, obstructive jaundice, endocrine disease, and certain malignant diseases) as well as by skin disease (ichthyosis, eczema, urticaria, and scabies). Where possible the underlying causes should be treated.

There is no really effective antipruritic. Calamine preparations are widely prescribed. Emollient preparations (section 13.2.1) may also be of value. Oral antihistamines (section 3.4.1) should be used in allergic rashes.

Though widely prescribed, topical antihistamines and local anaesthetics should be avoided as they may cause sensitisation; moreover topical antihistamines are only marginally effective. Insect bites, though often treated with such preparations are best treated with calamine preparations or emollients.

Crotamiton (Eurax®) shows little evidence of greater effectiveness than calamine in the relief of pruritus.

For systemic treatment of pruritus and urticaria, see Antihistamines, section 3.4.1; also Hydroxyzine Hydrochloride, section 4.1.2 and Trimeprazine Tartrate, section 3.4.2.

CALAMINE

Indications: pruritus

Calamine Application, Compound, calamine 10%, zinc oxide 5%, zinc stearate 2.5%, wool fat 2.5%, yellow soft paraffin 25%, liquid paraffin 55%. Price 50 g = **A**
Calamine Cream, Aqueous, calamine 4%, zinc oxide 3%, arachis oil 30%, emulsifying wax 6%, freshly boiled and cooled purified water 57%. Price 50 g = **A**
Calamine Lotion, calamine 15%, zinc oxide 5%, glycerol 5%, bentonite 3%, sodium citrate 0.5%, liquefied phenol 0.5%, in freshly boiled and cooled purified water. Price 200 ml = **B**
Calamine Lotion, Oily, calamine 5%, arachis oil 50%, oleic acid 0.5%, wool fat 1%, in calcium hydroxide solution. Price 200 ml = **C**
Calamine Ointment, calamine 15%, in white soft paraffin. Price 25 g = **A**

CROTAMITON

Indications: pruritus, scabies
Cautions: avoid use near eyes
Contra-indications: acute exudative dermatoses
Administration: apply as required every 6–10 hours

Eurax® (Geigy)
Lotion, crotamiton 10%. Do not dilute. Price 150 ml = **C**; 1000 ml = **F**
Ointment, crotamiton 10%. Price 30 g = **B**; 100 g = **C**

LOCAL ANAESTHETICS

Indications: relief of local pain, see notes above. See section 15.2 for use in surface anaesthesia
Cautions: may cause hypersensitivity

Anethaine® (Farley) *cream*, amethocaine hydrochloride 1%. Price 25 g = **B**
Dermogesic® (MSD) *ointment*, benzocaine, calamine, hexylated *m*-cresol. Price 25 g = **B**
Locan® (DF) *cream*, amethocaine, amylocaine, cinchocaine. Price 30 g = **C**
Nestosyl® (Bengué) *ointment*, benzocaine, butyl aminobenzoate, hexachlorophane, resorcinol, zinc oxide. Price 30 g = **B**
Nupercainal® (Ciba) *ointment*, cinchocaine hydrochloride 1.1%. Price 30 g = **B**
Nupercaine® (Ciba) *cream*, cinchocaine hydrochloride 1.1%. Price 30 g = **B**
Xylocaine® (Astra) *ointment*, lignocaine 5%. Price 15 g = **C**
Xylodase® (Astra) *cream*, lignocaine, hyaluronidase. Price 15 g = **C**
Xylotox® (Pharm. Mfg Co.) *ointment*, lignocaine 5%. Price 15 and 30 g (both) = **C**

TOPICAL ANTIHISTAMINES

Indications: pruritus, urticaria, see notes above
Cautions: may cause hypersensitivity

Anthical® (M&B) *cream*, mepyramine maleate, zinc oxide. Price 25 g = **C**
Anthisan® (M&B) *cream*, mepyramine maleate. Price 25 g = **C**; 450 g = **E**
Caladryl® (P-D) *cream*, calamine, camphor, diphenhydramine hydrochloride. Price 42 g = **C**. *Lotion*, ingredients as for cream. Price 125 ml = **C**
Phenergan® (M&B) *cream*, dibromopropamidine isethionate, promethazine. Price 25 g = **C**

13.4 Topical corticosteroids

CHOICE OF PREPARATION. Topical preparations of corticosteroids are used for the treatment of inflammatory conditions of the skin other than those due to an infection, in particular the eczematous disorders. Corticosteroids suppress various components of the inflammatory reaction while in use and are in no sense curative. They are indicated for the relief of symptoms and for the suppression of signs of the disorder when potentially less harmful measures are ineffective.

Corticosteroids are of no value in the treatment of urticaria and are contra-indicated in rosacea as they worsen the condition. They should not be used indiscriminately in pruritus.

The preparation containing the **least potent** drug at the **lowest strength** which is effective is the one of choice, but extemporaneous dilution should be avoided whenever possible. However, the more potent corticosteroids may be indicated in certain disorders.

Topical corticosteroid preparations are divided into four groups in respect of potency. In ascending order these are:

	Potency	Examples
IV	Mild	Hydrocortisone 1% cream or ointment
III	Moderately potent	Clobetasone butyrate 0.05% cream or ointment (Eumovate®)
II	Potent	Betamethasone 0.1% (as valerate) (Betnovate®)
I	Very potent	Clobetasol propionate 0.05% cream, ointment, or scalp application (Dermovate®)

Intradermal corticosteroid injections (see section 10.1.2.2) are more effective than the highly potent topical corticosteroid preparations and they should be reserved for severe cases where topical treatment has failed. Their effects last for several weeks.

SIDE EFFECTS. Unlike groups I and II, groups III and IV are rarely associated with side-effects. The more potent the preparation the more care is required, as absorption through the skin can cause severe pituitary-adrenal-axis suppression and hypercorticism, both of which depend on the area of the body treated and the duration of the treatment. It must also be remembered that absorption is greatest from raw surfaces and intertriginous areas, and is increased by occlusion.

Local side-effects from the use of corticosteroids topically include:

(a) the spread and worsening of untreated local infection;
(b) thinning of the skin which may be restored over a period of time although the original structure may never return;
(c) irreversible striae atrophicae;
(d) increased hair growth;
(e) perioral dermatitis, an inflammatory papular disorder occurring on the face of young women;
(f) acne spots at the site of application in some patients; and
(g) mild depigmentation and growth of vellus hair.

USE IN CHILDREN. Children, especially babies, are particularly susceptible to side-effects. Fluorinated corticosteroids have no place in paediatric treatment; a mild corticosteroid such as hydrocortisone is useful for treating napkin rash and infantile eczemas.

COMPOUND PREPARATIONS. The advantages of including other substances with corticosteroids in topical preparations are debatable. The commonest ones used are the antibacterials and there is little evidence that inclusion of these has any therapeutic effect in most cases. They may however be of value in eczemas that have become secondarily infected and in seborrhoeic dermatitis. For information on compound preparations see the appropriate corticosteroid monograph.

HYDROCORTISONE and HYDROCORTISONE ACETATE

Indications: mild inflammatory skin disorders
Cautions: see notes above; also avoid prolonged use in infants and children, and on the face
Contra-indications: untreated bacterial, fungal, or viral skin lesions
Side-effects: see notes above
Administration: apply sparingly 2–3 times daily

Creams

Hydrocortisone Cream, hydrocortisone or hydrocortisone acetate 1%, chlorocresol 0.1%, cetomacrogol emulsifying ointment 30% in freshly boiled and cooled purified water. Price 15 g = **B**; 30 g = **C**; 50 g = **D**; 100 g = **E**. Potency IV

Alphaderm® (Eaton)
Cream, hydrocortisone 1%, urea 10%, in a powder-in-cream basis. Price 30 g = **D**; 100 g = **G**. Potency III

Calmurid HC® (Pharmacia)
Cream, hydrocortisone 1%, urea 10%, in a water-miscible basis. Diluent aqueous cream, life of diluted cream 14 days. Price 30 g = **E**. Potency III

Cobadex® (Cox-Continental)
Cream, hydrocortisone 0.5%, dimethicone '350' 20%, in a water-miscible basis. Price 20 g = **C**. Potency IV
Cream, hydrocortisone 1%, dimethicone '350' 20%, in a water-miscible basis. Price 20 g = **D**. Potency IV

Cortril® (Pfizer)
Topical ointment non-greasy (= cream), hydrocortisone 1%, in a water-miscible basis. Price 15 g = **B**; 50 g = **D**. Potency IV
Topical ointment non-greasy (= cream), hydrocortisone 2.5%, in a water-miscible basis. Price 15 g = **C**; 50 g = **F**. Potency IV

Dioderm® (Dermal)
Cream, hydrocortisone 0.1%, in a water-miscible basis. Price 30 g = **D**. Potency IV

Dome-Cort® (Dome)
Cream, hydrocortisone 0.125%, in a water miscible basis. Price 100 g = **F**. Potency IV

Efcortelan® (Glaxo)
Cream, hydrocortisone 0.5%, in a water-miscible basis. Diluent cetomacrogol cream (formula A), life of diluted cream 14 days. Price 15 g = **B**. Potency IV
Cream, hydrocortisone 1%, in a water-miscible basis. Diluent as above. Price 15 g = **B**; 50 g = **C**; 20 × 1-g single-use Flexules® = **F**. Potency IV
Cream, hydrocortisone 2.5%, in a water-miscible basis. Diluent as above. Price 15 g = **C**. Potency IV

Hydrocortistab® (Boots)
Cream, hydrocortisone acetate 1%, in a water-miscible basis. Price 15 g = **B**. Potency IV

Hydrocortisyl® (Roussel)
Cream, hydrocortisone 1%, in a water-miscible basis. Price 15 g = **B**. Potency IV

Hydrocortone® (MSD)
Cream, hydrocortisone acetate 1%, in a water-miscible basis. Price 15 g = **B**. Potency IV

Ointments

Hydrocortisone Ointment, hydrocortisone, in white soft paraffin or a mixture of this with liquid paraffin, with or without wool fat. Price 15 g (0.5 or 1%) = **B**; 30 g (1%) = **C**; 100 g (1%) = **E**. Potency IV

Cortril® (Pfizer)
Topical ointment greasy (= ointment), hydrocortisone 1%, in a paraffin basis. Price 15 g = **C**. Potency IV
Topical ointment greasy (= ointment), hydrocortisone 2.5%, in a paraffin basis. Price 15 g = **C**. Potency IV

Efcortelan® (Glaxo)
Ointment, hydrocortisone 0.5%, in an anhydrous greasy basis. Diluent white soft paraffin, life of diluted ointment 14 days. Price 15 g = **B**. Potency IV
Ointment, hydrocortisone 1%, in an anhydrous greasy basis. Diluent as above. Price 15 g = **B**; 30 g = **C**; 20 × 1-g single-use Flexules® = **F**. Potency IV
Ointment, hydrocortisone 2.5%, in an anhydrous greasy basis. Diluent as above. Price 15 g = **C**. Potency IV

Hydrocortistab® (Boots)
Ointment, hydrocortisone 1%, in an anhydrous greasy basis. Price 15 g = **B**. Potency IV

Hydrocortisyl® (Roussel)
Ointment, hydrocortisone 1%, in an anhydrous greasy basis. Price 15 g = **B**. Potency IV

Hydrocortone® (MSD)
Ointment, hydrocortisone 1%, in an anhydrous greasy basis. Price 15 g = **B**. Potency IV

Lotions and Sprays

Hydrocortisone Lotion, hydrocortisone 1%, chlorocresol 0.05%, self-emulsifying monostearin 4%, glycerol 6.3% in freshly boiled and cooled purified water; may be prepared with any other suitable basis. Price 20 ml = **B**. Potency IV

Cortril® (Pfizer)
Spray (= application), hydrocortisone 50 mg/30 ml, pressurised aerosol unit. Price 30 ml = **C**; 60 ml = **D**. Potency IV

Efcortelan® (Glaxo)
Lotion, hydrocortisone 1%. Do not dilute. Price 20 ml = **B**. Potency IV

Dressings

Cortacream® (S&N)
Impregnated bandage, hydrocortisone 1%, silicone 10%. Price 75 mm × 2 m bandage = **E**. Potency IV

Compound preparations containing hydrocortisone and hydrocortisone acetate

Hydrocortisone and Neomycin Cream, hydrocortisone 0.5%, neomycin sulphate 0.5%, in a water-miscible basis. Price 15 g = **B**. Potency IV

Barquinol HC® (Fisons)
Cream, clioquinol, hydrocortisone acetate. Price 15 g = **C**. Potency IV

Chymacort® (Armour)
Ointment, hydrocortisone acetate 1%, pancreatic enzymes (chymotrypsin and trypsin) 10000 Armour units/g, in a water-miscible basis. Price 15 g = **D**

Cobadex-Nystatin® (Cox-Continental)
Ointment, benzalkonium chloride, dimethicone 350, hydrocortisone, nystatin. Price 20 g = **D**. Potency IV

▼ **Daktacort®** (Janssen)
Cream, hydrocortisone, miconazole nitrate. Price 15 g = **D**; 30 g = **F**. Potency IV

Dioderm-C® (Dermal)
Cream, clioquinol, hydrocortisone. Price 30 g = **E**. Potency IV

Eczederm with Hydrocortisone® (Quinoderm)
Cream, hydrocortisone, calamine, starch. Price 25 g = **C**. Potency IV

Eurax-Hydrocortisone® (Geigy)
Cream, crotamiton, hydrocortisone. Price 30 g = **C**. Potency IV

Framycort® (Fisons)
Ointment, framycetin sulphate, hydrocortisone acetate. Price 15 g = **D**. Potency IV

Fucidin H® (Leo)
Gel. fusidic acid, hydrocortisone acetate. Price 10 g = **D**; 25 g = **E**. Potency IV.
Ointment, hydrocortisone acetate, sodium fusidate. Price 10 g = **D**; 25 g = **E**. Potency IV

Genticin HC® (Nicholas)
Cream, gentamicin sulphate, hydrocortisone acetate. Price 15 g = **D**. Potency IV.
Ointment, ingredients as for cream. Price 15 g = **D**. Potency IV

Gregoderm® (Unigreg)
Ointment, hydrocortisone, neomycin sulphate, nystatin, polymyxin B sulphate. Price 15 g = **D**. Potency IV

Hepacort Plus® (Rona)
Cream, heparin sodium, hydrocortisone acetate. Price 10 g = **C**. Potency IV. For use in superficial phlebitis

Hydroderm® (MSD)
Ointment, bacitracin zinc, hydrocortisone, neomycin sulphate. Price 5 g = **B**; 15 g = **C**. Potency IV

Neo-Cortef® (Upjohn)
Lotion, hydrocortisone acetate, neomycin sulphate. Price 15 ml = **E**. Potency IV.
Ointment, hydrocortisone acetate 1%, neomycin sulphate. Price 5 g = **C**; 20 g = **E**. Potency IV.
Ointment, hydrocortisone acetate 2.5%, neomycin sulphate. Price 20 g = **G**. Potency IV

Steroxin-Hydrocortisone® (Geigy)
Cream, chlorquinaldol, hydrocortisone. Price 20 g = **D**. Potency IV

Terra-Cortril® (Pfizer)
Topical ointment, hydrocortisone, oxytetracycline hydrochloride. Price 15 g = **D**; 30 g = **E**. Potency IV.
Spray, ingredients as for topical ointment (pressurised aerosol pack). Price 30-ml unit = **D**; 60-ml unit = **E**. Potency IV

Terra-Cortril Nystatin® (Pfizer)
Cream, hydrocortisone, nystatin, oxytetracycline calcium. Price 30 g = **F**. Potency IV

Timodine® (R&C)
Cream, benzalkonium chloride, dimethicone 350, hydrocortisone, nystatin. Price 30 g = **E**. Potency IV

Vioform-Hydrocortisone® (Ciba)
Cream, clioquinol 3%, hydrocortisone 1%. Price 30 g = **D**
Ointment, clioquinol 3%, hydrocortisone 1%. Price 30 g = **D**

BECLOMETHASONE DIPROPIONATE

Indications: severe inflammatory skin disorders such as eczema in patients unresponsive to less potent corticosteroids
Cautions; Contra-indications; Side-effects: see under Hydrocortisone and notes above
Administration: apply sparingly twice daily, reducing frequency as condition responds

Propaderm® (A&H)
Cream, beclomethasone dipropionate 0.025%. Diluent cetomacrogol cream (formula A), life of diluted cream 14 days. Price 15 g = **C**; 50 g = **E**. Potency II
Forte cream, beclomethasone dipropionate 0.5%. Diluent as above. Price 5 g = **D**. Potency I
Ointment, beclomethasone dipropionate 0.025%, in a propylene glycol-paraffin basis. Diluent white soft paraffin, life of diluted ointment 14 days. Price 15 g = **C**; 50 g = **E**. Potency II

Propaderm-A® (A&H)
Ointment, beclomethasone dipropionate, chlortetracycline hydrochloride. Price 15 g = **C**; 50 g = **E**. Potency II

Propaderm-C® (A&H)
Cream, beclomethasone dipropionate, clioquinol. Price 15 g = **C**. Potency II. *Ointment*, ingredients as for cream. Price 15 g = **C**. Potency II

BETAMETHASONE

Indications: severe inflammatory skin disorders such as eczema in patients unresponsive to less potent corticosteroids
Cautions; Contra-indications; Side-effects: see under Hydrocortisone and notes above
Administration: apply sparingly 2–3 times daily, reducing frequency as condition improves

Betnovate® (Glaxo)
Scalp application, betamethasone 0.1% (as valerate), in a thickened alcoholic basis. Price 30 ml = **D**; 100 ml = **G**. Potency II
Caution: inflammable
Cream, betamethasone 0.1% (as valerate), in a water-miscible basis. Diluent cetomacrogol cream (formula A), life of diluted cream 14 days. Price 15 g = **C**; 30 g = **D**; 100 g = **F**; 20 × 1-g single-use Flexules® = **F**. Potency II
Lotion, betamethasone 0.1% (as valerate). Do not dilute. Price 20 ml = **C**. Potency II
Ointment, betamethasone 0.1% (as valerate), in an anhydrous paraffin basis. Diluent white soft paraffin or a mixture of this with liquid paraffin, life of diluted ointment 14 days. Price 15 g = **C**; 30 g = **D**; 100 g = **F**; 20 × 1-g single-use Flexules® = **F**. Potency II

Betnovate-C® (Glaxo)
Cream, betamethasone valerate, clioquinol. Price 15 g = **D**; 30 g = **E**. Potency II. *Ointment*, ingredients as for cream. Price 15 g = **D**; 30 g = **E**. Potency II

Betnovate-N® (Glaxo)
Cream, betamethasone valerate, neomycin sulphate. Price 15 g = **D**; 30 g = **E**; 100 g = **G**. Potency II. *Lotion*, ingredients as for cream.

Price 20 ml = **D**. Potency II. *Ointment*, ingredients as for cream. Price 15 g = **D**; 30 g = **E**; 100 g = **G**. Potency II

Betnovate-RD® (Glaxo)

Cream, betamethasone 0.025% (as valerate) in a water-miscible basis (1 in 4 dilution of Betnovate cream). Price 100 g = **E**. Potency III

Ointment, betamethasone 0.025% (as valerate) in an anhydrous paraffin basis (1 in 4 dilution of Betnovate ointment). Price 100 g = **E**. Potency III

CLOBETASOL PROPIONATE

Indications: short-term treatment of severe exacerbations of inflammatory skin disorders such as severe eczema and discoid lupus erythematosus in patients unresponsive to less potent corticosteroids

Cautions; Contra-indications; Side-effects: see under Hydrocortisone and notes above

Administration: apply sparingly 1–2 times daily, reducing frequency as condition responds

Dermovate® (Glaxo)

Scalp application, clobetasol propionate 0.05%, in a thickened alcoholic basis. Price 25 ml = **E**; 100 ml = **I**. Potency I

Caution: inflammable

Cream, clobetasol propionate 0.05%, in a water-miscible basis. Diluents cetamacrogol cream (formula A), aqueous cream, buffered cream, life of diluted cream 14 days. Price 25 g = **E**; 100 g = **H**; 20 × 1-g single-use Flexules® = **F**. Potency I

Ointment, clobetasol propionate 0.05%, in an anhydrous paraffin basis. Diluent white soft paraffin or a mixture of this with liquid paraffin, life of diluted ointment 14 days. Price 25 g = **E**; 100 g = **H**; 20 × 1-g single-use Flexules® = **F**. Potency I

Dermovate-NN® (Glaxo)

Cream, clobetasol propionate, neomycin sulphate, nystatin. Price 25 g = **E**. Potency 1.

Ointment, ingredients as for cream. Price 25 g = **E**. Potency I

CLOBETASONE BUTYRATE

Indications: mild inflammatory skin disorders in patients unresponsive to hydrocortisone

Cautions; Contra-indications; Side-effects: see under Hydrocortisone and notes above

Administration: apply sparingly up to 4 times daily, reducing frequency as condition responds

Eumovate® (Glaxo)

Cream, clobetasone butyrate 0.05%, in a water-miscible basis. Price 25 g = **D**; 100 g = **G**; 20 × 1-g single-use Flexules® = **F**. Potency III

Ointment, clobetasone butyrate 0.05%, in an anhydrous paraffin basis. Price 25 g = **D**; 100 g = **G**; 20 × 1-g single-use Flexules® = **F**. Potency III

▼ **Trimovate®** (Glaxo)

Cream, clobetasone butyrate, nystatin, oxytetracycline calcium. Price 25 g = **E**. Potency III. *Ointment*, chlortetracycline hydrochloride, clobetasone butyrate, nystatin. Price 25 g = **E**. Potency III

DESONIDE

Indications: severe inflammatory skin disorders such as eczema in patients unresponsive to less potent corticosteroids

Cautions; Contra-indications; Side-effects: see under Hydrocortisone and notes above

Administration: apply sparingly 2–3 times daily

Tridesilon® (Dome)

Cream, desonide 0.05%, in a water-miscible basis. Diluents cetomacrogol cream (formula A or B) or aqueous cream, life of diluted cream not more than 3 months. Price 15 g = **D**; 30 g = **E**. Potency II

Ointment, desonide 0.05%, in a white soft paraffin basis. Diluent white soft paraffin, life of diluted ointment not more then 3 months. Price 30 g = **E**. Potency II

DIFLUCORTOLONE VALERATE

Indications: severe inflammatory skin disorders such as eczema in patients unresponsive to less potent corticosteroids; high strength preparations (0.3%), short term treatment of severe exacerbations

Cautions; Contra-indications; Side-effects: see under Hydrocortisone and notes above

Administration: apply sparingly 2–3 times daily, reducing frequency as condition responds

▼ **Nerisone®** (Schering)

Cream, diflucortolone valerate 0.1%, in a water-miscible basis. Diluent aqueous cream, life of diluted cream 14 days. Price 30 g = **E**. Potency II

Oily cream, diflucortolone valerate 0.1%, in a water-in-oil basis. Diluent hydrous ointment (oily cream), life of diluted cream 14 days. Price 30 g = **E**. Potency II

Forte oily cream, diflucortolone valerate 0.3%, in a water-in-oil basis. Diluent as above. Price 15 g = **D**. Potency I

Ointment, diflucortolone valerate 0.1%, in an anhydrous basis. Diluent white soft paraffin, life of diluted ointment 14 days. Price 30 g = **E**. Potency II

Forte ointment, diflucortolone valerate 0.3% in an anhydrous basis. Diluent as above. Price 15 g = **D**. Potency I

▼ **Temetex®** (Roche)

Cream, diflucortolone valerate 0.1%, in a water-miscible basis. Price 30 g = **E**. Potency II

Fatty ointment, diflucortolone valerate 0.1%, in an anhydrous basis. Price 30 g = **E**. Potency II

Ointment, diflucortolone valerate 0.1%, in a water-in-oil cream basis. Price 30 g = **E**. Potency II

FLUCLOROLONE ACETONIDE

Indications: severe inflammatory skin disorders such as eczema in patients unresponsive to less potent corticosteroids

Cautions; Contra-indications; Side-effects: see under Hydrocortisone and notes above

Administration: apply sparingly twice daily, reducing frequency as condition responds

Topilar® (Syntex)

Cream, flucloroIone acetonide 0.025%, in FAPG basis (fatty alcohols, propylene glycol), non-aqueous, water-miscible. Price 30 g = **D**; 100 g = **F**. Potency II

Ointment, flucloroIone acetonide 0.025%, in an ointment basis. Diluent white soft paraffin, life of diluted ointment 14 days. Price 30 g = **D**; 100 g = **F**. Potency II

FLUOCINOLONE ACETONIDE

Indications: inflammatory skin disorders, 0.01% preparations in milder conditions, 0.025% preparations in severe conditions, and 0.2% preparation in short-term treatment of severe exacerbations

Cautions; Contra-indications; Side-effects: see under Hydrocortisone and notes above

Administration: apply sparingly 2–3 times daily

Synalar® (ICI)

Cream, fluocinolone acetonide 0.025%, in a water-miscible basis. Diluent cetomacrogol cream (formula B), life of diluted cream 14 days. Price 5 g = **B**; 15 g = **C**; 30 g = **D**; 50 g = **E**. Potency II

Forte cream, fluocinolone acetonide 0.2%, in a water-miscible basis. Diluent as above. Price 5 g = **D**. Potency I

Gel, fluocinolone acetonide 0.025%, in a water-miscible basis. Price 30 g = **D**. For use as a scalp application. Potency II

Lotion, fluocinolone acetonide 0.025%. Diluent sterile water or a fluid non-ionic cream, for example one made from cetostearyl alcohol 2.5% and cetomacrogol '1000' 0.5% in sterile water, life of diluted lotion 14 days. Price 20 ml = **C**. Potency II

Ointment, fluocinolone acetonide 0.025%, in an anhydrous greasy basis. Diluents white or yellow soft paraffin or eye ointment basis, life of diluted ointment 14 days. Price 5 g = **B**; 15 g = **C**; 30 g = **D**; 50 g = **E**. Potency II

Synalar C (ICI) *cream*, clioquinol, fluocinolone acetonide. Price 15 g = **C**. Potency II. *Ointment*, ingredients as for cream. Price 15 g = **C**. Potency II

Synalar N (ICI) *cream*, fluocinolone acetonide, neomycin sulphate. Price 5 g = **B**; 15 g = **C**; 30 g = **D**; 50 g = **E**. Potency II. *Lotion*, ingredients as for cream. Price 20 ml = **C**. Potency II. *Ointment*, ingredients as for cream. Price 5 g = **B**; 15 g = **C**; 30 g = **D**; 50 g = **E**. Potency II

Synandone® (ICI)

Cream, fluocinolone acetonide 0.01%, in a water-miscible basis. Price 30 g = **C**; 50 g = **D**. Potency III

Ointment, fluocinolone acetonide 0.01%, in an anhydrous greasy basis. Price 30 g = **C**; 50 g = **D**. Potency III

FLUOCINONIDE

Indications: severe inflammatory skin disorders such as eczema in patients unresponsive to less potent corticosteroids

Cautions; Contra-indications; Side-effects: see under Hydrocortisone and notes above

Administration: apply sparingly 3–4 times daily, reducing frequency as condition responds

Metosyn® (Stuart)

FAPG cream, fluocinonide 0.05%, in a non-aqueous water-miscible basis. Price 25 g = **D**; 100 g = **F**. Potency II

Ointment, fluocinonide 0.05%, in paraffin basis. Diluent white soft paraffin, life of diluted ointment 14 days. Price 25 g = **D**; 100 g = **F**. Potency II

FLUOCORTOLONE

Indications: 0.25% preparations—severe inflammatory skin disorders such as eczema in patients unresponsive to less potent corticosteroids; 0.1% preparations—milder inflammatory skin disorders

Cautions; Contra-indications; Side-effects: see under Hydrocortisone and notes above

Administration: apply sparingly 2–3 times daily, reducing frequency as condition responds

Ultradil® (Schering)

Cream plain, fluocortolone hexanoate 0.1%, fluocortolone pivalate 0.1%, in a water-miscible basis. Diluent aqueous cream or Ultrabase®, life of diluted cream 14 days. Price 50 g = **E**; 100 g = **G**. Potency III

Ointment plain, fluocortolone hexanoate 0.1%, fluocortolone pivalate 0.1%, in a water-in-oil emulsion basis. Diluent hydrous ointment (oily cream), life of diluted ointment 14 days. Price 50 g = **E**; 100 g = **G**. Potency III

Ultralanum® (Schering)

Cream plain, fluocortolone hexanoate 0.25%, fluocortolone pivalate 0.25%, in a water-miscible basis. Diluent aqueous cream or Ultrabase®, life of diluted cream 14 days. Price 30 g = **E**; 50 g = **F**. Potency II

Ointment plain, fluocortolone 0.25%, fluocortolone hexanoate 0.25%, in a water-in-oil emulsion basis. Diluent hydrous ointment (oily cream), life of diluted ointment 14 days. Price 30 g = **E**; 50 g = **F**. Potency II

Ointment, fluocortolone, fluocortolone hexanoate, clemizole hexachlorophane. Price 30 g = **E**; 50 g = **F**. Potency II

FLURANDRENOLONE

Indications: 0.05% preparations—severe inflammatory skin disorders such as eczema in patients unresponsive to less potent corticosteroids; 0.0125% preparations—milder inflammatory skin disorders

Cautions; Contra-indications; Side-effects: see under Hydrocortisone and notes above

Administration: apply sparingly 2–3 times daily

Haelan® (Dista)

Cream, flurandrenolone 0.0125%, in a water-miscible basis. Diluent aqueous cream, life of diluted cream 14 days. Price 60 g = **E**. Potency III

Ointment, flurandrenolone 0.0125%, in an anhydrous greasy basis. Diluent white soft paraffin, life of diluted ointment 14 days. Price 60 g = **E**. Potency III

Haelan-C® (Dista)

Cream, clioquinol, flurandrenolone. Price 30 g = **D**. Potency III.

Ointment, ingredients as for cream. Price 30 g = **D**. Potency III

Haelan-X® (Dista)

Cream, flurandrenolone 0.05%, in a water-miscible basis. Diluent as above. Price 15 g = **C**. Potency II

Ointment, flurandrenolone 0.05%, in an anhydrous greasy basis. Diluent as above. Price 15 g = **C**. Potency II

HALCINONIDE

Indications: severe inflammatory skin disorders such as eczema in patients unresponsive to less potent corticosteroids

Cautions; Contra-indications; Side-effects: see under Hydrocortisone and notes above

Administration: apply sparingly 2–3 times daily

Halcicomb® (FAIR)

Cream, halcinonide, neomycin sulphate, nystatin. Price 10 g = **C**; 25 g = **D**. Potency II

Ointment, ingredients as for cream. Price 10 g = **C**; 25 g = **D**. Potency II

Halciderm Topical® (Squibb)

Cream, halcinonide 0.1%, in a water-miscible basis. Price 15 g = **C**; 30 g = **D**. Potency II

HYDROCORTISONE BUTYRATE

Indications: severe inflammatory skin disorders such as eczema in patients unresponsive to less potent corticosteroids

Cautions; Contra-indications; Side-effects: see under Hydrocortisone and notes above

Administration: apply sparingly 2–4 times daily

Locoid® (Brocades)

Cream, hydrocortisone butyrate 0.1%, in a water-miscible basis. Price 30 g = **D**; 100 g = **G**. Potency II

Scalp lotion, hydrocortisone butyrate 0.1%, in an aqueous isopropyl alcohol basis. Price 20 ml = **E**; 100 g = **H**. Potency II

Caution: inflammable

Ointment, hydrocortisone butyrate 0.1%, in an anhydrous greasy basis. Price 30 g = **D**; 100 g = **G**. Potency II

Locoid C® (Brocades)

Cream, chlorquinaldol, hydrocortisone butyrate. Price 30 g = **E**. Potency II

Ointment, ingredients as for cream. Price 30 g = **E**. Potency II

TRIAMCINOLONE ACETONIDE

Indications: severe inflammatory skin disorders such as eczema in patients unresponsive to less potent corticosteroids

Cautions; Contra-indications; Side-effects: see under Hydrocortisone and notes above

Administration: apply sparingly 2–4 times daily

Adcortyl® (Squibb)

Cream, triamcinolone acetonide 0.1%, in a water-miscible basis. Diluents cetomacrogol cream (formula B), or aqueous cream provided that chlorocresol content is increased to 0.2%, life of diluted cream 4 weeks. Price 30 g = **D**. Potency II

Ointment, triamcinolone acetonide 0.1%, in an anhydrous greasy basis. Diluent white soft paraffin, life of diluted ointment 14 days. Price 30 g = **D**. Potency II

Spray (= application), triamcinolone acetonide 3.3 mg/50 g, pressurised aerosol unit. Price 50 g = **C**. Potency II

Ledercort® (Lederle)

Cream, triamcinolone acetonide 0.1%, in a water-miscible basis. Diluent aqueous cream, life of diluted cream 14 days. Price 15 g = **D**; 250 g = **J**. Potency II

Ointment, triamcinolone acetonide 0.1%, in an anhydrous greasy basis. Diluent 1 part wool fat, 9 parts white soft paraffin, life of diluted ointment 14 days. Price 15 g = **D**; 250 g = **J**. Potency II

Compound preparations containing triamcinolone acetonide

Adcortyl with Graneodin® (Squibb)

Cream, gramicidin, neomycin sulphate, triamcinolone acetonide. Price 15 g = **D**. Potency II

Ointment, ingredients as for cream. Price 15 g = **D**. Potency II

Aureocort® (Lederle)

Cream, chlortetracycline, triamcinolone acetonide. Price 15 g = **E**. Potency II

Ointment, chlortetracycline hydrochloride, triamcinolone acetonide. Price 15 g = **E**. Potency II

Spray (= application), ingredients as for ointment but higher proportion of chlortetracycline (pressurised aerosol pack). Price 60-g unit = **F**. Potency II

Nystadermal® (Squibb)

Cream, nystatin, triamcinolone acetonide. Price 15 g = **E**. Potency II

Remiderm® (Squibb)

Cream, halquinol, triamcinolone acetonide. Price 15 g = **C**; 30 g = **D**. Potency II

Ointment, ingredients as for cream. Price 15 g = **C**; 30 g = **D**. Potency II
Spray (= application), ingredients as for cream (pressurised aerosol pack). Price 50-g unit = **E**. Potency II

Silderm® (Lederle)
Cream, neomycin sulphate, triamcinolone acetonide, undecylenic acid. Price 15 g = **D**; 30 g = **E**. Potency II

Tri-Adcortyl® (Squibb)
Cream, gramicidin, neomycin sulphate, nystatin, triamcinolone acetonide. Price 15 g = **D**; 30 g = **E**. Potency II
Ointment, ingredients as for cream. Price 15 g = **D**; 30 g = **E**. Potency II

Tricaderm® (Squibb)
Solution, benzalkonium chloride, salicylic acid, triamcinolone acetonide. Price 25 ml = **E**. Potency II

13.5 Preparations for psoriasis and eczema

Eczema (dermatitis) is due to a particular type of epidermal inflammation and is caused by a wide variety of factors; where possible the causative factors should be established and removed (see also Hyposensitisation, section 3.4.2). In many cases no underlying factor can be identified (atopic eczema).

Dry, fissured, scaly lesions are treated with bland **emollients** (section 13.2.1) which are often all that is necessary to allay irritation and permit healing. Preparations containing zinc oxide and calamine are particularly useful; zinc may have a weak anti-eczematous action. **Topical corticosteroids** are described in section 13.4. Perfumed soaps should be **avoided** and preparations such as **emulsifying ointment** used as soap substitutes and in the bath. **Keratolytics** such as salicyclic acid, followed by ichthammol or coal tar (see below) are used in chronic eczematous conditions where there is marked thickening of the skin and pronounced scaling.

Weeping eczemas may be treated with corticosteroids; they are however commonly secondarily infected. Wet dressings of **potassium permanganate** (0.01%) (section 13.11) are applied. If a large area is involved, potassium permanganate baths are taken. When necessary **topical antibacterials** are used (section 13.10.1) but those which are not given systemically should be chosen.

Psoriasis is characterised by epidermal thickening and scaling. It has less tendency to heal than eczema. For mild conditions, treatment, other than reassurance and an emollient, may be unnecessary. In more troublesome cases, local application of **salicylic acid**, **coal tar**, or **dithranol** have a temporary beneficial effect. Corticosteroids should be avoided because, although they are effective, subsequent treatment becomes more difficult, as tachyphylaxis may occur and they may induce or precipitate severe pustular psoriasis. In resistant cases an **immunosuppressant**, usually methotrexate, may be used (see section 8.1.3) but this must always be done under hospital supervision and the dose adjusted according to severity of the condition and in accordance with haematological and biochemical measurements; the usual dose is 15 to 25 mg of methotrexate weekly, usually by mouth. Tranquillizers, hypnotics, and rest may be of prophylactic value.

Salicylic acid is used in all hyperkeratotic conditions to enhance the rate of loss of surface scale. Preparations containing salicylic acid 2% are used initially and then gradually increased to concentrations of 3 to 6%. Side-effects are few but include allergic contact sensitivity, or, when large areas are treated, salicylism (see section 10.1.1.1).

Ichthammol has a milder action than coal tar and is useful in the less acute forms of eczema. It can be applied conveniently to flexures of the limbs as zinc paste and ichthammol bandage (Ichthopaste®, Icthaband®).

Coal tar is more active than salicylic acid and has antipruritic and keratolytic properties. It is used in psoriasis and eczema. Coal tar has superseded wood tar as it is more active. The formulation and strength chosen depends on patient acceptability and severity of the condition; the 'thicker' the patch of eczema or psoriasis the stronger the concentration of coal tar required. **Coal tar paste** or **zinc and coal tar paste** are generally suitable for most cases but are limited by their unpleasant appearance and smell and they may not be used on the face. Some of the newer preparations are less unsightly and may be preferred. Preparations such as Carbo-Dome® are suitable for treating the face. **Zinc paste and coal tar bandage** is useful for treating the limbs. Scalp preparations are described in section 13.9. When lesions are extensive coal tar baths are useful. Combinations of coal tar with zinc or salicylic acid have no advantage over the simpler preparations. Preparations containing hydrocortisone and coal tar are useful in eczemas.

Dithranol is used in psoriasis and is the most potent topical preparation available for this condition. Usual concentrations are 0.1–2% although in individual patients 5% or more may be used. Dithranol must be used with caution as it can cause quite severe skin irritation. For this reason it must be applied only to the lesions and it is customary to start with low concentrations and gradually build up to the maximum concentration which produces a therapeutic effect without irritation. Some patients are intolerant to dithranol in low concentrations and it is important to recognise them early in treatment. Fair skin is more sensitive than dark skin. **Dithranol paste** is often used. Proprietary preparations cause less staining and irritation than dithranol paste. Dithranol and urea combinations (Psoradrate®) may improve skin texture by rehydration. **Dithranol triacetate** (Exolan®) has no advantage over traditional preparations.

Ingram's method of applying dithranol is the

usual method used in hospitals. Dithranol paste is applied to the lesions after the patient has soaked in a warm bath containing coal tar solution 1 in 800 and after drying is exposed to ultraviolet radiation to produce a slight erythema; the procedure is repeated daily.

Etretinate is a newly introduced drug for the treatment of severe resistant or complicated psoriasis or some of the congenital disorders of keratinisation. It should be prescribed only by consultant dermatologists or under hospital supervision. It is a retinoid compound with marked effects on keratinising epithelia. A therapeutic effect occurs after 2 to 3 weeks with maximum benefit after 4 to 6 weeks. Etretinate should be administered continuously because it treats only manifestations not the ultimate causes of these diseases, but treatment should be limited to a period of 6 months as experience with this drug is limited. Most patients suffer from dryness and cracking of the lips. Other side-effects include mild transient alopecia, occasional generalised pruritus, paronychia, and nose bleeds. Etretinate is teratogenic and should be avoided in women who may become pregnant. Contraceptive measures should be taken during treatment and for one year after a course of the drug.

Bufexamac is used in mild inflammatory skin conditions.

COAL TAR

Indications: chronic eczema and psoriasis
Side-effects: skin irritation and acne-like eruptions, photosensitisation

Ointments and similar preparations

Calamine and Coal Tar Ointment (see Formulary). Price 25 g = **A**

Coal Tar and Salicylic Acid Ointment, (see Formulary). Price 25 g = **A**

Coal Tar Paint, coal tar 10%, in acetone. Price 25 ml = **A**
Caution: highly inflammable

Coal Tar Paste, strong coal tar solution 7.5%, in compound zinc paste. Price 25 g = **A**

Zinc and Coal Tar Paste, zinc oxide 6%, coal tar 6%, emulsifying wax 5%, starch 38%, yellow soft paraffin 45%. Price 25 g = **A**

Alphosyl® (Stafford-Miller)
Cream, allantoin 2%, coal tar extract 5% in a water-miscible basis. Price 75 g = **D**
Lotion, allantoin 2%, coal tar extract 5%. Price 250 ml = **E**
Apply liberally 2–4 times daily

Carbo-Dome® (Dome)
Cream, coal tar solution 10%, in a water-miscible basis. Price 30 g = **C**; 100 g = **F**
Apply 2–3 times daily

▼ **Meditar®** (Brocades)
Application, coal tar 5% in wax stick. Price 20 g = **E**

Pragmatar® (SK&F)
Cream, cetyl alcohol-coal tar distillate 4%, salicylic acid 3%, sulphur 3%. Price 25 g = **C**
Apply sparingly daily; for scalp apply weekly

Psoriderm® (Dermal)
Cream, coal tar 6%, lecithin 0.4%. Price 225 ml = **E**
Apply 1–2 times daily

Impregnated dressings

Zinc Paste and Coal Tar Bandage, bandage impregnated with paste containing zinc oxide and coal tar. Price 75 mm × 6 m bandage = **D**

Coltapaste® (S&N)
Impregnated bandage, zinc paste and coal tar bandage. Price 75 mm × 6 m bandage = **C**

Tarband® (Seton)
Impregnated banadge, zinc paste and coal tar bandage. Price 75 mm × 6 m bandage = **C**

Bath preparations

Coal Tar Solution, coal tar 20%, polysorbate '80' 5%, in alcohol. Price 100 ml = **B**
Use 100 ml in a bath

Polytar Emollient—section 13.2.2

Psoriderm® (Dermal)
Bath emulsion, coal tar 40%. Price 200 ml = **D**
Use 30 ml in a bath and soak for 5 minutes

Shampoo preparations
Section 13.9

Coal tar and corticosteroid preparations

Alphosyl HC® (Stafford-Miller)
Cream, allantoin 2%, coal tar extract 5%, hydrocortisone 0.5% in a water-miscible basis. Price 30 g = **D**; 45 g = **E**. Potency IV
Apply 2–4 times daily

Carbo-Cort® (Dome)
Cream, coal tar solution 3%, hydrocortisone 0.25%. Price 30 g = **E**. Potency IV
Apply 2–3 times daily

Cor-Tar-Quin® (Dome)
Cream, coal tar solution 2%, di-iodohydroxyquinoline 1%, hydrocortisone 0.5%. Price 15 g = **E**. Potency IV
Apply 2–3 times daily

Tarcortin® (Stafford-Miller)
Cream, alcoholic extract of coal tar 5%, hydrocortisone 0.5%. Price 30 and 45 g (both) = **D**. Potency IV
Apply 3–4 times daily

BUFEXAMAC

Indications: local inflammation
Side-effects: skin irritation
Administration: apply sparingly 2–3 times daily

Parfenac® (Lederle)
Cream, bufexamac 5%, in a water-miscible basis. Do not dilute. Price 15 g = **C**; 30 g = **E**

DITHRANOL

Indications: subacute and chronic psoriasis, see notes above
Cautions: avoid use near eyes
Contra-indications: hypersensitivity; acute psoriasis
Side-effects: local burning sensation, stains skin, hair, and clothing
Administration: apply sparingly to the lesions, preferably at night; avoid contact with normal skin and broken or inflamed surfaces; wash hands thoroughly after use; initiate treatment with 0.1% preparations

Dithranol Ointment, dithranol, in yellow soft paraffin. Usual strengths 0.1 and 1% of dithranol. Part of basis may be replaced by hard paraffin if a stiffer preparation is required. Price 25 g = **A**
Dithranol Paste, dithranol in zinc and salicylic acid (Lassar's) paste. Usual strengths 0.1% ('weak dithranol paste') and 1% ('strong dithranol paste') of dithranol. Price 25 g = **A**
▼ **Antraderm Mild®** (Brocades)
Application, dithranol 0.5% in wax stick. Price 8 g = **E**
▼ **Antraderm®** (Brocades)
Application, dithranol 1% in wax stick. Price 8 g = **E**
▼ **Antraderm Forte®** (Brocades)
Application, dithranol 2% in wax stick. Price 8 g = **E**
Dithrocream® (Dermal)
Cream, dithranol 0.1%, in a water-miscible basis. Price 50 g = **E**
Cream, dithranol 0.25%, in a water-miscible basis. Price 50 g = **E**
Forte cream, dithranol 0.5%, in a water-miscible basis. Price 50 g = **E**
Dithrolan® (Dermal)
Ointment, dithranol 0.5%, salicylic acid 0.5%. Price 90 g = **F**
Psoradrate® (Eaton)
Cream, dithranol 0.1%, in a powder-in-cream basis containing hypermolar urea. Price 30 g = **D**; 100 g = **G**
▼ *Cream*, dithranol 0.2%, in a powder-in-cream basis containing hypermolar urea. Price 30 g = **E**; 100 g = **G**
Stie-Lasan® (Stiefel)
Ointment, dithranol 0.4%, salicylic acid 0.4%. Price 110 g = **F**

DITHRANOL TRIACETATE

Indications; Cautions; Contra-indications; Side-effects: see under Dithranol; see also notes above
Administration: see under Dithranol

Exolan® (Dermal)
Cream, dithranol triacetate 1% in a water-miscible basis. Price 50 g = **E**
Lotion, dithranol triacetate 0.1%, coal tar extract 5%, lecithin 0.4%. Price 200 ml = **E**

ETRETINATE

Indications; Cautions; Contra-indications; Side-effects: see notes above. Monitor liver function and plasma lipids (in patients with hypertriglyceridaemia) 1 month after initiating treatment and then at 3-monthly intervals
Dose: initially 0.5–1 mg/kg daily in two divided doses adjusted according to response

▼ **Tigason®** (Roche)
Capsules, yellow, etretinate 10 mg. Price 20 caps = **G** (Hosp. only)
Capsules, orange/yellow, etretinate 25 mg. Price 20 caps = **J** (Hosp. only)

ICHTHAMMOL

Indications: chronic eczema
Cautions: avoid application to broken or inflamed skin
Side-effects: skin irritation and sensitisation

Ichthammol Ointment, ichthammol 10%, yellow soft paraffin 45%, wool fat 45%. Price 25 g = **A**
Zinc and Ichthammol Cream, ichthammol 5%, cetostearyl alcohol 3%, wool fat 10%, in zinc cream. Price 100 g = **B**
Zinc Paste and Ichthammol Bandage, bandage impregnated with paste containing zinc oxide and ichthammol. Price 75 mm × 6 m bandage = **D**
Ichthopaste® (S&N)
Impregnated bandage, zinc paste and ichthammol bandage. Price 75 mm × 6 m bandage = **D**
Icthaband® (Seton)
Impregnated bandage, zinc paste and ichthammol bandage. Price 75 mm × 6 m bandage = **D**

SALICYLIC ACID

Indications: hyperkeratoses
Cautions: avoid broken or inflamed skin
Side-effects: irritation, systemic effects after prolonged use (see section 10.1.1.1)

Salicylic Acid Ointment, salicylic acid 2%, in wool alcohols ointment. Price 25 g = **A**
Zinc and Salicylic Acid Paste (Lassar's Paste), zinc oxide 24%, salicylic acid 2%, starch 24%, white soft paraffin 50%. Price 25 g = **A**

13.6 Preparations for acne

Most topical preparations are intended for removing follicular plugs and reducing skin flora. The skin is usually cleansed two or more times daily with detergent solutions, for example cetrimide solution (section 13.11). Abrasive agents may also be used but their effectiveness is uncertain.

Cleansing is followed by application of **antiseptics** and **keratolytics**. Preparations usually contain benzoyl peroxide, potassium hydroxyquinoline sulphate, sulphur, salicylic acid, or tretinoin. Many of these irritate the skin but it is doubtful if a therapeutic effect can be obtained without some degree of irritation. Topical application of **tretinoin** (Retin-A®) has been shown to be useful in treating acne but patients should be warned that some redness and skin peeling may occur after application for several days. Tretinoin is a vitamin A derivative.

Thick greasy preparations are generally **contra-indicated** in acne. Topical antibiotics are also used but their value is uncertain and they may cause sensitisation, particularly with neomycin. Preparations containing resorcinol should be avoided as prolonged application may interfere with thyroid function. Topical corticosteroids should not be used in acne. Systemic antibacterial treatment is useful. Tetracycline, erythromycin, and occasionally co-trimoxazole are used. The usual dosage regimen for tetracycline and erythromycin, taken before meals, is 250 mg 3 times daily for 1–4 weeks and then reduced to twice daily until improvement occurs. Maximum improvement usually occurs after three or four months but in resistant cases treatment may need to be continued for two or more years. As pseudomembranous colitis has been reported with tetracycline, caution is necessary in long term administration.

ABRASIVE AGENTS

Indications: cleansing in acne vulgaris
Cautions: avoid contact with eyes; discontinue use temporarily if skin becomes irritated

Brasivol® (Stiefel)
Paste No. 1, aluminium oxide 38.09% in fine particles, in a soap-detergent basis. Price 115 g = **E**
Paste No. 2, aluminium oxide 52.2% in medium particles, in a soap-detergent basis. Price 135 g = **E**
Paste No. 3, aluminium oxide 65.2% in coarse particles, in a soap-detergent basis. Price 150 g = **E**
Use instead of soap 1–3 times daily, starting with fine grade and progressing to coarser grades if required

Ionax Scrub® (Alcon)
Gel, polyethylene granules 21.9%, benzalkonium chloride 0.25%. Price 50 g = **D**; 100 g = **E**. ACBS: see Appendix 3
Use instead of soap 1–2 times daily

BENZOYL PEROXIDE

Indications: acne vulgaris
Cautions: avoid contact with eyes, mouth, and mucous membranes; may bleach fabrics
Administration: apply once daily to clean skin, starting treatment with lower-strength preparations

Acetoxyl® (Stiefel)
2.5 gel, benzoyl peroxide 2.5%, in an aqueous-acetone-gel basis. Price 40 g = **D**
5 gel, benzoyl peroxide 5%, in an aqueous-acetone-gel basis. Price 40 g = **D**

Acnegel® (Kirby-Warrick)
Gel, benzoyl peroxide 5%. Price 50 g = **D**
Forte gel, benzoyl peroxide 10%. Price 50 g = **D**

Benoxyl® (Stiefel)
5 cream, benzoyl peroxide 5%, in a water-miscible basis. Price 40 g = **D**
5 lotion, benzoyl peroxide 5%. Price 30 ml = **C**
10 lotion, benzoyl peroxide 10%. Price 30 ml = **C**

Panoxyl® (Stiefel)
5 acne gel, benzoyl peroxide 5%. Price 40 g = **D**
10 acne gel, benzoyl peroxide 10%. Price 40 g = **D**

SULPHUR

Indications: acne vulgaris
Administration: apply to clean skin 1–2 times daily

Sulphur Lotion, Compound, precipitated sulphur 4% (see Formulary). Price 100 ml = **B**
Sulphur Ointment, precipitated sulphur 10%, in simple ointment. Price 25 g = **A**

TRETINOIN

Indications: acne vulgaris
Cautions: avoid contact with eyes, mouth, and mucous membranes; do not use with other peeling agents or with ultra-violet lamps
Contra-indications: eczema, broken skin
Side-effects: irritation, erythema, desquamation, changes in pigmentation, photosensitivity
Administration: apply to clean skin 1–2 times daily

Retin-A® (Ortho)
Cream, tretinoin 0.05%. Price 60 g = **F**
Gel, tretinoin 0.025%. Price 60 g = **F**
Lotion, tretinoin 0.025%. Price 80 ml = **F**

COMPOUND PREPARATIONS FOR ACNE

Resorcinol and Sulphur Paste, resorcinol 5%, precipitated sulphur 5%, emulsifying ointment 50%, zinc oxide 40%. Price 25 g = **A**
Salicylic Acid and Sulphur Cream, salicylic acid 2%, precipitated sulphur 2%, in aqueous cream. Price 50 g = **A**
Salicylic Acid and Sulphur Ointment, salicylic acid 3%, precipitated sulphur 3%, in hydrous ointment (oily cream). Price 25 g = **A**
Zinc Sulphide Lotion, zinc sulphate 5%, sulphurated potash 5% (see Formulary). Price 100 ml = **A**
Acnil® (Fisons) *cream*, cetrimide, resorcinol, precipitated sulphur. Price 25 g = **C**
Actinac® (Roussel) *lotion*, allantoin, butoxyethyl nicotinate, chloramphenicol, hydrocortisone acetate, precipitated sulphur, powder for reconstitution. Price 2 × 5-g bottles of powder and 2 × 16-ml bottles of solvent = **F**. Potency IV

Benoxyl® (Stiefel)
5 with sulphur cream, benzoyl peroxide 5%, sulphur 2% in a water-miscible basis. Price 40 g = **D**

10 with sulphur cream, benzoyl peroxide 10%, sulphur 5% in a water-miscible basis. Price 40 g = **D**
5 with sulphur lotion, benzoyl peroxide 5%, sulphur 2%. Price 30 ml = **C**
10 with sulphur lotion, benzoyl peroxide 10%, sulphur 5%. Price 30 ml = **C**

Dome-Acne® (Dome) *cream*, resorcinol monoacetate, sulphur. Price 30 g = **D**. *Lotion*, ingredients as for cream. Price 50 ml = **D**. *Medicated cleanser* (= application), salicylic acid, sulphur. Price 100 g = **E**

Eskamel® (SK&F) *cream*, resorcinol, sulphur. Price 25 g = **C**

Medrone® (Upjohn) *acne lotion*, aluminium chlorhydroxide, methylprednisolone acetate, sulphur. Price 25 ml = **E**; 75 ml = **G**. Potency IV

Neo-Medrone® (Upjohn) *acne lotion*, aluminium chlorhydroxide complex, methylprednisolone acetate, neomycin sulphate, sulphur. Price 25 ml = **E**; 75 ml = **G**. Potency IV

Quinoderm® (Quinoderm)
Cream, benzoyl peroxide, potassium hydroxyquinoline sulphate. Price 25 g = **C**.
Lotio-gel (= lotion), ingredients as for cream. Price 30 ml = **C**.
Cream with hydrocortisone, other ingredients as above. Price 30 g = **C**. Potency IV

Vanair® (Carter-Wallace)
Cream, benzoyl peroxide 10%, sulphur 2.5% in a water-miscible basis. Price 30 g = **C**

13.7 Preparations for warts and calluses

The least destructive method possible should be chosen to treat these lesions as they are self-limiting and all viral warts including those on the soles (verrucas) eventually disappear spontaneously. **Salicylic acid** preparations are suitable, either salicylic acid collodion or one of the proprietary preparations, Duofilm® or Salactol®.

Podophyllin preparations may also be useful. Compound podophyllin paint, in concentrations of between 5 and 20% is employed for the treatment of anogenital warts. The paint should be allowed to stay on the treated area for not longer than 6 hours and then washed off. Care should be taken to avoid splashing the surrounding skin during application. Where there are a large number of warts only a few should be treated at any one time as severe toxicity caused by absorption of podophyllin has been reported. It should also be used with caution in pregnancy. Posalfilin® is suitable for treating plantar warts or horny warts on the fingers or palms.

Preparations containing formaldehyde, glutaraldehyde, and bromine are also available but their effects are unpredictable.

Ointments and liquid preparations are applied to the warts or callus, avoiding contact with surrounding skin, and covered with a plaster. Dead skin may be removed at intervals by rubbing with a pumice stone.

PODOPHYLLUM RESIN

Indications: anogenital and plantar warts
Cautions: irritant to skin and mucous membranes
Contra-indications: genital warts in pregnancy
Administration: see notes above

Podophyllin Paint, Compound, podophyllum resin 15% (see Formulary). Price 25 ml = **C**. For warts, including anogenital warts

Posalfilin® (Norgine)
Ointment, podophyllum resin 20%, salicylic acid 25%. Price 10 g = **D**. For plantar warts

BROMINE COMPOUNDS

Indications: warts, particularly plantar warts
Cautions: avoid contact with eyes

Callusolve® (Dermal)
Paint, benzalkonium chloride-bromine adduct 25%. Price 10 ml = **D**. For warts, particularly plantar warts

FORMALDEHYDE

Indications: warts, particularly plantar warts
Cautions: avoid broken skin

Formaldehyde Lotion, formaldehyde solution 3% in water (see Formulary). Price 100 ml = **A**
Soak affected area for 15 minutes daily

Veracur® (Typharm)
Gel, formaldehyde solution 1.5% in a water-miscible gel basis. Price 15 g = **C**. For plantar warts
Apply daily

GLUTARALDEHYDE

Indications: warts (except anogenital and facial warts)
Cautions: stains skin brown

Glutarol® (Dermal)
Solution (= application), glutaraldehyde 10%. Price 10 ml = **D**. For plantar warts
Apply twice daily

Verucasep® (Galen)
Gel, glutaraldehyde 10%. Price 15 g = **E**. For plantar warts
Apply twice daily

SALICYLIC ACID

Indications: removal of warts and hard skin
Cautions: avoid face and anogenital region
Side-effects: inflammation of surrounding skin

Salicylic Acid Adhesive Plaster 20% or 40%. Price 10 plasters 75 mm × 45 mm = **D**

Salicylic Acid Collodion, salicylic acid 12%, in flexible collodion. Price 5 ml = **A**

Duofilm® (Stiefel)
Paint, salicylic acid 16.7%, lactic acid 16.7% in flexible collodion. Price 15 ml = **E**. For plantar and refractory warts
Apply daily

Salactol® (Dermal)
Paint, salicylic acid 16.7%, lactic acid 16.7%, in flexible collodion. Price 10 ml = **D**. For warts, particularly plantar warts
Apply daily

13.8 Sunscreens and camouflaging preparations

13.8.1 Sunscreening preparations

Ultraviolet radiation may be harmful in certain diseases, for example lupus erythematosus, photosensitive dermatitis, and rosacea. Protection may also be required in patients who have already developed signs of chronic solar damage in the skin. Certain individuals are naturally sensitive to the sun's rays, while others are sensitised by systemic drugs, for example, protein-bound tetracyclines, benoxaprofen, chlorpromazine, and nalidixic acid.

There are two types of preparation which protect the skin from ultraviolet radiation. One type merely places an opaque barrier between the sun's rays and the skin; this is thick and greasy and not very acceptable to the patient. The second type is more useful. It contains substances that absorb the erythema-producing portions of the ultraviolet spectrum, for example **aminobenzoic acid, mexenone** (Uvistat®) and **padimate** (Spectraban®).

For maximum benefit these preparations must be applied frequently. Because they filter out only a proportion of harmful rays, burning may still occur in intense sunlight and patients with light-sensitive skin should spend as little time as possible exposed to sunlight. Unfortunately no preparation exists which specifically blocks the range of sunlight responsible for some photosensitive reactions, particularly the porphyrias and drug-induced sensitivity.

Sunscreen preparations containing bergamot oil (which contains 5-methoxypsoralen) may cause or promote skin cancers.

AMINOBENZOIC ACID

Indications: sunscreen
Cautions: may stain clothing

Aminobenzoic Acid Lotion, aminobenzoic acid 5 g, glycerol 20 ml, industrial methylated spirit 60 ml, purified water, freshly boiled and cooled, to 100 ml. Price 200 ml = **B**. Apply undiluted and allow to dry before exposure; repeat every 2 hours if necessary

MEXENONE

Indications: sunscreen
Administration: apply twice daily or more frequently to exposed areas of skin

Uvistat® (WBP)
Cream, mexenone 4%, in a water-miscible basis. Price 50 g = **C**; 100 g = **D**. ACBS: see Appendix 3
L-application, mexenone 4%, in a solid basis, for application to the lips. Price 5-g stick = **B**. ACBS: see Appendix 3

PADIMATE

Indications: sunscreen
Side-effects: rashes or skin irritation
Administration: apply once daily; renew after bathing or excessive sweating

Spectraban 4® (Stiefel)
Lotion, padimate 2.5%, in an alcoholic basis. Price 150 ml = **E**. ACBS: see Appendix 3
Caution: inflammable

Spectraban 15® (Stiefel)
Lotion, aminobenzoic acid 5%, padimate 2.5%, in an alcoholic basis. Price 150 ml = **E**. ACBS: see Appendix 3
Caution: inflammable

13.8.2 Camouflaging preparations

Disfigurement of the skin can be very embarrassing to patients and have a marked psychological effect. In skilled hands, or with experience, these preparations can be very effective in concealing scars, areas of discoloration, and birthmarks.

Boots Covering Cream® (Boots)
Cream, pigments and opacifying agents (4 shades) in a cream basis. Price 20 g = **C**. ACBS: see Appendix 3

Covermark® (Medexport)
Cream rouge (= cream), pigment, titanium dioxide, waxes and other ingredients (3 shades). Price 8 g = **F**. ACBS: see Appendix 3
Spotstick (= application), ingredients as above (7 shades). Price 3.5 g = **F**. ACBS: see Appendix 3
Grey toner (= cream), ingredients as above, in cream basis. Price 8 g = **F**. ACBS: see Appendix 3
Masking cream, ingredients as above (10 shades), in cream basis. Price 25 g = **F**. ACBS: see Appendix 3
Shading cream, ingredients as above, in cream basis. Price 8 g = **F**. ACBS: see Appendix 3
Finishing powder, ingredients as above, in dusting-powder basis. Price 50 g = **E**; 250 g = **H**. ACBS: see Appendix 3

Keromask® (Sterling Industrial)
Base cream, ochre pigments, titanium dioxide (3 shades). Price 15 ml = **D**. ACBS: see Appendix 3
Toning cream, ochre pigments, titanium dioxide (5 shades). Price 15 ml = **D**. ACBS: see Appendix 3

13.9 Scalp preparations

The treatment of choice in dandruff (*Pityriasis capitis*) is the frequent use of a mild detergent shampoo generally once or twice weekly. Shampoos containing tar extracts, for example Polytar® are also popular. Where this is insufficient for dealing with dandruff, a preparation containing **salicylic acid 2%** and **sulphur 2%** for example salicylic acid and sulphur cream is frequently helpful. Lotions or gels containing weak **corticosteroids** (section 13.4) applied to the scalp may also be useful in treating some of the more severe cases. Shampoos containing **selenium sulphide** are of little value in dandruff. Cradle cap in infants may be treated with application of **olive oil** before shampooing.

See also section 13.5 (psoriasis and eczema), section 13.10.4 (scabies), and section 13.10.2 (ringworm).

Salicylic Acid Lotion, salicylic acid 2% (see Formulary). Price 100 ml = **A**
Caution: highly inflammable

Alphosyl® (Stafford-Miller)
Application PC, allantoin 0.2%, refined alcoholic extract of coal tar 5%, in a shampoo basis. Price 60 g = **B**. ACBS: see Appendix 3

Betadine® (Napp)
Shampoo solution, povidone-iodine 4%, in a surfactant solution containing lanolin. Price 100 ml = **C**. ACBS: see Appendix 3

Capitol® (Dermal)
Gel (= shampoo application), benzalkonium chloride 0.5%. Price 120 g = **D**. ACBS: see Appendix 3

Ceanel® (Quinoderm)
Concentrate (= shampoo application), cetrimide 10%, undecenoic acid 1%, phenethyl alcohol 7.5%. Price 50 ml = **C**; 500 ml = **F**. ACBS: see Appendix 3

Cetavlon® (ICI)
P.C. solution (= shampoo application), cetrimide 17.5%. Price 125 ml = **B**. ACBS: see Appendix 3

Genisol® (Fisons)
Solution (= shampoo application), purified coal tar fractions 0.25%, sodium sulphosuccinated undecylenic monoalkylolamide 1%. Price 58 ml = **B**; 250 ml = **E**; 600 ml = **F**. ACBS: see Appendix 3

Ionil T® (Alcon)
Shampoo (= application), benzalkonium chloride 0.2%, coal tar solution 4.25%, salicylic acid 2% in a shampoo basis. Price 120 and 240 ml (both) = **D**. ACBS: see Appendix 3

Polytar® (Stiefel)
Liquid (= shampoo application), arachis oil extract of crude coal tar 0.3%, cade oil 0.3%, coal tar solution 0.1%, oleyl alcohol 1%, tar 0.3%. Price 65 ml = **C**; 150 ml = **D**; 350 ml = **E**. ACBS: see Appendix 3
Liquid plus (= shampoo application), ingredients as above with hydrolysed animal protein 3%. Price 150 ml = **C**; 350 ml = **E**. ACBS: see Appendix 3

Psoriderm® (Dermal)
Scalp lotion (= shampoo application), coal tar 2.5%, lecithin 0.3%. Price 112 ml = **E**

Synogist® (Maltown)
Shampoo solution, sodium sulphosuccinated undecylenic monoalkylolamide 2%. Price 100 ml = **D**

SELENIUM SULPHIDE

Indications: pityriasis capitis, seborrhoeic dermatitis
Cautions: avoid contact with the eyes and broken skin; do not apply within 48 hours of using hair colouring or permanent waving preparations
Administration: use as a shampoo twice weekly for 2 weeks, once weekly for 2 weeks, then every 3–6 weeks; wash hands thoroughly after use

Lenium® (Winthrop)
Cream (= shampoo application), selenium sulphide 2.5%. Price 9-g sachet = **A**; 42-g tube = **B**; 100-g tube = **C**

Selsun® (Abbott)
Shampoo application, selenium sulphide 2.5%. Price 50 ml = **B**; 100 ml = **C**; 150 ml = **D**

13.10 Treatment of skin infections

13.10.1 Antibacterial preparations

For many skin infections systemic antibacterial treatment is the method of choice because the infection is too deeply sited for adequate penetration of topical preparations. For details of preparations and suitable treatment see section 5.1.

Although there are a great many antibacterial drugs presented in topical preparations they are potentially hazardous and frequently their use is not necessary if adequate hygienic measures can be taken. Moreover not all skin conditions that are oozing, crusted, or characterised by pustules are actually infected. To minimise the development of resistant organisms it is advisable to limit the choice of drugs to be applied topically to those not used systemically. Unfortunately some of these drugs, for example neomycin, may cause sensitisation and, if large areas of skin are being treated, ototoxicity may be a hazard, particularly in the elderly. Resistant organisms are more common in hospitals, and whenever possible swabs for examination should be taken before beginning treatment. Topical preparations containing a corticosteroid are included in section 13.4.

Mafenide (Sulfamylon®) and **silver sulphadiazine** (Flamazine®) are useful in the treatment of infected burns.

13.10.1.1 ANTIBACTERIAL PREPARATIONS ONLY USED TOPICALLY

CHLORAMPHENICOL

Indications: skin infections
Side-effects: local hypersensitivity reactions

Chloramphenicol Cream (Drug Tariff Formula), chloramphenicol 1%, macrogol '4000' 49%, propylene glycol 50%. Price 50 g = **B**

FRAMYCETIN SULPHATE

Indications; Side-effects: see under Neomycin Sulphate

Framygen® (Fisons)
Cream, framycetin sulphate 0.5%, in a water-miscible basis. Price 15 g = **D**

Soframycin® (Roussel) *cream*, framycetin sulphate, gramicidin. Price 15 g = **D**. *Ointment*, ingredients as for cream. Price 15 g = **D**

Sofra-Tulle® (Roussel)
Impregnated dressing, framycetin sulphate 1%. Price 10 dressings (100 mm × 100 mm) = **D**; 10 dressings (300 mm × 100 mm) = **G**

MAFENIDE

Indications: pseudomonal infection of second- and third-degree burns
Cautions: pulmonary dysfunction
Side-effects: allergic reactions including rashes and erythema multiforme, metabolic acidosis

Sulfamylon® (Winthrop)
Cream, mafenide 8.5% (as acetate), in a water-miscible basis. Price 500 g = **J**

NEOMYCIN SULPHATE

Indications: skin infections, but see notes above
Side-effects: hypersensitivity reactions

Neomycin Cream, neomycin sulphate 0.5%, cetomacrogol emulsifying ointment 30%, chlorocresol 0.1%, disodium edetate 0.01%, freshly boiled and cooled purified water 69.39%. Price 100 g = **E**

Neomycin Ointment, neomycin sulphate 0.5% in an anhydrous greasy basis. Price 15 g = **A**; 28.4 g = **C**

Cicatrin® (Calmic)
Aerosol powder (= application), bacitracin zinc, L-cysteine, glycine, neomycin sulphate (pressurised aerosol pack). Price 3-g unit = **G**.
Cream, ingredients as above with threonine. Price 15 g = **E**; 30 g = **F**.
Dusting-powder, ingredients as for cream. Price 15 g = **E**; 50 g = **G**

Dispray Antibiotic® (Stuart)
Aerosol (= application), bacitracin zinc, neomycin sulphate, polymyxin B sulphate (pressurised aerosol pack). Price 110-g unit = **E**

Graneodin® (Squibb)
Ointment, gramicidin, neomycin sulphate. Price 15 g = **B**

Myciguent® (Upjohn)
Ointment, neomycin sulphate 0.5%, in an anhydrous greasy basis. Price 28.4 g = **C**

Neo-Medrone® (Upjohn) *cream*, methylprednisolone acetate, neomycin sulphate. Price 15 g = **D**. Potency IV

Nivemycin® (Boots)
Ointment, neomycin sulphate 0.5%, in an anhydrous greasy basis. Price 15 g = **A**

Polybactrin® (Calmic)
Spray, bacitracin zinc, neomycin sulphate, polymyxin B sulphate (sterile powder in pressurised aerosol pack). Price 110-g pack = **I**

Tribiotic® (Riker)
Application, bacitracin zinc, neomycin sulphate, polymyxin B sulphate (pressurised aerosol pack). Price 110-g unit = **G**

NITROFURAZONE

Indications: skin infections
Side-effects: local sensitisation

Furacin® (Eaton)
Soluble ointment (= cream), nitrofurazone 0.2%, in a water-soluble macrogol basis. Price 25 g = **C**
Solution, nitrofurazone 0.2%, in a water-miscible vehicle. Price 100 ml = **D**; 500 ml = **H**

POLYMYXIN B SULPHATE

Indications; Side-effects: see under Neomycin Sulphate

Polyfax® (Calmic)
Ointment, bacitracin zinc 500 units, polymyxin B sulphate 10 000 units. Price 20 g = **E**

POLYNOXYLIN

Indications: bacterial and fungal skin infections

Anaflex® (Geistlich)
Aerosol (= application), polynoxylin 2%, in a pressurised aerosol unit. Price 100 g = **E**
Cream, polynoxylin 10%, in a water-miscible basis. Price 50 g = **D**
Dusting-powder, polynoxylin 10%. Price 10 g = **C**; 30 g = **E**
Paste, polynoxylin 10%. For application to moist areas. Price 20 g = **C**

Ponoxylan® (Berk)
Gel, polynoxylin 10%. Price 25 g = **C**

SILVER SULPHADIAZINE

Indications; Cautions; Side-effects: see under Mafenide

Flamazine® (S&N Pharm.)
Cream, silver sulphadiazine 1%, in a water-soluble basis. Price 50 g = **E**; 250 g = **G**; 500 g = **I**

TRICLOCARBAN
Indications: skin infections

Cutisan® (Dales)
Dusting-powder, triclocarban 1%. Price 80 g = **E**
Ointment (= cream), triclocarban 2%, in a water-miscible basis. Price 30 g = **D**
Solution, triclocarban 1%, in a water-miscible vehicle. Price 45 ml = **E**

13.10.1.2 ANTIBACTERIAL PREPARATIONS ALSO USED SYSTEMICALLY

CHLORTETRACYCLINE HYDROCHLORIDE
Indications: skin infections, but see notes above; impetigo, see section 5.1, table 1
Cautions: overgrowth with non-susceptible organisms may occur
Side-effects: rarely local hypersensitivity reactions

Aureomycin® (Lederle)
Cream, chlortetracycline hydrochloride 3% as chlortetracycline. Price 30 g = **D**
Ointment, chlortetracycline hydrochloride 3%. Diluent wool fat 10% in white soft paraffin. Price 30 g = **D**

COLISTIN SULPHATE
Indications: skin infections
Side-effects: transient irritation

Colomycin® (Pharmax)
Powder, sterile, for making topical preparations, colistin sulphate. Price 1- and 5-g vial (both) = **J**

FUSIDIC ACID
Indications: staphylococcal skin infections and abscesses
Cautions: avoid contact with eyes
Side-effects: rarely hypersensitivity reactions

Fucidin® (Leo)
Cream, fusidic acid 2%. Price 10 g = **D**
Gel, fusidic acid 2%. Price 10 g = **D**; 25 g = **E**
Caviject gel, fusidic acid 2% in single-dose unit (7g) fitted with elongated nozzle. For treatment of abscesses. Price 1 unit = **D**
Intertulle (= impregnated dressing), sodium fusidate 2%. Price 10 dressings (100 mm × 100 mm) = **D**
Ointment, sodium fusidate 2%, in an anhydrous greasy basis. Price 10 g = **D**; 25 g = **E**

GENTAMICIN
Indications; Side-effects: see under Neomycin Sulphate (section 13.10.1.1)

Cidomycin® (Roussel)
Cream, gentamicin 0.3% (as sulphate), in a water-miscible basis. Do not dilute. Price 15 g = **D**; 30 g = **E**
Ointment, gentamicin 0.3% (as sulphate), in an anhydrous greasy basis. Do not dilute. Price 15 g = **D**; 30 g = **E**

Genticin® (Nicholas)
Cream, gentamicin 0.3% (as sulphate), in a water-miscible basis. Price 15 g = **D**; 100 g = **H**
Ointment, gentamicin 0.3% (as sulphate), in an anhydrous greasy basis. Price 15 g = **D**; 100 g = **H**

OXYTETRACYCLINE
Indications; Cautions; Side-effects: see under Chlortetracycline Hydrochloride

Terramycin® (Pfizer)
Ointment, oxytetracycline 3% (as hydrochloride). Price 15 g = **C**

TETRACYCLINE HYDROCHLORIDE
Indications; Cautions; Side-effects: see under Chlortetracycline Hydrochloride

Achromycin® (Lederle)
Ointment, tetracycline hydrochloride 3%. Price 30 g = **D**

13.10.2 Antifungal preparations

Ideally, skin scrapings should be examined to confirm the diagnosis before treatment has begun. Localised infections are treated with the topical preparations described in this section but widespread or intractable dermatophyte infections are treated systemically with griseofulvin or ketoconazole (section 5.2).

Tinea unguium (nail ringworm) and *T. capitis* (scalp ringworm) infections are best treated by systemic **griseofulvin** but other ringworm infections such as athlete's foot can be treated by topical application.

Compound benzoic acid ointment (Whitfield's ointment) is quite effective but not as elegant as the more modern, and more expensive, preparations. Of these, **clotrimazole** (Canesten®), **econazole** (Ecostatin®, Pevaryl®), and **miconazole** (Daktarin®, Dermonistat®), are commonly used. These preparations can also be used for candidal infections but preparations of **amphotericin** or **nystatin** are as effective.

BENZOIC ACID
Indications: mild fungal infections

Benzoic Acid Ointment, Compound, benzoic acid 6%, salicylic acid 3%, in emulsifying ointment. Price 25 g = **A**

AMPHOTERICIN
Indications: fungal infections, especially due to *Candida albicans*

Fungilin® (Squibb)
Cream, amphotericin 3%, in a water-miscible basis. Do not dilute. Price 15 g = **D**
Ointment, amphotericin 3%, in Plastibase®. Do not dilute. Price 15 g = **D**

CHLORPHENESIN

Indications: fungal infections, especially of the feet
Side-effects: rarely sensitivity

Mycil® (Farley)
Dusting-powder, chlorphenesin 1%. Price 55 g = **C**
Ointment, chlorphenesin 0.5% in a water-in-oil cream basis. Price 30 g = **C**

CLOTRIMAZOLE

Indications: fungal skin infections
Side-effects: occasional local irritation

Canesten® (Bayer)
Cream, clotrimazole 1%, in a water-miscible basis. Price 20 g = **D**; 50 g = **F**
Dusting-powder, clotrimazole 1%. Price 30 g = **D**
Solution (= application), clotrimazole 1% in macrogol 400. Price 20 ml = **E**
Spray, clotrimazole 1%, in 30% isopropyl alcohol. Price 40 ml = **F**

ECONAZOLE NITRATE

Indications; Side-effects: see under Clotrimazole

Econazole Nitrate Cream, econazole nitrate 1% in a water-miscible basis. Price 15 g = **D**; 30 g = **E**
Econazole Nitrate Lotion, econazole nitrate 1%. Price 30 ml = **E**
▼ **Ecostatin®** (FAIR)
Cream, econazole nitrate 1%, in a water-miscible basis. Price 15 g = **D**; 30 g = **E**
Dusting-powder, econazole nitrate 1%. Price 30 g = **E**
Spray-powder, econazole nitrate 1%. Price 200-g unit = **E**
Lotion, econazole nitrate 1%. Price 30 ml = **E**
Spray, econazole nitrate 1% in alcoholic solution. Price 150 g = **F**
▼ **Pevaryl®** (Ortho)
Cream, econazole nitrate 1% in a water-miscible basis. Price 30 g = **E**
Spray-powder, econazole nitrate 1%. Price 200-g unit (20 g powder) = **E**
Lotion, econazole nitrate 1%. Price 30 ml = **E**

GRISEOFULVIN

See section 5.2

KETOCONAZOLE

See section 5.2

MICONAZOLE NITRATE

Indications; Side-effects: see under Clotrimazole

Miconazole Nitrate Cream, miconazole nitrate 2% in a water-miscible basis. Price 30 g = **E**
Daktarin® (Janssen)
Cream, miconazole nitrate 2%, in a water-miscible basis. Price 30 g = **E**
Twin pack, 1 × 30 g pack of cream, with 1 × 30 g dusting-powder miconazole nitrate 2%. Price (complete) = **F**
Dermonistat® (Ortho)
Cream, miconazole nitrate 2%, in a water-miscible basis. Price 30 g = **E**

NATAMYCIN

Indications: fungal infections, especially due to *Candida* spp.

Pimafucin® (Brocades)
Cream, natamycin 2%, in a water-miscible basis. Price 25 g = **D**

NYSTATIN

Indications: skin infections due to *Candida* spp.

Multilind® (FAIR)
Ointment, nystatin 100 000 units/g, zinc oxide 5%. Price 30 g = **D**; 100 g = **F**. For napkin rash
Nystaform® (Dome)
Cream, clioquinol, nystatin. Price 30 g = **E**.
Ointment, ingredients as for cream. Price 30 g = **E**
Nystaform-HC® (Dome) *cream*, ingredients as for Nystaform with 3 times the amount of clioquinol and, in addition, hydrocortisone. Price 15 g = **D**; 30 g = **E**. Potency IV. *Lotion*, ingredients as for cream. Price 30 ml = **F**. Potency IV. *Ointment*, ingredients as for cream. Price 15 g = **D**; 30 g = **E**. Potency IV
Nystan® (Squibb)
Cream, nystatin 100 000 units/g, in a water-miscible basis. Price 15 g = **D**; 30 g = **E**
Dusting-powder, nystatin 100 000 units/g. Price 15 g = **C**
Gel, nystatin 100 000 units/g. Price 30 g = **E**
Ointment, nystatin 100 000 units/g, in Plastibase®. Price 15 g = **C**; 30 g = **E**
Tinaderm-M® (Kirby-Warrick)
Cream, nystatin, tolnaftate. Price 20 g = **D**. For fungal infection of skin and nails

PECILOCIN

Indications: topical ringworm infections
Contra-indications: ineffective against *Candida* spp.
Side-effects: rarely hypersensitivity reactions

Variotin® (Leo)
Ointment, pecilocin 3000 units/g. Price 10 g = **C**

SALICYLIC ACID

Section 13.5

TOLNAFTATE

Indications; Contra-indications; Side-effects: see under Pecilocin

Tinaderm® (Kirby-Warrick)
Cream, tolnaftate 1%, in a water-miscible basis. Price 15 g = **B**
Dusting-powder, tolnaftate 1%. Price 50 g = **C**
Solution, tolnaftate 1%. Price 20 ml = **C**

UNDECENOATES

Indications: topical ringworm infections

Zinc Undecenoate Dusting-powder, zinc undecenoate 10%, undecenoic acid 2%, pumilio pine oil 0.5%, starch 50%, in light kaolin. Price 50 g = **A**
Zinc Undecenoate Ointment, zinc undecenoate 20%, undecenoic acid 5%, in emulsifying ointment. Price 50 g = **B**
Monphytol® (LAB) *paint*, boric acid, chlorbutol, methyl salicylate, methyl undecenoate, propyl undecenoate, salicylic acid. Price 18 ml = **B**
Mycota® (Crookes Products)
Cream, zinc undecenoate 20%, undecenoic acid 5%. Price 25 g = **B**
Dusting-powder, zinc undecenoate 20%, undecenoic acid 2%. Price 70 g = **B**
Spray (= application), dichlorophen, hexachlorophane, undecenoic acid (pressurised aerosol pack). Price 200 g = **B**
Tineafax® (Wellcome)
Dusting-powder, zinc undecenoate 10%. Price 50 g = **C**
Ointment, zinc naphthenate, zinc undecenoate. Price 25 g = **B**

OTHER PREPARATIONS FOR FUNGAL INFECTIONS

Phortinea® (Philip Harris) *liquid* (= paint), 4-nitrophenol 2%. Price 15 ml (with applicator) = **B**
Phytex® (Pharmax) *paint*, borotannic complex, methyl salicylate, salicylic acid. Price 20 ml = **D**
Phytocil® (Rorer)
Cream, 2-*p*-chlorophenoxyethanol, menthol, 1-phenoxypropan-2-ol, salicylic acid. Price 25 g = **B**.
Dusting-powder, 2-*p*-chlorophenoxyethanol, 1-phenoxypropan-2-ol, zinc undecenoate. Price 50 g = **B**
Phytodermine® (M&B)
Dusting-powder, methyl hydroxybenzoate, salicylic acid. Price 50 g = **C**
Quinoped® (Quinoderm)
Cream, benzoyl peroxide, potassium hydroxyquinoline sulphate. Price 25 g = **B**

13.10.3 Antiviral preparations

Idoxuridine solution (5% in dimethyl sulphoxide) is used for severe herpetic infections of the skin. Both *Herpes simplex* and *zoster* seem to respond well to frequent applications if started early and continued for 3 to 4 days.

IDOXURIDINE IN DIMETHYL SULPHOXIDE

Indications: see notes above
Cautions: avoid contact with the eyes and mucous membranes
Side-effects: stinging on application, changes in taste; overuse may cause maceration
Administration: apply 5% solution to lesions 4 times daily for 3–4 days

Herpid® (WBP)
Solution (= application), idoxuridine 5% in dimethyl sulphoxide. Price 5 ml (with brush) = **H**
Iduridin® (Ferring)
Application, idoxuridine 5% in dimethyl sulphoxide. Price 5 ml with applicator = **G**
Application, idoxuridine 40% in dimethyl sulphoxide. Price 5 ml with applicator and 20 ml with dropper (both) = **J**
Apply on lint to the affected area daily for 4 days

13.10.4 Parasiticidal preparations

In the treatment of *scabies*, two applications of **benzyl benzoate** to all members of the affected household is still probably the most widely used treatment. Benzyl benzoate is a skin irritant with a characteristic odour, and **gamma benzene hexachloride** in a 1% cream is preferable for children as it is less irritant.

Monosulfiram lotion (Tetmosol®) diluted just before use with 2 or 3 parts of water is a most useful application for scabies and may be repeated daily for 2 or 3 days, preferably after a hot bath. It is also effective against fleas, lice, ticks, and most pathogenic fungi. Patients under treatment should not take alcohol because monosulfiram acts like disulfiram. **Crotamiton** (section 13.3) is also used for scabies.

Gamma benzene hexachloride is a well-established treatment for *pediculosis* (lice), but **malathion** and **carbaryl** are becoming accepted more widely, perhaps even as the treatment of choice.

The itch of scabies persists long after the infestation has been eliminated and antipruritic treatment may be required.

BENZYL BENZOATE

Indications: scabies, pediculosis
Cautions: avoid contact with the eyes
Side-effects: slight local irritation

Benzyl Benzoate Application, benzyl benzoate 25 g, emulsifying wax 2 g/100 ml, in purified water, freshly boiled and cooled. Price 150 ml = **B**
Directions for use: scabies—apply over the whole body, omitting the head and neck, after a hot bath. The application should be repeated after 5 days
Pediculosis—apply to affected area for 24 hours, remove by washing; in severe cases repeat 2–3 times

Ascabiol® (M&B)
Emulsion (= application), benzyl benzoate 25%. Price 200 ml = **D**
Directions as above

CARBARYL

Indications: pediculosis
Cautions; Side-effects: see under Benzyl Benzoate
Administration: shampoo—leave on hair for 2 minutes, rinse, comb, repeat procedure; lotion—apply to dry hair, allow to dry naturally, comb, wash 12 hours later

Carylderm® (Napp)
Gel shampoo, carbaryl 1%. Price 40 g = **B**
Lotion, carbaryl 0.5%, in an alcoholic basis. Price 55 ml = **B**
Caution: highly inflammable
Derbac® (Bengué)
Shampoo solution, carbaryl 0.5% in a shampoo basis. Price 50 ml = **B**

CROTAMITON

Indications: scabies
Cautions; Contra-indications: section 13.3
Administration: apply over the whole body omitting the head and neck, preferably after a hot bath, and remove by washing on the following day. The application may be repeated 24 hours later

Preparations
Section 13.3

GAMMA BENZENE HEXACHLORIDE

Indications: pediculosis, scabies
Cautions; Side-effects: see under Benzyl Benzoate

Gamma Benzene Hexachloride Application, gamma benzene hexachloride 100 mg, emulsifying wax 4 g, lavender oil 1 ml, xylene (of commerce) 15 ml/100 ml, in purified water, freshly boiled and cooled. Price 50 ml = **A**
Pediculosis—rub about one tablespoonful with the fingers into the hair and roots of the hair. Do not wash the head during the next 24 hours
Esoderm® (Priory)
Lotion, dicophane 1%, gamma benzene hexachloride 1%. For scabies and pediculosis. Price 55 ml = **B**. *Shampoo* (= application), ingredients as for lotion. For pediculosis. Price 40 g = **B**; 300 g = **D**
Lorexane® (ICI)
Cream, gamma benzene hexachloride 1%, in a water-miscible basis. Price 50 g = **B**. For scabies and pediculosis
No.3, medicated shampoo, gamma benzene hexachloride 2% in detergent basis, for use with water in pediculosis. Price 50 g = **B**
Quellada® (Stafford-Miller)
Application PC, gamma benzene hexachloride 1%, in a shampoo basis. Price 100 ml = **C**; 500 ml = **E**. For pediculosis
Lotion, gamma benzene hexachloride 1%, in a lotion basis. Price 100 ml = **C**; 500 ml = **E**. For scabies

MALATHION

Indications: pediculosis, scabies
Cautions; Side-effects: see under Benzyl Benzoate
Administration: see under Carbaryl

Derbac® (Bengué)
Liquid (= application), malathion 0.5%. Price 50 ml = **B**; 155 ml = **C**
Prioderm® (Napp)
Cream shampoo, malathion 1%. Price 40 g = **B**
Lotion, malathion 0.5%, in an alcoholic basis. Price 55 ml = **B**
Caution: highly inflammable

MONOSULFIRAM

Indications: scabies
Cautions; Side-effects: see under Benzyl Benzoate and notes above
Administration: see notes above

Tetmosol® (ICI)
Solution, monosulfiram 25%, in industrial methylated spirit. Price 100 ml = **C**. ACBS: see Appendix 3
Caution: highly inflammable

13.10.5 Preparations for minor skin infections

These preparations are used in minor burns, napkin rash, and abrasions. They are applied as necessary. Preparations containing hydrargaphen and sulphonamides should be **avoided**. Magnesium sulphate paste is now rarely used to treat carbuncles and boils as these are best treated with antibiotics.

Sprays and paints are also used in minor infections and are described in section 13.11.

Cetrimide Cream, cetrimide 0.5% in a suitable water-miscible basis such as cetostearyl alcohol 5%, liquid paraffin 50% in freshly boiled and cooled purified water. Price 50 g = **A**
Magnesium Sulphate Paste, dried magnesium sulphate 38%, phenol 0.5%, in anhydrous glycerol. Price 25 g = **A**
Proflavine Cream, proflavine hemisulphate 0.1%, yellow beeswax 2.5%, chlorocresol 0.1%, liquid paraffin 67.3%, freshly boiled and cooled purified water 25%, wool fat 5%. Price 100 ml = **B**
Bactrian® (Loveridge)
Cream, cetrimide 1%. Price 45 g = **B**
Betadine® (Napp)
Ointment, povidone-iodine 10%, in a water-miscible basis. Price 60 g = **D**; 500 g = **F**
Brulidine® (M&B)
Cream, dibromopropamidine isethionate 0.15%, in a water-miscible basis. Price 25 g = **C**
Cetavlex® (ICI)
Cream, cetrimide 0.5%, in a water-miscible basis. Price 50 g = **B**; 500 g = **E**

Conotrane® (WBP) *cream*, dimethicone 350, hydrargaphen. Price 60 g = **C**; 500 g = **F**

Drapolene® (Calmic)
Cream, benzalkonium chloride, cetrimide. Price 55 g = **B**; 100 g = **E**

Hibitane® (ICI)
Cream, chlorhexidine gluconate solution 5% (1% chlorhexidine gluconate), in a water-miscible basis. Price 50 g = **B**

Ilonium® (Ilon) *abscess salve* (= ointment), colophony, phenol, turpentine oil, larch turpentine, thymol. Price 30 g = **B**; 100 g = **D**

Kamillosan® (Norgine)
Ointment, extract of chamomile, volatile oil of chamomile, hexylresorcinol. Price 20 g = **D**

Madecassol® (Rona)
Ointment, centella 1%, in water-miscible basis. Price 10 g = **C**

M&B Antiseptic Cream (M&B)
Cream, propamidine isethionate 0.15%. Price 25 g = **C**

Miol® (Comprehensive)
Cream, alcloxa, calcium chloride, camphor, chlorphenesin, magnesium chloride, sodium chloride. Price 30 g = **D**.
Lotion, same ingredients except chlorphenesin. Price 100 ml = **D**

Morhulin® (Priory)
Ointment, sodium hypochlorite solution, cod-liver oil, zinc oxide. Price 50 g = **B**; 350 g = **E**

Morsep® (Priory)
Cream, cetrimide, sodium hypochlorite solution, vitamin A, ergocalciferol. Price 40 g = **A**; 300 g = **D**

Septex® (Norton) *No. 2 cream*, boric acid, sulphathiazole, zinc oxide. Price 50 g = **B**

Steroxin® (Geigy)
Ointment, chlorquinaldol 3%, in a non-greasy basis. Price 30 g = **B**

13.11 Antiseptics and skin disinfectants

These are used for preparation of the skin prior to surgery, as part of the treatment of infected skin conditions, for cleansing wounds and ulcers, and in the treatment of acne (section 13.6). Solutions of cetrimide, chlorhexidine, and sodium hypochlorite are no less effective than the more recent preparations such as povidone-iodine (Betadine®).

Topical preparations of hexachlorophane have been associated with severe neurotoxicity and should be used with caution in neonates and should not be used on large raw areas in infancy.

Astringent preparations precipitate protein and may assist in sealing an exuding surface. They include **aluminium acetate lotion** and **potassium permanganate solution** and are useful in treating eczematous reactions and suppurating wounds. **Silver nitrate lotion** is also used to treat suppurating lesions but causes black staining of the skin and toxic effects if used for longer than 1 or 2 days.

Aluminium Acetate Lotion, aluminium acetate approximately 0.65%, in water (see Formulary). To be used undiluted. Price 500 ml = **B**

Benzalkonium Chloride Solution, benzalkonium chloride 50%. Price 50 ml = **B**

Brilliant Green and Crystal Violet Paint, brilliant green 0.5%, crystal violet 0.5%, alcohol (90%) 50%, in water for preparations. Price 25 ml = **A**

Cetrimide Solution, yellow, cetrimide 1% in purified water freshly boiled and cooled. Price 100 ml = **A**

Strong Cetrimide Solution, yellow, cetrimide 40%, with alcohol (95%) 7.5%, tartrazine 0.0075%. It may be perfumed. Used for preparation of cetrimide solutions. Price 100 ml = **B**

Chloroxylenol Solution, chloroxylenol 5%, alcohol about 20%, terpineol 10%, in a soap solution. Price 100 ml = **B**

Crystal Violet Paint, crystal violet 0.5%, in water for preparations. Price 25 ml = **A**

Potassium Permanganate Solution, potassium permanganate 0.1%, in water (see Formulary). Price 500 ml = **B**
One part diluted with 7 parts of water contains potassium permanganate 1 in 8000

Silver Nitrate Lotion, silver nitrate 0.5%, in water (see Formulary). To be used undiluted. Price 50 ml = **A**

Surgical Spirit. Price 100 ml = **A**
Caution: inflammable

Zinc Sulphate Lotion, zinc sulphate 1%, with amaranth, in water (see Formulary). Price 200 ml = **A**

Betadine® (Napp)
Aerosol (= application), povidone-iodine 5%, in a pressurised aerosol unit. Price 88-ml unit = **E**
Paint, povidone-iodine 10% in alcoholic solution. Price 8 ml = **C**
Alcoholic solution, povidone-iodine 10%. Price 100 ml = **B**
Antiseptic solution, povidone-iodine 10% in aqueous solution. Price 100 ml = **B**
Scalp and skin cleanser solution, povidone-iodine 7.5%, in a surfactant basis. Price 100 ml = **C**. ACBS: see Appendix 3
Skin cleanser solution, povidone-iodine 4%, in a surfactant basis. Price 50 and 100 ml (both) = **C**. ACBS: see Appendix 3
Skin cleanser foam, povidone-iodine 7.5%, in a pressurised aerosol unit. Price 100-g unit = **F**. ACBS: see Appendix 3
Surgical scrub, povidone-iodine 7.5%, with non-ionic surfactants. Price 500 ml = **D**

Cetavlon® (ICI)
Solution, cetrimide 40%; to be diluted before use. Price 100 ml = **B**

Cyteal® (Concept)
Solution, chlorhexidine gluconate, chlorocresol, hexamidine isethionate. Price 500 ml = **D**

Dettol® (R&C)
Lotion (formerly antiseptic cream), chloroxylenol 1.3%. Price 113 g = **B**

Disadine DP® (Stuart)
Dry powder spray (= application), povidone-iodine 0.5%, in a pressurised aerosol unit. Price 150-g unit = **E**

Dispray 1 Quick Prep® (Stuart)
Aerosol (= application), chlorhexidine gluconate solution 2.5% (≡ 0.5% chlorhexidine gluconate), alcohol 70% in a pressurised aerosol unit. Price 400-ml unit = **D**
Caution: highly inflammable

Hibidil® (ICI)
Solution, pink, chlorhexidine gluconate 0.05%. Price 25 × 25-ml sachets = **E**; 6 × 100-ml sachets = **D**

Hibiscrub® (ICI)
Solution, red, chlorhexidine gluconate solution 20% (≡4% chlorhexidine gluconate), perfumed. Price 250 ml = **D**; 500 ml = **E**

Hibisol® (ICI)
Solution, blue, chlorhexidine gluconate solution 2.5% (≡0.5% chlorhexidine gluconate) in 70% isopropyl alcohol, with emollients. Price 250 and 500 ml (both) = **D**

Hibitane® (ICI)
Obstetric cream, chlorhexidine gluconate solution 5% (≡ 1% chlorhexidine gluconate), in a pourable water-miscible basis. Price 210 ml = **C**
Gluconate 20% solution, chlorhexidine gluconate solution 20%, aqueous solution. Price 500 ml = **G**
5% concentrate solution, red, chlorhexidine gluconate solution 25% (≡ 5% chlorhexidine gluconate), perfumed aqueous solution. Price 50 × 10-ml sachet = **F**; 500 ml = **D**

Merthiolate® (Lilly)
Tincture, thiomersal 0.1% with alcohol 50%. Price 100 ml = **A** (Hosp. only)

Noxyflex® (Geistlich)
Solution, powder for reconstitution, noxythiolin 2.5 g, amethocaine hydrochloride 10 mg. Price per vial = **F**

Noxyflex S® (Geistlich)
Solution, powder for reconstitution, noxythiolin. Price 2.5-g vial = **F**

pHiso-MED® (Winthrop)
Emulsion, hexachlorophane 3%. Price 150 ml = **E**

Roccal® (Winthrop)
Solution, blue, benzalkonium chloride 1%. Price 250 ml = **C**; 500 ml = **D**

Rotersept® (FAIR)
Spray (= application), chlorhexidine gluconate 0.2% in a pressurised aerosol unit. Price 284 g unit = **D**

Savloclens® (ICI)
Solution, yellow, cetrimide, chlorhexidine gluconate. Price 100-ml sachet = **A**

Savlodil® (ICI)
Solution, yellow, cetrimide, chlorhexidine gluconate. Price 25 × 25-ml sachets = **D**; 6 × 100-ml sachet = **C**

Savlon® (ICI)
Hospital concentrate (= solution), orange, ingredients as for Savlodil solution, for dilution before use. Price 50 × 10-ml sachets = **E**; 25 × 25 ml sachets = **D**; 1 litre = **E**

Ster-Zac® (Hough)
Bath concentrate solution, triclosan 2%. Price 28.5 ml = **B**; 500 ml = **E**. ACBS: see Appendix 3

Ster-Zac DC® (Hough)
Skin cleanser, hexachlorophane 3%. Price 150 ml = **E**

Steribath® (Stuart)
Solution, iodine-nonoxynol complex (4.5% available iodine). Price 14-ml sachet = **A**

13.12 Antiperspirants

Aluminium chloride 20% lotion (Anhydrol Forte®) is a potent antiperspirant used in the treatment of severe hyperhidrosis.

ALUMINIUM CHLORIDE

Indications: hyperhidrosis
Cautions: avoid contact with eyes; do not shave axilla or use depilatories within 12 hours of use
Side-effects: skin irritation—may require treatment with hydrocortisone cream
Administration: apply at night, wash off on following morning—do not bathe immediately before use

Anhydrol Forte® (Dermal)
Solution (= application), aluminium chloride hexahydrate 20%, 10-ml bottle with roll-on applicator. Price complete unit = **E**

Driclor® (Stiefel)
Application, aluminium chloride hexahydrate 20%, 60-ml bottle with roll-on applicator. Price complete unit = **E**

13.13 Preparations for wounds and ulcers

Preparations for ulcers are second-line treatment and the underlying causes should be treated. The main beneficial effect of local treatment is removal of slough and clot and the ablation of local infection. Preparations which absorb or help promote the removal of exudate may also help. It should be noted that substances applied to an open area are easily absorbed and perilesional skin is easily sensitised. Stasis dermatitis may be due to neomycin or lanolin sensitivity. Enzyme preparations such as streptokinase-streptodornase (Varidase®) or alternatively dextranomer (Debrisan®) are designed for sloughing ulcers and may help.

Usually all that is required is washing with an antiseptic solution such as dilute sodium hypochlorite solution, cetrimide, or potassium permanganate (section 13.11) and covering the lesion with an adequate dressing.

Cleansing preparations

Chlorinated Lime and Boric Acid Solution (Eusol), chlorinated lime 1.25%, boric acid 1.25%, water for preparations to 100 ml. Not less than 0.25% available chlorine. It must be freshly prepared. Price 100 ml = **A**

Chlorinated Soda Solution, Surgical (Dakins Solution), boric acid, chlorinated lime, sodium carbonate, sufficient of each to provide a solution containing 0.5% of available chlorine in water. Price 500 ml = **B**

Soap Spirit, soft soap 65%. Price 100 ml = **B**

Aserbine® (Bencard)
Cream, benzoic acid, malic acid, propylene glycol, salicylic acid. Price 100 g = **C**.
Solution, ingredients as for cream, approximately 6 times the strength. Price 100 ml = **B**

Benoxyl 20® (Stiefel)
Lotion, benzoyl peroxide 20%. For cutaneous ulcers. Price 100 ml = **F**

Debrisan® (Pharmacia)
Beads 100-300 μm diameter, dextranomer. For absorption of exudate. Price 7 × 4-g sachet = **J**; 60 g = **J**

Hioxyl® (Quinoderm)
Cream, hydrogen peroxide (stabilised) 1.5%. Price 25 g = **C**; 100 g = **F**

Lacticare® (Stiefel)
Lotion lactic acid, sodium pyrrolidonecarboxylate. Price 150 ml = **E**

Malatex® (Norton)
Cream, benzoic acid, malic acid, propylene glycol, salicylic acid. Price 100 and 125 g (both) = **C**.
Lotion, ingredients as for cream. Price 500 ml = **C**

Varidase Topical® (Lederle)
Powder, streptokinase 100 000 units, streptodornase 25 000 units. For preparing solutions for topical use. Price per vial = **G**

Dressings

Zinc Paste Bandage, bandage impregnated with paste containing zinc oxide. Price 75 mm × 6 m bandage = **D**

Calaband® (Seton)
Impregnated bandage, zinc paste and calamine. Price 75 mm × 6 m bandage = **C**

Quinaband® (Seton)
Impregnated bandage, zinc oxide, calamine, clioquinol. Price 75 mm × 6 m bandage = **C**

Rikospray Balsam® (Riker)
Application, benzoin, prepared storax (pressurised aerosol pack). Price 150-g unit = **E**

Stuart Tinct. Benz. Co. Spray® (Stuart)
Spray application, compound benzoin tincture 15% (pressurised aerosol spray). Price 150 g = **C**

Varihesive® (Squibb)
Dressing, gelatin 20%, pectin 20%, polyisobutylene 40%, sodium carboxymethylcellulose 20%. Price 5 dressings (100 mm × 100 mm) = **F**

Viscopaste® (S&N)
Impregnated bandage, zinc paste bandage (gelatinous paste). Price 75 mm × 6 m bandage = **D**

Viscopaste PB7® (S&N)
Impregnated bandage, zinc paste bandage (emulsifying basis). Requires additional bandaging. Price 75 mm × 6 m bandage = **D**

Zincaband® (Seton)
Impregnated bandage, zinc paste bandage (gelatinous paste). Price 75 mm × 6 m bandage = **D**

Oral preparations

Zincomed® (Medo)
Capsules, blue/white, zinc sulphate 220 mg. Price 20 caps = **A** (Hosp. only)
Dose: 1 capsule 3 times daily after meals

13.14 Topical preparations for circulatory disorders

These preparations are used to improve circulation in conditions such as chilblains and varicose veins but are of little value. Sclerotherapy in varicose veins is described in section 2.13.

Rubefacients are described in section 10.3.2.

Akrotherm® (Priory) *cream*, acetylcholine chloride, histamine acid phosphate, oxycholesterol. For chilblains. Price 40 g = **C**

Hirudoid® (Luitpold-Werk) *cream*, a heparinoid. Price 40 g = **D**. *Gel*, a heparinoid. For varicose veins and soft-tissue injuries. Price 40 g = **D**

Lasonil® (Bayer) *ointment*, heparinoid, hyaluronidase. For varicose conditions and haemorrhoids. Price 14 g = **B**; 40 g = **D**

Pernomol® (LAB) *paint*, camphor, chlorbutol, phenol, soap spirit, tannic acid. For chilblains. Price 2.5 ml = **B**

Secaderm® (Rorer) *salve* (= ointment), colophony, melaleuca oil, phenol, terebene, turpentine oil. For chilblains, boils, etc. Price 15 g = **B**

Vita-E® (Bioglan)
Ointment, tocopheryl acetate. For intermittent claudication. Price 50 g = **C**

14: Immunological products and VACCINES

In this chapter, immunisation is discussed under the following headings:

14.1 Active immunity

Vaccines are designed to produce specific protection against a given disease. They may consist of

1. an attenuated form of an infective agent, as in the vaccines which are used against virus diseases such as poliomyelitis and measles, or BCG used against tuberculosis,
2. inactivated preparations of the virus or bacteria, as in influenza, pertussis (whooping-cough), or typhoid vaccines, or
3. extracts of or exotoxins produced by a micro-organism, as tetanus vaccine.

Vaccines stimulate the production of protective antibody and other immune mechanisms. They are given by injection, with the exception of live attenuated poliomyelitis vaccines given by mouth, and vaccinia which is given transdermally.

In the case of vaccines consisting of living agents, immunisation is generally achieved with a single dose, but 3 doses are required in the case of oral poliomyelitis vaccine. Live virus multiplies in the body and usually produces a durable immunity but not always as long as that of the natural infection.

Inactivated vaccines usually require a primary series of doses of vaccine to produce an adequate antibody response and in certain cases reinforcing or 'booster' injections are required. The duration of immunity following the use of inactivated vaccines varies from months to many years.

SIDE-EFFECTS. Some vaccines such as poliomyelitis vaccines produce virtually no reactions, while others, as in the case of measles vaccine, may produce a very mild form of the disease. Some of the inactivated bacterial vaccines may produce mild discomfort at the site of injection and mild fever and malaise. Occasionally there are more serious untoward reactions which should always be reported in the usual way to the Committee on Safety of Medicines.

CONTRA-INDICATIONS. Most vaccines may have some contra-indications to their use, and the manufacturer's leaflet accompanying the vaccine should always be consulted. In general, vaccines should not be given to individuals if they have a febrile illness or if any active infection is present or suspected.

Many vaccines contain traces of various antibiotics used in their preparation and vaccine may need to be withheld from individuals who are sensitive to the antibiotic which it contains.

Live virus vaccines, especially rubella vaccine, should not be routinely offered to pregnant women because of possible harm to the foetus. They should not be given to individuals with impaired immune responsiveness, whether occurring naturally or as a result of radiotherapy or treatment with corticosteroids or other immunosuppressive drugs. They should not be given to those suffering from malignant conditions or other tumours of the reticulo-endothelial system. When two live virus vaccines are required they should be given either simultaneously or with an interval of at least 3 weeks.

14.2 Passive immunity

Defence or immediate protection against certain infective organisms can be obtained by injecting preparations made from the serum of immune individuals with adequate levels of antibody to the disease for which protection is sought.

Antibodies of human origin are usually termed immunoglobulins. The term antiserum is applied to material prepared in animals. Because of the serum sickness reactions that may follow injections of antisera, this therapy has been replaced wherever possible by the use of immunoglobulins, as in the case of tetanus. In this particular instance, tetanus vaccine or tetanus vaccine, adsorbed, should also be given if protection is needed as a result of injury (section 14.4.13).

Diphtheria antitoxin prepared in horses is still used, and serum sickness is common after administration of this preparation. (Reactions are theoretically possible after injection of human immunoglobulins but must be extraordinarily uncommon.)

14.3 Storage and reconstitution of immunological products

Care must be taken to store all vaccines and other immunological products under the conditions recommended by the manufacturer in the literature accompanying the vaccine, otherwise the preparation may become denatured and totally ineffective. **Refrigerated storage** is usually necessary. Opened multidose vials which have not been fully used should be discarded within one hour if no preservative is present (most live virus vaccines) or within 3 hours or at the end of a session when vaccines containing a preservative are used; this category includes poliomyelitis vaccine (oral).

Particular attention must be paid to the instructions on the use of diluents where these are provided (usually with freeze-dried preparations of the vaccines), and ampoules of vaccine should always be adequately shaken before use to ensure uniformity of the material to be injected.

14.4 Prevention and treatment of disease

AVAILABILITY OF VACCINES AND OTHER IMMUNOLOGICAL PRODUCTS. Anthrax, rabies (human diploid cell), smallpox (freeze-dried), and yellow fever vaccines, botulinum antitoxin, and snake venom antitoxins are available from local designated holding centres. Poliomyelitis vaccine (inactivated) is available on request to the Department of Health and Social Security, Room 416, 14 Russell Square, London WC1B 5EP, telephone 01-636 6811, extn 3117. Most other vaccines and other immunological products are available commercially. Enquiries for vaccines not available commercially should be made to the Department of Health and Social Security, address and telephone number above. In Scotland information about availability of vaccines can be obtained from the Chief Administrative Pharmaceutical Officer of the local Health Board.

14.4.1 Anthrax

A vaccine is available for anyone subject to heavy exposure to anthrax, such as those exposed to infected hides and carcasses and to imported bonemeal, fishmeal, and feeding stuffs. The vaccine is prepared from a culture of *Bacillus anthracis* and, following the primary course of injections, reinforcing doses should be given at about yearly intervals.

Anthrax Vaccine
Dose: initial course 3 doses of 0.5 ml by intramuscular injection at intervals of 3 weeks followed by a 4th dose after an interval of 6 months
Reinforcing doses: 0.5 ml by intramuscular injection annually
Availability and supply—section 14.4

14.4.2 Cholera

Vaccines against cholera contain killed Inaba and Ogawa serotypes and may also contain the El Tor biotype that became prevalent in 1961. Although an international certificate of vaccination is still required for entry to some countries, it is now recognised that while cholera vaccine may provide some individual protection for about 6 months it cannot control the spread of the disease. Reinforcing injections are required every 6 months for those living in endemic areas.

Patients who travel in a country where cholera exists should be warned that attention to the hygiene of food and water is still essential, even after vaccination.

Cholera Vaccine Cho/Vac. Price 1-ml amp = **C**; 1.5-ml amp = **D**; 10-ml vial = **D**; 50-ml vial = **G**
Dose: as specified on the label, usually 0.5 ml by subcutaneous or intramuscular injection followed after at least a week and preferably 4 weeks by a second dose of 1 ml

Vibriomune® (DF)
Cholera vaccine. Price 1-ml amp = **C**; 10-ml vial = **D**
Dose: 0.5 ml by subcutaneous injection followed after at least a week and preferably 4 weeks by a second dose of 1 ml

14.4.3 Diphtheria

Protection against diphtheria is essentially due to the presence in the blood stream of antitoxin, the production of which is stimulated by toxoid vaccines prepared from the toxin of *Corynebacterium diphtheriae*. This toxoid is more effective if adsorbed onto a mineral carrier, and adsorbed diphtheria vaccines are generally used for the routine immunisation of babies and given in the form of a triple vaccine, Adsorbed Diphtheria, Tetanus, and Pertussis Vaccine. A dose of Poliomyelitis Vaccine, Live (Oral) is generally given at the time of each of the doses of the triple vaccine (see schedule, section 14.6). Adsorbed Diphtheria and Tetanus Vaccine is used in place of the triple vaccine when it is decided not to immunise against whooping-cough. A reinforcing dose of adsorbed diphtheria and tetanus vaccine is recommended at the age of school entry, even though a full course of the triple vaccine or of diphtheria and tetanus vaccine has been given initially. Further reinforcing doses of diphtheria vaccine are not recommended except in the case of those who work in units where there is a potentially high risk of infection such as those employed in infectious disease units, hospitals for the mentally handicapped, or microbiology laboratories. It is possible that a special vaccine may be made available for this purpose, but in the meantime such staff should always be Schick tested in the first place and only those who are positive should be offered immunisation.

Diphtheria and Tetanus Vaccine DT/Vac/FT. A mixture of diphtheria formol toxoid and tetanus formol toxoid. Price 5-ml vial = **E**

Dose: reinforcing dose for children, 0.5 or 1 ml as stated on the label by intramuscular or deep subcutaneous injection

Diphtheria and Tetanus Vaccine, Adsorbed DT/Vac/Ads. Prepared from diphtheria formol toxoid and tetanus formol toxoid with a mineral carrier (aluminium hydroxide, aluminium phosphate, or calcium phosphate). Used for primary immunisation (see schedule, section 14.6) and reinforcing doses. Price 0.5-ml amp = **B**; 5-ml vial = **D**

Dose: 0.5 or 1 ml as stated on the label by intramuscular or deep subcutaneous injection; in adults 0.2 ml may be given

Diphtheria Antitoxin Dip/Ser. (Derived from equine serum). For passive immunisation and treatment of diphtheria.

Dose: prophylactic 500 to 2000 units by intramuscular injection; therapeutic 10 000 to 30 000 units by intramuscular injection; *or* 40 000 to 100 000 units by intravenous injection

Diphtheria, Tetanus, and Pertussis Vaccine DTPer/Vac. A mixture of diphtheria formol toxoid, tetanus formol toxoid, and pertussis vaccine. Used for reinforcing doses. Price 0.5-ml amp = **B**; 5-ml vial = **E**

Dose: 0.5 or 1 ml as stated on the label by intramuscular or deep subcutaneous injection

Diphtheria, Tetanus, and Pertussis Vaccine, Adsorbed DTPer/Vac/Ads. Prepared from diphtheria formol toxoid, tetanus formol toxoid, and pertussis vaccine with a mineral carrier (aluminium hydroxide, aluminium phosphate, or calcium phosphate). Used for primary immunisation (see schedule, section 14.6). Price 0.5-ml = **B**

Dose: 0.5 or 1 ml as stated on the label by intramuscular or deep subcutaneous injection

Diphtheria Vaccine Dip/Vac/FT. Consists of diphtheria formol toxoid. Used in reinforcing doses for children who do not require immunisation against tetanus or whooping-cough

Dose: the volume stated on the label by intramuscular or deep subcutaneous injection

Diphtheria Vaccine, Adsorbed Dip/Vac/Ads. Prepared from diphtheria formol toxoid with a mineral carrier (aluminium hydroxide, aluminium phosphate, or calcium phosphate). Used for primary immunisation of children who do not require immunisation against tetanus or whooping-cough. Price 0.5-ml amp = **B**

Dose: the volume stated on the label by intramuscular or deep subcutaneous injection

Diphtheria Vaccine TAF Dip/Vac/TAF. A suspension of floccules prepared from diphtheria vaccine (formol toxoid) and diphtheria antitoxin. Used for the immunisation of Schick-positive adults and children over 10 years. *Contra-indicated* in sensitivity to horse serum. Price 5-ml vial = **D**

Dose: for primary immunisation 3 doses of 0.5 ml by intramuscular or deep subcutaneous injection with an interval of 6–8 weeks between the first and second doses and 4–6 months between the second and third

Reinforcing dose: 0.5 ml by intramuscular or deep subcutaneous injection

Schick Test Toxin. Prepared from a sterile filtrate of a culture of *Corynebacterium diphtheriae*. Price 1-ml vial with 1-ml vial of Schick control = **G**

Dose: diagnostic, 0.1 or 0.2 ml as stated on the label, by intracutaneous injection

Trivax® (Wellcome)

Diphtheria, tetanus, and pertussis vaccine. For primary vaccination (see schedule, section 14.6). Price 0.5-ml amp = **C**; 5-ml vial = **E**

Dose: 0.5 ml by intramuscular or deep subcutaneous injection

Trivax-AD® (Wellcome)

Diphtheria, tetanus, and pertussis vaccine, adsorbed. For primary vaccination (see schedule, section 14.6). Price 0.5-ml amp = **C**; 5-ml vial = **E**

Dose: 0.5 ml by intramuscular or deep subcutaneous injection

14.4.4 Influenza

While most viruses are antigenically stable, the influenza viruses A and B (especially A) are constantly altering their antigenic structure as indicated by changes in the haemagglutinins (H) and neuraminidases (N) on the surface of the viruses. It is essential that influenza vaccines in use contain the H and N components of the prevalent strain or strains.

There are no influenza vaccines that will control the spread of epidemics and there is little evidence of the efficacy of live influenza vaccines in this respect. The recommended virus strains for vaccine production are grown in the allantoic cavity of developing chick embryos (and are therefore **contra-indicated** in those who are sensitive to eggs). The allantoic fluid is purified and the vaccines containing the haemagglutinin and neuraminidase of the strain expected to become prevalent are harvested. The World Health Organization makes recommendations as to what strains should be included in the vaccines and recently there have been two strains in circulation, one of them (H_1N_1) which was prevalent between 1947 and 1956 and the other (H_3N_2) which has been in circulation with minor changes since 1968. If the H and N of the anticipated strain are different from that of recent strains it may be that 2 doses of vaccine will be required; on the other

C = 51-100p, **D** = 101-180p, **E** = 181-300p, **F** = 301-450p, **G** = 451-650p, **H** = 651-900p, **I** = 901-1200p, **J** = over 1200p.

hand if an individual has been immunised against the strain which is still prevalent, it is doubtful if yearly immunisation against that strain is of any particular value. Individuals under the age of 27 in 1982 should receive 2 doses of influenza vaccine.

Since the influenza vaccines will not control epidemics they are recommended only for those at high risk, particularly the elderly, those with chronic infection of the cardiovascular and respiratory systems, for those in contact with the sick—doctors, nurses, etc., and for those living in closed institutions where opportunites for contact and spread are great.

Purified surface-antigen vaccines should be used in children aged 4–12 years; older children and adults may be vaccinated with influenza vaccine (inactivated) or surface-antigen vaccine.

Influenza Vaccine, Inactivated Flu/Vac. Used for active immunisation against epidemic influenza (see notes above). Also available as adsorbed vaccine (Flu/Vac/Ads)
Dose: 0.5 ml by deep subcutaneous or intramuscular injection during the autumn

Influenza Vaccine, Inactivated (Surface Antigen) Flu/Vac/SA. Used for active immunisation against epidemic influenza (see notes above).
Dose: 0.5 ml by deep subcutaneous or intramuscular injection

Fluvirin® (DF)
Inactivated influenza vaccine, surface antigen (purified). Price 0.5-ml syringe = **E**; 5- and 25-ml vial (both) = **J**

Influvac® (Duphar)
Inactivated influenza vaccine (whole virus vaccine). Price 0.5-ml amp or syringe = **D**; 5-ml vial = **J**

MFV-Ject® (Servier)
Inactivated influenza vaccine (disrupted virus vaccine). Price 0.5-ml syringe = **E**; 5- and 25-ml vial (both) = **J**

14.4.5 Measles

Measles vaccine consists of an attenuated strain of measles virus grown in chick-embryo fibroblast-tissue cultures. It should be offered to all children in the second year of life and may be expected to produce a durable immunity.

Administration of this vaccine to children may be associated with a mild measles-like syndrome with a measles-like rash and pyrexia which come on about a week after the injection of the vaccine. Much less commonly, convulsions and, rarely, encephalitis have been reported as being associated with measles vaccines. Convulsions in babies are relatively common and may occur by chance following any immunisation procedure; they are certainly much less frequently associated with measles vaccine than with other conditions leading to febrile episodes.

Serious neurological complications following the vaccine are extremely rare, perhaps of the order of 1 in 87 000 vaccinees and probably about 12–20 times less common than such complications associated with natural infections of measles, but it is difficult to get exact figures because of variable criteria of what is diagnosed as a serious neurological condition. Subacute sclerosing panencephalitis follows measles infection at a rate of approximately 5 to 10 cases for every million children who have developed measles. This condition may be associated with live measles vaccine at a rate of 0.5–1.0 case per million doses of vaccine distributed, and so it appears that measles vaccination to some extent protects against subacute sclerosing panencephalitis.

Unfortunately, measles vaccine is taken up by only about 50% of those eligible. This is said to be due to the fact that some doctors and parents do not consider that measles is now a serious disease. It is possible that, when there is a partial coverage of the susceptible members of population with vaccine, wild measles virus does not spread so readily, which means that in vaccinated communities, many children will grow up susceptible and may be subject to an attack of measles as adolescents or adults when the disease may be more serious.

Measles vaccine may also be used in the control of outbreaks and should be offered to school and playstreet contacts as soon as possible after the diagnosis of the index case.

If there is a history of convulsions or of epilepsy, it is generally considered wise to delay immunisation with measles vaccine until the child is 2 to 3 years of age and some recommend that an antiepileptic should be given for a fortnight following the immunisation in children with such a history.

Because of the generally poor uptake of this vaccine in the second year of life, it would seem wise to offer the vaccine also to children at entry to nursery or primary school. Again it would seem sensible to offer vaccine to any child entering secondary school who has not had either a natural infection or a previous dose of vaccine.

Children with a history of convulsions should be given measles vaccine only with simultaneous administration of specially diluted normal immunoglobulin supplied for use with measles vaccine.

Measles Vaccine, Live Meas/Vac(Live). Freeze-dried stabilised aqueous suspension of an approved strain of live attenuated measles virus grown in culture of chick-embryo cells. Used for active immunisation against measles (see schedule, section 14.6)

Mevilin-L® (DF)
Measles vaccine, live, Schwarz strain. Price 0.5-ml amp = **D**
Dose: 0.5 ml by subcutaneous or intramuscular injection

Rimevax® (SK&F)
Measles vaccine, live, Schwarz strain. Price 0.5-ml amp = **D**
Dose: 0.5 ml by subcutaneous or intramuscular injection

14.4.6 Mumps

Mumps vaccine consists of an attenuated strain of virus grown in chick-embryo tissue culture. Since mumps and its complications are very rarely serious there is little indication for the routine use of mumps vaccine

Mumpsvax® (Morson)
Mumps vaccine (Jeryl Lynn strain) Single-dose vial with syringe containing solvent. Price complete unit = **F**
Dose: ADULT or CHILD over 1 year, the contents of a vial by subcutaneous injection

14.4.7 Pertussis (whooping-cough)

Pertussis vaccine is usually given combined with diphtheria and tetanus vaccine starting after the third month of life (see schedule, section 14.6) but may also be given as a simple vaccine.

Pertussis-containing vaccines may give rise to local reactions at the site of injection, mild pyrexia, and irritability. With some vaccines available in the early 1960s persistent screaming and collapse were reported but these reactions are rarely observed with the vaccines now available.

Convulsions and encephalopathy have been reported as rare complications, but such conditions may arise from other causes and be falsely attributed to the vaccine. A 3-year study of children aged 2 months–3 years who were admitted to hospitals in Great Britain suffering from serious neurological illness of the type likely to be attributed to whooping-cough vaccine has been carried out. Out of the first 1000 cases notified to the study, only 35 children had received pertussis vaccine within 7 days before becoming ill. Of these 35 children, 32 had no previous neurological abnormality and on follow-up of these children 1 year later, 2 had died and 9 had developmental retardation, while 21 were normal.

It is advisable to postpone vaccination if the child is suffering from any acute febrile illness, particularly if it is respiratory, until fully recovered. Minor infections without fever or systemic upset are not regarded as contra-indications. Vaccination should not be carried out in children who have

(1) a history of any severe local or general reaction, *including a neurological reaction*, to a preceding dose; or
(2) a history of cerebral irritation or damage in the neonatal period, or who have suffered from fits or convulsions.

There are certain groups of children in whom whooping-cough vaccination is not absolutely contra-indicated but who require special consideration as to its advisability. These groups are

(1) children whose parents or siblings have a history of idiopathic epilepsy;
(2) children with developmental delay thought to be due to a neurological defect; and
(3) children with neurological disease

For these groups the risk of vaccination may be higher than in normal children but the effects of whooping-cough may be more severe, so that the benefits of vaccination would also be greater. The balance of risk and benefit should be assessed with special care in each individual case.

Allergy, according to much informed medical opinion, is not a contra-indication to the administration of pertussis vaccine.

Pertussis Vaccine Per/Vac. Used for active immunisation against whooping-cough when simultaneous immunisation against diphtheria and tetanus is not required (see schedule, section 14.6)
Dose: 0.5 or 1 ml as specified on the label by intramuscular or deep subcutaneous injection

14.4.8 Pneumococcal pneumonia

A polyvalent pneumonia vaccine is available for the immunisation of persons for whom the risk of contracting pneumococcal pneumonia is unusually high, for example patients who have had a splenectomy. It is effective in a single dose if the types of pneumonia in the community are reflected in the polysaccharides contained in the vaccine. Revaccination at intervals not less than 3 years is recommended. The vaccine should not be given to children under 2 years, in pregnancy, or when there is infection. It should be used with caution in cardiovascular or respiratory disease. Hypersensitivity reactions may occur.

▼ Pneumovax® (Morson)
A polyvalent vaccine prepared from the capsules of pneumococci. Used for immunisation against infections caused by pneumococci (see notes). Price 0.5-ml syringe = **G**
Dose: 0.5 ml by subcutaneous or intramuscular injection

14.4.9 Poliomyelitis

There are two types of poliomyelitis vaccine, namely poliomyelitis vaccine, inactivated, and poliomyelitis vaccine, live (oral). The oral vaccine, consisting of a mixture of attenuated strains of virus types 1, 2, and 3 is at present generally used.

INITIAL COURSE. Poliomyelitis vaccine, live (oral) is given on 3 occasions, usually at the same time as routine immunisation against diphtheria, tetanus, and pertussis (see schedule, section 14.6).

REINFORCEMENT. A reinforcing dose of oral poliomyelitis vaccine is recommended at school entry at which time children should also receive a reinforcing dose of diphtheria and tetanus vaccine. Oral poliomyelitis vaccine is also recommended at school leaving at the same time as a dose of tetanus vaccine.

Young parents who are having their babies immunised should be offered vaccine at the same time because of a tiny risk of infection of parents from vaccine virus which may have increased in neurovirulence following replication in the gut of their baby. Contact vaccine-associated poliomyelitis such as this is rare, and so is vaccine-associated poliomyelitis in those who actually received the vaccine. (These adverse effects occur about once in one or more millions of vaccinated persons.)

Contra-indications to the use of oral poliomyelitis vaccine include diarrhoea and hypogammaglobulinaemia which encourages excessive excretion of live vaccines.

TRAVELLERS. It is most important to ensure that adult travellers to areas of high endemicity are given a dose of oral poliomyelitis vaccine if they have not had immunisation against poliomyelitis in the past. Young adults and any children who have never been immunised should be given a complete course.

At the present time **poliomyelitis vaccine (inactivated)** may be used for those in whom poliomyelitis vaccine (oral) is contra-indicated and also for pregnant women, but in the future it might again come into routine use.

Poliomyelitis Vaccine, Inactivated Pol/Vac (Inact). An inactivated suspension of suitable strains of poliomyelitis virus, types 1, 2, and 3. Used for active immunisation when the oral vaccine cannot be used.

Dose: the volume stated on the label by subcutaneous or intramuscular injection; for primary immunisation 3 doses are required (see schedule, section 14.6)

Availability and supply—section 14.4

Poliomyelitis Vaccine, Live (Oral) Pol/Vac (Oral). A suspension of suitable live attenuated strains of poliomyelitis virus, types 1, 2, and 3. Used for active immunisation

Dose: the volume stated on the label; for primary immunisation 3 doses are required (see schedule, section 14.6)

14.4.10 Rabies

Since the time of Pasteur there have been a number of rabies vaccines in which the virus has been grown in nervous tissue of various animals. All of these vaccines have been associated with a greater or lesser degree of postvaccinal allergic encephalomyelitis. Other vaccines made from virus grown in animal tissue cultures or in embryonated duck eggs have tended to be of low antigenicity as measured by the levels of circulating antibodies achieved.

Recently, a human diploid cell vaccine has been developed. This vaccine has been shown to be life saving in trials carried out in Iran in people who had been bitten by infected wolves. It should be offered prophylactically to those at high risk—those working in quarantine stations, animal handlers, veterinary surgeons, and field workers who may be exposed to bites of wild animals. A detailed list is given in Health Circular HC(77)29. This vaccine produces a good antibody response when given in a 2-dose schedule with an interval of one month between doses and a reinforcing dose when required.

For post-exposure treatment a course of 4 injections should be given in the first 14 days after exposure followed by reinforcing doses at 1 and 3 months. The course may be discontinued if it is proved that the patient was not at risk. There are no known contra-indications to this diploid vaccine and its use should be considered whenever a patient has been attacked by an animal in a country where rabies is endemic, even if there is no direct evidence of rabies in the attacking animal.

Staff in attendance on a patient who is highly suspected of, or known to be suffering from, rabies should be offered vaccination. Four intracutaneous doses of human diploid cell vaccine given on the same day has been sugested for this purpose.

Advice on the use of rabies vaccine for pre-exposure prophylaxis and on the use of vaccine and immunoglobulin (section 14.5.2) for post-exposure use is given in Department of Health and Social Security, *Memorandum on Rabies*, London, HMSO, 1977. Advice on the treatment of rabies is available from the Duty Medical Officer, Central Public Health Laboratory, Colindale Avenue, Colindale, London NW9 5HT, telephone 01-205 7041.

Rabies Vaccine (Rab/Vac.). An inactivated suspension of suitable strains of rabies virus grown in cell cultures.

Availability and supply—section 14.4.

▼Merieux Inactivated Rabies Vaccine® (Servier)

Freeze-dried human diploid cell rabies vaccine prepared from Wistar strain PM/WI 38 1503-3M. For prevention and treatment of rabies. Price 1-ml vial with syringe = **J**

Dose: prophylactic, 1 ml by subcutaneous injection, followed by a second dose after 1 month and a third after 6–12 months

Therapeutic, 1 ml on the first, third, seventh and fourteenth day and after 1 and 3 months

14.4.11 Rubella

The introduction of a vaccine to protect a foetus, as yet not conceived, was a totally new idea. Rubella (German measles) as a childhood disease is of little moment, but rubella infection in the mother has a marked effect on the growth of the foetus which is more severe the earlier in pregnancy the infection occurs.

Rubella vaccines are prepared in tissue-culture cells of rabbit kidney or duck embryo, or human diploid cell lines. Contra-indications with regard to sensitivities or antibiotics vary from one vaccine to another and as always the literature accompanying the package should be consulted. But the main contra-indication at present applying to all of the available vaccines is pregnancy.

Rubella vaccine is recommended for prepubertal girls aged 10 to 13 years and for women of childbearing age, particular targets being those who may be at high risk of infection (for example school teachers) as well as those who might put pregnant women at risk of infection (for example nurses and doctors in obstetric units). It is recommended practice to offer vaccine to those women who are found to be seronegative to rubella virus.

The important point is that women offered vaccine should **not** become pregnant for 3 months after immunisation. If this cannot be assured then vaccine should at present be withheld. At the same time more and more evidence is accumulating which suggests that rubella vaccine virus may present less risk to the foetus than was originally thought compared with the serious risk of wild rubella virus in pregnant women. For short-term interim contraception at the time of vaccination medroxyprogesterone acetate (section 7.3.2) may be suitable.

In addition to offering vaccine to schoolgirls and those at special risk, vaccine is also being offered to previously unvaccinated and seronegative post-partum women. Again they must avoid pregnancy for 3 months. Immunising susceptible post-partum women a few days after delivery is important as far as the overall reduction of congenital abnormalities in the UK is concerned, for about 60% of these abnormalities occur in multiparous women.

In the long term it is hoped that the routine immunisation of schoolgirls will produce an immune adult female population but in order to prevent congenital abnormalities due to rubella it may require an acceptance of vaccine of more than 90% and this has rarely been generally achieved with other vaccines. Acceptance amongst schoolgirls might be greater if the effort was concentrated among 10-year-olds, but even so, with a high acceptance rate the efficacy of this programme will not be evident until the end of the century. The problem could be rapidly solved if it were shown that in fact vaccine virus is harmless to the developing foetus or if an inactivated vaccine could be produced, because patients could then be vaccinated routinely in their first pregnancy. At the same time the damage which is done by wild rubella virus must be kept in perspective, for it is responsible for perhaps only about 1% of all congenital abnormalities.

Rubella Vaccine, Live Rub/Vac (Live). A freeze-dried suspension of a suitable live attenuated strain of rubella virus grown in suitable cell cultures. Used for active immunisation against rubella (see schedule, section 14.6 and notes above). Price 0.5-ml amp = **D**; 5-ml vial = **G**

Dose: 0.5 ml by subcutaneous or intramuscular injection. Not to be given to any woman who may be pregnant. Advise women not to become pregnant within 3 months of vaccination

Almevax® (Wellcome)

Rubella vaccine, live, prepared from Wistar RA 27/3 strain propagated in human diploid cells. Used for active immunisation against rubella. Price 0.5-ml amp = **E**; 5-ml vial = **J**

Dose: 0.5 ml by subcutaneous injection. Not to be given to any woman who may be pregnant. Advise women not to become pregnant within 3 months of vaccination

Cendevax® (SK & F)

Rubella vaccine, live, prepared from Cendehill strain propagated in primary rabbit kidney cells. Used for active immunisation against rubella. Price 0.5-ml amp = **D**; 5-ml vial = **I**

Dose: 0.5 ml by subcutaneous injection. Not to be given to any woman who may be pregnant. Advise women not to become pregnant within 3 months of vaccination

14.4.12 Smallpox

Smallpox vaccination is no longer recommended routinely in the UK and most other countries because global eradication of smallpox has now been certified. The vaccine is offered to a small number of doctors and other health workers who may be called upon to deal with suspected cases of smallpox. Otherwise the only requirement for smallpox vaccination is for a few workers in institutions dealing with pox viruses and for travellers to a few countries that still insist on vaccination. This requirement changes from time to time and the up-to-date position in relation to the requirements of any particular country should be sought from the Department of Health and Social Security, Fleming House, London SE1 6BY, telephone 01-407 5522, or from the embassy or legation of the country concerned. Contra-indications to elective smallpox vaccine are pregnancy, babies under 1 year, any illness at the time of vaccination, eczema in the vaccinees or in members of their households; the vaccine is also contra-indicated in patients with impaired immune responsiveness, whether occurring naturally or as a result of radiotherapy or treatment with corticosteroids or other immunosuppressive drugs.

Smallpox Vaccine Var/Vac. Consists of vaccine lymph produced on the skin of living animals, supplied in freeze-dried form with diluent.

Dose: 0.02 ml by multiple pressure inoculation or through a single linear scratch not more than 2–3 mm long
Availability and supply—section 14.4

14.4.13 Tetanus

Tetanus vaccine stimulates the production of the protective antitoxin. It is offered routinely to babies in combination with diphtheria vaccine (DT/Vac/Ads) and more usually also combined with killed *Bordetella pertussis* organisms as Diphtheria, Tetanus, and Pertussis Vaccine (DT Per/Vac) or as an adsorbed vaccine (DT Per/Vac/Ads). In general, adsorption on aluminium hydroxide, aluminium phosphate, or calcium phosphate improves the antigenicity of diphtheria and tetanus toxoids or of diphtheria and tetanus mixtures but in the case of the triple antigen the pertussis acts as an adjuvant and there is little evidence that with this combination the adsorbent makes any significant difference to the antigenicity of the vaccine. The combined vaccines are described under Diphtheria (section 14.4.3).

Of the monovalent tetanus vaccines the adsorbed tetanus vaccine is to be preferred to the simple vaccine except in patients who have reacted abnormally to a previous dose of adsorbed toxoid and are considered to be at such high risk as to make further doses of tetanus vaccine necessary. Adsorbed vaccine must not be given intracutaneously.

In children, the triple vaccine or a course of adsorbed diphtheria and tetanus vaccine not only gives protection against tetanus in childhood but also gives the basic immunity for subsequent reinforcing doses of tetanus vaccine at school entry and at school leaving and also when a potentially tetanus-contaminated injury has been received. Normally, tetanus vaccine should not be given to anyone who has received a reinforcing dose within the previous year because of the possibility that hypersensitivity reactions may develop. In the case of clean minor wounds, no tetanus vaccine is indicated unless more than 5 years have elapsed since the last reinforcing dose of tetanus toxoid was given.

Active immunisation is important for persons in older age groups for they may never have had the routine courses of immunisation when younger. In these persons a course of tetanus vaccine (adsorbed) may be given.

For serious, potentially contaminated wounds antitetanus immunoglobulin injection (section 14.5.2) should be selectively used in addition to wound toilet, tetanus vaccine, and penicillin or another antibiotic.

Tetanus Vaccine Tet/Vac/FT. Tetanus formol toxoid. Used for active immunisation against tetanus (see notes). Price 0.5-ml amp = **B**; 5-ml vial = **E**
Dose: 0.5 ml or as stated on the label, by intramuscular or deep subcutaneous injection followed after 6–12 weeks by a second dose and after a further 4–12 months by a third

Tetanus Vaccine, Adsorbed Tet/Vac/Ads. Prepared from tetanus formol toxoid with a mineral carrier (aluminium hydroxide, aluminium phosphate, or calcium phosphate). Price 0.5-ml amp = **B**; 5-ml vial = **E**
Dose: as for Tetanus Vaccine

14.4.14 Tuberculosis

BCG (Bacillus Calmette-Guérin) is a live attenuated strain derived from bovine *Mycobacterium tuberculosis* which stimulates the development of hypersensitivity to *M. tuberculosis*. The vaccine is given by intracutaneous injection or it may be given by multiple puncture. 0.1 ml of the vaccine (reconstituted immediately before use) is injected intracutaneously just above the insertion of the deltoid muscle raising a wheal of about 8 mm in diameter. If it is injected too high, too far forward, or too far backward, the adjacent lymph glands may become involved and tender. After about 1 week a small swelling appears at the injection site which progresses to a papule or to a benign ulcer about 10 mm in diameter after 3 weeks and heals in 6–12 weeks. No dressing should be used unless there is much discharge from the ulcer.

Normally, BCG is offered routinely to tuberculin-negative children of 10–13 years. BCG vaccination should also be strongly recommended to those living in crowded conditions in urban communities and to all immigrants and their children from countries with a high incidence of tuberculosis. They should be tuberculin tested before vaccination with the exception of newborn babies who should be vaccinated without delay. With babies great care must be taken to ensure that the inoculation is given intracutaneously in a dose of 0.05 ml; if BCG is accidentally given subcutaneously to babies it may give rise to a troublesome persistent local reaction.

Bacillus Calmette-Guérin Vaccine. BCG Vaccine, Dried Tub/Vac/BCG. A freeze-dried preparation of live bacteria of a strain derived from the bacillus of Calmette and Guérin. Used for active immunisation.
Dose: 0.1 ml by intracutaneous injection

Bacillus Calmette-Guérin Vaccine, Percutaneous Tub/Vac/BCG(Perc). A preparation of live bacteria of a strain derived from the bacillus of Calmette and Guérin. Used for active immunisation (see notes) and administered by the percutaneous route with a suitable instrument.
Dose: 0.02 ml by percutaneous administration

DIAGNOSTIC REAGENTS. In the *Mantoux test* the initial dose is 1 unit of tuberculin PPD in 0.1 ml and in subsequent tests 10 units in 0.1 ml and finally 100 units in 0.1 ml. In the *Heaf test* (multiple puncture) a solution containing 100 000 units in 1 ml is used. For the *Tine*, *Imotest*, and other similar tests a special device impregnated with tuberculin is used.

Tuberculin PPD. The active principle of old tuberculin, 100 000 units/ml. Price 1-ml vial = **E**; 5-ml vial = **I**. Also available diluted 1 in 100 (1000 units/ml), 1 in 1000 (100 units/ml), and 1 in 10 000 (10 units/ml). Price 1 ml (all) = **D**
Dose: see notes above

14.4.15 Typhoid

Typhoid vaccination is no substitute for personal precautions in avoiding typhoid fever in countries where the disease is endemic; green salads and uncooked vegetables should be avoided and only fruits which can be skinned may be eaten. Only suitable bottled water or water treated with sterilising tablets should be used for drinking purposes.

Typhoid vaccine (monovalent typhoid vaccine) is now available and because it contains no paratyphoid components it is less likely to produce the local and systemic reactions which have, in the past, been so commonly associated with TAB. These local reactions which consist of swelling, pain, and tenderness appear about 2–3 hours after the subcutaneous or intramuscular injection of the vaccine. Systemic reactions which consist of fever, malaise, and headache may also occur and usually last for about 48 hours after injection. These reactions are virtually absent if the vaccine is given intracutaneously in a dose of 0.1–0.2 ml. There is no clear evidence that giving vaccine in a dose of 0.1 ml intracutaneously is as effective as a dose of 0.5 ml subcutaneously, which is the usual recommended dose. Normally, 2 doses should be given at 4–6 weeks interval for primary immunisation, with reinforcing doses about every 2 or 3 years on continued exposure.

Typhoid Vaccine Typhoid/Vac. A suspension of killed *Salmonella typhi* organisms. Used for active immunisation against typhoid. Price 1.5-ml vial = **D**
Dose: the volume stated on the label by subcutaneous injection, repeated after 4–6 weeks

14.4.16 Typhus

The vaccine consists of formalin-inactivated *Rickettsia prowazekii* grown in the yolk sac of embryonated hens' eggs and is effective against louse-borne typhus. This vaccine is not necessary for travellers visiting countries where the disease is endemic if they will be staying in urban accommodation but it could be of value for those living in close personal contact with the indigenous population of such areas. However the vaccine is no longer distributed in the United Kingdom.

14.4.17 Yellow Fever

Yellow fever vaccine consists of an attenuated yellow fever virus (17D strain) grown in developing chick embryos. It is available only at designated centres, but should not be given to children under 9 months of age since it may cause them to develop encephalitis. Vaccine should not be given to individuals who are sensitive to eggs without adequate precautions, otherwise there are no contra-indications except pregnancy and reactions are few. The immunity which probably lasts for life is officially accepted for 10 years starting from 10 days after primary vaccination and for a further 10 years immediately after revaccination.

Yellow Fever Vaccine, Live Yel/Vac. A suspension of chick embryo proteins containing attenuated 17D strain virus. Used for active immunisation against yellow fever.
Dose: the volume indicated on the label by subcutaneous injection
Availability and supply—section 14.4

Arilvax® (Wellcome)
Freeze-dried yellow fever vaccine, live.

14.5 Immunoglobulins

The injection of immunoglobulins produces immediate protection. Normally, when foreign immunoglobulins are injected, antibodies develop and this presents problems of hypersensitivity when, for example, horse antiserum is used against tetanus; these properties of horse and other animal sera have led to virtual abandonment of animal immunoglobulins for passive protection and human immunoglobulins have taken their place.

There are essentially two types of human immunoglobulin preparation: human **normal immunoglobulin** (HNIG, gamma globulin) prepared from the plasma of at least 1000 donors, and **specific immunoglobulins** for tetanus, rabies, vaccinia, etc. which are prepared by pooling the blood of convalescent patients or of immunised donors who have recently been specifically boosted.

Human normal immunoglobulin is presented in 2 size vials in the UK, 250 mg in 1.7 ml and 750 mg in 5 ml. Normal immunoglobulin and the specific immunoglobulins are available from the Public Health Laboratory Service laboratories and Regional Blood Transfusion Centres in England and Wales with the exception of antitetanus immunoglobulin which is distributed through Regional Blood Transfusion Centres to hospitals and is also available to general medical practitioners.

In Scotland all immunoglobulins are available from Blood Transfusion Centres. Antitetanus immunoglobulin is distributed by Blood Transfusion Centres to hospitals and general medical practitioners on demand. Normal immunoglobulin injection and anti-tetanus immunoglobulin injection are also available commercially.

14.5.1 Normal immunoglobulin

HEPATITIS A (infective hepatitis). At the time of writing there are no suitable techniques available for growing hepatitis A virus in quantities which would make vaccine preparation possible. Control depends on good hygiene and many studies have also shown the value of normal immunoglobulin in the prevention and control of outbreaks of this disease. It is recommended for controlling infection in contacts in closed institutions and also, under certain conditions, in school and home contacts and for travellers going to areas where the disease is highly endemic.

HEPATITIS B. At the present time a vaccine has been developed for trial consisting of hepatitis B surface antigen (HBsAg) prepared from human blood. Meanwhile, specific antihepatitis B virus immunoglobulin may be available for the prevention of infection in laboratory and other personnel who have accidently become contaminated with hepatitis B virus and for pregnant women and babies born to mothers who have become infected with this virus in pregnancy.

MEASLES. Normal immunoglobulin may be used to modify or prevent measles in the few babies in whom an attack of measles must be avoided and also to moderate the reactions to measles vaccine in children with a history of convulsions. The dose in both situations is critical and the leaflet accompanying the immunoglobulin should be consulted.

Normal Immunoglobulin Injection (HNIG). Immunoglobulin prepared from pools of at least 1000 donations of human plasma, available in liquid form or as a freeze-dried preparation for reconstitution. Used for the protection of susceptible contacts against hepatitis A virus (infectious hepatitis), measles and, to a lesser extent, rubella and poliomyelitis. Also used in hypogammaglobulinaemia and other immune deficiency states.

14.5.2 Specific immunoglobulins

RABIES. Following exposure to a suspected rabid animal, specific antirabies immunoglobulin, if possible of human origin, should be injected at the site of the bite and also given intramuscularly.

Antirabies Immunoglobulin Injection. Used for protection of persons who have been bitten by rabid animals or otherwise exposed to infection.
Dose: 20 units/kg by intramuscular injection and infiltration around wounds

TETANUS. Antitetanus immunoglobulin of human origin (HTIG) should be selectively used in addition to wound toilet, vaccine, and penicillin (or another antibiotic) for the more seriously contaminated wounds but is rarely required for those who have an established immunity in whom protection may be achieved by a reinforcing dose of vaccine. The administration of antitetanus immunoglobulin should be considered for patients not known to have received active immunisation (a) whose wound was sustained more than 6 hours before treatment was received and (b) with puncture wounds or wounds potentially heavily contaminated with tetanus spores, septic, or with much devitalised tissue. A dose of adsorbed toxoid should be given at the same time as the antitetanus immunoglobulin and the course of toxoid subsequently completed.

Antitetanus Immunoglobulin Injection (HTIG). Used for the protection of unimmunised persons when there is a specific risk of tetanus.
Dose: 250 units by intramuscular injection
Humotet® (Wellcome)
Antitetanus immunoglobulin injection 250 units/ml. Price 1-ml vial = **I**

VACCINIA. Antivaccinia immunoglobulin is available for the prevention and treatment of the complications of smallpox vaccination, as when vaccination is necessary in an individual for whom there are contra-indications to vaccination. It is also used in familial and other close contacts exposed to smallpox.

Antivaccinia Immunoglobulin Injection. Used to treat patients with generalised vaccinia or with localised vaccinial infection that endangers the eye.
Dose: by intramuscular injection, 1.5–2 g; CHILD under 1 year 500 mg, 1 to 6 years 1 g, and 7 to 14 years 1.5 g

OTHER SPECIFIC IMMUNOGLOBULINS (such as antivaricella/zoster immunoglobulin, antiherpes simplex immunoglobulin) are in limited supply and others are under study, but their availability and evaluation requires the cooperation of general practitioners to provide blood from patients who are convalescent from these and other specific viral infections in order to prepare specific immunoglobulin preparations.

14.5.3 Anti-D (Rh_0) immunoglobulin

Anti-D immunoglobulin is available to prevent a rhesus-negative mother from forming antibodies to foetal rhesus-positive cells which may pass into the maternal circulation during childbirth or abortion. It must be injected within 72 hours of the birth or abortion. The objective is to protect any further child from the hazard of haemolytic disease.

Anti-D (Rh_0) Immunoglobulin Injection. See notes (above).
Dose: for rhesus-negative women, 250–500 units by intramuscular injection following the birth of a rhesus-positive infant; after transfusion, up to 5000 units

Table: Schedule of vaccination and immunisation procedures (children and adults)

Age	Vaccine	Interval	Notes
During the first year of life	DTPer/Vac/Ads *and* Pol/Vac (Oral) (1st dose)		The first doses should be given at 3 months of age. If pertussis vaccine is contra-indicated or the parents decline, DT/Vac/Ads should be given
	DTPer/Vac/Ads *and* Pol/Vac (Oral) (2nd dose)	Preferably after an interval of 6–8 weeks	
	DTPer/Vac/Ads *and* Pol/Vac (Oral) (3rd dose)	Preferably after an interval of 4–6 months	
During the second year of life	Meas/Vac (Live)		
At school entry or entry to nursery school	DT/Vac/Ads *and* Pol/Vac (Oral)	Preferable to allow an interval of at least 3 years after completing basic course	
Between 11 and 13 years of age	Tub/Vac/BCG	Leave an interval of not less than 3 weeks between BCG and rubella vaccination	For tuberculin-negative children. For tuberculin-negative contacts at any age
Between 10 and 13 years of age (girls only)	Rub/Vac (Live)		All girls of this age should be offered rubella vaccine regardless of a past history of an attack of rubella
On leaving school or before employment or entering further education	Pol/Vac (Inact) *or* Pol/Vac (Oral); *and* Tet/Vac/Ads		
Adult life	Pol/Vac (Inact) *or* Pol/Vac (Oral) for previously unvaccinated adults	3 doses with an interval of 6–8 weeks between the first and second doses and of 4–6 months between the second and third	For travellers to countries where polio is endemic. Unvaccinated parents of a child being given oral vaccine should also be offered a course of Pol/Vac (Oral)
	Rub/Vac (Live) for susceptible women of child-bearing age		Adult females of child-bearing age should be tested for rubella antibodies and those sero-negative offered rubella vaccination. Pregnancy must first be excluded and the patient warned not to become pregnant for 3 months after immunisation
	Active immunisation against tetanus (Tet/Vac/Ads) for previously unvacinated adults	For previously unvaccinated adults: 2 doses at an interval of 6–8 weeks followed by a third dose 6 months later	

14.6 Vaccination programmes for children

A recent revised schedule promulgated by the Department of Health and Social Security proposes that the course of adsorbed diphtheria, tetanus and pertussis vaccine, together with poliomyelitis vaccine (oral) should commence at 3 months. The previous recommendation was more flexible and proposed that it should commence within the first 6 months and that it was preferable to start at about the sixth month. The revised schedule CMO(78)15—in Scotland SHHD/CAMO(78)18, on vaccination and immunisation procedures is set out in the Table. The principal points of difference from the previous schedule are as follows:

1. The basic course of triple vaccine, or diphtheria and tetanus vaccine, together with oral poliomyelitis vaccine should commence at the age

of 3 months. The intervals between the 3 doses of the basic course should remain the same as those previously recommended, that is 6–8 weeks between the first and second doses and 4–6 months between the second and third doses.
2. An alternative basic course which completes the protection against pertussis at an earlier age is described but for use only in the event of a whooping-cough epidemic. If this alternative is followed a booster dose of diphtheria and tetanus vaccine is necessary at 12–18 months of age to achieve a satisfactory level of immunity to these diseases.
3. It is recommended that a vaccine containing a pertussis component should not normally be offered after the age of 3 years.

Recently, some parents, who had chosen not to include a pertussis component in the basic immunisation of their infants, have changed their minds because of the greater prevalence of whooping-cough. The Joint Committee on Vaccination and Immunisation has advised that 3 doses of single pertussis vaccine (either plain or adsorbed) can be given at monthly intervals to provide protection in these cases. Where the basic course against diphtheria and tetanus is incomplete triple vaccine may be used to begin or complete the course against whooping-cough so that the infant is not given more injections than necessary.

Poliomyelitis vaccine, live (oral) is at present issued in 10-dose containers. The vaccine should be stored unopened at 4° but once the containers are opened the vaccine may lose its potency however it is stored. For this reason any vaccine remaining in the containers at the end of an immunisation session should be discarded. There is particular need to conserve supplies of vaccines, which in any case are expensive. As far as possible immunisation sessions should therefore be arranged to avoid undue wastage of vaccines, although it is recognised that it will not always be possible to muster those to be vaccinated in groups of 10. The practicability of dispensing vaccines in smaller doses is being considered.

14.7 International travel

No particular immunisation is required for travellers to the United States, Northern Europe, Australia, or New Zealand. In Southern Europe and particularly in those areas surrounding the Mediterranean, in Africa, the Middle East, Asia, and South America, certain special precautions are required. Mention has already been made of the personal precautions which should be taken in the prevention of **typhoid** (section 14.4.15); these also apply to **cholera** and other diarrhoeal diseases (including travellers' diarrhoea). Immunisation against typhoid is indicated for travellers to those countries where typhoid is endemic, and it would seem that the monovalent typhoid vaccine is acceptable, although it has not been subjected to detailed double-blind trials. Long-term travellers to areas that have a high incidence of **poliomyelitis** or **tuberculosis** should be immunised with the appropriate vaccine.

Cholera vaccine is no substitute for personal hygiene but has some protective value for about 6 months in preventing individual infections. It is required for travellers by some countries and must be certified on an International Certificate.

Stamped certificates supplied to general medical practitioners by Family Practitioner Committees (in Scotland by Health Boards) do not require to be authenticated by health authorities.

Smallpox vaccination may still be required for travel to some parts of the world and again as in the case of **cholera** and **yellow fever** vaccines, International Certificates are still required for travel to much of Africa and South America. The Health Departments of the UK have issued a leaflet, *Notice to Travellers—Health Protection*, which can usually be obtained from travel agents or from local authorities; it gives information on vaccination centres, etc. for overseas travellers.

Reference should also be made to the DHSS booklet, *Communicable Diseases Contracted Outside Great Britain*.

15: Drugs used in ANAESTHESIA

This chapter describes briefly drugs used in anaesthesia in minor and major surgery in hospitals, outpatient clinics, and general practice. The reader is referred to other sources for more detailed information on techniques of anaesthesia. This chapter is divided into two sections: general anaesthesia (15.1) and local anaesthesia (15.2).

15.1 General anaesthesia

Note: The drugs in section 15.1 should be used only by experienced personnel and in premises where adequate resuscitative equipment is available.

Except for short minor procedures, the use of single anaesthetic agents to produce general anaesthesia has now been superseded by balanced anaesthesia.

BALANCED ANAESTHESIA. In this procedure, low doses of several drugs with different actions are given to produce a state of balanced anaesthesia. By making use of drug interactions, light anaesthesia can be maintained with minimal toxicity to the patient, and recovery of the protective reflexes is possible within a few minutes of the end of the operation.

A typical sequence is to induce loss of consciousness for 2–3 minutes with thiopentone sodium or other intravenous anaesthetic (section 15.1.1) and maintain anaesthesia with nitrous oxide–oxygen mixtures supplemented, when necessary, with halothane or other potent inhalational anaesthetic (section 15.1.2), or with a narcotic analgesic. The action of the anaesthetic is enhanced by the narcotic analgesic and overall anaesthetic requirements are reduced. The narcotic may be given both as premedication and during the operation to provide analgesia after the operation. Narcotics may cause respiratory depression and prolong apnoea.

Adequate muscle relaxation is ensured by giving a neuromuscular blocking drug (section 15.1.5). Controlled or assisted respiration is necessary when muscle relaxants are used.

Persistent respiratory depression may be due to the residual effects of the narcotic analgesic. Narcotic antagonists may be used to reverse the depression but will also reverse the analgesia.

For certain procedures controlled hypotension may be required. Labetalol (see section 2.4), sodium nitroprusside (see section 2.5.1), and trimetaphan camsylate (see section 2.5.6) are used.

Beta-adrenoceptor blocking drugs (see section 2.4) may be used to control arrhythmias during anaesthesia.

15.1.1 Intravenous anaesthetics

Intravenous anaesthetics are mainly used for the rapid induction of anaesthesia which is then maintained with an appropriate inhalational drug such as nitrous oxide–oxygen (section 15.1.2), or by intermittent or continuous infusion. They may also be used alone to produce a light level of narcosis for short surgical procedures, particularly those performed with the aid of local anaesthetics.

In effective doses all the intravenous anaesthetics except ketamine, diazepam and other benzodiazepines, and the neuroleptic-narcotic mixtures, will produce loss of consciousness in one arm-brain circulation time.

Apart from ketamine, all the intravenous drugs depress cerebral function and can cause respiratory depression and hypotension. Adequate resuscitative facilities must be available.

Large doses of intravenous anaesthetics should be avoided in obstetrics as they rapidly cross the placenta and may affect the foetus.

In any dose they are **contra-indicated** in patients where there is no direct access to the airway or whose unprotected airways are likely to become obstructed during the procedure, as in mouth or throat surgery and in patients with a full stomach.

Dosage should be reduced when narcotic analgesics or central nervous depressant drugs are given concurrently. Narcotic analgesics are often given to reduce the dose of the intravenous anaesthetic.

There is a great individual variation in response to intravenous anaesthetics. Some, but not all, of this can be explained by lower tolerance of poor-risk patients or the increased requirements of those who have become tolerant to other cerebral depressants such as alcohol or sleeping tablets.

In order to assess individual requirements, the estimated dose should be injected over 20 seconds and a further 20–30 seconds allowed to assess its full effect before giving a supplementary dose. Intravenous drugs should not be given in sufficiently large doses to produce muscle relaxation, except for brief procedures. For tracheal intubation they should be followed by an inhalational sequence or by a neuromuscular blocking drug.

Thiopentone sodium (Intraval®) is used for the induction of anaesthesia and also as sole anaesthetic for minor operations and electroconvulsive treatment. It is the most widely used intravenous anaesthetic but also one of the most toxic and it has no analgesic properties. Induction is generally smooth and takes 10–30 seconds. Aqueous solutions prepared for injection are not stable, particularly when exposed to air. Solutions are given intravenously as they are irritant to subcutaneous tissue and arterial injection is particularly dangerous. Thiopentone sodium is usually given as a 2.5% solution.

Thiopentone should **not** be given to known or suspected porphyriacs and should be avoided in patients with a raised blood urea. It is best avoided in patients with marked congestive cardiac failure, but with preoxygenation and slow injection, small doses can be given to patients with other cardiac conditions. Thiopentone does not affect the intensity or duration of action of neuromuscular blocking agents.

Occasionally, induction may be accompanied by extraneous muscle movement, but this is not normally troublesome. Laryngospasm may also occur following induction; this is usually a reflex response and occurs most frequently in patients with upper respiratory disease who have not been premedicated with atropine.

Recovery from thiopentone is slow and its effects often persist for 6–8 hours. Return of consciousness does not imply return of full mental faculties. Patients are particularly susceptible to alcohol for up to 24 hours after administration.

Given by intermittent injection or by infusion, thiopentone has a marked cumulative effect which should be allowed for by reducing dosage. Dosage should be further reduced when anaesthesia is supplemented with narcotic analgesics.

Methohexitone sodium (Brietal Sodium®) is preferred to thiopentone sodium for outpatient and dental procedures because recovery is more rapid. It is less irritant to the tissues than thiopentone and solutions for injection are more stable.

Like all barbiturates, it is difficult with methohexitone to maintain a light level of sleep such as is required for conservative dentistry. Its use in this field should be considered as general anaesthesia rather than sedation.

Disadvantages associated with its use are that induction is less smooth than with thiopentone: hiccup, tremor, and involuntary movements occur more frequently. Opiate premedication may reduce their incidence but is not usually given because it increases recovery time.

Alphaxalone–alphadolone acetate (Althesin®) is a useful alternative to thiopentone for the induction of anaesthesia and is also used as sole agent for minor surgical operations. Recovery is quicker than with thiopentone sodium but slower than with methohexitone sodium. The main disadvantage is that it causes a high incidence of hypersensitivity reactions, usually seen as sudden profound hypotension, bronchospasm, and occasionally flushing. This may be caused by Cremophor EL® in the vehicle. Treatment consists of rapid infusion of electrolyte solutions and, if necessary, sympathomimetic drugs (see section 2.7.1). Alphaxalone–alphadolone should be avoided in patients who have a history of hypersensitivity reactions and used with caution in hepatic impairment.

Alphadolone acetate contributes little activity and is added together with Cremophor EL®, to solubilise alphaxalone in the aqueous injection. However, the injection is viscous and is difficult to inject through small bore needles.

Etomidate (Hypnomidate®) is a relatively new agent from which recovery is rapid and cardiovascular effects are slight. It appears to cause frequent extraneous muscle movements which precludes its use as sole anaesthetic agent. It seems that a consistently acceptable quality of anaesthesia is only possible when premedication with a narcotic analgesic such as fentanyl has been used. Etomidate causes a high incidence of pain and in some cases venous thrombosis on injection.

Propanidid (Epontol®) is the only available ultra-short acting intravenous anaesthetic. It is especially suited to very short outpatient procedures but, on account of its toxicity, its use is limited to situations where its very short action and lack of hangover effect offer real advantages over other drugs. Toxic effects include a high incidence of hypersensitivity reactions, particularly bronchoconstriction, which may be caused by the solubilising agent Cremophor EL® in the vehicle, and, with high doses, marked hypotension. It causes a transient stimulation of respiration which is then followed by respiratory depression. It also prolongs the action of suxamethonium.

Ketamine (Ketalar®) is used mainly as an induction agent for paediatric anaesthesia, particularly where repeated administration is likely. Its action is too prolonged for use in outpatient clinics. Ketamine, even in sub-hypnotic doses, has good analgesic properties. It is the only agent of this group which may be given by *intramuscular injection* and it is unique in producing catalepsy accompanied by increased muscle tone and cardiovascular stimulation. It is therefore a useful aid for maintaining airways patency, but is unsuitable for procedures requiring muscle relaxation, for example abdominal operations.

In adults its use is associated with an unacceptably high incidence of hallucinations and other transient psychotic sequelae which occur to a much lesser extent in children. Psychotic sequelae occur most often after short operations or if premedicating agents such as droperidol or intravenous diazepam have been omitted; such agents prolong the action of ketamine. It should not be used in adults with hypertension or in patients with a history of mental illness.

Diazepam is sometimes used by intravenous injection for the induction of anaesthesia. However, it differs from thiopentone in two respects. Firstly, there is a delay of up to 3 minutes before the peak effect occurs, and secondly there is a great individual variation in dose; some patients may not fall asleep even with a dose as high as 1 mg/kg.

MINOR SURGERY AND OUTPATIENT PROCEDURES. The level of narcosis required may vary from light sedation for unpleasant procedures such as endoscopy, to full anaesthesia. Agents used in minor surgery and outpatients should ideally give rapid recovery with minimal hangover thus enabling the protective reflexes to be regained, and the patient to become fully awake again, almost as soon as the procedure is over. Outpatients receiving anaesthetics should not be allowed home unaccompanied and alcohol should be avoided for 24 hours.

Diazepam is used by intravenous injection to produce light sedation with amnesia for unpleasant procedures or for operations under local anaesthesia. Its action starts in about 2 minutes. The 'sleep' dose shows great individual variation, from 200 to 500 micrograms/kg by intravenous injection, but if 20 mg is insufficient, an inhalational anaesthetic should be added. Diazepam has good amnesic properties. The patient will not usually recall application of the face mask but tracheal intubation or suxamethonium 'twitching' may be remembered. Its disadvantage in outpatients is that drowsiness persists for about 6 hours after the procedures. It is also used in sub-anaesthetic doses as a mild sedative in dentistry and allows retention of the pharyngeal reflexes while a local block is performed.

Diazepam injection is irritant to tissues and is followed by a high incidence of venous thrombosis which may not be noticed until a week after injection.

See also section 4.8.2 for its use in status epilepticus.

Lorazepam (Ativan®) is used similarly to diazepam. It is not fully evaluated but it appears to cause less respiratory depression and greater amnesia than diazepam. Its onset of action is much slower than that of diazepam and it takes up to 20 minutes to exert its full effect; for this reason it is not suitable for induction of anaesthesia.

THIOPENTONE SODIUM

Indications: induction of general anaesthesia; anaesthesia of short duration in minor surgical procedures

Cautions; Contra-indications; Side-effects: see notes above

Dose: *by intravenous injection*, in fit premedicated adults, initially 100–150 mg (4–6 ml of 2.5% solution) over 10–15 seconds, repeated if necessary according to the patient's response after 20–30 seconds; *or* up to 4 mg/kg; CHILD, induction 4–8 mg/kg

By continuous intravenous infusion, as a 0.2–0.4% solution, according to the patient's response

Intraval Sodium® (M&B)

Injection 2.5%, powder for reconstitution, thiopentone sodium. Price 500-mg amp = **C**; 2.5-g vial = **E**

Injection 5%, powder for reconstitution, thiopentone sodium. Price 0.5- and 1-g amp (both) = **C**; 5-g vial = **F**

ALPHAXALONE–ALPHADOLONE ACETATE

Indications: induction and maintenance of anaesthesia

Cautions; Side-effects: see notes above

Dose: as an injection containing alphaxalone 9 mg and alphadolone acetate 3 mg/ml

By slow intraveous injection, for induction, 0.05–0.075 ml/kg over 30 seconds; maintenance, incremental doses of 0.5–1 ml, repeated according to the patient's response; CHILD, induction 0.05–0.075 ml/kg

By intravenous infusion, for maintenance as a 10% dilution of the injection in sodium chloride or dextrose intravenous infusion, 10–20 ml/hour

Althesin® (Glaxo)

Injection, alphaxalone 9 mg and alphadolone acetate 3 mg/ml. Price 5-ml amp = **D**; 10-ml amp = **E**

DIAZEPAM

Indications: sedation with amnesia; as premedication. For use in status epilepticus see section 4.8.2

Cautions; Side-effects: see notes above and section 4.1.2

Dose: *by mouth*, 5 mg at night, 5 mg on waking, and 5 mg 2 hours before minor or dental surgery

By slow intravenous injection, 10–20 mg over 2–4 minutes as sedative cover for minor surgical and medical procedures; premedication 100–200 micrograms/kg

Oral preparations: see section 4.1.2

Parenteral preparations

Diazemuls® (KabiVitrum)

Injection (emulsion), diazepam 5 mg/ml. For intravenous injection or infusion. Price 2-ml amp = **B**

Valium® (Roche)

Injection, diazepam 5 mg/ml in solvent. Price 2- and 4-ml amp (both) = **B**

ETOMIDATE

Indications: induction of anaesthesia
Cautions; Side-effects: see notes above
Dose: *by slow intravenous injection*, induction 300 micrograms/kg; maintenance, 100–200 micrograms/kg according to the patient's response

▼ **Hypnomidate®** (Janssen)
Injection, etomidate 2 mg/ml in propylene glycol 35%. Price 10-ml amp = **C**
Concentrate for intravenous infusion, etomidate 125 mg (as hydrochloride)/ml. To be diluted with at least 50 volumes of dextrose intravenous infusion (5%) or sodium chloride intravenous infusion (0.9%) before use. Price 1-ml amp = **F**

KETAMINE

Indications: induction and maintenance of anaesthesia
Cautions; Side-effects: see notes above
Dose: *by slow intravenous injection*, 1–2 mg/kg over 60 seconds, repeated according to the patient's response
By deep intramuscular injection, 4–10 mg/kg, repeated according to the patient's response

Ketalar® (P-D)
Injection, ketamine 10 mg (as hydrochloride)/ml. Price 20-ml vial = **E**
Injection, ketamine 50 mg (as hydrochloride)/ml. Price 10-ml vial = **G**
Injection, ketamine 100 mg (as hydrochloride)/ml. Price 5-ml vial = **G**

LORAZEPAM

Indications: sedation with amnesia; as premedication
Cautions; Side-effects: as for Diazepam
Dose: *by mouth*, 2–3 mg at night, then 2–4 mg 1–2 hours before minor surgery or medical procedures
By slow intravenous injection, preferably diluted with an equal volume of sodium chloride intravenous infusion or water for injections, 50 micrograms/kg
By slow intramuscular injection, diluted as above, 50 micrograms/kg 1–1½ hours before operation

Oral preparations: see section 4.1.2

Parenteral preparations
Ativan® (Wyeth)
▼ *Injection*, lorazepam 4 mg/ml in solvent. Price 1-ml amp = **B**

METHOHEXITONE SODIUM

Indications: induction and maintenance of anaesthesia for short procedures
Cautions; Side-effects: see notes above
Dose: *by slow intravenous injection*, as a 1 or 2% solution, 50–120 mg over 25–60 seconds *or* 1–1.5 mg/kg, according to the patient's response; maintenance, 20–40 mg (2–4 ml of 1% solution) every 4–7 minutes; CHILD, induction 1–2 mg/kg
By continuous intravenous infusion, as a 0.1–0.2% solution in sodium chloride or dextrose intravenous infusion, according to the patient's response

Brietal Sodium® (Lilly)
Injection, powder for reconstitution, methohexitone sodium. Price 100 mg in 10-ml vial = **B**
Injection, powder for reconstitution, methohexitone sodium. Price 500 mg in 50-ml vial = **D**
Injection, powder for reconstitution, methohexitone sodium. Price 2.5 g in 17.5-ml vial = **F**
Injection, powder for reconstitution, methohexitone sodium. Price 2.5 g in 250-ml vial = **G**
Injection, powder for reconstitution, methohexitone sodium. Price 5 g in 35-ml vial = **H**

PROPANIDID

Indications: induction and maintenance of anaesthesia for short procedures
Cautions; Side-effects: see notes above
Dose: *by intravenous injection*, 5–10 mg/kg, usually 5–7 mg/kg, or 3–4 mg/kg in the frail or elderly; CHILD 7–10 mg/kg

Epontol® (Bayer)
Injection, propanidid 50 mg/ml. Price 10-ml amp = **B**

15.1.2 Inhalational anaesthetics

Gaseous and volatile anaesthetic agents are mainly used for *maintenance* of anaesthesia after induction with an intravenous induction agent (section 15.1.1). They are usually employed as part of a balanced anaesthesia technique (see section 15.1). Some inhalational anaesthetics, e.g. halothane and nitrous oxide, have a rapid onset of action and may be used for *induction* purposes. Others such as methoxyflurane and trichloroethylene are too slow acting for this purpose.

Gaseous agents require suitable equipment for storage under pressure, reduction to operating pressure, and monitoring of gas flow-rate. Most volatile agents are metered by calibrated vaporisers, using air, oxygen, or nitrous oxide–oxygen as carriers, though some can be given by direct drip on to a pad and vaporised by the patient's breath.

To prevent hypoxia, the gaseous agents must be given with an adequate concentration of oxygen.

Nitrous oxide is used for induction and maintenance of anaesthesia. It is a weak anaesthetic agent with marked analgesic properties and is relatively non-toxic. It is widely used as a background anaesthetic and a carrier gas for other volatile agents in general anaesthesia. The usual concentration is 70 to 75% with 20% oxygen during induction of anaesthesia and 30% oxygen during maintenance. More powerful inhalational and intravenous anaesthetic agents and narcotic analgesics are given to increase its weak action when necessary. Nitrous oxide–oxygen and thiopentone sodium are commonly used together and muscle relaxants are also given when required (section 15.1.5).

When used as an induction agent, nitrous oxide has a rapid action (2 to 3 minutes) but, except for short procedures, it is not used as the sole agent because hypoxic mixtures, for example nitrous oxide 90%–oxygen 10%, are needed to produce adequate anaesthesia and even this may be insufficient in resistant patients. A volatile or parenteral supplement should then be added: lower concentrations of nitrous oxide with 20–30% oxygen are often used with halothane, trichloroethylene, or other volatile agents.

A mixture of nitrous oxide and oxygen (Entonox®) containing 50% of each gas is used in sub-anaesthetic doses for its analgesic properties in obstetrics and painful procedures such as wound and burn dressing. Nitrous oxide should not be used to provide muscle relaxation and suitable neuromuscular blocking drugs should be used if necessary. It should not be used in patients with an air-containing closed space, such as a tension pneumothorax, as pressure will build up as nitrous oxide diffuses into the space. Prolonged use is associated with a fall in the white-cell count.

Halothane (Fluothane®) is the most widely used of the volatile agents. Its advantages are that induction is smooth and rapid, that the vapour is non-irritant, pleasant to inhale, and does not induce coughing or breath-holding, and there is a low incidence of postoperative vomiting.

It is used for the maintenance of anaesthesia in major surgery and to supplement the anaesthetic action of nitrous oxide–oxygen mixtures in balanced anaesthesia (section 15.1).

Halothane should be used only for the induction of anaesthesia in children and in short procedures where rapid recovery is needed. Induction is slow (about 5 minutes) and so it is often used with thiopentone sodium, but halothane alone is the induction agent of choice for patients with poor veins. Concentrations of up to 5% mixed with at least 25% oxygen are used alone or with nitrous oxide–oxygen mixtures. It may be used in a similar way for anaesthesia in outpatient procedures. Recovery is less prolonged than with the intravenous anaesthetic agents. Halothane will produce moderate muscular relaxation but specific muscle relaxants should be used when additional relaxation is necessary.

Disadvantages of using halothane are that hypercarbia or adrenaline injections must be avoided because they may cause ventricular arrhythmias. Should adrenaline be necessary during halothane anaesthesia, pretreatment with a small intravenous dose of beta-adrenoceptor blocking drug is advisable. Hypercarbia should be avoided by assisting respiration.

Postural hypotension resulting from halothane-induced bradycardia and vasodilatation is proportional to the administered concentration of the anaesthetic. Hypotension is an advantage in operations where controlled hypotension is required; it reduces capillary bleeding and gives a relatively bloodless field. High concentrations of halothane (5%) are used to induce hypotension; controlled ventilation is then necessary.

Where possible, halothane should not be used more than once in 4 to 6 months as there is some evidence that disturbances of liver function and, rarely, jaundice may occur, sometimes after discharge from hospital, especially in obese patients. The risk is greater when the interval between administrations is less than 6 weeks.

Cyclopropane is a potent anaesthetic which is used for induction and maintenance of anaesthesia. It is administered using a suitable closed-circuit system. It is a useful agent for rapid induction in obstetrics but otherwise its use has declined since the introduction of balanced anaesthesia. When used for induction purposes with oxygen it is effective in a lower concentration than nitrous oxide and is therefore less likely to cause hypoxia. It is often advocated for use in poor risk patients for this reason.

When used in maintenance anaesthesia it is sufficiently potent to be used for producing deep levels of anaesthesia. Assisted respiration is required when cyclopropane is used in concentrations capable of causing muscle relaxation.

The disadvantages of cyclopropane are its explosive and inflammable nature, the potent respiratory depressant action which occurs at all concentrations, and the ventricular dysrhythmias associated with its use. These are aggravated by hypercarbia and adrenaline injections which should be avoided, as for halothane. Recovery, although rapid, may be associated with postoperative vomiting.

Methoxyflurane (Penthrane®) is declining in use because it causes a dose-related renal toxicity which is attributed to free fluoride ions. Low concentrations of methoxyflurane (0.2 to 0.5%) may be administered for periods of up to 1 hour as part of the balanced technique but thereafter an alternative agent should be used. The main use of methoxyflurane is in maintenance of anaesthesia in patients who have had recent exposure to halothane, or in patients likely to require adrenaline during the operation. It is also used to produce controlled hypotension in certain operations such as plastic surgery. It has good analgesic properties and is used in sub-anaesthetic doses to provide analgesia in a similar way to trichloroethylene.

Methoxyflurane has the slowest onset of action of the anaesthetic agents and is therefore not suitable for use in induction. Recovery time is long, but there is a low incidence of postoperative vomiting.

Trichloroethylene (Trilene®) is a weak anaesthetic but it has useful analgesic properties. It is used in sub-anaesthetic doses from special vaporisers to provide analgesia in painful obstetric procedures and in burn and wound dressing. It is often included as an analgesic in low concentrations in mixtures for maintenance of anaesthesia (see section 15.1 for balanced anaesthesia). It is unsuitable for induction and is usually given with other anaesthetic agents because it is not potent enough for use alone except in procedures such as body-surface operations. It is commonly used with nitrous oxide–oxygen mixtures.

Disadvantages associated with its use are that recovery is often delayed, partly because trichloroethylene is retained in the tissues, and partly because some of its metabolites are active. Postoperative vomiting occurs frequently. It should not be used in apparatus requiring soda lime absorption.

Enflurane (Ethrane®) is a recently introduced inhalational anaesthetic and its place in anaesthesia is not yet fully evaluated. It is considered to be a useful alternative to halothane and, when used as part of a balanced technique, the action of the two agents is virtually indistinguishable. It has two advantages over halothane: adrenaline can be injected during enflurane anaesthesia without the risk of ventricular ectopic beats or fibrillation, and enflurane is eliminated more rapidly from the body than halothane thus allowing shorter exposure to its effects. Preliminary results indicate that liver dysfunction occurs less frequently after a second administration than with halothane. Disadvantages are that induction may not be as smooth or rapid as with halothane and there may be a higher incidence of extraneous muscle movement and respiratory disturbance.

Ether, Anaesthetic (diethyl ether) is rarely used as an anaesthetic agent because of its inflammability and irritant effect on the respiratory tract. It is not suitable for induction and produces a high incidence of nausea and vomiting. It is occasionally used in paediatrics as a supplement to nitrous oxide–oxygen mixtures.

CYCLOPROPANE

Indications; Cautions; Side-effects: see notes above

Dose: using a suitable closed-circuit anaesthetic apparatus, for light *anaesthesia* 7–10% in oxygen, for moderate to deep anaesthesia 20–30%

ENFLURANE

Indications; Cautions; Side-effects: see notes above

Dose: using a suitable calibrated vaporiser, *induction*, increased gradually from 1% to 4% in air, oxygen, or nitrous oxide–oxygen, according to the patient's response

Maintenance, 0.5 to 3%

▼ **Ethrane®** (Abbott)
Enflurane. Price 250 ml = **J**

ETHER, ANAESTHETIC

Indications; Cautions; Side-effects: see notes above

Dose: from an open mask or a suitable vaporiser, *induction*, up to 20% in air

Maintenance, 3–10% in air

Price 500 ml = **E**

HALOTHANE

Indications; Cautions; Side-effects: see notes above

Dose: using a suitable vaporiser, *induction*, increased gradually to 2–5% in air, oxygen, or nitrous oxide–oxygen; CHILD 1.5–2%

Maintenance, adults and children, 0.5–2%

Halothane (M&B)
Price 250 ml = **G**

Fluothane® (ICI)
Halothane. Price 250 ml = **G**

METHOXYFLURANE

Indications; Cautions; Side-effects: see notes above

Dose: *maintenance*, 0.2–0.5% using a suitable vaporiser

Analgesic, 0.35% from a preset vaporiser

Penthrane Inhalation® (Abbott)
Methoxyflurane. Price 125 ml = **G**

NITROUS OXIDE

Indications; Cautions; Side-effects: see notes above

Dose: using a suitable anaesthetic apparatus, a mixture with 20–30% oxygen for *induction* and *maintenance* of light anaesthesia

Analgesic, as a mixture with 50% oxygen, according to the patient's needs

TRICHLOROETHYLENE

Indications; Cautions; Side-effects: see notes above; must not be used with soda lime in closed circuits

Dose: *maintenance* of light anaesthesia, 0.2–2% using a suitable vaporiser

Analgesic, 0.35–0.5% using a suitable vaporiser

Trilene® (ICI)
Trichloroethylene. Price 250 ml = **D**

15.1.3 Anticholinergic premedication drugs

Anticholinergic premedication agents, usually **atropine, hyoscine** (scopolamine), or **glycopyrronium** (Robinul®), are used to dry bronchial and salivary secretions which are increased by intubation and the inhalational anaesthetics. They are also used to prevent excessive bradycardia and hypotension caused by halothane, cyclopropane, thiopentone, methohexitone, suxamethonium, and neostigmine.

Atropine is the most commonly used. Intravenous administration immediately before anaesthesia is generally preferred to intramuscular injection (which should be given 30–60 minutes before the operation) because it ensures that the patient is adequately atropinised even if the operation is delayed. The pre-operative discomfort of dry mouth is also avoided.

Hyoscine is a less effective drying agent than atropine but provides a higher degree of amnesia. A disadvantage is that it may slow the heart rate.

Phenothiazine derivatives have too little activity to be effective drying agents when used alone.

ATROPINE SULPHATE

Indications: drying secretions, reversal of hypotension with excessive bradycardia; with neostigmine for reversal of competitive neuromuscular block

Cautions: cardiovascular disease, glaucoma, paralytic ileus

Side-effects: tachycardia

Dose: premedication, *by intravenous injection*, 300–600 micrograms immediately before induction of anaesthesia, and for reversal of hypotension with bradycardia

By intramuscular injection, 300–600 micrograms 30–60 minutes before induction; CHILD 20 micrograms/kg

For control of muscarinic side-effects of neostigmine in reversal of competitive neuromuscular block, *by intravenous injection*, 0.6–1.2 mg

Atropine Sulphate Injection—see section 2.3.2

Morphine and Atropine Injection—see under Morphine Salts (section 15.1.4.1)

GLYCOPYRRONIUM BROMIDE

Indications; Cautions; Side-effects: see under Atropine Sulphate

Dose: premedication, *by intramuscular or intravenous injection,* 200–400 micrograms, *or* 4–5 micrograms/kg to a max. of 400 micrograms; CHILD, *by intramuscular or intravenous injection*, 4–8 micrograms/kg to a max. of 200 micrograms; intra-operative use, *by intravenous injection*, as for premedication

For control of muscarinic side-effects of neostigmine in reversal of competitive neuromuscular block, *by intravenous injection*, 10–15 micrograns/kg with 50 micrograms/kg neostigmine; CHILD, 10 micrograms/kg with 50 micrograms/kg neostigmine

▼ Robinul® (Robins)

Injection, glycopyrronium bromide 200 micrograms/ml. Price 1-ml amp = **B**; 3-ml amp = **C**

HYOSCINE HYDROBROMIDE

(Scopolamine Hydrobromide)

Indications: drying secretions, amnesia

Cautions: see under Atropine Sulphate; may slow heart; avoid in the elderly

Dose: premedication, *by subcutaneous injection*, 200–600 micrograms 30–60 minutes before induction of anaesthesia, usually with papaveretum; CHILD 15 micrograms/kg

Hyoscine Injection, hyoscine hydrobromide 400 and 600 micrograms/ml. Price 1-ml amp (both) = **B**

Papaveretum and Hyoscine Injection, see under Papaveretum (section 15.1.4.1)

15.1.4 Sedative premedication drugs

Sedative premedication agents include the **narcotic analgesics, anxiolytics**, and **neuroleptics**. These drugs are used to alleviate pre-operative anxiety and provide some degree of postoperative amnesia. They also facilitate induction and diminish overall anaesthetic requirements by enhancing the effects of the anaesthetic agents. Large doses should be avoided as they also enhance the respiratory depressant and hypotensive effects of anaesthetics.

The most common premedication agents are the narcotic analgesics **morphine, papaveretum**, or **pethidine** (with atropine or hyoscine), usually given about an hour before the operation. There is a trend towards the use of *oral* premedication agents, such as the benzodiazepines **diazepam** and **lorazepam**, given the night before and on the morning of the operation. Chlordiazepoxide is rarely used for this purpose.

Alternatively, phenothiazine derivatives may be used. **Promethazine, trimeprazine**, or **chlorpromazine** is generally given. They have a useful anti-emetic action which may prevent postoperative sickness, but like the narcotic analgesics they increase respiratory depression and hypotension; large doses should therefore be avoided. The butyrophenone **droperidol** is less frequently used but it should not be given alone, except in very small doses, as it causes extrapyramidal side-effects. Haloperidol is rarely used in anaesthesia. **Barbiturates** should be **avoided**, especially where pain is present, as they cause restlessness and confusion.

PREMEDICATION IN CHILDREN. Oral or rectal administration is preferred to parenteral injection where possible but is not altogether satisfactory. Oral **trimeprazine** is widely used but when given alone it may cause postoperative restlessness when pain is present. An alternative is **diazepam**.

Narcotic analgesics also provide additional analgesia *during* surgery and postoperatively. Fentanyl, pentazocine, pethidine, or phenoperidine may be given intravenously when necessary. **Piritramide** (see section 4.7.2) is used in postoperative analgesia.

15.1.4.1 NARCOTIC ANALGESICS

FENTANYL

Indications: analgesia during operation, neuroleptanalgesia, enhancement of anaesthetics; respiratory depressant in assisted respiration

Cautions: myasthenia gravis, postoperative respiratory depression from doses above 200 micrograms require assisted respiration (effects may be terminated with naloxone or doxapram). Drug interactions: see Appendix 1

Side-effects: transient hypotension, bradycardia, nausea and vomiting

Dose: *by intravenous injection*, with spontaneous respiration, 100–200 micrograms, then 50 micrograms every 20–30 minutes as required; CHILD 3–5 micrograms/kg

With assisted respiration, up to 600 micrograms; CHILD 10–15 micrograms/kg

CD **Sublimaze®** (Janssen)

Injection, fentanyl 50 micrograms (as citrate)/ml. Price 2-ml amp = **B**; 10-ml amp = **E**

CD **Thalamonal®** (Janssen)

Injection, fentanyl 50 micrograms (as citrate), droperidol 2.5 mg/ml. Price 2-ml amp = **C**

Dose: by intramuscular or intravenous injection 1–2 ml to a max. of 8 ml; CHILD, by intramuscular injection 0.4–1.5 ml

MORPHINE SALTS

Indications: analgesia during and after operation; enhancement of anaesthetics; pre-operative sedation

Cautions; Contra-indications; Side-effects: see section 4.7.2 and notes above. Drug interactions: see Appendix 1

Dose: *by subcutaneous or intramuscular injection*, 10–15 mg 1–1½ hours before operation; CHILD, *by intramuscular injection*, 150 micrograms/kg. See also section 4.7.2 for analgesia

CD **Morphine Sulphate Injection,** morphine sulphate, 10, 15, and 20 mg/ml. Price 1-ml amp (all) = **A**. Morphine sulphate 30 mg/ml. Price 1- and 2-ml amp (both) = **B**

CD **Morphine and Atropine Injection,** morphine sulphate 10 mg, atropine sulphate 600 micrograms/ml. Price 1-ml amp = **A**

Dose: by subcutaneous injection, 0.5–1 ml

PAPAVERETUM

Indications: analgesia during and after operation; enhancement of anaesthetics; pre-operative sedation

Cautions; Contra-indications; Side-effects: see section 4.7.2 and notes above. Drug interactions: see Appendix 1

Dose: *by mouth or by intramuscular, intravenous, or subcutaneous injection*, 10–20 mg 45–60 minutes before anaesthesia; CHILD 200–300 micrograms/kg

Note: Papaveretum contains anhydrous morphine 50% as hydrochloride with the hydrochlorides of other opium alkaloids. 10 mg papaveretum is equivalent in morphine content to about 6.25 mg of morphine sulphate

CD **Papaveretum Injection,** papaveretum 10 mg/ml, price 1-ml amp = **B**; 20 mg/ml, price 1-ml amp = **A**

CD **Papaveretum and Hyoscine Injection,** papaveretum 20 mg, hyoscine hydrobromide 400 micrograms/ml. Price 1-ml amp = **A**

Dose: by subcutaneous or intramuscular injection, 1 ml

CD **Omnopon®** (Roche)

Tablets, buff, papaveretum 10 mg. Price 20 tabs = **B**

Injection, papaveretum 20 mg/ml. Price 1-ml amp = **A**

CD **Omnopon-Scopolamine®** (Roche)

Injection, papaveretum 20 mg, hyoscine hydrobromide 400 micrograms/ml. Price 1-ml amp = **A**

Dose: by subcutaneous or intramuscular injection, 1 ml

PETHIDINE HYDROCHLORIDE

Indications: analgesia before, during, and after operation, enhancement of anaesthetics, for basal narcosis with phenothiazines; respiratory depressant in prolonged assisted respiration

Cautions; Contra-indications; Side-effects: see section 4.7.2 and notes above. Drug interactions: see Appendix 1

Dose: premedication, *by intramuscular injection*, 50–100 mg 1 hour before operation; CHILD 4.5 mg/kg

Adjunct to nitrous oxide–oxygen, *by intravenous injection*, 25 mg repeated when required

CD **Pethidine Injection,** pethidine hydrochloride 10 mg/ml. Price 5- and 10-ml amp (both) = **B**. Pethidine hydrochloride 50 mg/ml. Price 1- and 2-ml amp (both) = **A**

CD **Pamergan P100®** (M&B)

Injection, pethidine hydrochloride 50 mg, promethazine hydrochloride 25 mg/ml. Price 2-ml amp = **B**

Dose: 2 ml by intramuscular injection or, diluted to 10 ml, by intravenous injection, 1–1½ hours before operation; CHILD, by intramuscular injection, 8–12 years 0.75 ml, 13–16 years 1 ml

CD **Pamergan AP100/25®** (M&B)

Injection, pethidine hydrochloride 100 mg, atropine sulphate 600 micrograms, promethazine hydrochloride 25 mg/ml. Price 1-ml amp = **B**

Dose: 1 ml by intramuscular injection or, diluted to 10 ml, by intravenous injection; CHILD, by intramuscular injection, 8–12 years 0.4 ml, 13–16 years 0.5 ml

CD Pethilorfan® (Roche)

Injection, pethidine hydrochloride 50 mg, levallorphan tartrate 625 micrograms/ml. Price 1- and 2-ml amp (both) = **A**

Dose: premedication, 2 ml by subcutaneous, intramuscular or intravenous injection 1 hour before operation; adjunct to nitrous oxide–oxygen 0.5–1 ml by intravenous injection; CHILD ¼–½ adult dose

PHENOPERIDINE HYDROCHLORIDE

Indications: analgesia during operation, neuroleptanalgesia, enhancement of anaesthetics; respiratory depressant in prolonged assisted respiration

Cautions; Contra-indications; Side-effects: see under Pethidine Hydrochloride and Fentanyl. Doses above 1 mg cause respiratory depression and require assisted respiration (effects may be terminated with naloxone or doxapram)

Dose: *by intravenous injection*, with spontaneous respiration, 0.5–1 mg, then 500 micrograms every 40–60 minutes as required; CHILD 30–50 micrograms/kg

With assisted respiration, 2–5 mg, then 1 mg as required; CHILD 100–150 micrograms/kg

CD Operidine® (Janssen)

Injection, phenoperidine hydrochloride 1 mg/ml. Price 2-ml amp = **C**

15.1.4.2 ANXIOLYTICS AND NEUROLEPTICS

CHLORPROMAZINE HYDROCHLORIDE

Indications: anti-emetic, pre-operative sedation, enhancement of anaesthetics, sedatives, and analgesics; induction of hypothermia

Cautions; Contra-indications; Side-effects: see section 4.2.1.

Dose: premedication, *by intramuscular injection*, 20–50 mg 60 minutes before operation

Largactil® (M&B)

Solution 1% (= injection), chlorpromazine hydrochloride 10 mg/ml. Price 5-ml amp = **A**

Solution 2.5% (= injection), chlorpromazine hydrochloride 25 mg/ml. Price 1- or 2-ml amp = **A**

DIAZEPAM

Indications: pre-operative sedation, amnesia

See section 15.1.1

DROPERIDOL

Indications: anti-emetic, pre-operative sedation; neuroleptanalgesia

Cautions; Contra-indications; Side-effects: see notes above and section 4.2.1

Dose: premedication, *by intramuscular injection*, 10 mg 60 minutes before operation; CHILD 300–600 micrograms/kg

Neuroleptanalgesia, *by intravenous injection*, up to 15 mg with a narcotic analgesic; CHILD 200–300 micrograms/kg

Droleptan® (Janssen)

Injection, droperidol 5 mg/ml. Price 2-ml amp = **C**

Thalamonal®—see under Fentanyl (section 15.1.4.1)

HALOPERIDOL

Indications: anti-emetic, pre-operative sedation

Cautions; Contra-indications; Side-effects: see notes above and section 4.2.1

Dose: premedication, *by intramuscular injection*, 1–5 mg 1–8 hours before operation

Haldol® (Janssen)

Injection, haloperidol 5 mg/ml. Price 1-ml amp = **B**; 2-ml amp = **C**

Serenace® (Searle)

Injection, haloperidol 5 mg/ml. Price 1-ml amp = **B**

Injection, haloperidol 10 mg/ml. Price 2-ml amp = **C**

LORAZEPAM

Indications: pre-operative sedation, amnesia

See section 15.1.1

PERPHENAZINE

Indications: anti-emetic, pre-operative sedation

Cautions; Contra-indications; Side-effects: see section 4.2.1. Drug interactions: see Appendix 1

Dose: premedication, *by intramuscular injection*, 5 mg 1 hour before operation

Fentazin® (A&H)

Injection, perphenazine 5 mg/ml. Price 1-ml amp = **A**

PROMETHAZINE HYDROCHLORIDE

Indications: anti-emetic, pre-operative sedative and anticholinergic agent

Cautions; Side-effects: see section 4.6 and notes above

Dose: premedication, *by mouth,* CHILD 6–12 months 10 mg, 1–5 years 15–20 mg, 6–10 years 20–25 mg

By deep intramuscular injection, 25–50 mg 1 hour before operation; CHILD 5–10 years, 6.25–12.5 mg

Pamergan—see under Pethidine Hydrochloride (section 15.1.4.1)

Phenergan—see section 3.4.1

TEMAZEPAM

Indications: premedication; anxiety before investigatory procedures

Cautions; Side-effects; Dose; Preparations: see section 4.1.1

TRIMEPRAZINE TARTRATE

Indications: pre-operative sedation, anti-emetic; also used in pruritus

Cautions: avoid alcohol. Drug interactions: see Appendix 1. See also notes above

Side-effects: drowsiness, dryness of the mouth, allergic skin reactions

Dose: premedication, 3–4.5 mg/kg 1–2 hours before operation; CHILD 2–7 years 2–4 mg/kg
Pruritus, 10–40 mg daily in divided doses; CHILD 7.5–25 mg daily in 3 or 4 divided doses

Vallergan® (M&B)

Tablets, blue, s/c, trimeprazine tartrate 10 mg. Price 20 tabs = **B**

Syrup (= paediatric elixir), yellow, trimeprazine tartrate 7.5 mg/5 ml. Diluent syrup without preservative, life of diluted elixir 14 days. Price 125 ml = **C**

Syrup forte (= strong paediatric elixir), pink, trimeprazine tartrate 30 mg/5 ml. Diluent syrup (without preservative), life of diluted elixir 14 days. Price 125 ml = **D**

15.1.5 Muscle relaxants

Muscle relaxants used in anaesthesia are also known as **neuromuscular blocking drugs** or **myoneural blocking drugs**. By specific blockade of the neuromuscular junction they enable light levels of anaesthesia to be employed with adequate relaxation of the muscles of the abdomen and diaphragm. They also relax the vocal cords and allow the passage of an endotracheal tube. Their action differs from the muscle relaxants acting on the spinal cord or brain which are used in musculoskeletal disorders (see section 10.2.2).

Patients who have received a muscle relaxant should **always** have their respiration assisted or controlled until the drug has been inactivated or antagonised (section 15.1.6). As they may cause painful muscle spasm they should be given after induction of anaesthesia.

NON-DEPOLARISING OR COMPETITIVE MUSCLE RELAXANTS. Drugs of this group include alcuronium, fazadinium, gallamine, pancuronium, and tubocurarine. They cause blockade by competing with acetylcholine at the receptor site at the neuromuscular junction. These drugs are best suited to the production of paralysis of long duration. They have a slower, less complete action than the depolarising muscle relaxants and should be avoided in myasthenia gravis.

The action of the competitive muscle relaxants may be reversed with anticholinesterases such as neostigmine (section 15.1.6).

Tubocurarine may be regarded as the standard non-depolarising muscle relaxant but in recent years its use has declined. It starts to act between 3–5 minutes and lasts for about 30 minutes after injection. It often causes an erythematous rash on the chest and neck and this is probably caused by histamine release (bronchoconstriction does not occur). Onset of blockade is invariably associated with hypotension and this, though transient, is dangerous in poor-risk patients.

Pancuronium (Pavulon®) has replaced tubocurarine as the drug of choice for major surgery. It has the advantages of a quicker onset of action and of not causing significant histamine release or significant changes in blood pressure; there is no evidence that it causes ganglionic blockade.

Gallamine (Flaxedil®) has a more rapid onset of action and recovery than tubocurarine or pancuronium. It causes undesirable tachycardia by its vagolytic action. It should be avoided in patients with severe renal disease.

Alcuronium (Alloferin®) appears to have no significant advantages over tubocurarine or pancuronium. Its duration of action is similar to tubocurarine and it may lower arterial pressure.

Fazadinium (Fazadon®) is the newest of the competitive muscle relaxants and although it is the most rapid in action and acts for about 40 minutes it does not provide the fast and complete relaxation characteristic of suxamethonium and therefore offers no advantage. It causes marked tachycardia and should be avoided in patients with severe renal disease.

DEPOLARISING MUSCLE RELAXANTS. **Suxamethonium** is the only commonly used drug of this group. With a 5-minute duration of action it is the ideal agent for passage of an endotracheal tube but may be used in repeated dosage for longer procedures. **Suxethonium** is occasionally used.

They act by mimicking the action of acetylcholine at the neuromuscular junction but cause blockade. Depolarisation is prolonged since their disengagement from the receptor site and subsequent breakdown is slower than for acetylcholine.

These drugs produce rapid, complete, and predictable paralysis, and recovery is spontaneous. Unlike the non-depolarising muscle relaxants (above) their action cannot be reversed and their clinical application is therefore limited.

Paralysis is usually preceded by muscle fasciculation. There is a sharp rise in plasma potassium and creatine phosphokinase and there may be muscle pains postoperatively. Suxamethonium is **contra-indicated** in severe liver disease and in burned patients. Premedication with atropine is desirable.

Prolonged muscle paralysis may occur in patients with low or atypical plasma pseudocholinesterase enzymes. Prolonged paralysis may also occur in **dual block**, which occurs after repeated doses of suxamethonium have been used and is caused by the development of a non-depolarising block following the primary depolarising block. Artificial ventilation should be continued until muscle function is restored. Dual block is diagnosed by giving a short-acting anticholinesterase such as edrophonium; if an improvement occurs the block is treated with neostigmine (section 15.1.6).

PANCURONIUM BROMIDE

Indications: non-depolarising muscle relaxant of medium duration

Cautions; Side-effects: see notes above; caution where tachycardia could be dangerous. Reduce dose in obesity and following suxamethonium. Drug interactions: see Appendix 1

Dose: *by intravenous injection*, initially for intubation 50–100 micrograms/kg then 10–20 micrograms/kg according to the patient's response; CHILD initially 60–100 micrograms/kg, then 10–20 micrograms/kg, neonate 30–40 micrograms/kg initially then 10–20 micrograms/kg

Intensive care, *by intravenous injection*, 60 micrograms/kg every 1–1½ hours; *by intramuscular injection*, 30–60 micrograms every 1–2 hours

Pavulon® (Organon-Teknika)
Injection, pancuronium bromide 2 mg/ml. Price 2-ml amp = **C**

SUXAMETHONIUM SALTS

Indications: depolarising muscle relaxant of short duration

Cautions; Side-effects: see notes above. Drug interactions: see Appendix 1

Dose: expressed as suxamethonium chloride

By intravenous injection, 20–100 mg, according to the patient's needs. CHILD, initially 1–1.5 mg/kg, then ⅓rd of the initial dose

By intravenous infusion, as a 0.1% solution in dextrose intravenous infusion (5%) or sodium chloride intravenous infusion (0.9%), 2–5 mg/minute (2–5 ml/minute)

Suxamethonium Chloride Injection, suxamethonium chloride 50 mg/ml. Price 2-ml amp = **B**; 10-ml vial = **E**

Anectine® (Calmic)
Injection, suxamethonium *chloride* 50 mg/ml. Price 2-ml amp = **B**

Brevidil M® (M&B)
Injection, suxamethonium *bromide* 67 mg (equivalent to about 50 mg of suxamethonium chloride), powder for reconstitution before use with water for injections or dextrose intravenous infusion (5%) or sodium chloride intravenous infusion (0.9%). Price 67-mg amp = **C**

Scoline® (DF)
Injection, suxamethonium *chloride* 50 mg/ml. Price 2-ml amp = **B**; 10-ml vial = **E**

ALCURONIUM CHLORIDE

Indications: non-depolarising muscle relaxant of medium duration

Cautions; Side-effects: see notes above. Drug interactions: see Appendix 1

Dose: *by intravenous injection*, initially 200–250 micrograms/kg, then ⅙th–¼th of the initial dose, according to the patient's response; CHILD, initially, 125–200 micrograms/kg, then ⅓rd of the initial dose

Alloferin® (Roche)
Injection, alcuronium chloride 5 mg/ml. Price 2-ml amp = **B**

FAZADINIUM

Indications: non-depolarising muscle relaxant of long duration

Cautions; Side-effects: see notes above. Drug interactions: see Appendix 1

Dose: *by intravenous injection*, 0.75–1 mg/kg, then increments of up to 15 mg, according to the patient's response

Fazadon® (DF)
Injection, fazadinium 15 mg (as bromide)/ml. Price 5-ml amp = **C**

GALLAMINE TRIETHIODIDE

Indications: non-depolarising muscle relaxant of medium duration

Cautions; Side-effects: see notes above. Drug interactions: see Appendix 1

Dose: *by intravenous injection*, 80–120 mg, then 20–40 mg according to the patient's response; CHILD, initially, 1.5 mg/kg, then ⅓rd of the initial dose

Flaxedil® (M&B)
Injection, gallamine triethiodide 40 mg/ml. Price 2- and 3-ml amp (both) = **B**

SUXETHONIUM

Indications; Cautions; Side-effects: see under Suxamethonium salts (above)

Dose: *by intravenous injection*, adults and children, suxethonium 1–1.25 mg/kg, repeated according to the patient's response

Brevidil-E® (M&B)
Injection, suxethonium 100 mg (as suxethonium bromide 150 mg), powder for reconstitution before use with water for injections. Price per amp = **C**

TUBOCURARINE CHLORIDE

Indications: non-depolarising muscle relaxant of medium to long duration

Cautions; Side-effects: see notes above. Drug interactions: see Appendix 1

Dose: *by intravenous injection*, initially 10–15 mg, then supplements, according to the patient's response, of 5 mg, to a max. of 40 mg; CHILD, initially 330 micrograms/kg, then ⅓rd of the initial dose

Tubocurarine Injection, tubocurarine chloride 10 mg/ml. Price 1.5-ml amp = **C**

Jexin® (DF)
Injection, tubocurarine chloride 10 mg/ml. Price 1.5-ml amp = **C**

Tubarine Miscible® (Calmic)
Injection, tubocurarine chloride 10 mg/ml. Price 1.5-ml amp = **D**

15.1.6 Anticholinesterases used in surgery

Anticholinesterase drugs reverse the effects of the non-depolarising (competitive) muscle relaxant drugs such as tubocurarine but they prolong the action of the depolarising muscle relaxant drug suxamethonium.

Edrophonium (Tensilon®) has a transient action and is used to diagnose dual block caused by suxamethonium (section 15.1.5).

Neostigmine has a longer duration of action than edrophonium. It is the specific drug for reversal of non-depolarising (competitive) blockade. It acts within one minute of intravenous injection and lasts for 20 to 30 minutes; a second dose may then be necessary. A suitable dose is 1 mg per 20 kg body-weight. It is also used in the treatment of dual block.

Before neostigmine is used **atropine** should be given to prevent excessive salivation, bradycardia, and other muscarinic actions of neostigmine. A suitable dose is 0.6 to 1.2 mg of atropine sulphate by intravenous injection.

For drugs used in myasthenia gravis see section 10.2.1.

EDROPHONIUM CHLORIDE

Indications: brief reversal of non-depolarising neuromuscular blockade; diagnosis of dual block (section 15.1.5)

Cautions; Side-effects: see section 10.2.1 and notes above. Atropine should also be given

Dose: reversal of blockade, *by intravenous injection*, 10 mg (after or with atropine sulphate 0.6–1.2 mg), repeated at intervals of 10 minutes according to the patient's response
Diagnosis of dual block, *by intravenous injection*, 10 mg (with atropine)

Tensilon® (Roche)
Injection, edrophonium chloride 10 mg/ml. Price 1-ml amp = **B**

NEOSTIGMINE METHYLSULPHATE

Indications: reversal of non-depolarising neuromuscular blockade

Cautions; Side-effects: see section 10.2.1 and notes above. Atropine should also be given

Dose: *by intravenous injection*, 1–5 mg *or* 1 mg/20 kg, after or with atropine sulphate 0.6–1.2 mg

Prostigmin® (Roche)
Injection, neostigmine methylsulphate 500 micrograms/ml. Price 1-ml amp = **A**
Injection, neostigmine methylsulphate 2.5 mg/ml. Price 1-ml amp = **A**

15.1.7 Antagonists for respiratory depression

The narcotic antagonists **levallorphan** (Lorfan®) and **naloxone** (Narcan®) are used at the end of an operation to reverse respiratory depression caused by narcotic analgesics. Unless the dosage is carefully adjusted, analgesia may also be reversed. For respiratory stimulants see section 3.5. **Doxapram** is a respiratory stimulant which does not reverse the other effects of narcotic analgesics.

DOXAPRAM HYDROCHLORIDE

Indications: postoperative respiratory depression

Contra-indications; Side-effects: see section 3.5

Dose: *by intravenous injection* 1–15 mg/kg repeated if necessary after 1 hour

Preparations
See section 3.5

LEVALLORPHAN TARTRATE

Indications: reversal of narcotic-induced respiratory depression

Side-effects: drowsiness, coma, sweating, restlessness, bradycardia, hypotension, and miosis indicate overdosage

Dose: *by intravenous injection*, 0.5–1 mg, repeated after 3—5 minutes if necessary

Lorfan® (Roche)
Injection, levallorphan tartrate 1 mg/ml. Price 1-ml amp = **A**

NALOXONE HYDROCHLORIDE

Indications: reversal of narcotic-induced respiratory depression

Cautions; Contra-indications: see under Emergency Treatment of Poisoning, section 13

Dose: *by intravenous injection*, 100–200 micrograms (1.5–3 micrograms/kg), adjusted according to the response, then 100 micrograms every 2 minutes; CHILD, 5–10 micrograms/kg
Neonate, *by intravenous, intramuscular, or subcutaneous injection*, 10 micrograms/kg, repeated every 2 minutes *or* 200 micrograms (60 micrograms/kg) *by intramuscular injection* as a single dose

Preparations
See under Emergency Treatment of Poisoning, section 13

15.1.8 Antagonists for malignant hyperthermia

Dantrolene (Dantrium®) is the only drug available for the reversal of malignant hyperthermia caused by inhalational anaesthetics and muscle relaxants.

DANTROLENE SODIUM

Indications: malignant hyperthermia
Cautions: avoid extravasation
Dose: by rapid intravenous injection, 1 mg/kg, repeated to a max. of 10 mg/kg

▼ **Dantrium Intravenous®** (Eaton)
Injection, powder for reconstitution, dantrolene sodium, with mannitol. Price 20-mg vial = **J** (Hosp. only)

15.2 Local anaesthesia

The use of local anaesthetics by injection or by application to mucous membranes to produce local analgesia is discussed in this section.

The following sections also include information on local anaesthetics acting on the sites shown:

1.7 Colon and rectum
11.7 Eye
12.3 Oropharynx
13.3 Skin

USE OF LOCAL ANAESTHETICS

Local anaesthetic drugs act by causing a reversible block to conduction along nerve fibres. The smaller the nerve fibre the more sensitive it is so that a differential block may occur where the smaller fibres carrying pain sensation and automatic impulses are blocked, sparing coarse touch and movement. The drugs used vary widely in their potency, toxicity, duration of action, stability, solubility in water, and ability to penetrate mucous membranes. These variations determine their suitability for surface infiltration, regional, epidural, and spinal anaesthesia.

ADMINISTRATION. In estimating the safe dosage of these drugs it is important to take account of the rate at which they are absorbed and excreted as well as their potency. The patient's age, weight, physique, and clinical condition, the degree of vascularity of the area to which the drug is to be applied, and the duration of administration are other factors which must be taken into account.

Local anaesthetics do not rely on the circulation to transport them to their sites of action, but uptake into the general circulation is important in terminating their action. Following most regional anaesthetic procedures, maximum arterial blood concentrations of anaesthetic develop within about 10 to 25 minutes, so careful surveillance for toxic effects is necessary during the first 30 minutes after injection.

TOXICITY. Toxic effects associated with the local anaesthetics are usually a result of excessively high blood concentrations. The main effects are excitation of the central nervous system (nervousness, nausea, and convulsions) followed by depression. Less commonly the cardiovascular system is depressed. Hypersensitivity reactions occur mainly with the ester-type local anaesthetics such as amethocaine, benzocaine, cocaine, and procaine.

USE OF VASOCONSTRICTORS. Toxicity may occur with repeated dosages due to accumulation of the drug, and reducing doses should therefore be given. Toxic effects may also occur if the injection is too rapid. Local anaesthetics should **not** be injected into inflamed or infected tissues nor should they be applied to the traumatised urethra. Under these conditions the drug may be so rapidly absorbed that a systemic rather than a local reaction is produced.

Most local anaesthetics, with the exception of mepivacaine, cause dilatation of blood vessels. The addition of a vasoconstrictor such as **adrenaline** diminishes local blood flow, slows the rate of absorption of the local anaesthetic, and prolongs its local effect. Care is necessary when using adrenaline for this purpose because, in excess, it may produce ischaemic necrosis.

Adrenaline should **not** be added to injections used in digits and appendages. When adrenaline is included in an injection of lignocaine or procaine the final concentration should be 1 in 200 000 (500 micrograms/100 ml). In dental surgery, up to 1 in 80 000 (1.25 mg/100 ml) of adrenaline is used with local anaesthetics. Higher concentrations are occasionally used but there is no justification for so doing.

The total dose of adrenaline should **not** exceed 500 micrograms and it is essential not to exceed a concentration of 1 in 200 000 if more than 50 ml of the mixture is to be injected.

Local anaesthetics containing adrenaline and noradrenaline should not be used in patients taking tricyclic antidepressants because of an increased risk of cardiac arrhythmias and hypertension. Prilocaine with felypressin may be used instead. This restriction does not apply to patients on monoamine-oxidase inhibitors.

LOCAL ANAESTHETIC DRUGS

Lignocaine is the most widely used local anaesthetic drug. It acts more rapidly and is more stable than most other local anaesthetics. It is effectively absorbed from mucous membranes and is a useful surface anaesthetic in concentrations of 2 to 4%. It is used in lower concentrations than procaine because it diffuses more quickly. Except for surface anaesthesia, solutions should not usually exceed 1% in strength. The duration of the block (with adrenaline) is about 1½ hours.

The great advantage of **bupivacaine** (Marcain®) over other local anaesthetics is its duration of action of up to 8 hours when used for nerve blocks. It has a slow onset of action, taking up to 30 minutes for full effect. It is often used in lumbar epidural blockade and is particularly suitable for continuous epidural analgesia in labour; it then has a 2- to 3-hour duration of action. The maximum dose is 150 mg in any 4-hour period.

Mepivacaine (Chlorocain®) is similar in action to lignocaine but it has a slightly longer duration of action. It is a useful local anaesthetic for spinal anaesthesia and is used for this purpose as a 4% hyperbaric solution which produces analgesia lasting for about 1½ hours. It is also used in dental anaesthesia. Mepivacaine is the only local anaesthetic that does not have vasodilator properties and therefore need not be given with adrenaline.

Prilocaine (Citanest®) is a local anaesthetic of low toxicity which is similar to lignocaine. It can be used for infiltration, regional nerve block, and spinal anaesthesia and regional intravenous analgesia. The maximum adult dose is 400 mg, or 600 mg if adrenaline or felypressin is added. If used in high doses, methaemoglobinaemia may occur which can be treated with intravenous methylene blue 1% injection using a dose of 75–100 mg.

Amethocaine is an effective local anaesthetic for topical application. Because of its toxicity, use of amethocaine by injection has been largely replaced by the safer bupivacaine. It is rapidly absorbed from mucous membranes and should **never** be applied to inflamed, traumatised, or highly vascular surfaces. It should **never** be used to provide anaesthesia for bronchoscopy or cystoscopy, as lignocaine is a safer alternative. Hypersensitivity to amethocaine has been reported.

Benzocaine is a local anaesthetic of low potency and toxicity. Its only use is in surface anaesthesia for the relief of pain and irritation in the oropharynx (see section 12.3.1) and around the anus (see section 1.7.1).

Cinchocaine is a potentially toxic drug and is generally only used for surface anaesthesia.

Cocaine readily penetrates mucous membranes and is an effective surface anaesthetic but it has now been replaced by less toxic alternatives. It potentiates the action of adrenaline and possesses vasoconstrictor and mydriatic properties and should therefore **not** be used with adrenaline. It should **never** be given by injection because of its toxicity and only up to 100 mg should be applied to mucous membranes. It stimulates the central nervous system and is a drug of addiction. In hypersensitive patients it may cause collapse due to cardiac depression and it is therefore prudent to test patients initially before application of cocaine.

Concentrations of 5 to 20% (50–200 mg/ml) are applied to the nose, throat, and larynx.

For the use of cocaine in ophthalmology see section 11.7.

Procaine is now seldom used. It is as potent an anaesthetic as lignocaine but has a shorter duration of action. It provides less intense analgesia because it has less tendency to spread through the tissues. It is poorly absorbed from mucous membranes and is of no value as a surface anaesthetic. When used for infiltration or regional anaesthesia, adrenaline 1 in 200 000 (500 micrograms/100 ml) is generally added. Its metabolite para-aminobenzoic acid inhibits the action of the sulphonamides.

LIGNOCAINE HYDROCHLORIDE

Indications: local anaesthesia by surface, infiltration, regional, epidural, and caudal routes; dental anaesthesia

Cautions: epilepsy, hepatic impairment, impaired cardiac conduction, bradycardia. Reduce dose in elderly or debilitated patients. Resuscitative equipment should be available. See section 2.3.3 for effects on heart

Contra-indications: myasthenia gravis, hypovolaemia, complete heart block. Do not use solutions containing adrenaline for anaesthesia in appendages

Side-effects: hypotension, bradycardia, cardiac arrest. CNS effects include agitation, euphoria, respiratory depression, convulsions. See also notes above

Dose: adjusted according to the site of operation and response of the patient

By injection, max. dose 200 mg, or 500 mg with solutions which also contain adrenaline. Max. dose of adrenaline 500 micrograms

Infiltration anaesthesia, 0.25–0.5%, with adrenaline 1 in 200 000, using 2–50 ml of a 0.5% solution in minor surgery and up to 60 ml in more extensive surgery

Nerve blocks, with adrenaline 1 in 200 000, 1% to a max. of 50 ml, 2% to a max. of 25 ml

Epidural and caudal block, with adrenaline 1 in 200 000, 1% to a max. of 50 ml, 2% to a max. of 25 ml

Surface anaesthesia, usual strengths 2–4%. Mouth, throat, and upper gastro-intestinal tract, 1–4%, to a max. of 200 mg

Lignocaine Hydrochloride Injections (Plain)

Lidothesin® (Pharm. Mfg Co.)

Injection 0.5%, lignocaine hydrochloride 5 mg/ml. Price 2-, 5-, and 10-ml amp (all) = **A**; 20-ml vial = **B**; 20-ml amp and 50-ml vial (both) = **C**

Injection 1%, lignocaine hydrochloride 10 mg/ml. Price 2-, 5-, and 10-ml amp (all) = **A**; 20-ml vial = **B**; 20-ml amp and 50-ml vial (both) = **C**

Injection 1.5%, for epidural use, lignocaine hydrochloride 15 mg/ml. Price 20-ml amp = **C**

Injection 2%, lignocaine hydrochloride 20 mg/ml. Price 2-, 5-, and 10-ml amp (all) = **A**; 20-ml vial = **B**; 20-ml amp and 50-ml vial (both) = **C**

Injection 5%, lignocaine hydrochloride 50 mg/ml. Price 10-ml amp = **A**

Xylocaine® (Astra)

Injection 0.5%, anhydrous lignocaine hydrochloride 5 mg/ml. Price 10-ml amp = **B**; 20- and 50-ml vial (both) = **C**

Injection 1%, anhydrous lignocaine hydrochloride 10 mg/ml. Price 2-ml amp = **A**; 10-ml amp = **B**; 20- and 50-ml vial (both) = **C**
Injection 1.5%, for epidural use, anhydrous lignocaine hydrochloride 15 mg/ml. Price 25-ml amp = **D**
Injection 2%, anhydrous lignocaine hydrochloride 20 mg/ml. Price 5-ml amp = **B**; 20- and 50-ml vial (both) = **C**

Lignocaine and Adrenaline Injections
Lidothesin® (Pharm. Mfg Co.)
Injection 0.5% with adrenaline 1 in 200 000, lignocaine hydrochloride 5 mg/ml, adrenaline 1 in 200 000 (500 micrograms/100 ml). Price 20-ml vial = **B**; 50-ml vial = **C**
Injection 1% with adrenaline 1 in 100 000, lignocaine hydrochloride 10 mg/ml, adrenaline 1 in 100 000 (1 mg/100 ml). Price 5- and 10-ml amp = **A**; 20-ml vial = **B**; 50-ml vial = **C**
Injection 2% with adrenaline 1 in 100 000, lignocaine hydrochloride 20 mg/ml, adrenaline 1 in 100 000 (1 mg/100 ml). Price 2-, 5-, and 10-ml amp = **A**; 20-ml vial = **B**; 50-ml vial = **C**
Xylocaine® (Astra)
Injection 0.5% with adrenaline 1 in 200 000, anhydrous lignocaine hydrochloride 5 mg/ml, adrenaline 1 in 200 000 (500 micrograms/100 ml). Price 50-ml vial = **C**
Injection 1% with adrenaline 1 in 200 000, anhydrous lignocaine hydrochloride 10 mg/ml, adrenaline 1 in 200 000 (500 micrograms/100 ml). Price 10-ml amp = **B**; 20- and 50-ml vial (both) = **C**
Injection 2% with adrenaline 1 in 200 000, anhydrous lignocaine hydrochloride 20 mg/ml adrenaline 1 in 200 000 (500 micrograms/100 ml). Price 20- and 50-ml vial (both) = **C**

Lignocaine Injections for Dental Use
A large variety of lignocaine injections, plain or with adrenaline or noradrenaline, is also available in dental cartridges under the names **Lidothesin, Lignostab, Neo-Lidocaton, Xylocaine,** and **Xylotox.**

Lignocaine for Surface Anaesthesia
Lignocaine Gel, lignocaine hydrochloride 1% or 2% with chlorhexidine gluconate solution 0.25% or hydroxybenzoates in a sterile lubricant water-miscible basis. Price 15 ml(both) = **B**
Instillagel® (Rimmer)
Gel, lignocaine hydrochloride 2%, chlorhexidine gluconate solution 0.25% in a lubricant basis in disposable syringe. Price 6- and 11-ml syringe (both) = **B**
Dose: 6–11 ml into urethra
Lidothesin® (Pharm. Mfg Co.)
Antiseptic gel, lignocaine hydrochloride 1% or 2% chlorhexidine gluconate solution 0.25% in a sterile lubricant water-miscible basis. Price 15 ml (both) = **B**
Topical 4% (=sterile solution for topical use), lignocaine hydrochloride 40 mg/ml. Price 25-ml bottle = **C**
Xylocaine® (Astra)
Gel, anhydrous lignocaine hydrochloride 2% in sterile lubricant water-miscible basis. Price 20 g = **C**
Antiseptic gel, lignocaine hydrochloride 2%, chlorhexidine gluconate solution 0.25% in a sterile lubricant water-miscible basis. Price 15 ml = **B**
Ointment, lignocaine 5% in a water-miscible basis. Price 15 g = **C**
Spray (=aerosol spray), lignocaine 10% (100 mg/g) with cetylpyridinium chloride 0.01% in a metered spray container supplying 10 mg lignocaine/dose; 800 spray doses per container. With sterilisable spray nozzles. Price 80-g bottle = **F**
Topical 4% (=solution for topical use), anhydrous lignocaine hydrochloride 40 mg/ml. Price 25-ml bottle = **C**
Dose: up to 5 ml
Xylocaine Viscous® (Astra)
Oral solution 2%, anhydrous lignocaine hydrochloride 20 mg/ml, for surface anaesthesia of the upper digestive tract. Price 150 ml = **D**
Dose: 5–15 ml to a max. of 30 ml in 24 hours with a minimum of 4 hours between successive doses
Xylodase® (Astra)
Cream, lignocaine 50 mg, hyaluronidase 150 micrograms (50 units)/g. For application to mucous membranes of mouth. Price 15 g = **C**
Xylotox® (Pharm. Mfg Co.)
Jelly (=gel), lignocaine hydrochloride 2% in a lubricant water-miscible basis. Price 15 g = **B**; 30 g = **C**
Ointment (=cream), lignocaine 5% in a water-miscible basis. Price 15 and 30 g (both) = **C**
Oral solution 2%, red, lignocaine hydrochloride 20 mg/ml in a viscous basis, for surface anaesthesia of upper digestive tract. Price 200 ml = **D**
Dose: 5–15 ml to a max. of 45 ml in 24 hours, with a minimum of 4 hours between successive doses
Topical solution 4%, lignocaine hydrochloride 40 mg/ml, adrenaline 1 in 50 000 (20 micrograms/ml). Price 25-ml bottle = **C**
Dose: up to 5 ml applied to the gums, larynx, and pharynx
Spray (=aerosol spray), lignocaine 10% (100 mg/g) with cetrimide 0.05% in a metered spray container supplying 10 mg lignocaine/dose. With sterilisable spray nozzles. Price 85-g bottle = **F**
Dose: up to 20 doses/24 hours

BUPIVACAINE HYDROCHLORIDE
Indications: prolonged local anaesthesia by regional nerve block; epidural block
Cautions; Contra-indications; Side-effects: see under Lignocaine Hydrochloride and notes above
Dose: adjusted according to the site of operation and response of the patient

By injection, up to 2 mg/kg in any 4-hour period as a 0.25 or 0.5% solution, with or without adrenaline

Marcain Plain® (DF)

Injection 0.25%, bupivacaine hydrochloride 2.5 mg/ml. Price 10-ml amp = **C**

Injection 0.5%, bupivacaine hydrochloride 5 mg/ml. Price 10-ml amp = **C**

Marcain with Adrenaline® (DF)

Injection 0.25%, bupivacaine hydrochloride 2.5 mg/ml, adrenaline 1 in 400 000 (250 micrograms/100 ml). Price 10-ml amp = **C**

Injection 0.5%, bupivacaine hydrochloride 5 mg/ml, adrenaline 1 in 200 000 (500 micrograms/100 ml). Price 10-ml amp = **C**

MEPIVACAINE HYDROCHLORIDE

Indications: local anaesthesia by spinal route; dental anaesthesia

Cautions; Side-effects: see under Lignocaine Hydrochloride and notes above

Dose: spinal anaesthesia, 20–80 mg, adjusted according to the site of operation and the response of the patient

Chlorocain® (Pharm. Mfg Co.)

Hyperbaric injection 4%, mepivacaine hydrochloride 40 mg/ml, dextrose 9.5% for spinal anaesthesia. Price 2-ml amp = **B**

PRILOCAINE HYDROCHLORIDE

Indications: local anaesthesia by infiltration, regional, spinal and surface routes; dental anaesthesia

Cautions; Contra-indications; Side-effects: see under Lignocaine Hydrochloride and notes above

Dose: adjusted according to the site of operation and response of patient, to a max. of 400 mg used alone, or 600 mg if used with adrenaline or felypressin

Citanest® (Astra)

Injection 0.5%, prilocaine hydrochloride 5 mg/ml. Price 20- and 50-ml vial (both) = **C**

Injection 1%, prilocaine hydrochloride 10 mg/ml. Price 20- and 50-ml vial (both) = **C**

Citanest with Octapressin® (Astra)

Injection 3%, prilocaine hydrochloride 30 mg/ml, felypressin 0.03 unit/ml. Price 2-ml cartridge and self-aspirating cartridge (both) = **A**

PROCAINE HYDROCHLORIDE

Indications: local anaesthesia by infiltration and regional routes

Cautions; Side-effects: see notes above

Dose: adjusted according to the site of operation and the patient's response

By injection, up to 1 g (200 ml of 0.5% solution or 100 ml of 1%) with adrenaline 1 in 200 000 (to a max. of 500 micrograms)

Procaine Injection, procaine hydrochloride 1 or 2% (10 or 20 mg/ml) in sodium chloride intravenous infusion. Price 2-ml amp (both) = **B**

Appendix 1: Drug Interactions

When two or more drugs are given at the same time they may exert their effects independently or they may interact. The result of the interaction may be potentiation or antagonism of one drug by another, or occasionally some other effect. Adverse drug interactions should be reported to the Committee on Safety of Medicines in the same way as other adverse drug reactions.

Drug interactions may be **pharmacodynamic** or **pharmacokinetic.**

Pharmacodynamic interactions

These are interactions between drugs which have similar or antagonistic pharmacological effects or side-effects. They may be due to competition at receptor sites, or occur between drugs acting on the same physiological system. They are usually predictable from a knowledge of the pharmacology of the interacting drugs and, in general, interactions demonstrated with one drug are likely to occur with related drugs. They occur to a greater or lesser extent in most patients who receive the interacting drugs.

Pharmacokinetic interactions

These occur when one drug alters the absorption, distribution, metabolism, or excretion of another, thus increasing or reducing the amount of drug available to produce its pharmacological effects. They are not easily predicted and many of them affect only a small proportion of patients taking the combination of drugs. Pharmacokinetic interactions occurring with one drug cannot be assumed to occur with related drugs unless their pharmacokinetic properties are known to be similar.

Pharmacokinetic interactions are of several types:

1. Interactions affecting drug absorption

Either the rate of drug absorption or the amount of drug absorbed can be altered by drug interactions. Delayed absorption is rarely of clinical importance unless high peak blood concentrations are required, as, for example, may be the case when giving an analgesic. A reduction in the total amount of drug absorbed is more likely to result in ineffective therapy.

2. Interactions due to changes in protein binding of drugs

Most drugs are loosely bound, to a variable extent, to plasma proteins. Protein-binding sites are non-specific and one drug can displace another thereby increasing the proportion of drug free to diffuse out of the plasma to its site of action. This will produce a detectable increase in effect only if the drug is extensively bound (more than 90%) and is not widely distributed throughout the body. Even for such drugs displacement rarely produces more than a transient potentiation because the increased concentration of free drug results in an increased rate of elimination tending to restore the free concentration to its original level.

Displacement from protein binding plays a part in the potentiation of warfarin by phenylbutazone, sulphonamides, and tolbutamide but the importance of these interactions is due mainly to the fact that warfarin metabolism is also inhibited.

3. Interactions affecting drug metabolism

Many drugs are inactivated by metabolism in the liver. One drug can increase the rate of metabolism of another by enzyme induction of the hepatic microsomal enzyme system. This results in lower blood concentrations and a reduced effect of the drug. On withdrawal of the inducer blood levels increase and toxicity may occur. The most important enzyme inducers in man are the barbiturates, dichloralphenazone, some antiepileptics, and rifampicin. Drugs affected include warfarin and the oral contraceptives.

The opposite effect is seen when one drug inhibits the metabolism of another producing higher blood concentrations, an increased effect and a risk of toxicity. Some drugs which potentiate the effect of warfarin and of phenytoin do so by this mechanism.

4. Interactions affecting the renal excretion of drugs

Drugs are eliminated through the kidney both by glomerular filtration and by active tubular secretion. Competition occurs between drugs which share active transport mechanisms in the proximal tubule. Thus probenecid delays the excretion of many drugs including penicillins, some cephalosporins, indomethacin, and dapsone; aspirin may increase the toxicity of methotrexate by a similar mechanism.

Relative importance of interactions

Many drug interactions are harmless; many of those which are potentially harmful occur in only a small proportion of patients given the interacting drugs; and the result of an interaction may be more serious in one patient than another. The drugs most often involved in serious interactions are those with a small therapeutic ratio, such as phenytoin, and those where the dose must be carefully controlled according to the response, as with anticoagulants, antihypertensives, and antidiabetics. Patients at increased risk from drug interactions include the elderly and those with impaired renal or liver function.

The table lists potentially harmful interactions which are likely to have clinical importance at least in some patients. The drug whose action is affected is listed in column 1, column 2 contains the interacting drugs and column 3 gives the result of the interaction.

Table: Drug Interactions

Drug affected	Drug interacting	Effect
1: Gastro-intestinal system		
Metoclopramide	Anticholinergic drugs such as atropine, benzhexol, propantheline	Antagonism
2: Cardiovascular system		
Anti-arrhythmic drugs	Any combinations of 2 or more	Increased myocardial depression
Disopyramide, Quinidine	Diuretics—bumetanide, ethacrynic acid, frusemide, thiazides	Toxicity increased by hypokalaemia
Lignocaine, Mexiletine, Tocainide	Diuretics—bumetanide, ethacrynic acid, frusemide, thiazides	Antagonised by hypokalaemia
Mexiletine	Atropine, narcotic analgesics	Delayed absorption
	Acetazolamide, antacids	Reduced excretion and higher blood concentrations
Verapamil	Beta-adrenoceptor blocking drugs	Asystole
Antihypertensive drugs	Anti-inflammatory analgesics such as indomethacin, phenylbutazone; carbenoxolone, corticosteroids, corticotrophin; oestrogens, oral contraceptives	Reduced effect
	Alcohol, antidepressants, hypnotics, sedatives, tranquillisers; fenfluramine; levodopa; vasodilators, nitrates	Potentiation
Bethanidine, Debrisoquine, Guanethidine	Sympathomimetic amines (including some common cold remedies); mazindol, pizotifen; tricyclic antidepressants	Antagonism
Clonidine	Beta-adrenoceptor blocking drugs	Increased risk of clonidine withdrawal hypertension
	Prazosin, tricyclic antidepressants	Antagonism
Beta-adrenoceptor blocking drugs	Ergotamine	Peripheral vasoconstriction
	Nifedipine	Heart failure, worsening angina, precipitation of myocardial infarction
	Prenylamine	Increased myocardial depression
	Sympathomimetic amines such as adrenaline, amphetamines, phenylephrine	Severe hypertension reported
Propranolol	Cimetidine	Potentiation because of decreased hepatic metabolism

Drug affected	Drug interacting	Effect
Digoxin and other cardiac glycosides	Carbenoxolone; diuretics—bumetanide, ethacrynic acid, frusemide, thiazides	Increased toxicity
	Cholestyramine	Reduced absorption
	Phenobarbitone, rifampicin	Inhibition (digitoxin only)
	Quinidine	Potentiation. Halve maintenance dose of digoxin
Digoxin	Amiodarone	Potentiation. Halve maintenance dose of digoxin
Diuretics	Anti-inflammatory analgesics such as indomethacin; carbenoxolone, corticosteroids, corticotrophin; oestrogens	Antagonism
Bumetanide, Frusemide, Thiazides	Acetazolamide, carbenoxolone, corticosteroids, corticotrophin	Hypokalaemia
	Trilostane	Decreased potassium loss
Amiloride, Potassium canrenoate, Spironolactone, Triamterene	Captopril, potassium supplements	Hyperkalaemia
Heparin	Aspirin, dipyridamole	Potentiation
Oral anticoagulants		
Coumarins such as warfarin	Barbiturates, carbamazepine, dichloralphenazone, glutethimide, griseofulvin, oral contraceptives, primidone, rifampicin, vitamin K	Inhibition
	Alcohol, amiodarone, anabolic steroids, aspirin, azapropazone, bezafibrate, chloral hydrate, chloramphenicol, cimetidine, clofibrate, co-trimoxazole, danazol, dextrothyroxine, dipyridamole, mefenamic acid, metronidazole, neomycin, oxyphenbutazone, phenylbutazone, sulphonamides, thyroxine	Potentiation
	Allopurinol; diflunisal, feprazone, piroxicam, sulindac and possibly other anti-inflammatory analgesics; cholestyramine, dextropropoxyphene, indomethacin, nalidixic acid, phenytoin, sulphinpyrazone, tetracyclines	Potentiation may occur
Phenindione	Oral contraceptives, vitamin K	Inhibition
	Anabolic steroids, aspirin, bezafibrate, cholestyramine, clofibrate, dipyridamole, neomycin, thyroxine	Potentiation
Vasoconstrictors	Tricyclic antidepressants	Potentiation
Adrenaline, Noradrenaline	Beta-adrenoceptor blocking drugs	Potentiation of hypertensive effect

Drug affected	Drug interacting	Effect
4: Central nervous system		
Analgesics		
Aspirin	Metoclopramide	Potentiation
Diflunisal	Antacids	Reduced absorption
Naproxen	Probenecid	Increased blood concentrations
Paracetamol	Cholestyramine	Reduced absorption
	Metoclopramide	Potentiation
Antiepileptics	Antidepressants, phenothiazine derivatives	Antagonism
Carbamazepine	Dextropropoxyphene	Potentiation
Phenobarbitone, Primidone	Phenytoin, sodium valproate	Increased sedation
Phenytoin	Chloramphenicol, cimetidine, co-trimoxazole, diazepam, dicoumarol, disulfiram, isoniazid, pheneturide, phenylbutazone, sulphaphenazole, sulphinpyrazone, sulthiame, viloxazine	Potentiation
	Aspirin, sodium valproate	Transient potentiation
Sodium valproate	Carbamazepine, phenobarbitone, phenytoin, primidone	Reduced blood concentrations of valproate
Drugs for parkinsonism	Haloperidol, phenothiazine derivatives; methyldopa, metoclopramide, reserpine	These have extra-pyramidal side-effects
Anticholinergic drugs such as benzhexol etc.	Amantadine, antidepressants, antihistamines, disopyramide, phenothiazine derivatives	Increased side-effects, dry mouth, urine retention, confusional states, etc.
Levodopa	Chlordiazepoxide, diazepam	Antagonism—occasionally
	Metoclopramide	Increased blood concentrations of levodopa
	Pyridoxine	Antagonism (does not occur if dopa decarboxylase inhibitor also given)
Hypnotics and sedatives	Alcohol, antidepressants, antihistamines, narcotic analgesics	Potentiation
Diazepam	Cimetidine	Potentiation because of decreased hepatic metabolism
Monoamine-oxidase inhibitors	Sympathomimetic amines such as amphetamine, common cold remedies, ephedrine; fencamfamin, fenfluramine, levodopa, oxypertine	Hypertensive crisis. N.B. can occur up to 2 weeks after stopping MAOI
	Narcotic analgesics, reserpine, tricyclic antidepressants	CNS excitation, hypertension
	Tryptophan	CNS excitation. Reduce dose of tryptophan

Drug affected	Drug interacting	Effect
Tricyclic antidepressants	Alcohol	Potentiation of sedative effect
	Oral contraceptives	Reduced effect
Miscellaneous		
Betahistine	Antihistamines	Antagonism
Chlorpromazine	Antacids	Reduced absorption
Haloperidol, Phenothiazine derivatives	Metoclopramide	Increased risk of extrapyramidal effects
Lithium carbonate	Diuretics, sodium depletion; diclofenac, indomethacin, phenylbutazone	Potentiation
	Acetazolamide, aminophylline, sodium bicarbonate	Increased lithium excretion
	Haloperidol	Increased risk of extrapyramidal effects
5: Infections		
Aminoglycosides Gentamicin etc.	Ethacrynic acid, frusemide	Increased ototoxicity
Cephaloridine, Cephalothin	Ethacrynic acid, frusemide; gentamicin	Increased nephrotoxicity
Chloramphenicol	Phenobarbitone	Reduced blood concentrations
Dapsone	Probenecid	Reduced excretion—increased side-effects
Furazolidone, Metronidazole	Alcohol	'Antabuse' reaction
Griseofulvin	Phenobarbitone	Antagonism
Ketoconazole	Antacids, anticholinergic drugs, cimetidine	Decreased absorption
Lincomycin	Kaolin mixtures	Reduced absorption
Nitrofurantoin	Probenecid	Reduced excretion—increased side-effects
Phenoxymethylpenicillin	Neomycin	Reduced absorption
Vancomycin	Cholestyramine	Antagonism
Tetracyclines	Antacids, dairy products, oral iron, zinc sulphate	Reduced absorption
Doxycycline	Barbiturates, carbamazepine, phenytoin	Reduced blood concentrations
Tetracycline	Cimetidine	Decreased absorption
6: Endocrine system		
Antidiabetic drugs (oral and insulin)	Alcohol; beta-adrenoceptor blocking drugs; monoamine-oxidase inhibitors	Potentiation
	Corticosteroids, corticotrophin; diazoxide; diuretics—bumetanide, frusemide, thiazides; oral contraceptives	Antagonism

Drug affected	Drug interacting	Effect
Metformin, Phenformin	Alcohol	Increased risk of lactic acidosis
Sulphonylureas—Chlorpropamide, Tolbutamide	Bezafibrate, chloramphenicol, clofibrate, co-trimoxazole, dicoumarol, oxyphenbutazone, phenylbutazone, sulphaphenazole	Potentiation
Chlorpropamide	Alcohol	Flushing in susceptible patients
Chlorpropamide, Tolbutamide	Rifampicin	Reduced effect
Corticosteroids, corticotrophin	Carbenoxolone; diuretics—ethacrynic acid, frusemide, thiazides	Increased potassium loss
Cortisone, Dexamethasone, Hydrocortisone, Prednisolone, Prednisone	Barbiturates, phenytoin, primidone, rifampicin	Reduced effect
Thyroxine	Cholestyramine	Reduced absorption
	Fenclofenac, phenylbutazone, phenytoin	False low total serum-thyroxine concentration
7: Obstetrics and gynaecology		
Oral contraceptives	Aldosterone antagonists, barbiturates, carbamazepine, dichloralphenazone, griseofulvin, phenytoin, primidone, rifampicin	Reduced effect
	Oral antibiotics such as ampicillin, tetracycline	Reduced effect—risk probably small
8: Malignant disease and immunosuppression		
Azathioprine, Mercaptopurine	Allopurinol	Potentiation—increased toxicity
Methotrexate	Aspirin, phenylbutazone, probenecid	Delayed excretion—increased toxicity
	Antiepileptics; co-trimoxazole, pyrimethamine	Increased anti-folate effect
Procarbazine	Alcohol	'Antabuse' reaction
9: Nutrition and blood		
Oral iron	Magnesium trisilicate; tetracyclines	Reduced absorption
10: Musculoskeletal and joint diseases		
Indomethacin	Probenecid	Increased blood concentrations
Penicillamine	Oral iron, zinc sulphate	Reduced absorption
Phenylbutazone	Cholestyramine	Reduced absorption
Probenecid, Sulphinpyrazone	Aspirin	Inhibition

Drug affected	Drug interacting	Effect
15: Anaesthesia		
Anaesthetics	Antihypertensive drugs; beta-adrenoceptor blocking drugs; chlorpromazine	Potentiation of hypotensive effect
	Adrenaline, isoprenaline, levodopa	Arrhythmias with halothane, cyclopropane, trichloroethylene
Thiopentone	Sulphonamides	Potentiation
Muscle relaxants	Colistin, polymyxin B; lithium, propranolol, quinidine	Potentiation
Competitive neuromuscular blocking drugs such as tubocurarine	Aminoglycosides, clindamycin, lincomycin; magnesium salts	Potentiation
Depolarising neuromuscular blocking drugs such as suxamethonium	Cyclophosphamide, ecothiopate eye-drops, neostigmine, propanidid, thiotepa	Potentiation
	Digoxin	Arrhythmias

Appendix 2: Intravenous Additives

Addition of medication to infusion fluids

Drugs may be added to a container of infusion fluid and given by slow intravenous infusion (see Table 1). This method is of value when it is desirable to maintain constant blood concentrations or when the injection of a more concentrated solution is dangerous, but owing to the possibility of instability, incompatibility, and bacterial growth the method should be considered only when it is clearly beneficial. The advantages and limitations of direct addition to infusion containers are given below.

In some cases drugs may be given intermittently through the giving set or directly into the drip tubing (see Tables 2 and 3).

INTRAVENOUS ADDITIVE POLICIES. Health Circular HC(76)9 recommends that a local policy on the addition of drugs to intravenous fluids should be drawn up by a multi-disciplinary team in each Health District and issued as a document to the members of staff concerned.

Centralised additive services are provided in a number of hospital pharmacy departments and should be used when available in preference to making additions in hospital wards.

The information in the following section should be read in conjunction with any appropriate local policy documents.

Direct addition of medication to infusion containers

Basic guidelines

1. Drugs should only be added to infusion containers when constant blood concentrations are needed or when the administration of a more concentrated solution would be harmful.
2. In general only one drug should be added to any infusion container and the components should be of known compatibility (see Table 1). Ready-prepared solutions should be used whenever possible. Drugs should not normally be added to blood products, mannitol, or sodium bicarbonate. Only specially prepared additives should be used with fat emulsions or amino-acid solutions.
3. Solutions should be thoroughly mixed by shaking and checked for absence of particulate matter before use.
4. Strict asepsis should be maintained using appropriate techniques throughout and in general the same giving set should not be used for more than 24 hours.
5. The infusion container should be labelled with the date and time the addition was made, the name and quantity of additive, and the name of the patient. When possible, containers should be retained for a period after use in case they are needed for investigation.
6. It is good practice to examine intravenous infusions from time to time while they are running. If cloudiness, crystallisation, change of colour, or any other sign of interaction or contamination is observed the infusion should be discontinued.

Problems involving additives

Several problems may arise when adding drugs to intravenous infusions.

MICROBIAL CONTAMINATION. The accidental entry and subsequent growth of micro-organisms converts the infusion fluid pathway into a potential vehicle for infection with micro-organisms, particularly species of *Candida, Enterobacter*, and *Klebsiella*. Ready-prepared infusions containing the additional drugs, or infusions prepared by an additive service (when available) should therefore be used in preference to making extemporaneous additions to infusion containers on wards etc. However, when this is necessary strict aseptic procedure should be followed.

INCOMPATIBILITY. Physical and chemical incompatibilities may occur with loss of potency, increase in toxicity, or other adverse effect. The solutions may become opalescent or precipitation may occur, but in many instances there is no visual indication of incompatibility. Interaction may take place at any point in the infusion fluid pathway, and the potential for incompatibility is also increased when more than one substance is added to the infusion fluid. Information on compatibility is given in the accompanying tables. The suitability of additions may also be checked by reference to manufacturer's literature and additional information is usually available in hospital pharmacies.

Common incompatibilities. Precipitation reactions are numerous and varied and may occur as a result of pH, concentration changes, 'salting-out' effects, complexation or other chemical changes. Precipitation or other particle formation must be avoided since, apart from lack of control of dosage on administration, it may initiate or exacerbate adverse effects. This is particularly important in the case of drugs which have been implicated in either thrombophlebitis (e.g. diazepam) or in skin sloughing or necrosis caused by extravasation (e.g. sodium bicarbonate, thiopentone sodium and certain cytotoxic drugs such as doxorubicin, methotrexate and fluorouracil). It is also especially important to effect solution of colloidal drugs and to prevent their subsequent precipitation in order to avoid a pyrogenic reaction (e.g. amphotericin).

It is considered undesirable to mix beta-lactam antibiotics such as semi-synthetic penicillins and cephalosporins with proteinaceous materials on the grounds that immunogenic and allergenic conjugates could be formed.

A number of preparations undergo significant loss of potency when added singly or in combination to large volume infusions. Examples include ampicillin in infusions that contain carbohydrates or lactates, mustine hydrochloride in isotonic saline and gentamicin/carbenicillin combinations. The breakdown products of dacarbazine have been implicated in adverse effects.

Blood. Because of the large number of incompatibilities, drugs should not normally be added to blood and blood products for infusion purposes. Examples of incompatibility with blood include hypertonic mannitol solutions (irreversible crenation of red cells), dextrans (rouleaux formation and interference with cross-matching), dextrose (clumping of red cells), metaraminol tartrate (haemolysis), and oxytocin (inactivation of the additive).

If the giving set is not changed after the administration of blood, but used for other infusion fluids, a precipitate of fibrin may be formed which, apart from physically blocking the set, increases the likelihood of microbial growth.

Blood should always be taken for grouping and cross-matching before infusing dextrans.

Intravenous fat emulsions may break down with coalescence of fat globules and separation of phases when additions such as antibiotics or electrolytes are made, thus increasing the possibility of embolism. Only specially formulated items such as Vitlipid® may be added to appropriate intravenous fat emulsions.

Other infusions that frequently give rise to incompatibility include amino acids, mannitol, and sodium bicarbonate.

Bactericides such as chlorocresol 0.1% or phenylmercuric nitrate 0.001% are present in some injection solutions. The total volume of such solutions added to a container for infusion on one occasion should not exceed 15 ml.

Method of making additions to infusion solutions

Ready-prepared infusions should be used when they are available. **Potassium chloride** is usually available in concentrations of 20, 27 and 40 mmol/litre in sodium chloride intravenous infusion (0.9%), dextrose intravenous infusion (5%) or sodium chloride and dextrose intravenous infusion. **Lignocaine hydrochloride** is usually available in concentrations of 0.1 or 0.2% in dextrose intravenous infusion (5%).

When addition is required to be made extemporaneously, any product reconstitution instructions such as those relating to concentration, vehicle, mixing, and handling precautions should be strictly followed using an aseptic technique throughout. Once the product has been reconstituted, addition to the infusion fluid should be made immediately in order to minimise accidental microbial contamination and, with certain products, to prevent degradation or other formulation change which may occur; for example reconstituted ampicillin injection on standing degrades rapidly and also may form polymers which could cause sensitivity reactions.

It is also important in certain instances that an infusion fluid of certain pH be used. **Amphotericin** injection (Fungizone®) requires dilution in dextrose injection of pH greater than 4.2 and **frusemide** injection (Lasix®) should be added to certain infusions the pH of which should be greater than 5.5.

When drug additions are made into the infusion container it is important to effect thorough mixing; additions should not be made to an infusion container that has been hung and connected to an administration set as mixing is hampered. If the solutions are not thoroughly mixed a concentrated layer of drug product may form owing to differences in density of the product and infusion. **Potassium chloride** is particularly prone to this 'layering' effect when added without adequate mixing to infusions packed in non-rigid infusion containers, and if such a mixture is administered an insidious effect on the heart may result.

A time limit between addition of the additive to the infusion and completion of administration must be imposed for certain admixtures to guarantee satisfactory drug potency and compatibility. For admixtures in which degradation occurs without the formation of toxic substances, an acceptable limit is the time taken for 10% decomposition of the drug ($t_{10\%}$). When toxic substances are produced stricter limits may be imposed.

Certain injections must be protected from light during continuous infusion to minimise oxidation, for example amphotericin, dacarbazine, and sodium nitroprusside.

CONTINUOUS INFUSION. Table 1 lists a number of intravenous drug preparations which must be diluted in a large volume infusion and which are administered by continuous infusion. Pencillins may be given by continuous infusion but intermittent infusion is usually preferred. Dilution with a small volume of an appropriate vehicle and administration using a motorised infusion pump is advocated for preparations such as heparin where strict control over administration is required. In this case the appropriate dose may be dissolved in 10 to 20 ml of sodium chloride intravenous infusion (0.9%).

Intermittent infusion

Table 2 lists a number of intravenous preparations that are both compatible and clinically suitable for administration when given by intermittent infusion in a relatively small volume of infusion over a short period of time, for example 100 ml in 30 minutes. This method is applicable where the product is incompatible or is unstable over the normal period necessary for continuous infusion or where adequate serum and tissue concentrations are not produced by continuous infusion. The limited stability of ampicillin or amoxycillin in large volume infusions containing carbohydrate or lactate may be overcome using this method.

Carbenicillin, dacarbazine, and ticarcillin may be given by intermittent infusion in order to achieve satisfactory serum and tissue concentrations. Gentamicin may be administered similarly, although it is normally given by direct intravenous bolus injection for the same reason.

An in-line burette may be used for intermittent infusion techniques in order to achieve strict control over the time and rate of administration of a bolus injection, especially for infants and children and in intensive care units. Intermittent infusion may also make use of the 'piggy-back' technique provided that no additions are made to the primary infusion. In this method the drug is added to a small secondary container connected to a Y-type injection site on the primary infusion administration set; the secondary solution is usually infused within 30 minutes. A third method is to inject the solution through the rubber septum of the drip tubing injection site using an aseptic technique.

Addition through the drip-tubing

Addition of drug preparations aseptically via the rubber septum of the injection site of a fast-running infusion is indicated for a number of cytotoxic drugs in order to minimise extravasation.

In general, drug preparations intended for a bolus effect should be given directly into a separate vein where possible. Failing this, administration may be made via the drip-tubing provided that the preparation is compatible with the infusion fluid when given in this manner. A number of preparations which are suitable for such administration are listed in Table 3. Drug preparations which should **not** be given in this way include frusemide.

Table 1. Compatible infusion admixtures suitable for continuous infusion

Additive[1]	Intravenous infusion	Comments
Acetylcysteine *Parvolex®*	Dextrose 5%	
Alphaxalone/alphadolone acetate *Althesin®*	Dextrose 5%; Sodium chloride 0.9%	
Aminophylline	Dextrose 5%; Sodium chloride 0.9%	
Amoxycillin sodium *Amoxil®*	Sodium chloride 0.9%; Ringer's solution; Sodium lactate M/6; Sodium lactate, compound (Hartmann's solution)	Reconstituted solutions should be diluted and administered without delay. The maximum period between addition and completion of administration is 6 hours.
Amphotericin sodium deoxycholate complex[2] *Fungizone®*	Dextrose 5%	Dissolve thoroughly at reconstitution stage. The pH of the dextrose intravenous infusion must not be below 4.2. Check each container. Protect infusion from light. Suggested infusion time 6 hours.
Ampicillin sodium *Penbritin®*	Sodium chloride 0.9%; Ringer's solution; Sodium lactate M/6; Sodium lactate, compound (Hartmann's solution)	Reconstituted solutions should be diluted and administered without delay. Maximum period between addition and completion of administration 6 hours.
Ancrod *Arvin®*	Sodium chloride 0.9%	Suggested volume 50–500 ml.
Aprotinin *Trasylol®*	Dextrose 5%; Sodium chloride 0.9%; Sodium chloride and dextrose; Ringer's solution	
Benzylpenicillin sodium	Dextrose 5%; Sodium chloride 0.9%	When given in dextrose 5% the maximum period between addition and completion of administration is 6 hours.
Betamethasone sodium phosphate *Betnesol®*	Dextrose 5%; Sodium chloride 0.9%; Sodium chloride and dextrose	

Table 1. Compatible infusion admixtures suitable for continuous infusion (*continued*)

Additive[1]	Intravenous infusion	Comments
Calcium gluconate	Dextrose 5%; Sodium chloride 0.9%; Sodium chloride and dextrose	Avoid solutions containing bicarbonates, phosphates, or sulphates.
Cefoxitin sodium *Mefoxin®*	Dextrose 5%; Sodium chloride 0.9%; Sodium chloride and dextrose; Sodium lactate M/6; Sodium lactate, compound (Hartmann's solution)	
Cephaloridine *Ceporin®*	Dextrose 5%; Sodium chloride 0.9%	Maximum period between addition and completion of administration 6 hours.
Cephamandole nafate *Kefadol®*	Dextrose 5% or 10%; Sodium chloride 0.9%; Sodium chloride and dextrose; Sodium lactate M/6	
Cephazolin sodium *Kefzol®*	Dextrose 5% or 10%; Sodium chloride 0.9%; Sodium chloride and dextrose; Sodium lactate, compound (Hartmann's solution)	
Cephradine *Velosef®*	Dextrose 5%; Sodium chloride 0.9%; Sodium lactate M/6	Reconsituted solution should be diluted and administered without delay; maximum period between addition and completion of administration 8 hours.
Cisplatin *Neoplatin®*	Sodium chloride 0.9%; Sodium chloride and dextrose	Suggested infusion time 6–8 hours.
Clindamycin phosphate *Dalacin C®*	Dextrose 5%; Sodium chloride 0.9%; Sodium chloride and dextrose	
Cloxacillin sodium *Orbenin®*	Dextrose 5%; Sodium chloride 0.9%; Ringer's solution; Sodium lactate M/6; Sodium lactate, compound (Hartmann's solution); Dextrans	Suggested infusion time 6 hours.
Colistin sulphomethate sodium *Colomycin®*	Dextrose 5%; Sodium chloride 0.9%; Ringer's solution; Laevulose; Dextrans	Maximum period between addition and completion of administration 6 hours
Co-trimoxazole sodium *Septrin®* for infusion *Bactrim®* for infusion	Dextrose 5%; Sodium chloride 0.9%; Ringer's solution; Laevulose; Dextrans	Ampoule solution has a pH of about 10. Suggested infusion time 1½ hours.
Cytarabine *Cytosar®*	Dextrose 5%; Sodium chloride 0.9%; Water for injections	
Desferrioxamine mesylate *Desferal®*	Dextrose 5%; Sodium chloride 0.9%	Reconstituted with Water for injections.
Dexamethasone sodium phosphate *Decadron®*; *Oradexon®*	Dextrose 5%; Sodium chloride 0.9%	

Table 1. Compatible infusion admixtures suitable for continuous infusion (*continued*)

Additive[1]	Intravenous infusion	Comments
Diazepam[3] *Valium®*	Dextrose 5%; Sodium chloride 0.9%	Dilute to a strength of not more than 40 mg in 500 ml. Maximum period between addition and completion of administration 6 hours.
Diazemuls®	Dextrose 5%; Dextrose 10%	May be diluted to a maximum strength of 200 mg in 500 ml. Maximum period between addition and completion of administration 6 hours.
Dinoprost *Prostin F2 alpha®*	Dextrose 5%; Sodium chloride 0.9%	
Dinoprostone *Prostin E2®*	Dextrose 5%; Sodium chloride 0.9%	
Dopamine hydrochloride *Intropin®*	Dextrose 5%; Sodium chloride 0.9%; Sodium chloride and dextrose; Sodium lactate M/6; Sodium lactate, compound (Hartmann's solution)	
Erythromycin lactobionate *Erythrocin®*	Dextrose 5%; Sodium chloride 0.9%	Reconstitute with water for injections; pH of dextrose infusion should be adjusted with sodium bicarbonate to above 5·5
Ethanol	Dextrose 5%; Sodium chloride 0.9%; Sodium chloride and dextrose; Ringer's solution; Sodium lactate, compound (Hartmann's solution)	
Flucloxacillin sodium *Floxapen®*	Dextrose 5%; Sodium chloride 0.9%; Ringer's solution; Sodium lactate M/6; Sodium lactate, compound (Hartmann's solution)	Suggested infusion time 6 hours
Folinic acid (calcium salt) *Calcium Leucovorin®*	Sodium chloride 0.9%	
Frusemide (sodium salt) *Dryptal®*; *Lasix®*	Sodium chloride 0.9%; Ringer's solution	pH of infusion must be above 5.5. Dextrose solutions are unsuitable.
Glyceryl trinitrate *Tridil®*	Dextrose 5%; Sodium chloride 0.9%	Incompatible with polyvinyl chloride infusion containers such as Viaflex® or Steriflex®. Use glass or polyethylene containers or give via syringe pump.
Heparin sodium	Dextrose 5%; Sodium chloride 0.9%; Sodium chloride and dextrose	Administration with a motorised pump may be advisable.
Hydralazine hydrochloride *Apresoline®*	Sodium chloride 0.9%; Sodium lactate M/6	Suggested volume 500 ml
Hydrocortisone sodium phosphate *Efcortesol®*	Dextrose 5%; Sodium chloride 0.9%; Sodium chloride and dextrose	
Hydrocortisone sodium succinate *Efcortelan Soluble®*	Dextrose 5%; Sodium chloride 0.9%	

Table 1. Compatible infusion admixtures suitable for continuous infusion (*continued*)

Additive[1]	Intravenous infusion	Comments
Hydrocortisone sodium succinate (*continued*)		
Solu-Cortef®	Sodium chloride and dextrose	
Insulin[3]	Sodium chloride 0.9%; Sodium lactate, compound (Hartmann's solution)	See section 6.1.3.
Isoprenaline hydrochloride[2] *Saventrine IV®*	Dextrose 5%; Sodium chloride and dextrose	pH of the infusion must be below 5. Suggested minimum volume 500 ml.
Isosorbide dinitrate *Cedocard IV®*; *Isoket®*	Dextrose 5%; Sodium chloride 0.9%	Incompatible with polyvinyl chloride infusion containers such as Viaflex® or Steriflex®. Use glass or polyethylene containers or via a syringe pump
Isoxsuprine hydrochloride *Duvadilan®*	Sodium chloride 0.9%	
Lignocaine hydrochloride[2,4] *Lidothesin 5%®*; *Xylocard 20%®*	Dextrose 5%	Use ready prepared solutions when available.
Lincomycin hydrochloride[2] *Lincocin®*	Dextrose 5%; Sodium chloride 0.9%	Minimum period of infusion 1 hour. Suggested minimum volume 250 ml.
Melphalan *Alkeran®*	Sodium chloride 0.9%	Use the diluent provided to reconstitute. The maximum period between addition and completion of administration is 8 hours.
Metaraminol tartrate *Aramine®*	Dextrose 5%; Sodium chloride 0.9%	
Methicillin sodium *Celbenin®*	Dextrose 5%; Sodium chloride 0.9%; Ringer's solution; Sodium lactate M/6; Sodium lactate, compound (Hartmann's solution); Dextrans	The maximum period between addition and completion of administration is 4 hours.
Methotrexate sodium[2,4] 500 mg	Sodium chloride 0.9%	The product is irritant to tissues. Avoid contamination of eyes or skin. Methotrexate powder for injection 50 mg is unsuitable for continuous infusion.
Methylprednisolone sodium succinate *Solu-Medrone®*	Dextrose 5%; Sodium chloride 0.9%; Sodium chloride and dextrose	
Mexiletine hydrochloride *Mexitil®*	Dextrose 5%; Sodium chloride 0.9%	
Miconazole *Daktarin®*	Dextrose 5%; Sodium chloride 0.9%	Minimum period of infusion 30 minutes.
Noradrenaline solution, strong sterile[2] *Levophed®*	Dextrose 5%; Sodium chloride and dextrose	pH of the infusion solution must be below 6.
Oxpentifylline *Trental®*	Dextrose 5%; Sodium chloride 0.9%; Laevulose	Suggested volume 250–500 ml. To be given over 1½–3 hours.

Table 1. Compatible infusion admixtures suitable for continuous infusion (*continued*)

Additive[1]	Intravenous infusion	Comments
Oxytocin[2] *Syntocinon®*	Dextrose 5%; Sodium chloride 0.9%; Ringer's solution; Sodium lactate M/6; Dextrans	
Polymyxin B sulphate *Aerosporin®*	Dextrose 5%	Suggested volume 200–500 ml. To be given over 1–1½ hours.
Potassium chloride[2]	Dextrose 5%; Sodium chloride 0.9%; Sodium chloride and dextrose	Mix thoroughly to avoid 'layering' especially in non-rigid infusion containers. Use ready prepared solutions when possible.
Prednisolone sodium phosphate *Codelsol®*	Dextrose 5%; Sodium chloride 0.9%	
Quinine dihydrochloride	Sodium chloride 0.9%	To be given over 4 hours.
Ritodrine hydrochloride[2] *Yutopar®*	Dextrose 5%; Sodium chloride 0.9%; Sodium chloride and dextrose	
Salbutamol sulphate[2,4] *Ventolin®* for intravenous infusion	Dextrose 5%; Sodium Chloride 0.9%; Sodium chloride and dextrose	To be given over not less than 2 hours.
Sodium calciumedetate *Ledclair®*	Dextrose 5%; Sodium chloride 0.9%	Suggested volume 250–500 ml.
Sodium fusidate *Fucidin®*	Dextrose 5%; Sodium chloride 0.9%; Sodium chloride and dextrose; Laevulose	Use the buffer solution provided to reconstitute.
Sodium nitroprusside *Nipride®*	Dextrose 5%	Suggested volume 500–1000 ml. Use the diluent provided to reconstitute. Protect the infusion from light. The maximum period between addition and completion of administration is 4 hours.
Streptokinase *Kabikinase®*	Dextrose 5%; Sodium chloride 0.9%	
Sulphadiazine sodium	Sodium chloride 0.9%	Ampoule solution has a pH of over 10.
Suxamethonium salts *Anectine®*; *Brevidil M®*; *Scoline®*	Dextrose 5%; Sodium chloride 0.9%	
Terbutaline sulphate *Bricanyl®*	Dextrose 5%; Sodium chloride 0.9%; Sodium chloride and dextrose	Suggested volume 500 ml. To be given over 8–10 hours.
Tetracycline hydrochloride *Achromycin®*	Dextrose 5%; Sodium chloride 0.9%; Sodium chloride and dextrose; Sodium lactate, compound (Hartmann's solution)	Minimum volume 100 ml. To be given over not more than 8 hours.
Trimethoprim lactate *Syraprim®*	Dextrose 5%; Sodium lactate M/6; Laevulose	
Trisodium edetate *Limclair®*	Dextrose 5%; Sodium chloride 0.9%	Give over 2–3 hours.
Urea *Ureaphil®*	Dextrose 5%	

Table 1. Compatible infusion admixtures suitable for continuous infusion (*continued*)

Additive[1]	Intravenous infusion	Comments
Urokinase *Abbokinase®*; *Urokinase*	Sodium chloride 0.9%	
Verapamil hydrochloride *Cordilox®*	Dextrose 5%; Sodium chloride 0.9%; Sodium chloride and dextrose; Laevulose	

1 The proprietary forms indicated in the tables have been shown to be suitable. If other forms are used suitability should be checked with the manufacturer.
2 Preparation must be given diluted in a large-volume infusion.
3 This method of administration is not reliable because the drug is adsorbed to some extent by the plastics of the infusion set.
4 Different formulations are available for bolus injection.

Table 2. Intravenous admixtures suitable for administration by intermittent infusion

Additive	Intravenous infusion	Volume suggested	To be given over (minutes)
Amikacin sulphate *Amikin®*	Sodium chloride 0.9%; Sodium lactate, compound (Hartmann's solution)		30
Amoxycillin sodium *Amoxil®*	Dextrose 5%; Sodium chloride 0.9%	100 ml	30–60
Ampicillin sodium *Penbritin®*	Dextrose 5%; Sodium chloride 0.9%	100 ml	30–60
Ampicillin/cloxacillin (sodium salts) *Ampiclox®*	Dextrose 5%; Sodium chloride 0.9%	100 ml	30–60
Ampicillin/flucloxacillin (sodium salts) *Magnapen®*	Dextrose 5%; Sodium chloride 0.9%	100 ml	30–60
Azlocillin sodium *Securopen®*	Dextrose 5% or 10%; Sodium chloride 0.9%; Ringer's solution; Laevulose		20–30
Benzylpenicillin sodium	Dextrose 5%; Sodium chloride 0.9%	100 ml	30–60
Bleomycin sulphate	Sodium chloride 0.9%	200 ml	To be given slowly
Bumetanide *Burinex®*	Dextrose 5%; Sodium chloride 0.9%; Sodium chloride and dextrose	500 ml	30–60
Carbenicillin sodium *Pyopen®*	Dextrose 5%; Water for injections	100 ml	30–40
Carmustine *BiCNU®*	Dextrose 5%; Sodium chloride 0.9%		60–120
Cefotaxime sodium *Claforan®*	Dextrose 5%; Sodium chloride 0.9%; Water for injections	40–100 ml	20–60
Cefoxitin sodium *Mefoxin®*	Dextrose 5%; Sodium chloride 0.9%; Sodium chloride and dextrose; Sodium lactate, compound (Hartmann's solution)		

Table 2. Intravenous admixtures suitable for administration by intermittent infusion (*continued*)

Additive	Intravenous infusion	Volume suggested	To be given over (minutes)
Cefuroxime *Zinacef®*	Dextrose 5%; Sodium chloride 0.9%	50–100 ml	30
Cephaloridine *Ceporin®*	Dextrose 5%; Sodium chloride 0.9%;	50–100 ml	30–60
Cephalothin sodium *Keflin®*	Dextrose 5%; Sodium chloride 0.9%; Sodium chloride and dextrose		
Cephamandole nafate *Kefadol®*	Dextrose 5%; Dextrose 10%; Sodium chloride 0.9%; Sodium chloride and dextrose; Sodium lactate M/6		
Cephazolin sodium *Kefzol®*	Dextrose 5%; Dextrose 10%; Sodium chloride 0.9%; Sodium chloride and dextrose		
Chloramphenical sodium succinate *Kemicetine®*	Dextrose 5%; Sodium chloride 0.9%		
Cimetidine *Tagamet®*	Dextrose 5%; Sodium chloride 0.9%	250 ml	120
Clindamycin phosphate *Dalacin C®*	Dextrose 5%; Sodium chloride 0.9%; Sodium chloride and dextrose		
Clomipramine *Anafranil®*	Dextrose 5%; Sodium chloride 0.9%	125–500 ml	45–120
Clonazepam *Rivotril®*	Dextrose 5%; Sodium chloride 0.9%	250 ml	
Cloxacillin sodium *Orbenin®*	Dextrose 5%; Sodium chloride 0.9%	100 ml	30–60
Colistin sulphomethate sodium *Colomycin®*	Dextrose 5%; Sodium chloride 0.9%; Ringer's solution; Laevulose; Dextrans		
Cyclophosphamide *Endoxana®*	Water for injections	50–100 ml	5–15
Dacarbazine *DTIC®*	Dextrose 5%; Sodium chloride 0.9%	250 ml	Not more than 30 Protect infusion from light
Dexamethasone sodium phosphate *Decadron®* *Oradexon®*	Dextrose 5%; Sodium chloride 0.9%		
Dinoprostone *Prostin E2®*	Dextrose 5%; Sodium chloride 0.9%		
Disopyramide phosphate *Norpace®* *Rythmodan®*	Dextrose 5%; Sodium chloride 0.9%; Ringer's solution; Sodium lactate, compound (Hartmann's solution)		
Dobutamine hydrochloride *Dobutrex®*	Dextrose 5%; Sodium chloride 0.9%; Sodium lactate M/6		

Table 2. Intravenous admixtures suitable for administration by intermittent infusion (*Continued*)

Additive	Intravenous infusion	Volume suggested	To be given over (minutes)
Etoposide *Vepesid®*	Sodium chloride 0.9%		Not less than 30
Flucloxacillin sodium *Floxapen®*	Dextrose 5%; Sodium chloride 0.9%	100 ml	30–60
Fluorouracil sodium	Dextrose 5%	500 ml	240
Gentamicin sulphate *Cidomycin®* *Garamycin®* *Genticin®*	Dextrose 5%; Sodium chloride 0.9%	50–100 ml	20–120
Ifosfamide *Mitoxana®*	Sodium chloride and dextrose		30–120
Iron dextran *Imferon®*	Dextrose 5%; Sodium chloride 0.9%		
Kanamycin sulphate *Kannasyn®* *Kantrex®*	Dextrose 5%; Sodium chloride 0.9%		
Labetalol hydrochloride *Trandate®*	Sodium chloride and dextrose	200 ml	Adjust rate with in-line burette
Mecillinam *Selexidin®*	Dextrose 5%; Sodium chloride 0.9%		15–30
Methicillin sodium *Celbenin®*	Dextrose 5%; Sodium chloride 0.9%		30–60
Methohexitone sodium *Brietal Sodium®*	Dextrose 5%; Sodium chloride 0.9%	250–500 ml	
Methyldopate hydrochloride *Aldomet®*	Dextrose 5%	100 ml	30–60
Mezlocillin sodium *Baypen®* (5 g)	Dextrose 5%; Sodium chloride 0.9%; Water for injections	50 ml	15–20
Miconazole *Daktarin®*	Dextrose 5%; Sodium chloride 0.9%	200–500 ml	At least 30
Mithramycin *Mithracin®*	Dextrose 5%	1000 ml	240–360
Naftidrofuryl oxalate *Praxilene®*	Dextrose 5%; Dextrose 10%; Sodium chloride 0.9%; Dextrans; Laevulose	250–500 ml	90–120
Netilmicin sulphate *Netillin®*	Dextrose 5%; Sodium chloride 0.9%	50–200 ml	30–120
Orciprenaline sulphate *Alupent obstetric®*	Dextrose 5%	500 ml	
Phenoxybenzamine hydrochloride *Dibenyline®*	Sodium chloride 0.9%		Not less than 60
Phentolamine mesylate *Rogitine®*	Dextrose 5%; Sodium chloride 0.9%; Sodium chloride and dextrose		10 (diagnostic) 180 (therapy)
Phenylephrine hydrochloride	Dextrose 5%; Sodium chloride 0.9%		

Table 2. Intravenous admixtures suitable for administration by intermittent infusion (*continued*)

Additive	Intravenous infusion	Volume suggested	To be given over (minutes)
Prenalterol hydrochloride *Hyprenan®* *Varbian®*	Dextrose 5%; Sodium chloride 0.9%; Ringer's solution		
Ranitidine hydrochloride *Zantac®*	Dextrose 5%; Sodium chloride 0.9%; Sodium chloride and dextrose; Sodium lactate, compound (Hartmann's solution)		
Ticarcillin sodium *Ticar®*	Dextrose 5%; Water for injections	100–150 ml	30–60
Tobramycin sulphate *Nebcin®*	Dextrose 5%; Sodium chloride 0.9%	50–100 ml	20–60
Tocainide hydrochloride *Tonocard®*	Dextrose 5%; Sodium chloride 0.9%	50–100 ml	15–30
Trimetaphan camsylate *Arfonad®*	Dextrose 5%; Sodium chloride 0.9%; Sodium chloride and dextrose	100–500 ml	
Vancomycin hydrochloride *Vancocin®*	Dextrose 5%; Sodium chloride 0.9%	100–200 ml	20–30
Vitamins B & C *Pabrinex®* *Parentrovite®*	Dextrose 5%; Sodium chloride 0.9%		

Table 3. Injections which may be given via the drip-tubing of the administration set with infusions of dextrose 5%, sodium chloride 0.9%, or sodium chloride and dextrose

Actinomycin D (*Cosmegen Lyovac®*)
Amoxycillin sodium (*Amoxil®*)
Ampicillin sodium (*Penbritin®*)
Ampicillin/cloxacillin sodium salts (*Ampiclox®*)
Ampicillin/flucloxacillin sodium salts (*Magnapen®*)
Aprotinin (*Trasylol®*)
Cefoxitin sodium (*Mefoxin®*)
Cephamandole (*Kefadol®*)
Cephaloridine (*Ceporin®*)
Cephalothin sodium (*Keflin®*)
Cephazolin sodium (*Kefzol®*)
Cloxacillin sodium (*Orbenin®*)
Chloramphenicol sodium succinate (*Kemicetine®*)
Cyclophosphamide (*Endoxana®*)
Cytarabine (*Cytosar®*)
Dexamethasone sodium phosphate (*Decadron®*; *Oradexon®*)
Doxorubicin hydrochloride (*Adriamycin®*)
Ethacrynic acid sodium salt (*Edecrin®*)
Flucloxacillin sodium (*Floxapen®*)
Hydrocortisone sodium phosphate (*Efcortesol®*)
Hydrocortisone sodium succinate (*Efcortelan Soluble®*; *Solu-Cortef®*)
Ifosfamide (*Mitoxana®*)
Melphalan (*Alkeran®*)
Metaraminol tartrate (*Aramine®*)
Mustine hydrochloride
Tobramycin sulphate (*Nebcin®*)
Vinblastine (*Velbe®*)
Vincristine (*Oncovin®*)
Vindesine (*Eldisine®*)
Vitamins B and C injection (*Pabrinex®*; *Parentrovite®*)

Appendix 3: Borderline Substances

In certain conditions some foods (and toilet preparations) have characteristics of drugs and the Advisory Committee on Borderline Substances advises as to the circumstances in which such substances may be regarded as drugs. The Advisory Committee's recommendations are listed below. Prescriptions issued in accordance with the Committee's advice and endorsed 'ACBS' will normally not be investigated.

ALCOHOLIC BEVERAGES
(Wines, tonic wines and similar preparations)
Cannot be regarded as drugs. Where the therapeutic qualities of alcohol are required rectified spirit (suitably flavoured and diluted) should be prescribed.

ANTI-SMOKING PREPARATIONS
Should not be regarded as drugs.

DISINFECTANTS
Should be regarded as drugs only when ordered in such quantities and with such directions as are appropriate for the treatment of patients. Not to be regarded as drugs if ordered for general hygienic purposes.

VITAMIN PREPARATIONS
Should be regarded as drugs only when used for example in the management of actual or potential vitamin deficiency. Not to be regarded as drugs when used routinely.

DIETARY PRODUCTS

FOODS
The following are to be regarded as foods: Allergilac; Cantaflour; Complan; Devonsheer Rice Wafers; Energen starch reduced bran crispbread; Glucodin; Granogen; Linoleic acid; Malt extract with cod liver oil; Optimax powder; Rite-Diet gluten-free canned rich fruit cake and half-coated milk chocolate or sultana biscuits; Rite-Diet Soya Bran; Saxin; SMA Powder and Liquid; SMA Gold Cap Powder and Ready-to-feed; Safflower seed oils; Sweetex; Trufree Bread Mix, Pasta Mix, Plain Flour, and Sweet Biscuits.
Note: Neither gluten-free products nor those containing linoleic acid (e.g. sunflower and safflower seed oils) should be regarded as drugs in the management of *multiple sclerosis*.

DRUGS
The following are to be regarded as drugs but only when prescribed as specified:

Aglutella Azeta Cream Filled Wafers: for phenylketonuria, similar amino-acid abnormalities, renal failure, liver failure and liver cirrhosis.
Albumaid Complete: for malabsorption states where there is failure to hydrolyse and/or absorb protein.
Albumaid Complete, RVHB, and **X Methionine:** for homocystinuria.
Albumaid XP and **Concentrate:** for phenylketonuria.
Alembicol D: for steatorrhoea associated with cystic fibrosis of the pancreas, intestinal lymphangiectasis, surgery of the intestine, chronic liver disease, liver cirrhosis; other proven malabsorption syndromes and in a ketogenic diet in the management of epilepsy.
Aminex: for phenylketonuria, similar amino-acid abnormalities, liver cirrhosis, chronic renal failure, proven lactose with sucrose intolerance.
Aminogran Food Supplement: for phenylketonuria.
Aminogran Mineral Mixture: for phenylketonuria and as a mineral supplement for use with synthetic diets and those with severe restriction of natural food.
Aminutrin: for malabsorption states where there is failure to hydrolyse and/or absorb protein.
Calonutrin: for disaccharide intolerance (without isomaltose intolerance), amino acid (and other similar disorders) and/or whole protein intolerance, liver cirrhosis and in proven hypoglycaemia where there is no need to limit sodium and potassium intake, and other proven malabsorption states.
Caloreen: for renal failure, liver cirrhosis, disaccharide intolerance (without isomaltose intolerance), disorders of amino-acid metabolism (and other similar disorders), and/or whole protein intolerance, malabsorption states and other conditions, including proven hypoglycaemia, requiring a high energy, low fluid intake, whether or not sodium and/or potassium restriction is essential.
Carobel: for thickening feeds in the treatment of vomiting.
Casilan: for biochemically proven hypoproteinaemia.
Clinifeed and **Clinifeed Iso Vanilla:** for short bowel syndrome; intractable malabsorption; pre-operative preparation of patients who are undernourished; treatment for those with proven inflammatory bowel disease, following total gastrectomy and dysphagia.
Comminuted Chicken Meat: for carbohydrate intolerance in association with possible or proven intolerance of milk.
Corn Oil: *only* for familial hypercholesterolaemia.
Cow and Gate Formula S Soya Food: for milk intolerance and galactosaemia.
Cymogran: for phenylketonuria.
Dextrose: see glucose.
d.p. Low Protein Chocolate Flavoured Chip Cookies: for phenylketonuria, similar amino acid abnormalities, renal failure, liver failure and liver cirrhosis.
Edosol: for conditions requiring a minimal sodium intake.
Ensure: for short bowel syndrome, intractable malabsorption, pre-operative preparation of patients who are undernourished, treatment for

those with proven inflammatory bowel disease, treatment following total gastrectomy and dysphagia.

Flexical: for short bowel syndrome, intractable malabsorption, pre-operative preparation of patients who are undernourished and treatment following total gastrectomy.

Forceval Protein: for biochemically proven hypoproteinaemia and as a supplement for inflammatory bowel syndrome, intractable malabsorption, pre-operative preparation of patients who are undernourished, treatment of those with proven inflammatory bowel disease, treatment following gastrectomy and dysphagia, where a reduced salt intake is required.

Fructose: for proven glucose/galactose intolerance.

Galactomin Formula 17 and
Galactomin Formula 18: for lactose intolerance and proven galactosaemia or galactokinase deficiency.

Galactomin Formula 19: for glucose plus galactose intolerance.

Glucose: for glycogen storage disease and sucrose/isomaltose intolerance

Gluten-free Products: not necessarily low protein, lactose or sucrose free:

Aglutella Gentili—macaroni, spaghetti, spaghetti rings.
Aproten Products—anellini, biscuits, crispbread, ditalini, flour, rigatini, tagliatelle.
Bi-Aglut biscuits
Farley's biscuits
GF Brand crackers
Glutenex (Liga)
Juvela Gluten-free mix
Rite-Diet flour, bread mix, sweet (without chocolate or sultanas) and savoury (cheese) biscuits, gluten-free/protein-free bread, gluten-free bread with soya bran, low protein gluten-free cream filled wafers (vanilla flavour), low protein pasta (macaroni).
Tritamyl gluten-free flour
Trufree self-raising flour, Cantabread mix, and bread mix with rice bran
Verkade Dutch food biscuits
for gluten-sensitive enteropathies including steatorrhoea due to gluten-sensitivity, coeliac disease and dermatitis herpetiformis.

HF2: for histidinaemia.

Hycal: for renal failure, liver cirrhosis or other conditions requiring a high energy, low fluid, low electrolyte diet.

Isocal: for short bowel syndrome, intractable malabsorption, pre-operative preparation of patients who are undernourished, treatment for those with proven inflammatory bowel disease, treatment following total gastrectomy and dysphagia.

Liquigen: for steatorrhoea associated with cystic fibrosis of the pancreas, intestinal lymphangiectasis, surgery of the intestine, chronic liver disease, liver cirrhosis, other proven malabsorption syndromes, a ketogenic diet in the management of epilepsy and in Type 1 hyperlipoproteinaemia.

Locasol: for intolerance to calcium.

Lofenalac: for phenylketonuria.

Maxijul: for renal failure, liver cirrhosis, disaccharide intolerance (without isomaltose intolerance), disorders of amino-acid metabolism (and other similar disorders), and/or whole protein intolerance, malabsorption states and other conditions, including proven hypoglycaemia, requiring a high energy low fluid intake.

Maxijul LE: as above where sodium and/or potassium restriction is essential.

MCT(1) Powder: for steatorrhoea associated with cystic fibrosis of the pancreas, intestinal lymphangiectasis, chronic liver disease and surgery of the intestine in infants.

Medium Chain Triglyceride (MCT) Oil: for steatorrhoea associated with cystic fibrosis of the pancreas, intestinal lymphangiectasis, surgery of the intestine, chronic liver disease, liver cirrhosis, other proven malabsorption syndromes and in a ketogenic diet in the management of epilepsy, and in Type 1 hyperlipoproteinaemia.

Metabolic Mineral Mixture: as a mineral supplement in the dietary treatment of carbohydrate and amino acid disorders.

Minafen: for phenylketonuria.

MSUD Aid: for Maple Syrup Urine Disease.

Nestargel: for thickening feeds in the treatment of vomiting.

Nutramigen: for infants with galactosaemia, lactose intolerance without sucrose intolerance, and infants and children sensitive to whole protein.

PK Aid 1: for phenylketonuria.

Portagen: for lactose intolerance without sucrose intolerance but requiring MCT, steatorrhoea associated with cystic fibrosis of the pancreas, intestinal lymphangiectasis, surgery of the intestine, chronic liver disease, liver cirrhosis, other proven malabsorption syndromes.

Pregestimil: for sucrose and/or lactose intolerance in association with whole protein intolerance or where amino acids and peptides are indicated in conjunction with MCT. Also for proven malabsorption syndromes in which a reduced fat diet is indicated such as steatorrhoea associated with cystic fibrosis and surgery of the intestine.

Prosobee Liquid and Powder: for milk intolerance and galactosaemia.

Prosparol: for renal failure and other conditions requiring a high energy, low fluid, low electrolyte diet; disorders of amino acid metabolism or carbohydrate absorption; in a ketogenic diet in the management of epilepsy.

Protein-free Products

Aglutella Gentili—macaroni, semolina, spaghetti, spaghetti-rings.
Aproten Products—anellini, biscuits, crispbread, ditalini, flour, rigatini, tagliatelle.
Juvela low-protein mix.
Rite-Diet low-protein flour-mix, gluten-free/protein-free bread, low protein gluten-free cream filled wafers (vanilla flavour), low protein macaroni: for phenylketonuria, similar amino acid abnormalities, renal failure, liver failure, liver cirrhosis, gluten-sensitive enteropathies including steatorrhoea due to gluten-

sensitivity, coeliac disease and dermatitis herpetiformis.

Rite-Diet Low-Protein Gluten-free Biscuits: for phenylketonuria, similar amino-acid abnormalities, renal failure, liver failure, and liver cirrhosis.

Rite-Diet Low-Sodium Bread: for conditions in which a low-sodium diet is indicated.

Sunflower Oil: *only* for familial hypercholesterolaemia.

Triosorbon: for short bowel syndrome, intractable malabsorption, pre-operative preparation of patients who are undernourished, treatment for those with proven inflammatory bowel disease, treatment following total gastrectomy and dysphagia.

Tritamyl PK Flour: for phenylketonuria and similar amino-acid abnormalities, gluten-sensitive enteropathies including steatorrhoea due to gluten sensitivity, coeliac disease and dermatitis herpetiformis.

Velactin: for milk intolerance.

Vivonex: for short bowel syndrome, intractable malabsorption, preoperative preparation of patients who are undernourished and treatment following total gastrectomy, and dysphagia due to an incurable malignancy.

Wysoy: for milk intolerance and galactosaemia.

Topical preparations

TOILET PREPARATIONS

The following are to be regarded as toilet preparations: Acne Aid Bar; Atrixo; Aveeno Bar; Aveeno Bar Oilated; Cidal; Covermark Removing Cream; Dansac Skin Lotion; Derbac Soap; Gamophen; Genatosan; Ipsel Hygienic Baby Salve; Lacto-Calamine; Neutrogena; Nivea; Oilatum Bar; Prodermide Solid; Sebaveen; Simple Soap; United Skin Care Programme; Woodwards Baby Cream.

DRUGS

The following are to be regarded as drugs: Esoderm; Lenium; Lorexane No. 3; Oilatum Emollient; Selsun; Suleo-Shampoo.

The following are to be regarded as drugs only when prescribed as specified:

PRODUCTS FOR SKIN CARE AROUND STOMATA:

Colobase
Karaya Paste
Kerodex Double Seven
Translet Barrier Cream
Skin Gel

COVERING CREAMS:

Boots Covering Cream

Covermark Masking Cream, Spotstick, Cream Rouge, Shading Cream, Grey Toner, Finishing Powder (excluding **Removing Cream**)

Keromask: for concealment of birth marks, post-operative scars and other deformities and as adjunctive therapy in the relief of emotional disturbances due to mutilating skin disease.

DEODORANTS:

Atmocol Aerosol
Chironair Odour Control Liquid
Dor
No Roma
Ostobon
Ostosan

Stomogel: for patients with ileostomies or colostomies.

Translet Plus One and Two

EMOLLIENTS:

Polytar Emollient: for psoriasis, eczema, atopic and pruritic dermatoses.

SCALP CLEANSERS AND SHAMPOOS

Alphosyl: for psoriasis and other scaly disorders of the scalp.

Betadine: for seborrhoeic conditions of the scalp associated with excessive dandruff, pruritic scaling, exudation, erythema; pityriasis capitis; infected lesions of the scalp; pyodermas (recurrent furunculosis, infective folliculitis, impetigo).

Capitol: for pityriasis capitis and seborrhoeic dermatitis of the scalp.

Ceanel Concentrate: for psoriasis or seborrhoeic conditions.

Cetavlon PC: for seborrhoea capitis and seborrhoeic dermatitis.

Genisol: for psoriasis, eczema, and seborrhoea of the scalp

Ionil T: for seborrhoeic dermatitis of the scalp.

Polytar Liquid: for psoriasis, eczema and seborrhoea of the scalp.

Polytar Plus: for the treatment of scalp disorders such as dandruff, psoriasis, seborrhoea, eczema and pruritus and the removal of pastes and pomades used in the treatment of psoriasis.

SKIN CLEANSERS

Betadine Products—Skin Cleanser, Foam, Scalp and Skin Cleanser: for infective conditions of the skin.

Ionax Scrub: for the control and hygiene of acne and the cleansing of the skin prior to acne treatment.

Ster-Zac Bath Concentrate: for staphylococcal skin infections.

Tetmosol: for control of scabies.

SUN SCREENS

Piz Buin Creme Extreme No. 6

Spectraban: for protection of skin from ultraviolet radiation in photodermatoses.

Uvistat: for protection of skin from ultra violet radiation in photodermatoses, including those resulting from radiotherapy.

Formulary

Only the formulae of non-proprietary preparations mentioned in the classified notes and commonly dispensed extemporaneously are listed here for information. For further details of suitable methods of preparation, packaging, and labelling, see *The Pharmaceutical Codex* 11th Edition.

Obsolete formulae may be found in the *Compendium of Past Formulae 1933–1966* (1971) and *Supplement* (1979) issued by the National Pharmaceutical Association.

Ear-drops

10 ml to be dispensed unless otherwise directed
Labelling: in the absence of instructions by the prescriber state—3 or 4 drops to be put into the affected ear

Sodium Bicarbonate Ear-drops, BP

Sodium Bicarbonate		5	g
Glycerol		30	ml
Purified Water, freshly boiled and cooled	to	100	ml

It should be recently prepared

Elixirs

Dilution: see Guidance on Prescribing, general information

Chloral Elixir, Paediatric, BP

Chloral Hydrate		200	mg
Water for Preparations		0.1	ml
Black Currant Syrup		1	ml
Syrup	to	5	ml

It should be recently prepared
Diluent syrup. The diluted elixir must be freshly prepared

CD Diamorphine and Cocaine Elixir, BPC

Diamorphine Hydrochloride		5	mg
Cocaine Hydrochloride		5	mg
Alcohol (90%)		0.625	ml
Syrup		1.25	ml
Chloroform Water	to	5	ml

It must be freshly prepared
The proportion of diamorphine hydrochloride may be altered when specified by the prescriber

CD Diamorphine, Cocaine and Chlorpromazine Elixir, BPC

Diamorphine Hydrochloride		5	mg
Cocaine Hydrochloride		5	mg
Alcohol (90%)		0.625	ml
Chlorpromazine Elixir		1.25	ml
Chloroform Water	to	5	ml

It must be freshly prepared
The proportion of diamorphine hydrochloride may be altered when specified by the prescriber
5 ml contains 6.25 mg of chlorpromazine hydrochloride

Isoniazid Elixir, BPC

Isoniazid		50	mg
Citric Acid Monohydrate		12.5	mg
Sodium Citrate		60	mg
Concentrated Anise Water		0.05	ml
Compound Tartrazine Solution		0.05	ml
Glycerol		1	ml
Chloroform Water, Double-strength		2	ml
Water for Preparations	to	5	ml

Diluent chloroform water. The diluted elixir must be freshly prepared

Morphine and Cocaine Elixir, BPC

Morphine Hydrochloride		5	mg
Cocaine Hydrochloride		5	mg
Alcohol (90%)		0.625	ml
Syrup		1.25	ml
Chloroform Water	to	5	ml

It should be recently prepared
The proportion of morphine hydrochloride may be altered when specified by the prescriber. If above 13 mg per 5 ml the elixir becomes **CD**

Morphine, Cocaine and Chlorpromazine Elixir, BPC

Morphine Hydrochloride		5	mg
Cocaine Hydrochloride		5	mg
Alcohol (90%)		0.625	ml
Chlorpromazine Elixir		1.25	ml
Chloroform Water	to	5	ml

It should be recently prepared
The proportion of morphine hydrochloride may be altered when specified by the prescriber. If above 13 mg per 5 ml the elixir becomes **CD**
5 ml contains 6.25 mg of chlorpromazine hydrochloride

Phenobarbitone Elixir, BP

Phenobarbitone		30	mg
Compound Tartrazine Solution		0.1	ml
Compound Orange Spirit		0.24	ml
Alcohol (90%)		4	ml
Glycerol		4	ml
Water for Preparations	to	10	ml

Diluent syrup. The diluted elixir must be freshly prepared

Gargles

Labelling: in the absence of instructions by the prescriber, the directions for use given below the preparation should be stated

Phenol Gargle

Phenol Glycerin	5	ml
Amaranth Solution	1	ml
Water for preparations	to 100	ml

When diluted the gargle contains about 0.5% w/v of phenol
Directions for use: to be diluted with an equal quantity of warm water
300 ml to be dispensed unless otherwise directed

Inhalations

Labelling: in the absence of instructions by the prescriber, the directions for use given below the preparation should be stated

Menthol and Benzoin Inhalation, BP

Menthol	2	g
Benzoin Inhalation	to 100	ml

Directions for use: add 1 teaspoonful to a pint of hot, not boiling, water and inhale the vapour.
25 ml to be dispensed unless otherwise directed

Menthol and Eucalyptus Inhalation, BP

Menthol	2	g
Eucalyptus Oil	10	ml
Light Magnesium Carbonate	7	g
Water for Preparations	to 100	ml

Directions for use: add 1 teaspoonful to a pint of hot, not boiling, water and inhale the vapour
25 ml to be dispensed unless otherwise directed

Linctuses

Dilution: see Guidance on Prescribing, general information

Codeine Linctus, Paediatric, BPC

Codeine Linctus	1	ml
Syrup	to 5	ml

Diluent syrup
5 ml contains 3 mg of codeine phosphate

CD Diamorphine Linctus, BPC

Diamorphine Hydrochloride	3	mg
Compound Tartrazine Solution	0.06	ml
Glycerol	1.25	ml
Oxymel	1.25	ml
Syrup	to 5	ml

Diluent syrup. It must be freshly prepared

Opiate Squill Linctus, BP
(Gee's Linctus)

Camphorated Opium Tincture	
Squill Oxymel	
Tolu Syrup	of each, equal parts

Diluent syrup
5 ml contains 800 micrograms of anhydrous morphine

Opiate Squill Linctus, Paediatric, BP

Camphorated Opium Tincture	0.3	ml
Squill Oxymel	0.3	ml
Tolu Syrup	0.3	ml
Glycerol	1	ml
Syrup	to 5	ml

Diluent syrup
5 ml contains 150 micrograms of anhydrous morphine

Simple Linctus, BP

Citric Acid Monohydrate	125	mg
Concentrated Anise Water	0.05	ml
Amaranth Solution	0.075	ml
Chloroform Spirit	0.3	ml
Syrup	to 5	ml

Diluent syrup

Simple Linctus, Paediatric, BP

Simple Linctus	1.25	ml
Syrup	to 5	ml

Diluent syrup

Liniments

Methyl Salicylate Liniment, BP

Methyl Salicylate	25	ml
Arachis Oil	to 100	ml

It should be kept in airtight containers in a cool place
100 ml to be dispensed unless otherwise directed

Lotions

Labelling: in the absence of instructions by the prescriber, the directions for use, if any, given below the preparation should be stated

Aluminium Acetate Lotion

Aluminium Acetate Solution	5	ml
Purified Water, freshly boiled and cooled	to 100	ml

It contains about 0.65% of aluminium acetate.
It must be freshly prepared
To be used undiluted
500 ml to be dispensed unless otherwise directed

Formaldehyde Lotion

Formaldehyde Solution	3	ml
Water for Preparations	to 100	ml

It must be freshly prepared
100 ml to be dispensed unless otherwise directed

Salicylic Acid Lotion, BP

Salicylic Acid	2	g
Castor Oil	1	ml
Industrial Methylated Spirit	to 100	ml

Labelling: Caution: this preparation is inflammable. Do not use, or dry the hair, near a fire or naked flame
100 ml to be dispensed unless otherwise directed

Silver Nitrate Lotion

Silver Nitrate		500	mg
Purified Water, freshly boiled and cooled	to	100	ml

It must be freshly prepared, and protected from light
Directions for use: to be used undiluted
Labelling: this lotion will produce black stains on skin and clothing
50 ml to be dispensed unless otherwise directed

Sulphur Lotion, Compound, BPC

Precipitated Sulphur		4	g
Quillaia Tincture		0.5	ml
Glycerol		2	ml
Industrial Methylated Spirit		6	ml
Calcium Hydroxide Solution	to	100	ml

200 ml to be dispensed unless otherwise directed

Zinc Sulphate Lotion, BP

Zinc Sulphate		1	g
Amaranth Solution		1	ml
Water for Preparations	to	100	ml

200 ml to be dispensed unless otherwise directed

Zinc Sulphide Lotion, BPC

Sulphurated Potash		5	g
Zinc Sulphate		5	g
Camphor Water, Concentrated		2.5	ml
Water for Preparations	to	100	ml

It must be freshly prepared
100 ml to be dispensed unless otherwise directed

Mixtures

Dilution: see Guidance on Prescribing, general information
Labelling: mixtures, other than paediatric mixtures, and others with a dose of 5 ml, should be diluted with water before taking

Aluminium Hydroxide and Belladonna Mixture, BPC

Belladonna Tincture		0.5	ml
Chloroform Spirit		0.25	ml
Aluminium Hydroxide Mixture	to	5	ml

It must be freshly prepared

Ammonia and Ipecacuanha Mixture, BP

Ammonium Bicarbonate		200	mg
Ipecacuanha Tincture		0.3	ml
Concentrated Anise Water		0.05	ml
Concentrated Camphor Water		0.1	ml
Liquorice Liquid Extract		0.5	ml
Chloroform Water, Double-strength		5	ml
Water for Preparations	to	10	ml

It should be recently prepared

Ammonium Chloride Mixture, BP

Ammonium Chloride		1	g
Aromatic Ammonia Solution		0.5	ml
Liquorice Liquid Extract		1	ml
Water for Preparations	to	10	ml

It should be recently prepared

Ammonium Chloride and Morphine Mixture, BP

Ammonium Chloride		300	mg
Chloroform and Morphine Tincture		0.3	ml
Ammonium Bicarbonate		200	mg
Liquorice Liquid Extract		0.5	ml
Water for Preparations	to	10	ml

It should be recently prepared
10 ml contains 500 micrograms of anhydrous morphine

Belladonna Mixture, Paediatric, BPC

Belladonna Tincture		0.15	ml
Compound Orange Spirit		0.01	ml
Benzoic Acid Solution		0.1	ml
Glycerol		0.5	ml
Syrup		1	ml
Water for Preparations	to	5	ml

It should be recently prepared
Dose: up to 1 year 5 ml; 1–5 years 10 ml
5 ml contains 45 micrograms of belladonna alkaloids

Aromatic Chalk with Opium Mixture, BP

Chalk and Opium Mixture

Chalk		325	mg
Opium Tincture		0.5	ml
Sucrose		650	mg
Tragacanth, in powder		20	mg
Aromatic Ammonia Solution		0.5	ml
Catechu Tincture		0.5	ml
Compound Cardamom Tincture		1	ml
Chloroform Water, Double-strength		5	ml
Water for Preparations	to	10	ml

It should be recently prepared
10 ml contains 5 mg of anhydrous morphine

Chalk Mixture, Paediatric, BP

Chalk		100	mg
Tragacanth, in powder		10	mg
Concentrated Cinnamon Water		0.02	ml
Syrup		0.5	ml
Chloroform Water, Double-strength		2.5	ml
Water for Preparations	to	5	ml

It should be recently prepared
Dose: up to 1 year 5 ml; 1–5 years 10 ml

Chloral Mixture, BP

Chloral Hydrate		1	g
Syrup		2	ml
Water for Preparations	to	10	ml

It should be recently prepared
Diluent syrup 1 part with water 4 parts. The diluted mixture must be freshly prepared
Labelling: to be taken well diluted with water

Ferrous Sulphate Mixture, Paediatric, BP

Ferrous Sulphate	60	mg
Ascorbic Acid	10	mg
Orange Syrup	0.5	ml
Chloroform Water, Double-strength	2.5	ml
Purified Water, freshly boiled and cooled to	5	ml

It should be recently prepared
Dose: up to 1 year 5 ml; 1–5 years 10 ml
Labelling: to be taken well diluted with water

Gentian Mixture, Alkaline, BP

Concentrated Compound Gentian Infusion	1	ml
Sodium Bicarbonate	500	mg
Chloroform Water, Double-strength	5	ml
Water for Preparations to	10	ml

It should be recently prepared

Ipecacuanha and Morphine Mixture, BP

Ipecacuanha Tincture	0.2	ml
Chloroform and Morphine Tincture	0.4	ml
Liquorice Liquid Extract	1	ml
Water for Preparations to	10	ml

It should be recently prepared
10 ml contains 700 micrograms of anhydrous morphine

Ipecacuanha Emetic Mixture, Paediatric, BP

Ipecacuanha Liquid Extract	0.7	ml
Hydrochloric Acid	0.025	ml
Glycerol	1	ml
Syrup to	10	ml

Kaolin and Morphine Mixture, BP

Light Kaolin, or Light Kaolin (Natural)	2	g
Sodium Bicarbonate	500	mg
Chloroform and Morphine Tincture	0.4	ml
Water for Preparations to	10	ml

It should be recently prepared, unless the kaolin has been sterilised
10 ml contains 700 micrograms of anhydrous morphine

Kaolin Mixture, BP

Light Kaolin, or Light Kaolin (Natural)	2	g
Light Magnesium Carbonate	500	mg
Sodium Bicarbonate	500	mg
Peppermint Emulsion, Concentrated	0.25	ml
Chloroform Water, Double-strength	5	ml
Water for Preparations to	10	ml

It should be recently prepared, unless the kaolin has been sterilised

Kaolin Mixture, Paediatric, BP

Light Kaolin, or Light Kaolin (Natural)	1	g
Amaranth Solution	0.05	ml
Benzoic Acid Solution	0.1	ml
Raspberry Syrup	1	ml
Chloroform Water, Double-strength	2.5	ml
Water for Preparations to	5	ml

It should be recently prepared, unless the kaolin has been sterilised
Dose: up to 1 year 5 ml; 1–5 years 10 ml

Magnesium Carbonate Mixture, BPC

Light Magnesium Carbonate	500	mg
Sodium Bicarbonate	800	mg
Peppermint Emulsion, Concentrated	0.25	ml
Chloroform Water, Double-strength	5	ml
Water for Preparations to	10	ml

It should be recently prepared

Magnesium Carbonate Mixture, Aromatic, BP

Light Magnesium Carbonate	300	mg
Sodium Bicarbonate	500	mg
Aromatic Cardamom Tincture	0.3	ml
Chloroform Water, Double-strength	5	ml
Water for Preparations to	10	ml

It should be recently prepared

Magnesium Sulphate Mixture, BP

Magnesium Sulphate	4	g
Light Magnesium Carbonate	500	mg
Peppermint Emulsion, Concentrated	0.25	ml
Chloroform Water, Double-strength	3	ml
Water for Preparations to	10	ml

It should be recently prepared

Magnesium Trisilicate and Belladonna Mixture, BPC

Belladonna Tincture	0.5	ml
Magnesium Trisilicate Mixture to	10	ml

It must be freshly prepared
5 ml contains 15 micrograms of belladonna alkaloids

Magnesium Trisilicate Mixture, BP

Magnesium Trisilicate	500	mg
Light Magnesium Carbonate	500	mg
Sodium Bicarbonate	500	mg
Peppermint Emulsion, Concentrated	0.25	ml
Chloroform Water, Double-strength	5	ml
Water for Preparations to	10	ml

It should be recently prepared

CD Methadone Mixture 1 mg/ml, DTF

Methadone Hydrochloride		5	mg
Green S and Tartrazine Solution		0.01	ml
Compound Tartrazine Solution		0.04	ml
Syrup		2.5	ml
Chloroform Water, Double-strength	to	5	ml

This preparation is 2½ times the strength of Methadone Linctus and is intended only for drug dependent persons for whom treatment is normally ordered on form FP10(H.P.)(ad)

The title includes the strength and prescriptions should be written accordingly

Potassium Citrate Mixture, BP

Potassium Citrate		3	g
Citric Acid Monohydrate		500	mg
Lemon Spirit		0.05	ml
Quillaia Tincture		0.1	ml
Syrup		2.5	ml
Chloroform Water, Double-strength		3	ml
Water for Preparations	to	10	ml

It should be recently prepared

Diluent syrup

Labelling: to be taken well diluted with water

Rhubarb and Soda Mixture, Ammoniated, BP

Rhubarb, in powder		250	mg
Sodium Bicarbonate		800	mg
Ammonium Bicarbonate		200	mg
Peppermint Emulsion, Concentrated		0.25	ml
Chloroform Water, Double-strength		5	ml
Water for Preparations	to	10	ml

It should be recently prepared

Rhubarb Mixture, Compound, BPC

Compound Rhubarb Tincture		1	ml
Light Magnesium Carbonate		500	mg
Sodium Bicarbonate		500	mg
Strong Ginger Tincture		0.3	ml
Chloroform Water, Double-strength		5	ml
Water for Preparations	to	10	ml

It should be recently prepared

Sodium Salicylate Mixture, BP

Sodium Salicylate		500	mg
Sodium Metabisulphite		10	mg
Concentrated Orange Peel Infusion		0.5	ml
Chloroform Water, Double-strength		5	ml
Water for Preparations	to	10	ml

It should be recently prepared

Sodium Salicylate Mixture, Strong, BP

Sodium Salicylate		1	g
Sodium Metabisulphite		10	mg
Peppermint Emulsion, Concentrated		0.25	ml
Chloroform Water, Double-strength		5	ml
Water for Preparations	to	10	ml

It should be recently prepared

Mouth-washes

Labelling: in the absence of instructions by the prescriber, the directions for use given under the preparation should be stated

Sodium Chloride Mouth-wash, Compound, BP

Sodium Chloride		1.5	g
Sodium Bicarbonate		1.0	g
Peppermint Emulsion, Concentrated		2.5	ml
Chloroform Water, Double-strength		50	ml
Water for Preparations	to	100	ml

It should recently prepared

Directions for use: to be used with an equal quantity of warm water

Nasal Drops

Ephedrine Nasal Drops BPC

Ephedrine Hydrochloride		500	mg
Chlorbutol		500	mg
Sodium Chloride		500	mg
Water for Preparations	to	100	ml

When Ephedrine Nasal Drops 1% is prescribed, nasal drops containing ephedrine hydrochloride 1 g/100 ml in the same vehicle is supplied

Ointments

25 g to be dispensed unless otherwise directed

Calamine and Coal Tar Ointment, BP

Calamine, finely sifted	12.5	g
Zinc Oxide, finely sifted	12.5	g
Strong Coal Tar Solution	2.5	g
Hydrous Wool Fat	25	g
White Soft Paraffin	47.5	g

Coal Tar and Salicylic Acid Ointment, BP

Coal Tar	2	g
Salicylic Acid	2	g
Emulsifying Wax	11.4	g
White Soft Paraffin	19	g
Coconut Oil	54	g
Polysorbate 80	4	g
Liquid Paraffin	7.6	g

Paraffin Ointment, BP

Hard Paraffin	3	g
White Soft Paraffin	90	g
White Beeswax	2	g
Cetostearyl Alcohol	5	g

Paints

Podophyllin Paint, Compound, BP

Podophyllum Resin		15	g
Compound Benzoin Tincture	to	100	ml

Caution: This paint is very irritant to the eyes
5 ml to be dispensed unless otherwise directed

Oral Powders

Sodium Chloride and Dextrose Oral Powder, Compound, BP

For each powder take:

Sodium Chloride	500 mg
Sodium Bicarbonate	750 mg
Potassium Chloride	750 mg
Dextrose	20 g

It may be flavoured
It should be dispensed in airtight containers
Note: Sodium Chloride and Dextrose Oral Powder, Compound, Small Size is available as a manufactured product—see section 9.2.1.3

Solutions

Labelling: in the absence of instructions by the prescriber, the directions for use, if any, given below the preparations should be stated

Potassium Permanganate Solution

Potassium Permanganate		100 mg
Water for Preparations	to	100 ml

It must be freshly prepared
One part to be diluted with 7 parts of water, or as directed
The diluted solution contains potassium permanganate about 1 in 8000
500 ml to be dispensed unless otherwise directed

Water for Preparations

Potable water drawn freshly from the supply of a public water undertaking and suitable for drinking. Water obtained from the supply via a local storage tank is unsuitable for this purpose. If such a water supply is not available, or if stored water is the only source of mains water, freshly boiled and cooled purified water should be used instead. It should also be used when the potable water in a district is unsuitable for a particular preparation

Dental Practitioners' Formulary

List of Dental Preparations

The following list has been approved by the appropriate Secretaries of State, and the preparations therein may be prescribed by dental practitioners on form FP14.

Capsules
- Amoxycillin Capsules, BP
- Ampicillin Capsules, BP
- Cephalexin Capsules, BP
- Chlordiazepoxide Capsules, BP
- Clindamycin Capsules, BP
- Mefenamic Acid Capsules, BP

Cream
- Hydrocortisone Cream, BPC

Elixirs
- Chloral Elixir, Paediatric, BP
- Diazepam Elixir, DPF
- Paracetamol Elixir, Paediatric, BP
- Promethazine Hydrochloride Elixir, BP
- Triclofos Elixir, BP

Gargle
- Phenol Gargle, BPC

Gels
- Any gel prepared for dental use and containing at least 1 per cent of chlorhexidine gluconate

Glycerin
- Compound Thymol Glycerin, BP

Inhalations
- Menthol and Benzoin Inhalation, BP
- Menthol and Eucalyptus Inhalation, BP

Injections
- Cephaloridine Injection, BP
- Lincomycin Injection, BP

Lozenges
- Amphotericin Lozenges, BPC
- Benzocaine Lozenges, DPF
- Hydrocortisone Lozenges, BPC

Mixtures
- Amoxycillin Mixture, DPF
- Amphotericin Mixture, DPF
- Ampicillin Mixture, BPC
- Clindamycin Mixture, Paediatric, DPF
- Co-trimoxazole Mixture, Paediatric, BPC
- Erythromycin Ethylsuccinate Mixture, DPF
- Magnesium Hydroxide Mixture, BP
- Nystatin Mixture, BPC

Mouth-bath
- Tetracycline Mouth-bath, DPF

Mouth-washes
- Chlorhexidine Mouth-wash, DPF
- Chlorhexidine Mouth-wash, Compound, DPF
- Hydrogen Peroxide Mouth-wash, DPF
- Phenol Mouth-wash, Alkaline, DPF
- Sodium Chloride Mouth-wash, Compound, BP
- Sodium Perborate Mouth-wash, Buffered, DPF
- Zinc Sulphate Mouth-wash, DPF

Nasal Drops
- Ephedrine Nasal Drops, BPC

Ointments
- Amphotericin Ointment, DPF
- Nystatin Ointment, BPC

Paints
- Brilliant Green and Crystal Violet Paint, BP
- Idoxuridine Paint, DPF

Pastes
- Carboxymethylcellulose Gelatin Paste, DPF whether or not containing amphotericin
- Choline Salicylate Dental Paste, DPF
- Triamcinolone Dental Paste, BPC

Oral Powder
- Amoxycillin Oral Powder, DPF

Solutions
- Formaldehyde Solution, BP
- Hydrogen Peroxide Solution (6 per cent), BP
- Iodine Solution, Weak, BP

Solution-tablets
- Mouth-wash Solution-tablets, BP
- Thymol Solution-tablets, Compound, BPC 1963

Tablets
- Ampicillin Tablets, Paediatric, BPC
- Ascorbic Acid Tablets, BP
- Aspirin Tablets, BP
- Aspirin Tablets, Dispersible, BP
- Aspirin, Paracetamol, and Codeine Tablets, DPF
- Carbamazepine Tablets, BP
- Cephalexin Tablets, BP
- Chlordiazepoxide Tablets, BP
- Chlorpheniramine Tablets, BP
- Codeine and Paracetamol Tablets, DPF
- Co-trimoxazole Tablets, BP
- Co-trimoxazole Tablets, Paediatric, BP
- Diazepam Tablets, BP
- Dihydrocodeine Tablets, BP
- Dihydrocodeine and Paracetamol Tablets, DPF
- Erythromycin Tablets, BP
- Metronidazole Tablets, BP
- Nitrazepam Tablets, BP
- Nystatin Tablets, BP
- Oxytetracycline Tablets, BP
- Paracetamol Tablets, BP
- Pentazocine Tablets, BP
- Promethazine Hydrochloride Tablets, BP
- Tetracycline Tablets, BP
- Triclofos Tablets, BP
- Vitamin B Tablets, Compound, Strong, BPC

Penicillin
- Benzylpenicillin Injection, BP
- Benzylpenicillin Tablets, BP
- Penicillin Triple Injection, BPC
- Penicillin VK Capsules, BP
- Penicillin V Elixir, BPC
- Penicillin V Mixture, BPC
- Penicillin VK Tablets, BP
- Injections of Procaine Penicillin, whether or not containing Benzylpenicillin; the following injections are included in the Dental Practitioners' Formulary:
  - Procaine Penicillin Injection, BP
  - Procaine Penicillin Injection, Fortified, BP

Preparations not included in the BP or BPC

Amoxycillin Mixture (proprietary product: *Amoxil Syrup*), amoxycillin 125 mg (as trihydrate)/5 ml when reconstituted with water for preparation

Amoxycillin Oral Powder (proprietary product: *Amoxil Sachets*) amoxycillin 3 g (as trihydrate)
Dose: amoxycillin 3 g in water as a single dose

Amphotericin Mixture (proprietary product: *Fungilin Suspension*), amphotericin 100 mg/ml

Amphotericin Ointment (proprietary product: *Fungilin Ointment*), amphotericin 3%, in Plastibase

Aspirin, Paracetamol, and Codeine Tablets (proprietary product: *Veganin Tablets*), aspirin 250 mg, paracetamol 250 mg, codeine phosphate 6.8 mg

Benzocaine Lozenges, benzocaine 10 mg. They are prepared by compression

Carboxymethylcellulose Gelatin Paste (proprietary product: *Orabase Paste*), gelatin, pectin, sodium carboxymethylcellulose, 16.58% of each in Plastibase

Choline Salicylate Dental Paste (proprietary products: *Bonjela Paste*; *Teejel Gel*), choline salicylate 8.7% in a gel basis

Chlorhexidine Gel (proprietary product: *Corsodyl Dental Gel*), chlorhexidine gluconate 1%

Chlorhexidine Mouth-wash (proprietary product: *Corsodyl Mouth-wash*), chlorhexidine gluconate 0.2%

Chlorhexidine Mouth-wash, Compound (proprietary product: *Eludril Mouth-wash*), chlorhexidine gluconate 0.1%, chlorbutol 0.1%

Clindamycin Mixture, Paediatric (proprietary product: *Dalacin C Paediatric Suspension*), clindamycin 75 mg (as hydrochloride palmitate)/5 ml when reconstituted with purified water, freshly boiled and cooled

Codeine and Paracetamol Tablets (proprietary product: *Panadeine Co Tablets*), codeine phosphate 8 mg, paracetamol 500 mg

Diazepam Elixir (proprietary product: *Valium Syrup*), diazepam 2 mg/5 ml

Dihydrocodeine and Paracetamol Tablets (proprietary product: *Paramol-118*), dihydrocodeine tartrate 10 mg, paracetamol 500 mg

Erythromycin Ethylsuccinate Mixture (proprietary product: *Erythroped Suspension*), erythromycin 250 mg (as ethylsuccinate)/5 ml when reconstituted with water for preparations

Hydrogen Peroxide Mouth-wash, consists of hydrogen peroxide solution (6%)
Directions for use: 15 ml to be used in half a tumblerful of warm water
200 ml to be dispensed unless otherwise directed

Idoxuridine Paint, consists of idoxuridine eye-drops; idoxuridine 0.1% in aqueous solution
Directions for use: to be painted on the lesion 4–5 times daily, unless otherwise directed
15 ml to be dispensed unless otherwise directed

Phenol Mouth-wash, Alkaline, liquified phenol 3 ml, amaranth solution 1 ml, potassium hydroxide solution 3 ml, water for preparations to 100 ml
Directions for use: to be used diluted with 10 times its volume of warm water
200 ml to be dispensed unless otherwise directed

Sodium Perborate Mouth-wash, Buffered (proprietary product: *Bocasan Mouth-wash*), sodium perborate monohydrate 68.6%, sodium hydrogen tartrate 29.4%, menthol, peppermint oil
Directions for use: the contents of one sachet to be dissolved in 30 ml of water

Tetracycline Mouth-bath, consists of tetracycline mixture; tetracycline equivalent to 125 mg of tetracycline hydrochloride/5 ml
Directions for use: 10 ml to be held in the mouth for 2–3 minutes 3 times daily, unless otherwise directed

Thymol Solution-tablets, Compound, BPC 1963, contain borax, phenol, sodium bicarbonate, thymol, and amaranth
Directions for use: 1 solution-tablet to be dissolved in half a tumblerful of warm water before use
12 solution-tablets to be dispensed unless otherwise directed

Zinc Sulphate Mouth-wash, consists of zinc sulphate lotion; zinc sulphate 1 g, amaranth solution 1 ml/100 ml in water for preparations
Directions for use: dilute 1 part with 4 parts of warm water
200 ml to be dispensed unless otherwise directed

New and Discontinued Preparations

New Preparations

Preparations added since the compilation of BNF 1981 no. 2

Antraderm
Apsin VK
Apsolox
Augmentin
Bactrian
Bezalip
Caplenal
Chymacort
Colobase
Coparvax
Cotrimox
Dextrolyte
Diatensec
Driclor
Emtexate
Formula S
Franolyn Expect
Givitol
Gluten-free Crackers
Hep-Rinse
Hyprenan
Ibu-Slo
Imotest
Indoflex
Meditar
Merocaine
Microlet
Miochol
Mucolex
Nanormon
Netillin
Pabrinex
Pendramine
Percutol
Regulan
Rimevax
Spectralgen
Tiempe
Tigason
Tonocard
Travogyn
Unisomnia
Unitrim
Vanair
Varbian
Vepesid
Wysoy
Zantac
Zincomed
Zovirax

Discontinued Preparations

Preparations discontinued since the compilation of BNF 1981 no. 2

Admune
Aluphos
Bidrolar
Complamex
Crasnitin
Femergin
Filon
Gastalar
Hydromycin-D
Isoxyl
Katorin
Kethamed
Majeptil
Mesontoin
Metilar
Milonorm
Noveril
Paramisan
Potensan Forte
Practo-Clyss
Protopan
Rona-Phyllin
Sinaxar
Tannex
Theonar
Throsil
Trescatyl
Trevintix
Triperidol
Typhus Vaccine
Ultandren
Uraband

Name Changes

Old	*New*	*Old*	*New*
Ostomy	Translet	Pulmodrine	Pholcomed Expectorant
Rona-Slophyllin	Slo-Phyllin	Redoxon	Roscorbic

Changes Since the Preparation of the Main Text

New Preparations

Introduced up to January 1982

Atrovent® (Boehringer Ingelheim)
Respirator solution, ipratropium bromide 0.025%. Price 20 ml = **D**

Cedocard® (Tillotts)
Tablets, pink, scored, isosorbide dinitrate 10 mg. Price 20 tabs = **B**

Cyklokapron® (KabiVitrum)
Syrup (= elixir), tranexamic acid 500 mg/5 ml. Price 250 ml = **I**

▼ **Demser®** (MSD)
Capsules, blue, metirosine 250 mg (Hosp. only)

▼ **Prostin VR®** (Upjohn)
Injection, alprostadil (prostaglandin E_1) 500 micrograms/ml in alcohol. To be diluted before use. Price 1-ml amp = **J**

▼ **Secadrex®** (M&B)
Tablets, f/c, acebutolol 200 mg (as hydrochloride), hydrochlorothiazide 12.5 mg. Price 20 tabs = **G**

Theo-Dur® (Fisons)
Tablets, s/r, scored, theophylline 200 mg. Price 20 tabs = **D**
Tablets, s/r, scored, theophylline 300 mg. Price 20 tabs = **D**
Dose: 200–300 mg twice daily, increased if necessary by 100–150 mg increments; CHILD up to 35 kg 100 mg twice daily, over 35 kg 200 mg twice daily, increased or decreased as necessary by 100 mg

Travasept 100® (Travenol)
Solution, cetrimide 0.15%, chlorhexidine acetate 0.015%. Price 500 ml and 1 litre (both) = **C**

Trimopan® (Berk)
Suspension (= mixture), trimethoprim 50 mg/5 ml. Price 100 ml = **D**

Preparations Discontinued

since the preparation of the main text

Envacar
Neovax
Sedatussin

Index of Manufacturers

Abbott
Abbott Laboratories Ltd,
Queenborough, Kent ME11 5EL.
Sheerness 663371

A&H
Allen & Hanburys Ltd,
Greenford, Middx UB6 0HD.
01-422 2331

Alcon
Alcon Laboratories (UK) Ltd,
Imperial Way, Watford WD2 4YR.
Watford 46133

Alembic Products
Alembic Products Ltd,
Oaklands House, Oaklands Drive, Sale, Manchester M33 1WS.
061-962 4423

Allergan
Allergan Ltd,
Fennels Lodge, St. Peter's Close, Loudwater, High Wycombe, Bucks HP11 1JT.
062-85 27778

American Hospital Supply
American Hospital Supply (UK) Ltd,
53 Church Rd, Ashford, Middx TW15 2TY.
Ashford (Middx) 47101

Andard-Mount
Andard-Mount (London) Ltd,
24 London Rd, Wembley, Middx HA9 7HD.
01-903 6388

Aplin & Barrett
Aplin & Barrett Ltd,
Bythesea Rd, Trowbridge, Wilts. BA14 8HS
022 14 3611

APS
Approved Prescription Services Ltd,
Whitcliffe House, Whitcliffe Rd, Cleckheaton, West Yorks BD19 3BZ.
Cleckheaton 876776

Armour
Armour Pharmaceutical Co. Ltd,
St. Leonards House,
St. Leonards Rd, Eastbourne, East Sussex BN21 3YG.
Eastbourne 641144

Ashe
Ashe Laboratories Ltd,
Ashetree Works, Kingston Rd, Leatherhead, Surrey KT22 7JZ.
Leatherhead 76151

Astra
Astra Pharmaceuticals Ltd,
St. Peter's House, 2 Bricket Rd, St. Albans, Herts AL1 3JW.
St. Albans 33241

Ayerst
Ayerst Laboratories Ltd,
South Way, Andover, Hants SP10 5LT.
Andover 58711

Bayer
Bayer UK Ltd,
Pharmaceutical Division, Burrell Rd, Haywards Heath, West Sussex RH16 1TP.
0444 414161

BDH
BDH Pharmaceuticals Ltd,
Lenten House, Lenten St, Alton, Hants GU34 1JD.
0420-88767

Beecham
Beecham Research Laboratories,
Beecham House, Great West Rd, Brentford, Middx TW8 9BD.
01-560 5151

Beecham Foods
Beecham Products,
Research and Development (Foods), 11 Stoke Poges Lane, Slough, Berks SL1 3NW
Slough 33433

Bencard
Bencard,
Great West Rd, Brentford, Middx TW8 9BE.
01-560 5151

Bengué
Bengué & Co. Ltd,
St. Ives House, St. Ives Rd, Maidenhead, Berks SL6 1RD.
Maidenhead 33191

Berk
Berk Pharmaceuticals Ltd,
St. Leonards House,
St. Leonards Road, Eastbourne, East Sussex BN21 3YG.
Eastbourne 641144

Bioglan
Bioglan Laboratories Ltd,
Spirella Building, Bridge Rd, Letchworth, Herts SG6 4ET.
Letchworth 74644

Boehringer Ingelheim
Boehringer Ingelheim Ltd,
Southern Industrial Estate, Bracknell, Berks RG12 4YS.
Bracknell 24600

Boots
The Boots Co. Ltd,
1 Thane Rd West, Nottingham NG2 3AA.
Nottingham 56111

Bristol
Bristol Cardiovascular,
Station Rd, Langley, Slough SL3 6EB.
Slough 44266

Brocades
Brocades (Great Britain) Ltd,
Brocades House, Pyrford Rd, West Byfleet, Weybridge, Surrey KT14 6RA.
Byfleet 45536

Burgess
Edwin Burgess Ltd,
Longwick Rd, Princes Risborough, Aylesbury, Bucks HP17 9RR.
Princes Risborough 6881

Calmic
Calmic Medical Division,
The Wellcome Foundation Ltd,
Crewe Hall, Crewe, Cheshire CW1 1UB.
Crewe 583151

Cantassium
The Cantassium Company,
Larkhall Laboratories, 225 Putney Bridge Rd, London SW15 2PY.
01-870 0971

Carlton
Carlton Laboratories (UK) Ltd,
4 Manor Parade, Salvington Rd, Durrington, Worthing,
West Sussex BN13 2JP.
Worthing 63235

Carnegie
Carnegie Medical,
1 Morley St, Loughborough, Leics LE11 1EP.
0509-68181

Carnrick
Carnrick Laboratories,
52 The Parade, Oadby, Leicester LE2 5BB.
Leicester 718001

Carter-Wallace
Carter-Wallace Ltd,
Wear Bay Rd, Folkestone, Kent CT19 6PG.
0303-57661

Chelsea
Chelsea Drug & Chemical Co. Ltd,
310 Old Brompton Rd, London SW5 9JQ.
01-370 4321

Ciba
CIBA Laboratories,
Wimblehurst Rd, Horsham, West Sussex RH12 4AB.
Horsham 50101

Coates & Cooper
Coates & Cooper Ltd,
Hill Farm Avenue, Watford WD2 7RA.
Garston 75255

Collins
L. D. Collins & Co. Ltd,
Sunray House, 9 Plantagenet Rd, New Barnet, Herts EN5 5JG.
01-440 1470

Coloplast
Coloplast Ltd,
Somersham Rd, St. Ives, Huntingdon PE17 4LN.
Huntingdon 62600

Colson & Kay
Colson & Kay Ltd,
Shentonfield Rd, Manchester
M22 4RW.
061-491 1980

Comprehensive
Comprehensive Pharmaceuticals
Ltd,
95 Frampton St, London NW8
8NA.
01-723 1107

Concept
Concept Pharmaceuticals Ltd,
59 High St, Rickmansworth,
Herts WD3 1EZ.
Rickmansworth 79388

Consolidated
Consolidated Chemicals Ltd,
The Industrial Estate, Wrexham,
Clwyd LL13 9PS.
Wrexham 61351

Cooper
Cooper Health Products Ltd,
Gatehouse Rd, Aylesbury, Bucks
HP19 3ED.
0296-32601

CooperVision
CooperVision Ltd,
21 The Avenue, Southampton
SO9 1WP.
Southampton 331231

Cow & Gate
Cow & Gate Ltd,
Cow & Gate House, Trowbridge,
Wilts BA14 8YX.
Trowbridge 68381

Cox-Continental
Cox-Continental Ltd,
Brookside Ave, Rustington,
West Sussex BN16 3LF.
Rustington 74231

Crookes
Crookes Laboratories Ltd,
PO Box 94, 1 Thane Rd West,
Nottingham NG2 3AA.

Crookes Products
Crookes Products Ltd,
PO Box 94, 1 Thane Rd West,
Nottingham NG2 3AA.
Nottingham 57431

Dales
Dales Pharmaceuticals Ltd,
Snaygill Industrial Estate,
Keighley Rd, Skipton, North
Yorkshire BD23 2RW.
0756 61311

DDSA
DDSA Pharmaceuticals Ltd,
310 Old Brompton Rd, London
SW5 9JQ.
01-373 7884

De Witt
De Witt International Ltd,
Seymour Rd, London E10 7LX.
01-539 3334

Delandale
Delandale Laboratories Ltd,
Delandale House, 37 Old Dover
Rd, Canterbury, Kent CT1 3JB.
Canterbury 66353

Dendron
Dendron Ltd,
94 Rickmansworth Rd, Watford
WD1 7JJ.
Watford 29251

Dermal
Dermal Laboratories Ltd,
Tatmore Place, Gosmore,
Hitchin, Herts SG4 7QR.
Hitchin 58866

Dermalex
Dermalex Co. Ltd,
146 Kilburn High Rd, London
NW6 4JD.
01-624 4686

DF
Duncan, Flockhart & Co. Ltd,
700 Oldfield Lane North,
Greenford, Middx UB6 0HD.
01-422 2331

Dista
Dista Products Ltd,
Kingsclere Rd, Basingstoke,
Hants RG21 2XA.
Basingstoke 52011

Dome
Dome/Hollister-Stier,
Division of Miles Laboratories
Ltd, Stoke Court, Stoke Poges,
Slough SL2 4LY.
Farnham Common 5151

Downs
Downs Surgical Ltd,
Church Path, Mitcham, Surrey
CR4 3UE.
01-648 6291

Duphar
Duphar Laboratories Ltd,
Gaters Hill, West End,
Southampton SO3 3JD.
West End (Hants) 6171

Eaton
Eaton Laboratories,
Regent House, The Broadway,
Woking, Surrey GU21 5AP.
Woking 71671

Evans
Evans Medical Ltd,
891 Greenford Rd, Greenford,
Middx UB6 0HE.
01-422 3434

FAIR
FAIR Laboratories Ltd,
Squibb House, 141 Staines Rd,
Hounslow, Middx TW3 3JA.
01-572 7422

Farillon
Farillon Ltd,
Bryant Ave, Romford, Essex
RM3 0PJ.
Ingrebourne 71136

Farley
Farley Health Products Ltd,
Torr Lane, Plymouth PL3 5UA.
0752-701621

Farmitalia Carlo Erba
Farmitalia Carlo Erba Ltd,
Kingmaker House, Station Rd,
Barnet, Herts EN5 1NU.
01-440 7171

Ferring
Ferring Pharmaceuticals Ltd,
11 Mount Road, Feltham, Middx
TW13 6JG.
01-898 8396

Fisons
Fisons Ltd,
Pharmaceutical Division, 12
Derby Rd, Loughborough, Leics
LE11 0BB.
Loughborough 63113

Galen
Galen Ltd,
19 Lower Seagoe Industrial
Estate, Portadown, Craigavon,
Armagh BT63 5QD.
0762-34974

Geigy
Geigy Pharmaceuticals,
Wimblehurst Rd, Horsham, West
Sussex RH12 4AB.
Horsham 50101

Geistlich
Geistlich Sons Ltd,
Newton Bank, Long Lane,
Chester CH2 3QZ.
Chester 47534

GF Supplies
GF Dietary Supplies Ltd,
Lowther Road, Stanmore, Middx
HA7 1EL.
01-206 0522

Glaxo
Glaxo Laboratories Ltd,
Greenford Rd, Greenford,
Middx UB6 0HE.
01-422 3434

Glenwood
Glenwood Laboratories Ltd,
19 Wincheap, Canterbury, Kent
CT1 3TB.
0227-60139

Henleys
Henleys Medical Supplies Ltd,
Alexandra Works, Clarendon
Road, London N8 0DL.
01-889 3151

Hoechst
Hoechst UK Ltd,
Pharmaceutical Division, Hoechst
House, Salisbury Rd, Hounslow,
Middx TW4 6JH.
01-570 7712

Hough
Hough, Hoseason & Co. Ltd,
22 Chapel St, Levenshulme,
Manchester M19 3PT.
061-224 3271

ICI
Imperial Chemical Industries Ltd,
Pharmaceuticals Division,
Alderley Park, Macclesfield,
Cheshire SK10 4TF.
Alderley Edge 582828

Ilon
Ilon Laboratories (Hamilton) Ltd,
Lorne St, Hamilton, Strathclyde ML3 9AB.
0698-285129

International Labs
International Laboratories Ltd,
Charwell House, Wilsom Rd,
Alton, Hants GU34 2TJ.
Alton 88174

Jackson
Ernest Jackson & Co. Ltd,
Crediton, Devon EX17 3AP.
Crediton 2251

Janssen
Janssen Pharmaceutical Ltd,
Janssen House, Chapel St,
Marlow, Bucks SL7 1ET.
Marlow 71744

K/L
K/L Pharmaceuticals Ltd,
25 Macadam Place, South
Newmoor Industrial Estate,
Irvine KA11 4HP.
0294 215951

KabiVitrum
KabiVitrum Ltd,
KabiVitrum House, Riverside
Way, Uxbridge, Middx UB8 2YF.
Uxbridge 51144

Kerfoot
Thomas Kerfoot & Co. Ltd,
Vale of Bardsley, Ashton-under-Lyne, Lancs OL7 9RR.
061-330 4531

Kerodex
Kerodex Ltd,
202 Terminus Rd, Eastbourne,
East Sussex BN21 3DF.
0323-639671

Keymer
Keymer Pharmaceuticals Ltd,
The Brow, Burgess Hill,
West Sussex RH15 9NE.
Burgess Hill 6011

Kirby-Warrick
Kirby-Warrick Pharmaceuticals Ltd,
Mildenhall, Bury St. Edmunds,
Suffolk IP28 7AX.
Mildenhall 716321

LAB
Laboratories for Applied Biology Ltd,
91 Amhurst Park, London N16 5DR.
01-800 2252

Labaz
Labaz: Sanofi UK Ltd,
Regent House, Heaton Lane,
Stockport SK4 1AG.
061-480 0895

Larkhall
Larkhall Laboratories,
225 Putney Bridge Rd, London SW15 2PY.
01-870 0971

Lederle
Lederle Laboratories,
Fareham Rd, Gosport, Hants PO13 0AS.
Fareham 236131

Leo
Leo Laboratories Ltd,
Longwick Rd, Princes
Risborough, Aylesbury, Bucks HP17 9RR.
Princes Risborough 7333

Lepetit
Lepetit Pharmaceuticals Ltd,
Meadowbank, Bath Rd,
Hounslow, Middx TW5 9QY.
01-759 9001

Lewis
Lewis Laboratories Ltd,
Lavender Walk, Leeds LS9 8JG.
0532-482032

Lilly
Eli Lilly & Co. Ltd,
Kingsclere Rd, Basingstoke,
Hants RG21 2XA.
Basingstoke 3241

Lipha
Lipha Pharmaceuticals Ltd,
Old Farm Rd, West Drayton,
Middx UB7 7LD.
West Drayton 49331

Loveridge
J. M. Loveridge Ltd,
6 Millbrook Rd, Southampton SO9 3LT.
Southampton 28411

Loxley
Loxley Medical,
Bessingby Estate, Bridlington,
North Humberside YO16 4SU.
Bridlington 75356

Luitpold-Werk
Luitpold-Werk (Munich),
Hayes Gate House, 27 Uxbridge
Rd, Hayes, Middx UB4 0JD.
01-561 8774

Lundbeck
Lundbeck Ltd,
Lundbeck House, Hastings St,
Luton LU1 5BE.
Luton 416565

Macarthys
Macarthys Laboratories Ltd,
Chesham House, Chesham
Close, Romford RM1 4JX.
Romford 46033

Maltown
Maltown Ltd,
PO Box 53, Harrogate, North
Yorks HG2 0NH.
0423-62593

Martindale
Martindale Pharmaceuticals Ltd,
Chesham House, Chesham
Close, Romford RM1 4JX.
Romford 46033

M&B
May & Baker Ltd,
Dagenham, Essex RM10 7XS.
01-592 3060

MCP
MCP Pharmaceuticals Ltd,
Simpson Parkway, Kirkton
Campus, Livingston, West
Lothian EH54 7BH.
Livingston 412512

Mead Johnson
Mead Johnson,
Station Rd, Langley, Slough SL3 6EB.
Slough 44266

Medexport
Medexport Ltd,
PO Box 25, Arundel, West
Sussex BN18 0SW.

Medo
Medo-Chemicals Ltd,
130 High St, Chesham, Bucks HP5 1EF.
0494 772071

Merck
E. Merck Ltd,
Winchester Rd, Four Marks,
Alton, Hants GU34 5HG.
Alton 64011

Merrell
Merrell Pharmaceuticals Ltd,
Rusham Park, Whitehall Lane,
Egham, Surrey TW20 9NW.
Egham 34422

Morson
Thomas Morson Pharmaceuticals,
Hertford Rd, Hoddesdon, Herts EN11 9BU.
Hoddesdon 67272

MSD
Merck Sharp & Dohme Ltd,
Hertford Rd,
Hoddesdon, Herts EN11 9BU.
Hoddesdon 67272

Napp
Napp Laboratories Ltd,
Hill Farm Ave, Watford WD2 7RA.
Garston 75255

Nestlé
Nestlé Co. Ltd,
St. George's House, Croydon CR9 1NR.
01-686 3333

Nicholas
Nicholas Laboratories Ltd,
PO Box 17, Slough SL1 4AU.
Slough 23971

Nordic
Nordic Pharmaceuticals Ltd,
11 Mount Road, Feltham, Middx TW13 6JC.
01-898 8665

Nordisk
Nordisk-UK,
Hurst House, 157 Walton Rd,
East Molesey, Surrey KT8 0DX.
01-941 4635

Norgine
Norgine Ltd,
59–62 High Holborn, London
WC1V 6EB.
01-405 3151

Norma
Norma Chemicals Ltd,
1a Frognal, London NW3 6AN.
01-435 7627

Norton
H. N. Norton & Co. Ltd,
Patman House, George Lane,
South Woodford, London E18
2LS.
01-530 6421

Novo
Novo Laboratories Ltd,
Ringway House, Bell Rd,
Daneshill East, Basingstoke,
Hants RG24 0QN.
Basingstoke 55055

Organon
Organon Laboratories Ltd,
Crown House, London Rd,
Morden, Surrey SM4 5DZ.
01-542 6611

Organon-Teknika
Organon-Teknika Ltd,
Teknika House, Cromwell Rd,
St. Neots, Huntingdon, Cambs
PE19 2HS.
0480-76963

Ortho
Ortho Pharmaceutical Ltd,
PO Box 79, Saunderton, High
Wycombe, Bucks HP14 4HJ.
Naphill 3541

P&B
Paines & Byrne Ltd,
Pabyrn Laboratories, 177 Bilton
Rd, Perivale, Greenford, Middx
UB6 7HG.
01-997 1143

P-D
Parke, Davis & Co.,
Usk Rd, Pontypool, Gwent NP4
0YH.
Pontypool 2468

Pfizer
Pfizer Ltd,
Sandwich, Kent CT13 9NJ.
Sandwich 613511

Pharm. Mfg Co.
Pharmaceutical Manufacturing
Co.,
Westhoughton, Bolton BL5 3SL.
0942-811567

Pharmacia
Pharmacia (Great Britain) Ltd,
Prince Regent Rd, Hounslow,
Middx TW3 1NE.
01-572 7321

Pharmax
Pharmax Ltd,
Bourne Rd, Bexley, Kent DA5
1NX.
Crayford 526551

Philip Harris
Philip Harris Medical Ltd,
Hazelwell Lane, Birmingham
B30 2PS.
021-458 2020

Phillips Yeast
Phillips Yeast Products Ltd,
Park Royal Rd, London NW10
7JX.
01-965 7533

Plough
Plough (UK) Ltd,
Penarth St, London SE15 1TR.
01-639 4363

Potter & Clarke
Potter & Clarke Ltd,
415 Limpsfield Rd, The Green,
Warlingham, Surrey CR3 9YS.
08832 5233

Priory
Priory Laboratories Ltd,
Hill Farm Ave, Watford WD2
7RA.
Garston 75255

Procea
Procea,
Alexandra Road, Dublin 1.
Dublin 741741

Quinoderm
Quinoderm Ltd,
Manchester Rd, Oldham, Lancs
OL8 4PB.
061-624 9307

Radiol
Radiol Chemicals Ltd,
Stepfield, Witham, Essex CM8
3AG.
Witham 12538

Raymed
Raymed,
Viaduct Rd, Leeds LS4 2BR.
Leeds 31862

R&C
Reckitt & Colman
Pharmaceutical Division,
Dansom Lane, Hull HU8 7DS.
Hull 26151

Regent
Regent Laboratories Ltd,
Cunard Road, London NW10
6PN.
01-965 3637

Riker
Riker Laboratories,
Morley St, Loughborough, Leics
LE11 1EP.
Loughborough 68181

Rimmer
Rimmer Bros,
18 Aylesbury St, Clerkenwell,
London EC1R 0DD.
01-251 6494

Robins
A. H. Robins Co. Ltd,
Redkiln Way, Horsham, West
Sussex RH13 5QP.
Horsham 60361

Roche
Roche Products Ltd,
PO Box 8, Welwyn Garden City,
Herts AL7 3AY.
Welwyn Garden 28128

Rona
Rona Laboratories Ltd,
Cadwell Lane, Hitchin, Herts
SG4 0SF.
Hitchin 51421

Rorer
Rorer Pharmaceuticals,
Stepfield, Witham, Essex CM8
3AG.
Witham 512538

Roussel
Roussel Laboratories Ltd,
Roussel House, North End Rd,
Wembley Park, Middx HA9
0NF.
01-903 1454

RP Drugs
RP Drugs Ltd,
RPD House, Yorkdale Industrial
Park, Braithwaite St, Leeds LS11
9XE.
0532-441400

Rybar
Rybar Laboratories Ltd,
25 Sycamore Rd, Amersham,
Bucks
Amersham 22741

Salt
Salt & Son Ltd,
220 Corporation St, Birmingham
B4 6QR.
021-233 1038

Sandoz
Sandoz Products Ltd,
Sandoz House, 98 The Centre,
Feltham, Middx TW13 4EP.
01-890 1366

Sanol Schwarz
Sanol Schwarz Pharmaceuticals
Ltd,
130 High Street, Chesham, Bucks
HP5 1EF.
0494 772071

SAS
SAS Chemicals Ltd,
Victoria House, Vernon Place,
London WC1B 4DR.
01-404 5711

Schering
Schering Chemicals Ltd,
Pharmaceutical Division, Burgess
Hill, West Sussex RH15 9NE.
Burgess Hill 6011

Scientific Hospital Supplies
Scientific Hospital Supplies Ltd,
38 Queensland St, Liverpool L7
3JG.
051-709 3588

Scotia
Scotia Pharmaceutical Products, 558 Cathcart Rd, Glasgow G42 8YG.
041-423 1856

Searle
Searle Pharmaceuticals, PO Box 53, Lane End Rd, High Wycombe, Bucks HP12 4HL.
High Wycombe 21124

Serono
Serono Laboratories (UK) Ltd, 2 Tewin Court, Welwyn Garden City, Herts AL7 1AU.
Welwyn Garden 31972

Servier
Servier Laboratories Ltd, Fulmer Hall, Windmill Rd, Fulmer, Slough, SL3 6HH.
Fulmer 2744

Seton
Seton Products Ltd, Tubiton House, Medlock St, Oldham, Lancs OL1 3HS.
061-652 2222

Simpla
Simpla Plastics Ltd, Phoenix Estate, Caerphilly Rd, Cardiff CF4 4XG.
Cardiff 62100

Sinclair
Sinclair Pharmaceuticals Ltd, Borough Rd, Godalming, Surrey GU7 2AB.
Godalming 28222

SK&F
Smith Kline & French Laboratories Ltd, Welwyn Garden City, Herts AL7 1EY.
Welwyn Garden 25111

Smith & Hill
Smith & Hill Ltd, 53 Cresswell Rd, Sheffield S9 4JZ.
0742-440321

S&N
Smith & Nephew Ltd, Bessemer Rd, Welwyn Garden City, Herts AL7 1HF.
Welwyn Garden 25151

S&N Pharm.
Smith & Nephew Pharmaceuticals Ltd, Bampton Rd, Harold Hill, Romford, Essex RM3 8SL.
Ingrebourne 49333

Spodefell
Spodefell Ltd, 5 Inverness Mews, London W2 3JQ.
01-229 9125

Squibb
E. R. Squibb & Sons Ltd, Squibb House, 141 Staines Rd, Hounslow, Middx TW3 3JA.
01-572 7422

Stafford-Miller
Stafford-Miller Ltd, Stafford-Miller House, The Common, Hatfield, Herts AL10 0NZ.
Hatfield 61151

STD Pharmaceutical
STD Pharmaceutical Products Ltd, 6 Broad St, Hereford HR4 9AE.
Hereford 2152

Sterling Health
Sterling Health, Surbiton, Surrey KT6 4PH.
01-399 5751

Sterling Industrial
Sterling Industrial, Chapeltown, Sheffield S30 4YP.
0742 467171

Sterling Research
Sterling Research Laboratories, Surbiton, Surrey KT6 4PH.
01-399 5252

Stiefel
Stiefel Laboratories (UK) Ltd, Wellcroft Rd, Slough SL1 4AQ.
Slough 37832

Stuart
Stuart Pharmaceuticals Ltd, Carr House, Carrs Rd, Cheadle, Cheshire SK8 2EG.
061-491 1444

Syntex
Syntex Pharmaceuticals Ltd, St. Ives House, St. Ives Rd, Maidenhead, Berks SL6 1RD.
Maidenhead 33191

Thames
Thames Laboratories Ltd, Thames Building, 206 Upper Richmond Rd West, London SW14 8AH.
01-876 4316

Tillotts
Tillotts Laboratories, Unit 24, Henlow Trading Estate, Henlow, Beds. SG16 6DS.
0462-813933

Tosara
Tosara Products (UK) Ltd, 59 Crosby Rd North, Liverpool L22 4QD.
051-920 0460

Travenol
Travenol Laboratories Ltd, Caxton Way, Thetford, Norfolk IP24 3SE.
Thetford 4581

Typharm
Typharm Ltd, 5 Cowley Road, Chantry Park, Nuffield Industrial Estate, Poole, Dorset.
020 13 3527

Unigreg
Unigreg Ltd, Spa House, 15–17 Worple Rd, Wimbledon, London SW19 4JS.
01-946 9871

Unimed
Unimed Pharmaceuticals Ltd, 24 Steynton Ave, Bexley, Kent DA5 3HP.
01-309 7003

Upjohn
Upjohn Ltd, Fleming Way, Crawley, West Sussex RH10 2NJ.
Crawley 31133

Vitabiotics
Vitabiotics Ltd, 122 Mount Pleasant, Alperton, Middx HA0 1UG.
01-903 5541

Wade
Wade Pharmaceuticals Ltd, Stepfield, Witham, Essex CM8 3AG.
Witham 512538

Wallace Mfg
Wallace Manufacturing Chemists Ltd, 1a Frognal, London NW3 6AN.
01-435 7627

Wander
Wander Pharmaceuticals, 98 The Centre, Feltham, Middx TW13 4EP.
01-890 1366

Warner
William R. Warner & Co. Ltd, Usk Rd, Pontypool, Gwent NP4 0YH.
Pontypool 2468

WBP
WB Pharmaceuticals Ltd, PO Box 23, Bracknell, Berks RG12 4YS.
Bracknell 50222

Weddel
Weddel Pharmaceuticals Ltd, Weddel House, 14 West Smithfield, London EC1A 9HY.
01-248 1212

Welbeck
Welbeck Medical Distributors Ltd, Sanofi UK Ltd, Regent House, Heaton Lane, Stockport SK4 1AG.
061-480 0895

Welfare Foods
Welfare Foods (Stockport) Ltd, 63 London Rd South, Poynton, Stockport, Cheshire SK12 1LA.
0625-877387

Wellcome
Wellcome Medical Division, The Wellcome Foundation Ltd, Crewe Hall, Crewe, Cheshire CW1 1UB.
Crewe 583151

Wilcox
Wilcox Laboratories Ltd, Calgary House, Tobermory, Isle

of Mull, Argyll TN38 0EG.
068-84 201

Winthrop
Winthrop Laboratories,
Sterling-Winthrop House,
Surbiton, Surrey KT6 4PH.
01-399 5252

Wyeth
Wyeth Laboratories,
Huntercombe Lane South,
Taplow, Maidenhead, Berks SL6 0PH.
Slough 28311

Zyma
Zyma (UK) Ltd,
Hurdsfield Industrial Estate,
Macclesfield, Cheshire SK10 2LY.
Macclesfield 21933

Index

E

H

I

J

K

L

N

O

Q

R

S

T

W

X

Y